Osteomyelitis of the Foot and Ankle

Osteomyelitis of the Foot and Ankle

Troy J. Boffeli

Editor

Osteomyelitis of the Foot and Ankle

Medical and Surgical Management

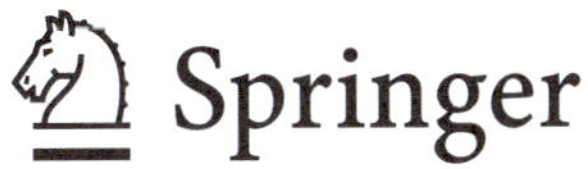 Springer

Editor
Troy J. Boffeli, DPM, FACFAS
Regions Hospital/HealthPartners
Institute for Education and Research
St. Paul, MN, USA

ISBN 978-3-319-35854-3   ISBN 978-3-319-18926-0   (eBook)
DOI 10.1007/978-3-319-18926-0

Springer Cham Heidelberg New York Dordrecht London
© Springer International Publishing Switzerland 2015
Softcover reprint of the hardcover 1st edition 2015

Printed on acid-free paper

Springer International Publishing AG Switzerland is part of Springer Science+Business Media (www.springer.com)

Preface

The onset of osteomyelitis in the foot or ankle is frequently the turning point where an otherwise stable wound, injury, or elective surgery becomes a serious medical condition. While largely associated with diabetic foot wounds, osteomyelitis also has a major impact on the outcome of decubitus ulcers, puncture wounds, septic arthritis, open fractures, and gangrene. A chronic wound can remain stable for months or even years without much more than topical treatment or occasional antibiotics for cellulitis. It is the onset of deep infection of the underlying bone and joint structures that frequently leads to hospitalization, emergency surgery, and amputation.

Lower extremity osteomyelitis is a daily occurrence in most hospitals around the world, yet there are limited resources to guide treatment of an individual patient. Evidence-based guidelines to help the surgeon determine what or when to amputate are lacking. Meaningful evidence is challenging due to highly variable patient presentation, including wound location, extent of osteomyelitis, vascular status, and associated deformities. This book was written to provide specific treatment protocols which can be individualized to a particular patient's condition after consideration of the entire clinical picture. The chapters are organized based on anatomic location of the wound and infection, allowing clinicians easy access to relevant treatment options.

This is a how-to book focusing on a variety of challenging and controversial situations related to the treatment of patients with osteomyelitis of the foot and ankle.

- How to diagnose osteomyelitis early in the course of disease without unnecessary tests or harmful biopsy procedures is covered in the early chapters.
- How to avoid excessive cost and side effects associated with antibiotics for conditions that are better treated surgically is carefully considered for various clinical presentations.
- How to minimize the risk of recurring wounds and infection yet preserve optimal foot function after surgery is a major focus of surgical treatment guidelines.
- How to incorporate advanced techniques like flap surgery, minimally invasive procedures, or local delivery of antibiotics is addressed using case examples that highlight alternative surgical approaches.

Our attempt to answer these challenging questions is the foundation of this book. Whether a seasoned foot and ankle surgeon looking for a new approach or a vascular surgeon searching for late-night guidance, the reader is likely to gain new insights. The effectiveness of shared decision-making between the patient, surgeon, infectious disease specialist, radiologist, and hospitalist or primary provider is largely dependent on knowledge of treatment options. This book is intended to provide the entire care team with practical guidelines to treat both chronic wounds with low-grade bone infection and acute limb-threatening infections.

The image-heavy format of this text is of real value, providing a unique look into the treatment protocols discussed. Rather than vague recommendations to "resect to viable, bleeding bone," pictures are used to fully describe the methods presented. To that end, treatment protocols for nearly every ulcer location or bone of the foot and ankle are laid out in a step-by-step pictorial format.

The reader might notice that there is no chapter on the definitive surgical treatment for diabetic foot infection. The surgeon should forget about the quest for definitive treatment and focus instead on planning ahead for future foot function and revision options should recurrent problems develop. This approach represents a philosophical shift away from radical resection and toward biomechanically sound methods that make foot function a priority. These methods often employ minimal resection techniques combined with biopsy-directed medical treatment in an effort to preserve structures of the foot and ankle which are important for gait. This conservative approach applies to ideal procedure selection, incision or flap design, extent of bone resection, and level of amputation.

Contributors were carefully selected based on expertise, background, and clinical focus. Authors are both thought leaders and clinicians who deal with foot and ankle osteomyelitis on a daily basis. The information contained here represents a number of major teaching institutions with the community of interest represented by a multidisciplinary panel of experts.

St. Paul, MN, USA   Troy J. Boffeli

Contents

Contributors

Kyle W. Abben, DPM, AACFAS Jamestown Regional Medical Center, Jamestown, ND, USA

Jill F. Ashcraft, DPM Harvard Medical School, Mount Auburn Hospital, Cambridge, MA, USA

David B. Banach, MD, MPH, MS Section of Infectious Diseases, Yale School of Medicine, Woodbridge, CT, USA

Peter A. Blume, DPM, FACFAS Yale New Haven Hospital, New Haven, CT, USA

Troy J. Boffeli, DPM, FACFAS Regions Hospital/HealthPartners Institute for Education and Research, St. Paul, MN, USA

Rachel C. Collier, FACFAOM Regions Hospital/HealthPartners Institute for Education and Research, St. Paul, MN, USA

Emily A. Cook, DPM, MPH, CPH, FACFAS Division of Podiatric Surgery, Department of Surgery, Mount Auburn Hospital, Cambridge, MA, USA

Jeremy J. Cook, DPM, MPH, CPH, FACFAS Division of Podiatric Surgery, Department of Surgery, Mount Auburn Hospital, Cambridge, MA, USA

Michael E. Edmonds, MD Diabetic Foot Clinic, Department of Diabetics, Kings College Hospital, London, UK

Professor of Surgery, Surgery Orthopedics and Rehabilitation Anesthesia, Yale New Haven Hospital, New Haven, CT, USA

Ralph J. Faville, Jr, MD Department of Pediatric Infections Disease, Gillette Childrens Specialty Healthcare, St. Paul, MN, USA

Corey M. Fidler, DPM MedStar Washington Hospital Center, Washington, DC, USA

Caitlin S. Garwood, DPM Department of Plastic Surgery, Center for Wound Healing & Hyperbaric Medicine, Georgetown University Hospital, Washington, DC, USA

Lindsay Gates, MD Yale New Haven Hospital, New Haven, CT, USA

Shelby B. Hyllengren, DPM Allina Health Cambridge Medical Center, Cambridge, MN, USA

Allen M. Jacobs, DPM, FACFAS St. Louis, MO, USA

Suzanne B. Keel, MD Department of Pathology, Regions Hospital, St. Paul, MN, USA

Paul J. Kim, DPM, MS, FACFAS Department of Plastic Surgery, Center for Wound Healing & Hyperbaric Medicine, Georgetown University Hospital, Washington, DC, USA

Kevin J. Mahoney, DPM Regions Hospital/HealthPartners Institute for Education and Research, St. Paul, MN, USA

Chris A. Manu, MBBS, BSc, MRCP Department of Diabetes, Kings College Hospital, London, UK

Noah G. Oliver, DPM, AACFAS Ochsner Medical Center, New Orleans, LA, USA

Matthew C. Peterson, DPM Fairview Health Services, Edina, MN, USA

Ryan R. Pfannenstein, DPM, FACFAS Regions Hospital/HealthPartners Institute for Education and Research, St. Paul, MN, USA

Laurence G. Rubin, DPM, FACFAS Richmond, VA, USA

Michael Sganga, DPM Mount Auburn Hospital, Cambridge, MA, USA

John S. Steinberg, DPM, FACFAS Department of Plastic Surgery, Georgetown University School of Medicine, Washington, DC, USA

Bauer E. Sumpio, MD Department of Diabetes, King's College Hospital, London, UK

Jessica A. Tabatt, DPM Essentia Health-Brainerd Medical Center, Brainerd, MN, USA

Jonathan C. Thompson, DPM, MHA, AACFAS Orthopedic Center, Mayo Clinic Health System, Eau Claire, WI, USA

Susan B. Truman, MD St. Paul Radiology and HealthPartners, St. Paul, MN, USA

Brett J. Waverly, DPM Regions Hospital/HealthPartners Institute for Education and Research, St. Paul, MN, USA

Relevance of Osteomyelitis to Clinical Practice

Caitlin S. Garwood and Paul J. Kim

Introduction

Osteomyelitis is one of the most devastating conditions of the foot and ankle, and it remains a challenge to the clinician in both diagnosis and treatment. The lower extremity tends to be more susceptible to infection due to thin soft tissue layers, potentially poor vascular supply, neuropathy, structural deformity, boney prominences, and poor fitting shoes. Trauma, diabetes, peripheral vascular disease, prosthetic implants, and bacteremia can all lead to debilitating infection within the bones of the lower extremity. Advances in diagnosis and treatment have helped promote limb salvage, but there is still a great risk of partial or complete limb loss once infection involves the skeletal framework. Osteomyelitis is considered to be one of the most difficult-to-treat infectious disease processes. Despite its devastating outcomes and relatively high prevalence, there is a wide disparity in its diagnosis and treatment. Thus, a consensus for the most appropriate modalities for diagnosis and the most effective methods for treatment is difficult to achieve. This chapter will introduce the topic of osteomyelitis of the foot and ankle and provide a broad construct for a more detailed discussion found in the remainder of this book. Osteomyelitis simply defined is inflammation of bone usually caused by an infectious source, as was first introduced by Nelaton in 1844 [1, 2]. When broken down into its components, "osteo-" means bone, "myelo-" means marrow, and "-itis" means inflammation. This very definition can cause confusion depending on the clinician's perspective and specialty. For example, a surgeon treating "osteomyelitis" assumes a clinical infectious process corroborated by the pathologist who diagnoses osteomyelitis histologically. The pathologist, however, is reporting elements of an inflammatory process and not necessarily infection. In other words, osteomyelitis can mean something different to each specialist. It is possible that the lack of consensus for definition of osteomyelitis can create an environment where necessary treatment may not be rendered. Further, other terms can add to the overall confusion in defining osteomyelitis or related diagnoses. In the literature, the term "osteitis" can be confused with osteomyelitis but usually refers to involvement of the cortex only, whereas osteomyelitis also invades the bone marrow. Similarly, "periosteitis" is an infectious process involving only the periosteum [1–4]. Osteomyelitis can involve only part of a single section of bone or may encompass multiple sections of a bone such as the periosteum, cortex, or marrow. It can also involve more than one bone, which is often the case when occurring from a septic joint, infected prostheses, or an infection resulting from Charcot neuroarthropathy.

Epidemiological data on osteomyelitis of the foot and ankle is not consistent or abundant. Most of the data available is focused on other parts of the body, such as the tibia or mandible. In addition, most of the research on foot and ankle osteomyelitis is developed around osteomyelitis present in diabetic foot ulcers, leaving minimal data related to trauma and other causes. The overall incidence of osteomyelitis is not generally high because healthy bone is normally resistant to infection. Waldvogel et al. in 1970 reported that 19 % of osteomyelitis cases were due to hematogenous spread, 47 % from contiguous-focus, and 34 % were associated with vascular insufficiency [5, 6]. Currently the incidence of new cases of hematogenous, pediatric osteomyelitis is 2.9–22 per 100,000 patients [7–9]. The overall incidence of bone and joint infections in adults is 54.6 per 100,000 as was reported in 2012 [10]. It is still thought that today the majority of cases, particularly in adults, are contiguous-focus osteomyelitis especially with the dramatic rise in the diabetic population. As far as posttraumatic osteomyelitis, 2–16 % of open fractures are associated with bone infection depending on the extent and severity of the injury [11–13].

C.S. Garwood, D.P.M. • P.J. Kim, D.P.M., M.S., F.A.C.F.A.S. (✉)
Department of Plastic Surgery, Center for Wound Healing
& Hyperbaric Medicine, Georgetown University Hospital,
3800 Reservoir Rd, NW, Bles 1st Floor, Washington,
DC 20007, USA
e-mail: caitlin.garwood@gmail.com;
paul.j.kim@gunet.georgetown.edu

© Springer International Publishing Switzerland 2015
T.J. Boffeli (ed.), *Osteomyelitis of the Foot and Ankle*, DOI 10.1007/978-3-319-18926-0_1

Currently 382 million people worldwide are living with diabetes [14]. The risk of foot ulceration in diabetic patients is as high as 25 % and approximately 20–68 % of these ulcerations are reported to be complicated by osteomyelitis [15–21]. Osteomyelitis brings a significant risk of amputation whether it is a single digit, total ray, transmetatarsal, or lower limb and the rate of amputation has been reported to be up to 66 % [16, 21–23].

Etiology and Classification

Ideally, classifying osteomyelitis should incorporate all possible etiologies as well as address the various timing of the disease. Further, it is helpful when a classification system includes suggestions for treatment. Due to the different types of osteomyelitis, several classification schemes have been developed.

Osteomyelitis is broadly categorized into acute, subacute, or chronic based on timing and presentation of the disease process. Acute bone infection develops over several days to weeks, with 2 weeks being the most accepted time frame [5, 6, 24]. Chronic osteomyelitis has been defined arbitrarily as evolving or lasting over several months, with 6 months being the most widely accepted period [5, 6, 25, 26]. Any infection lingering between 2 and 6 months would then be classified as subacute. The temporal definitions are imprecise and confusing especially when there might be evidence of necrotic and chronic changes in the bone only one week after presentation. Others have defined "acute" as the first presentation of osteomyelitis in a particular bone and "chronic" as a recurrence of the infection that had previously been treated. Categorizing osteomyelitis as "initial" and "recurrent" may be more useful for the clinician in terms of implementing a proper treatment regimen [2, 3].

Osteomyelitis can be classified based on the cause whether by direct extension, hematogenous spread through contamination of the bloodstream, or contiguous spread from a current site of infection [27]. Direct extension osteomyelitis encompasses bone infections that arise from either a puncture wound or elective surgery that exposes bone to an infectious contaminant. It has been reported in the literature that 2 % of puncture wounds lead to osteomyelitis [28, 29]. Hematogenous osteomyelitis occurs from the seeding of bacteria from a distant site or bacteremia that spreads through the vascular system [26, 30]. It is thought to be primarily a pediatric disease with 85 % of the cases occurring in patients 17 years of age or younger [31]. It can also occur in the elderly or intravenous drug abusers. The last etiology is contiguous spread which includes bone infections that start from a soft tissue infection including open fractures, decubitus ulcers, or diabetic foot ulcers.

Two classification systems are commonly used throughout the literature and are important in understanding osteomyelitis. Other classifications have been described but are not used in common practice (Table 1.1). Waldvogel in 1970 developed a classification based on the duration of the disease, the mechanism of infection, and presence or absence of vascular insufficiency [5, 32]. A short coming of this classification system is that it provides no therapeutic guidelines (Table 1.2). Cierny and Mader developed a classification that is most applicable to long and large bones and has been seen as difficult to apply to digital bones or other small bones in the foot. It is based on the area of bone infected and the physiological status of the host and also incorporates the dynamic nature of the disease, which is useful to the clinician (Table 1.3) [25, 32, 33].

Table 1.1 Classification schemes for osteomyelitis [5, 33, 121]

Reference	Classification	Overview

[5], see Table 1.2	"Waldvogel"	• Mechanism
		  – Hematogenous
		  – Contiguous
		  – Vascular compromise
		• Duration
		  – Acute
		  – Chronic

[33], see Table 1.3	"Cierny-Mader"	• Anatomic
		  – Medullary
		  – Superficial
		  – Localized
		  – Diffuse
		• Physiologic
		  – Normal host
		  – Compromised
		  – Prohibitive

[121]	"Buckholtz"	1. Wound induced 2. Mechanogenic infection 3. Physeal osteomyelitis 4. Ischemic limb disease 5. Combinations of 1–4 6. Osteitis with septic arthritis 7. Chronic osteitis/osteomyelitis

Table 1.2 Waldvogel classification of osteomyelitis [5, 6, 31]

	Type	Characteristics
Mechanism of bone infection	Hematogenous	Seeding of bacteria from a distance source that spreads through the bloodstream
	Contiguous	Infection from an adjacent site such as open fracture
	Associated with vascular compromise	Infections in patients with peripheral vascular disease or diabetes
Duration of infection	Acute	Initial diagnosis of osteomyelitis. Edema, abscess, vascular congestion, small vessel thrombosis
	Chronic	Prolonged or recurrence of acute case Ischemia, necrosis, sequestra

Table 1.3 Cierny-Mader staging system for osteomyelitis [26, 31–33]

	Stage	Name	Characteristics	Clinical example(s)
Anatomic type	I	Medullary	Infection restricted to the bone marrow	1. Infected intramedullary rod 2. Hematogenous osteomyelitis
	II	Superficial	Infection restricted to outer cortex	Diabetic foot ulcer with infection extending to bone
	III	Localized	Well demarcated, full-thickness lesion without instability	Progression from Stage I or II
	IV	Diffuse	Infection spread to entire bone circumference with instability	Progression from Stage I, II, or III
Physiologic class	A	Normal host	No comorbidities	
	B	Bs	Systemic compromise	Diabetes, malnutrition, renal failure, hepatic failure, malignancy, extremes of age, immune disease
		Bl	Local compromise	Smoking, chronic lymphedema, major or small vessel compromise, venous stasis, arthritis, large scars, neuropathy
		Bls	Systemic and local compromise	Combination of above factors
	C	Prohibitive/poor clinical conditions	Treatment has a higher risk than osteomyelitis itself	Patient who is not a surgical candidate or who cannot tolerate long-term antibiotics

Pathophysiology and Microbiology

The pathophysiology of osteomyelitis is complicated but a basic understanding can help in the diagnosis and treatment of this disease. Throughout the natural course of osteomyelitis osseous changes occur, biofilm forms, and neutrophils cause major defects. All forms of osteomyelitis begin by bacteria adhering to the bone matrix via receptors to fibronectin, fibrinogen, laminin, collagen, and proteins [4, 34–37]. The attached organisms cause an inflammatory response of the bone. As inflammation persists and intramedullary pressure rises, the vascular channels become obliterated causing patches of ischemia and bone necrosis. These areas of necrotic bone can detach from the bone and are called sequestra [4, 25, 26, 34–38]. As necrotic bone is forming, osteoclastic activity is stimulated by inflammatory factors such as interleukin-1 and tumor necrosis factor. This causes loss of bone and creates a destructive appearance of the bone. At the same time, a periosteal reaction begins and causes new bone formation. This surrounds and encases the sequestrum and is termed involucrum. During the process of bone formation and destruction cloaca form, which are openings in the involucrum that connect to the sequestrum. It is through the cloaca which exudate often extrudes [3, 38].

Bacteria are able to fend off host defenses as well as antibiotics through the formation of biofilm, and thus infections can persist even after medical or surgical treatments. Biofilms are colonies of pathogens that bind to the surfaces of wounds or implants. They are generally composed of 25–30 % pathogen and 70–75 % self-secreted amorphous matrix [34–39]. A wound bed is an ideal environment for biofilm to form since it is moist and nutritionally supportive. Biofilm also tends to form on devitalized tissue and bone, such as involucrum [38]. It has been reported that as rapidly as 10 h, many of the bacteria flora present on the skin can form a biofilm [40]. They generally are polymicrobial in nature with anaerobes, *Serratia*, *Staphylococcus*, and *Pseudomonas* being the most robust [38–41]. In addition to multiple species present, there are various mechanisms by which a biofilm inhibits wound healing and can make the host more susceptible to osteomyelitis. The matrix created by the biofilm itself creates a physical barrier that inhibits host inflammatory cells from ridding the body of the pathogens. Biofilms are highly resistant to antibiotics as they do not easily penetrate through this matrix. Also, there is a metabolically senescent nature of biofilm, which leads to further resistance since many antibiotics target rapidly dividing bacteria [35, 39, 41]. Thus, it has become increasingly important to treat and extinguish the biofilm in a wound, on the surface of hardware (screws, plates, suture, joint implants), or on exposed bone in order to fully treat or prevent osteomyelitis.

Most foot and ankle osteomyelitis is polymicrobial in nature, except hematogenous osteomyelitis, which is almost always monomicrobial [38]. As with soft tissue infections, the causative agent in bone infections is primarily bacterial but can also result from fungal, parasitic, viral, or mycobacterial infections (Table 1.4) [32, 42]. *Staphylococcus aureus* is the most prevalent causative organism in osteomyelitis [4, 43]. It accounts for the majority of hematogenous osteomyelitis in children and adults and is present in many other foot and ankle cases. *S. aureus* has a number of unique traits that make it particularly virulent. First, it contains factors that allow it to attach to extracellular matrix proteins contributing to early colonization of the host. *S. aureus* also has features such as toxins and capsular polysaccharides that make it less susceptible to host defenses. Osteolysis has been seen to occur rapidly from the increased osteoclastic activity due to the release of tumor necrosis factor-α, prostoglandins, and

Table 1.4 Most commonly associated microorganism and their clinical setting [4, 25, 32]

Common clinical setting	Etiology
Hematogenous, all ages	*Staphylococcus aureus*
Hematogenous, infants/children	*Haemophilus influenzae*
Diabetes mellitus, vascular insufficiency, contaminated open fracture	Polymicrobial: *Staphylococcus aureus*, *B-Hemolytic Streptococci*, *Enterococci*, aerobic gram-negative bacilli
Orthopedic implant devices, hardware, foreign bodies	*Staphylococcus aureus*, coagulase-negative staphylococci (*Staphylococcus epidermidis*)
Human or animal bites	*Pasteurella multocida*, *Eikenella corrodens*
Puncture wounds on the foot	*Pseudomonas aeruginosa*
Soil contamination	*Clostridium* sp., *Bacillus* sp., *Stenotrophomonas maltophilia*, *Nocardia* sp., atypical mycobacteria, *Aspergillus* sp., *Rhizopus* sp., *Mucor* sp.
Sickle-cell disease	*Salmonella* sp.
Intravenous drug users	*Pseudomonas aeruginosa*, *Staphylococcus aureus*, *Candida* sp.

interleukin-1. It is the combination of these factors that makes *S. aureus* a common culprit in chronic infections leading to osteomyelitis [25, 26, 32, 35, 38]. Of great importance in foot and ankle osteomyelitis is the increasing prevalence of methacillin-resistant *S. aureus* (MRSA). This pathogen is frequently encountered in hospitalized patients along with other multidrug-resistant organisms. In 2013, it was reported that the incidence of community acquired MRSA was 1.6–29.7 cases per 100,000 and 2.8–43 % of those were bone and joint infections [44]. It has also been reported to account for 15.3 % of osteomyelitis cases in diabetic foot infections [26, 45, 46]. This rise in incidence throughout the general population, not just diabetic patients, has prompted clinicians to use broad-spectrum antibiotics prior to culture results. The treatment of MRSA osteomyelitis can be more prolonged and complicated with increasing lengths of hospital stays and complications [44, 45].

Pseudomonas aeruginosa is another common organism seen in osteomyelitis of the foot. It is frequently seen as the infecting organism in plantar puncture wounds since it is present on the soles of shoes and its predilection for warm, moist environments. It has been reported that osteomyelitis complicates 1.8–6.4 % of puncture wounds sustained to the feet [2, 26, 47–49]. In 2.5–14.6 % of diabetic foot osteomyelitis, *P. aeruginosa* has been isolated and is associated with a higher rate of recurrence and amputation than *S. aureus* [26, 46]. Thus, *P. aeruginosa* may be a more problematic and underappreciated organism in osteomyelitis.

Populations at Risk

Osteomyelitis behaves differently in various patient populations as well as different anatomical locations. There are cohorts of patients that are at a higher risk of developing a bone infection and situations where the clinician needs a higher index of suspicion for the disease. Recognizing patients and clinical situations with a high predilection for developing osteomyelitis will help the clinician with early diagnosis and an appropriate treatment protocol.

As mentioned previously, hematogenous osteomyelitis most frequently occurs in children. Those with an even higher risk factor are children with sickle-cell disease [50]. Due to obstruction and damage to the spleen, they are at an extreme susceptibility to infection. Risk factors in adults include intravenous drug use as well as common causes of bacteremia. These include urinary tract infections, indwelling catheters, central intravenous lines, and hemodialysis [2].

Recent trauma or surgery can put a patient at a higher risk of developing osteomyelitis. Any foot and ankle surgery can lead to a deep infection involving the bone. An incisional dehiscence, if not treated appropriately and in a timely fashion, can cause a debilitating infection in the bone. Likewise, implanted devices including plates, joint implants, and external fixators bring a higher risk factor simply by introducing a foreign material into the body. These implanted devices due to its contact on the bone surface can provide an optimal environment for biofilm formation, which in turn can cause infection of the underlying bone [51]. Patients who sustain an open fracture are more susceptible to osteomyelitis until the bone is covered with a soft tissue envelope. The longer the bone is exposed, the more likely the chance of developing a complication [52]. It is recommended that definitive soft tissue reconstruction take place within 7 days of injury and ideally by day 3, to minimize the risk of reconstructive failure or deep infections [52–54]. Injuries to the nail plate can also increase the risk of bone infection, particularly in pediatric patients because of the lack of soft tissue between the nail and the underlying bone [2, 55, 56]. Puncture wounds to the foot as well as animal or human bites can predispose the bone to infection [48, 49].

Complicating factors such as peripheral neuropathy, peripheral vascular disease, and underlying immunocompromise can lead to foot ulcerations. Wound chronicity can eventually lead to deep ulcers that penetrate to the level of the bone. It is important for high-risk patients, such as diabetics, to minimize ulcerations by appropriate foot care and prevention [22, 23, 57]. Peripheral vascular disease (PVD), which is encountered in diabetic patients as well as tobacco abusers, is another risk factor. With decreased blood circulation to the foot or ankle, patients are at a higher risk of developing a wound [58]. The lack of blood flow creates a recalcitrant wound healing environment and the patients are at a higher risk for osteomyelitis. Often, patients will have both diabetes and PVD and have a 2- to 5.5-fold increase risk of ulceration leading to osteomyelitis [15, 59]. Patients with an impaired immune function may not have the ability to appropriately fight off an infection and thus are at a higher statistical risk of developing a deep bone infection. This includes patients taking corticosteroids for rheumatic or dermatologic diseases, patients receiving chemotherapy, organ transplant recipients, as well as systemic diseases like diabetes [25, 58, 60]. Uncontrolled diabetics live in a state of elevated glucose levels which impairs leukocyte function and can negatively affect the body's ability to respond to antimicrobials [60].

The lower extremity itself is a risk factor for developing osteomyelitis and is well known to be a hard-to-treat anatomical location. The foot and ankle has a relatively thin soft tissue envelope covering deep anatomical structures. This makes the lower extremity highly susceptible to repetitive trauma especially in areas of boney prominences. Once bone is exposed, soft tissue coverage can be challenging. There are very limited options for local tissue coverage in the lower extremity. Surgeons have thus turned to free tissue transfer to increase soft tissue girth, but the complexity of these procedures can lead to significant complications in many patients, especially in the elderly or patients with diabetes, peripheral vascular disease, end stage renal disease, or infection [61, 62]. In addition, instability is often created when bone is resected from the foot or when partial amputations are performed. This creates a dysfunctional lower extremity and can also lead to other problems including new ulcerations. As mentioned previously, many patients with foot osteomyelitis have poor vascular supply and the inability to heal. Rather than undergoing numerous limb salvage procedures when osteomyelitis is involved, patients may be better served with a below-knee or above-knee amputation [61–66].

Diagnosis

A unique challenge with osteomyelitis is *definitively* diagnosing the disease and making this diagnosis early. An accurate diagnosis is needed in order to formulate an appropriate treatment plan which is especially true for this progressive destructive process. There are several modalities used for identifying osteomyelitis including history, physical examination, laboratory values, imaging, microbiology, and bone biopsies (Fig. 1.1) [20, 67–81]. Ultimately, a combination of these modalities is needed to diagnose osteomyelitis. Each diagnostic modality has its own strengths and weaknesses with no single modality providing conclusive evidence of bone infection. To date, no single, robust, consensus-driven, diagnostic algorithm is available for clinicians to utilize for osteomyelitis. Since there is no standardized method available, ambiguous results and potentially failure of treatment can result.

An adequate history can be very informative for raising the suspicion and approaching a diagnosis of osteomyelitis. Frequent symptoms can include redness, swelling, pain, or drainage from a wound or surgical site. Often the pain is described as vague, deep, and chronic [4]. Any history of trauma or ulceration should be thoroughly investigated. Past medical history should be evaluated as well for systemic diseases and their current management and control. For example, it is important to evaluate glycemic control in diabetic patients. Other useful information includes nutritional status, ambulatory status, age, and presence of neuropathic or peripheral vascular symptoms [4, 26].

Physical examination and laboratory values for infection are two other commonly utilized modalities for the diagnosis of osteomyelitis. The physical signs of osteomyelitis are subjective in nature. This includes signs of infection of the overlying soft tissue envelope as well as the quality of the suspected area of bone infection. Fragmentation, necrosis, desiccation, and frank purulence of the bone are strong indicators of infection. However, these signs may not be specific for osteomyelitis. Fragmentation could be due to other factors including nutrition, age, Charcot neuro-osteoarthropathy, and trauma. Necrosis and desiccation could be the result of vascular compromise. Further, frank purulence may not be coming from the bone but from the surrounding soft tissue infection. The Grayson study recommended the "probe-to-bone" test for the diagnosis for osteomyelitis [19]. They reported a sensitivity of 66 %, specificity of 85 %, and a positive predictive value of 89 % with probe-to-bone test and presence of osteomyelitis. However, a subsequent study by Lavery et al. called into question the specificity for this test [68]. Their diagnosis had been confirmed with a bone culture and they found a sensitivity of 87 %, specificity of 91 %, positive predictive value of only 57 %, but a negative predictive value of 98 %. This shows that a negative probe-to-bone test may be more useful in excluding osteomyelitis than a positive test would be for confirming diagnosis. Elevated laboratory values including C-Reactive Protein, erythrocyte sedimentation rate, and white blood cell counts may be surrogate indicators of bone infection but lack specificity for osteomyelitis [82–84].

One of the major problems with diagnosing osteomyelitis is that imaging studies have low sensitivity to early detection and are non-specific. Plain radiographs, nuclear medicine studies, and magnetic resonance imaging are among the most

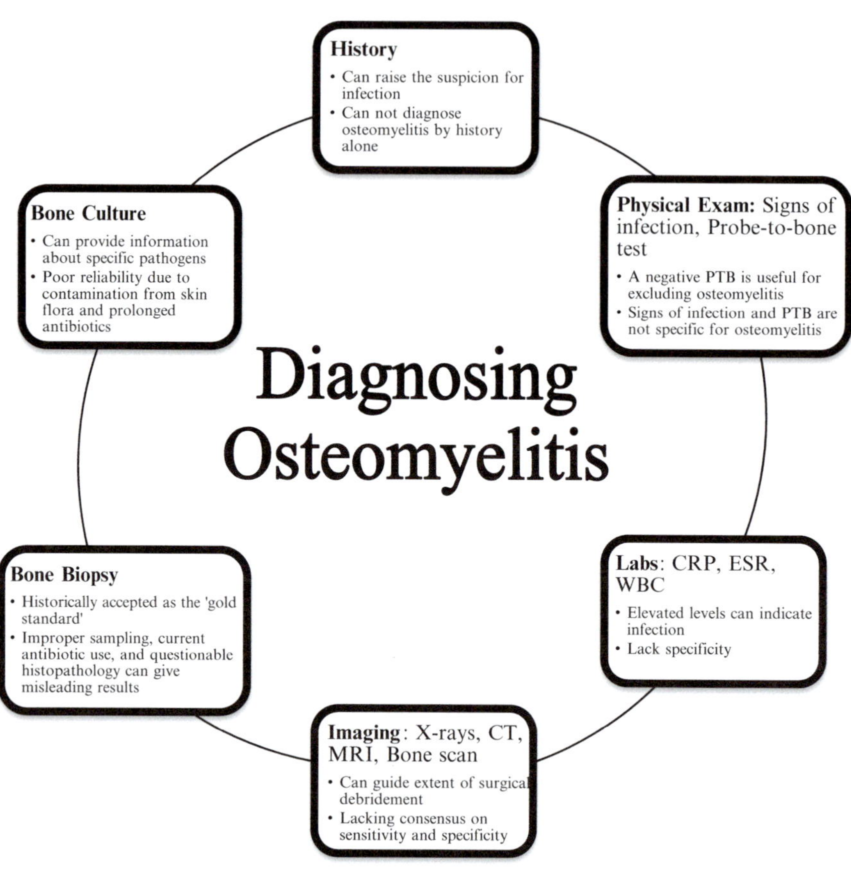

Fig. 1.1 Modalities used for diagnosing osteomyelitis. Each box represents a different modality with key points listed below. It is designed to represent the fact that several tools are used in combination to formulate the diagnosis of osteomyelitis [4, 19, 20, 26, 67–87]

commonly used imaging modalities for the diagnosis of osteomyelitis. Several studies have looked at the sensitivity and specificity of each without reaching a consensus on appropriate imaging [20, 67, 70–79, 85]. The second major issue is the difficulty in distinguishing between osteomyelitis and a different disease entity. This is especially troubling to the foot and ankle surgeon when dealing with diabetic patients. Sixty to seventy percent of diabetic patients have mild to moderate peripheral neuropathy and are at risk of developing neuro-osteoarthropathy [88, 89]. Charcot neuro-osteoarthropathy of the foot can often be mistaken for osteomyelitis both on physical examination as well as on imaging. Even more of a challenge is when both disease entities are present concomitantly.

Bone biopsy and bone culture are also commonly used to definitively diagnose osteomyelitis. In fact, it has long been purported that a bone biopsy is the gold standard for diagnosing osteomyelitis. However, it is not without its own challenges and problems due to improper sampling techniques, current use of antibiotics, or questionable histopathology results [80]. A study by Meyr et al. evaluated the reliability of histopathology of bone biopsies used for diagnosis of osteomyelitis in diabetic patients. They found a unanimous agreement between four board-certified pathologists for only 33.33 % of the specimens examined. Questionable results

where at least one pathologist diagnosed "no evidence of OM" and at least one other pathologist diagnosed "findings consistent with OM," occurred 41.03 % of the time [80]. Further, as discussed in a previous paragraph, osteomyelitis may be used as a descriptive histological term that may or may not indicate infection, rather than a diagnosis. Bone tissue cultures also pose an issue with specimen contamination and only specific bacteria being cultured [86, 87]. There is a risk of false-positive results from skin flora surrounding the bone, but also a risk of false-negative results due to prolonged release of antibiotics from bone [87]. Thus, there is poor reliability of bone cultures taken in the presence of a wound in determining the diagnosis of osteomyelitis as well as the infecting pathogen.

Management

The ideal management of osteomyelitis depends on several factors specific to each patient and circumstance. Both medical and surgical methods are available and often a combination of therapies is necessary (Fig. 1.2). The goal of treatment is to eliminate infection and to prevent the development of a chronic infection or recurrence. A team approach to treatment

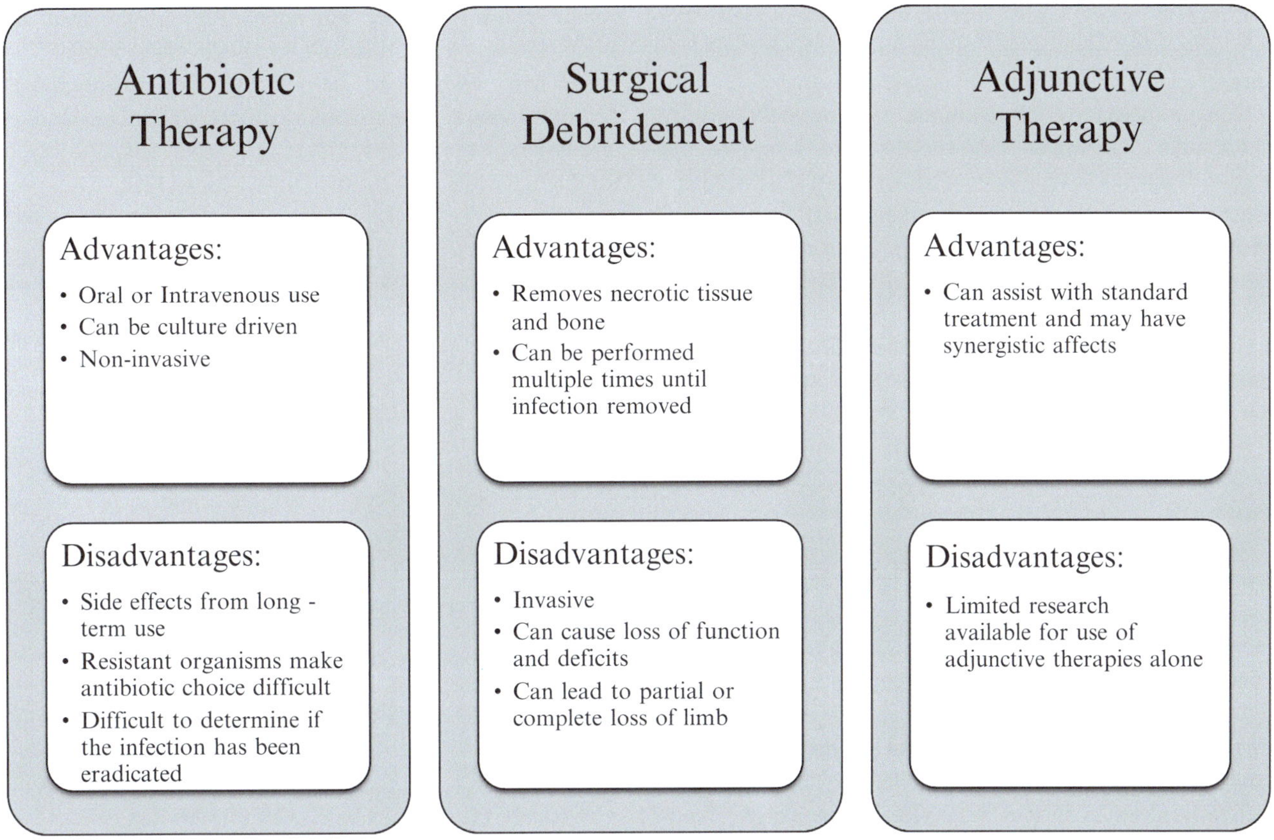

<table>
<tr>
<th>Antibiotic Therapy</th>
<th>Surgical Debridement</th>
<th>Adjunctive Therapy</th>
</tr>
<tr>
<td>

Advantages:

- Oral or Intravenous use
- Can be culture driven
- Non-invasive

</td>
<td>

Advantages:

- Removes necrotic tissue and bone
- Can be performed multiple times until infection removed

</td>
<td>

Advantages:

- Can assist with standard treatment and may have synergistic affects

</td>
</tr>
<tr>
<td>

Disadvantages:

- Side effects from long - term use
- Resistant organisms make antibiotic choice difficult
- Difficult to determine if the infection has been eradicated

</td>
<td>

Disadvantages:

- Invasive
- Can cause loss of function and deficits
- Can lead to partial or complete loss of limb

</td>
<td>

Disadvantages:

- Limited research available for use of adjunctive therapies alone

</td>
</tr>
</table>

Fig. 1.2 Management of osteomyelitis. The advantages and disadvantages of antibiotic therapy, surgical debridement, and adjunctive therapy [2, 25, 92–107]

is often employed and includes specialty care for wound management, surgical debridement, antibiotic therapy, vascular optimization, and soft tissue or limb reconstruction [18, 57, 90, 91].

It has long been accepted that 4–6 weeks of parenteral antibiotics is the standard course of treatment for osteomyelitis. This theory, however, was largely drawn from animal models as well as observational data with randomized patient trials lacking [2]. The choice of antibiotics should be pathogen-driven while taking into consideration bone penetration, long-term side effects, and cost-effectiveness. Oral antibiotics are now being seen as an acceptable alternative to parenteral treatment as several antibiotics have excellent oral bioavailability with good bone penetration. Some oral antibiotics with acceptable oral bioavailability commonly include linezolid, fluoroquinolones, and clindamycin. Many have also employed a combination therapy where parenteral antibiotics are initiated for approximately 2 weeks followed by a prolonged course of oral antibiotics [2, 25, 92–94]. A recent Cochrane Review showed no statistically significant difference in terms of remission for patients treated with oral versus parenteral antibiotics. They also found no or insufficient evidence in terms of optimal length of treatment or medication [93].

Surgical debridement of bone infection is of significant importance in situations in which antibiotic therapy is not adequate, abscess or necrotic tissue is present, or systemic illness or sepsis mandates surgical intervention. A surgical plan is formulated based on the site and extent of infection as well as preservation of a functional limb. A surgeon must remove all necrotic bone and soft tissue which can frequently leave large deficits of bone or lead to minor or major amputation. After adequate debridement, there may be the need for boney stabilization or soft tissue reconstruction and coverage [93, 95–97]. Antibiotic impregnated spacers are also used to elute antibiotics over time in an area where infected bone was resected [98]. It has been seen useful for salvage after osteomyelitis, most frequently in the forefoot, in patients who would have otherwise received an amputation [98–100].

Another adjunctive therapy is the use of hyperbaric oxygen (HBO) therapy for chronic osteomyelitis. HBO therapy increases the oxygen tension of tissue and bone and has been shown to have several proposed effects on wound healing and osteomyelitis including improved leukocyte function, increased osteoclastic activity, and neovascularization [2, 26, 101, 102]. Although there is some proven efficacy when used in conjunction with other treatment modalities, strong evidence is lacking on the success or efficacy of HBO therapy, especially when used alone and not with antibiotics or surgery [2, 101–107].

The combination of antibiotic therapy with surgical debridement has proven to be successful for long-term outcomes. It has not been proven whether surgical debridement alone would be adequate to prevent remission. Some authors believe that inadequate debridement is correlated with higher rates of recurrence [93, 96, 97, 108, 109]. Others report that antibiotic therapy can be shortened after debridement [110, 111]. Ultimately, a combination of therapies is most widely used and the clinician must make the decision based on each unique clinical situation.

Outlook

Unfortunately for patients affected by osteomyelitis of the foot and ankle, amputation can be an end result. This can include digital, partial ray, transmetatarsal, midfoot, below-knee or above-knee amputations. Amputations can have a great impact on a patient psychologically and in terms of their quality of life [112–116]. Digital and partial foot amputations alter the biomechanics of the foot and can lead to difficulty in ambulation or new ulcer formation and recurrence. Major amputations come wrought with complications as well including inability to ambulate, increased energy expenditure, and increase risk of mortality. It has been reported that a major leg amputation has a mortality rate of 52–70 % at 2 and 5 years [117, 118]. Every attempt should be made to preserve pedal function; however for some patients, the benefit of amputation out-weighs the risk of long-term antibiotics or multiple salvage surgeries. The overall recurrence rate of osteomyelitis remains at about 20–30 % in a patient's lifetime. In certain situations, such as with *P. aeruginosa*, the recurrence rate is as high as 50 % [93, 119, 120]. Patients who have osteomyelitis are considered to have a lifetime risk of recurrence at the same site of previous infection due to alterations to the bone surfaces and health.

Conclusion

Osteomyelitis of the foot and ankle is a major public health problem. With the rise in bacterial resistance to antibiotics as well as the lack of new antibiotics in the development pipeline, judicious use is required. However, there is a lack of consensus on the most appropriate methods for diagnosis and treatment of osteomyelitis. Thus, antibiotics may be used inappropriately. Surgical options for the treatment of osteomyelitis including resection, removal of hardware, and amputation also have problems. The lack of skeletal integrity compromises the functional capabilities of the foot and ankle. Experienced clinicians recognize that current diagnostic and treatment modalities fall short of providing a definitive answer. The following chapters provide a detailed discussion on the current evidence as well as valuable insight for the diagnosis and treatment of osteomyelitis.

References

1. Oloff L, Schulhofer S. Osteomyelitis. In: Banks A, Downy M, Martin D, Miller S, editors. McGlamry's comprehensive textbook of foot and ankle surgery. 3rd ed. Philadelphia: Lippincott, Williams & Wilkins; 2001.
2. Oloff LM, Heard GS. Osteomyelitis. In: Southerland JT, Boberg JS, Downey MS, Nakra A, Rabjohn LV, editors. McGlamry's comprehensive textbook of foot and ankle surgery. 4th ed. Philadelphia: Lippincott Williams & Wilkins; 2012.
3. Baltensperger M, Eyrich G. Osteomyelitis of the jaws. Lepzig: Springer; 2009.
4. Chihara S, Segreti J. Osteomyelitis. Dis Mon. 2010;56(1):5–31.
5. Waldvogel FA, Medoff G, Swartz MN. Osteomyelitis: a review of clinical features, therapeutic considerations and unusual aspects. N Engl J Med. 1970;282:198–206.
6. Waldvogel FA, Vasey H. Osteomyelitis: the past decade. N Engl J Med. 1980;303(7):360–70.
7. Blyth MJ, Kincaid R, Craigen MA, Bennet GC. The changing epidemiology of acute and subacute haematogenous osteomyelitis in children. J Bone Joint Surg Br. 2001;83(1):99–102.
8. Stoesser N, Pocock J, Moore CE, Soeng S, Hor P, Sar P, et al. The epidemiology of pediatric bone and joint infections in Cambodia, 2007–2011. J Trop Pediatr. 2013;59(1):36–42.
9. Grammatico-Guillon L, Maakaroun Vermesse Z, Baron S, Gettner S, Rusch E, Bernard L. Paediatric bone and joint infections are more common in boys and toddlers: a national epidemiology study. Acta Paediatr. 2013;102(3):e120–5.
10. Grammatico-Guillon L, Baron S, Gettner S, Lecuyer A, Gaborit C, Rosset P, et al. Bone and joint infections in hospitalized patients in France, 2008: clinical and economic outcomes. J Hosp Infect. 2012;82(1):40–8.
11. Browner BD. Skeletal trauma basic science, management, and reconstruction. In: Browner BD, editor. MD Consult. 4th ed. Philadelphia: Saunders/Elsevier; 2009.
12. Mader JT, Cripps MW, Calhoun JH. Adult posttraumatic osteomyelitis of the tibia. Clin Orthop Relat Res. 1999;360:14–21.
13. Roesgen M, Hierholzer G, Hax PM. Post-traumatic osteomyelitis. Pathophysiology and management. Arch Orthop Trauma Surg. 1989;108(1):1–9.
14. International Diabetes Federation. IDF diabetes atlas. 6th ed. Brussels, Belgium: International Diabetes Federation; 2013. http://www.idf.org/diabetesatlas.
15. Lavery LA, Armstrong DG, Wunderlich RP, Mohler MJ, Wendel CS, Lipsky BA. Risk factors for foot infections in individuals with diabetes. Diabetes Care. 2006;29:1288–93.
16. Singh N, Armstrong DG, Lipsky BA. Preventing foot ulcers in patients with diabetes. JAMA. 2005;293:217–28.
17. Lipsky BA, Berendt AR, Deery HG, et al. Diagnosis and treatment of diabetic foot infections. Clin Infect Dis. 2004;39(7):885–910.
18. Shank CF, Feibel JB. Osteomyelitis in the diabetic foot: diagnosis and management. Foot Ankle Clin. 2006;11(4):775–89.
19. Grayson ML, Gibbons GW, Balogh K, Levin E, Karchmer AW. Probing to bone in infected pedal ulcers. A clinical sign of underlying osteomyelitis in diabetic patients. JAMA. 1995;273(9): 721–3.

20. Newman LG, Waller J, Palestro CJ, Schwartz M, Klein MJ, Hermann G, et al. Unsuspected osteomyelitis in diabetic foot ulcers. Diagnosis and monitoring by leukocyte scanning with indium in 111 oxyquinoline. JAMA. 1991;266(9):1246–51.

21. Balsells M, Viade J, Millan M, Garcia JR, Garcia-Pascual L, del Pozo C, et al. Prevalence of osteomyelitis in non-healing diabetic foot ulcers: usefulness of radiologic and scintigraphic findings. Diabetes Res Clin Pract. 1997;38(2):123–7.

22. Hartemann-Heurtier A, Senneville E. Diabetic foot osteomyelitis. Diabetes Metab. 2008;34(2):87–95.

23. Game FL. Osteomyelitis in the diabetic foot: diagnosis and management. Med Clin North Am. 2013;97(5):947–56.

24. Hatzenbuehler J, Pulling TJ. Diagnosis and management of osteomyelitis. Am Fam Physician. 2011;84(9):1027–33.

25. Lew DP, Waldvogel FA. Osteomyelitis. Lancet. 2004;364(9431):369–79.

26. Lindbloom BJ, James ER, McGarvey WC. Osteomyelitis of the foot and ankle: diagnosis, epidemiology, and treatment. Forthcoming: Foot Ankle Clin N AM; 2014. http://dx.doi.org/10.1016/j.fcl.2014.06.012.

27. Harmer JL, Pickard J, Stinchcombe SJ. The role of diagnostic imaging in the evaluation of suspected osteomyelitis in the foot: a critical review. Foot (Edinb). 2011;21(3):149–53.

28. Ansari MA, Shukla VK. Foot infections. Int J Low Extrem Wounds. 2005;4(2):74–87.

29. Malizos KN, Gougoulias NE, Dailiana ZH, Varitimidis S, Bargiotas KA, Paridis D. Ankle and foot osteomyelitis: treatment protocol and clinical results. Injury. 2010;41:285–93.

30. Kelsey R, Kor A, Cordano F. Hematogenous osteomyelitis of the calcaneus in children: surgical treatment and use of implanted antibiotic beads. J Foot Ankle Surg. 1995;34(6):547–55.

31. Lima AL, Oliveira PR, Carvalho VC, Cimerman S, Savio E. Recommendations for the treatment of osteomyelitis. Braz J Infect Dis. 2014;18(5):526–34. http://dx.doi.org/10.1016/j.bjid.2013.12.005.

32. Sia IG, Berbari EF. Osteomyelitis. Best Pract Res Clin Rheumatol. 2006;20(6):1065–81.

33. Cierny 3rd G, Mader JT, Penninck JJ. A clinical staging system for adult osteomyelitis. Clin Orthop Relat Res. 2003;414:7–24.

34. Uçkay I, Pittet D, Vaudaux P, Sax H, Lew D, Waldvogel F. Foreign body infections due to *Staphylococcus epidermidis*. Ann Med. 2009;41(2):109–19.

35. Uckay I, Buchs NC, Seghrouchni K, Assal M, Hoffmeyer P, Lew D, Bacterial Osteomylitis: The Clinician's Point of View. Diagnostic imaging of infections and inflammatory diseases: a multidisciplinary approach. 1st ed. Geneva: Wiley; 2014.

36. Uckay I, Assal M, Legout L, Rohner P, Stern R, Lew D, et al. Recurrent osteomyelitis caused by infection with different bacterial strains without obvious source of reinfection. J Clin Microbiol. 2006;44(3):1194–6.

37. Sendi P, Proctor RA. Staphylococcus aureus as an intracellular pathogen: the role of small colony variants. Trends Microbiol. 2009;17(2):54–8.

38. Brady RA, Leid JG, Costerton JW, Shirtliff ME. Osteomyelitis: clinical overview and mechanisms of infection persistence. Clinical Microbiol. 2006;28(9):65–72.

39. Kim PJ, Steinberg JS. Wound care: biofilm and its impact on the latest treatment modalities for ulcerations of the diabetic foot. Semin Vasc Surg. 2012;25(2):70–4.

40. Harrison-Balestra C, Cazzaniga AL, Davis SC, et al. A wound-isolated Pseudomonas aeruginosa grows a biofilm in vitro within 10 hours and is visualized by light microscopy. Dermatol Surg. 2003;29(6):631–5.

41. Thomsen TR, Aasholm MS, Rudkjobing VB, Saunders AM, Bjarnsholt T, Givskov M, et al. The bacteriology of chronic venous leg ulcer examined by culture-independent molecular methods. Wound Repair Regen. 2010;18(1):38–49.

42. Bariteau JT, Waryasz GR, McDonnell M, Fischer SA, Hayda RA, Born CT. Fungal osteomyelitis and septic arthritis. J Am Acad Orthop Surg. 2014;22(6):390–401.

43. Dirschl DR, Almekinders LC. Osteomyelitis: common causes and treatment recommendations. Drugs. 1993;45(1):29–43.

44. Vardakas KZ, Kontopidis I, Gkegkes ID, Rafailidis PI, Falagas ME. Incidence, characteristics, and outcomes of patients with bone and joint infections due to community-associated methicillin-resistant Staphylococcus aureus: a systematic review. Eur J Clin Microbiol Infect Dis. 2013;32(6):711–21.

45. Aragon-Sanchez J, Lipsky BA, Lazaro-Martinez JL. Diagnosing diabetic foot osteomyelitis: is the combination of probe-to-bone and plain radiography sufficient for high-risk patients? Diabet Med. 2011;28(2):191–4.

46. Acharya S, Soliman M, Egun A, Rajbhandari SM. Conservative management of diabetic foot osteomyelitis. Diabetes Res Clin Pract. 2013;101(3):e18–20.

47. Corey SV, Butterworth ML. Puncture wounds. In: Southerland JT, Boberg JS, Downey MS, Nakra A, Rabjohn LV, editors. McGlamry's comprehensive textbook of foot and ankle surgery. 4th ed. Philadelphia: Lippincott Williams & Wilkins; 2012.

48. Laughlin RT, Reeve F, Wright DG, Mader JT, Calhoun JH. Calcaneal osteomyelitis caused by nail puncture wounds. Foot Ankle Int. 1997;18(9):575–7.

49. Weber EJ. Plantar puncture wounds: a survey to determine the incidence of infection. J Accid Emerg Med. 1996;13(4):274–7.

50. Onwubalili JK. Sickle cell disease and infection. J Infect. 1983;7(1):2–20.

51. Zimmerli W, Trampuz A, Ochsner PE. Prosthetic joint infections. N Engl J Med. 2004;351:1645–54.

52. Liu DS, Sofiadellis F, Ashton M, MacGill K, Webb A. Early soft tissue coverage and negative pressure wound therapy optimizes patient outcomes in lower limb trauma. Injury. 2012;43(6):772–8.

53. Gopal S, Majumder S, Batchelor AG, Knight SL, De Boer P, Smith RM. Fix and flap: the radical orthopaedic and plastic treatment of severe open fractures of the tibia. J Bone Joint Surg. 2000;82(7):959–66.

54. Hou Z, Irqit K, Strohecker KA, Matzko ME, Wingert NC, DeSantis JG, Smith WR. Delayed flap reconstruction with vacuum-assisted closure management of the open IIIB tibial fractures. J Trauma. 2011;71(6):1705–8.

55. Pinckney LE, Currarino G, Kennedy LA. The stubbed great toe: a cause of occult compound fracture and infection. Radiology. 1981;138(2):375–7.

56. Böhm E, Josten C. What's new in exogenous osteomyelitis. Pathol Res Pract. 1992;188(1–2):254–8.

57. Jeffcoate WJ, Lipsky BA. Controversies in diagnosing and managing osteomyelitis of the foot in diabetes. Clin Infect Dis. 2004;39 Suppl 2:s115–22.

58. Boyko EJ, Ahroni JH, Stensel V, Forsberg RC, Davignon DR, Smith DG. A prospective study of risk factors for diabetic foot ulcer. Diabetes Care. 1999;22(7):1036–42.

59. Peters EJ, Lavery LA, Armstrong DG. Diabetic lower extremity infection influence of physical, psychological, and social factors. J Diabetes Complications. 2005;19(2):107–12.

60. Shilling AM, Raphael J. Diabetes, hyperglycemia, and infections. Best Pract Res Clin Anaesthesiol. 2008;22(3):519–35.

61. Janis JE, Kwon RK, Attinger CE. The new reconstructive ladder: modifications to the traditional model. Plast Reconstr Surg. 2011;127 Suppl 1:205S–12.

62. Iorio ML, Shuck J, Attinger CE. Wound healing in the upper and lower extremities: a systematic review on the use of acellular dermal matrices. Plast Reconstr Surg. 2012;130(5 Suppl 2):232S–41.

63. Parrett BM, Pomahac B, Demling RH, Orgill DP. Fourth degree burns to the lower extremity with exposed tendon and bone: a ten-year experience. J Burn Care Res. 2006;27(1):34–9.

64. Parrett BM, Matros E, Pribaz JJ, Orgill DP. Lower extremity trauma: trends in the management of soft tissue reconstruction of open tibia-fibula fractures. Plast Reconstr Surg. 2006;117(4): 1315–22.

65. Ofer N, Baumeister S, Ohlbauer M, Germann G, Saurbier M. Microsurgical reconstruction of the burned upper extremity. Handchir Mikrochir Plast Chir. 2005;37(4):245–55.

66. Baumeister S, Koller M, Dragu A, Germann G, Sauerbier M. Principles of microvascular reconstruction in burn and electrical burn injuries. Burns. 2005;31:92–8.

67. Teh J, Berendt T, Lipsky BA. Investigating suspected bone infection in the diabetic foot. BMJ. 2009;339:b4690.

68. Lavery LA, Armstrong DG, Peters EJ, Lipsky BA. Probe-to-bone test for diagnosing diabetic foot osteomyelitis: reliable or relic? Diabetes Care. 2007;30:270–4.

69. Shone A, Burnside J, Chipchase S, Game F, Jeffcoate W. Probing the validity of the probe-to-bone test in the diagnosis of osteomyelitis of the foot in diabetes. Diabetes Care. 2006;29(4):945.

70. Dinh MT, Abad CL, Safdar N. Diagnostic accuracy of the physical examination and imaging tests for osteomyelitis underlying diabetic foot ulcers: meta-analysis. Clin Infect Dis. 2008;47(4):519–27.

71. Capriotti G, Chianelli M, Signore A. Nuclear medicine imaging of diabetic foot infection: results of meta-analysis. Nucl Med Commun. 2006;27(10):757–64.

72. Sanverti SE, Ergen FB, Oznur A. Current challenges in imaging of the diabetic foot. Diabet Foot Ankle. 2012;3:5. http://dx.doi. org/10.3402/dfa.v3i0.18754.

73. Morrison WB, Schweitzer ME, Batte WG, Radack DP, Russel KM. Osteomyelitis of the foot: relative importance of primary and secondary MR imaging signs. Radiology. 1998;207(3):625–32.

74. Collins MS, Schaar MM, Wenger DE, Mandrekar JN. T1-weighted MRI characteristics of pedal osteomyelitis. AJR Am J Roentgenol. 2005;185(2):386–93.

75. Rozzanigo U, Tagliani A, Vittorini E, Pacchioni R, Brivio LR, Caudana R. Role of magnetic resonance imaging in the evaluation of diabetic foot with suspected osteomyelitis. Radiol Med. 2009;114(1):121–32.

76. Gnanasegaran G, Chicklore S, Vijayanathan S, O'Doherty MJ, Fogelman I. Diabetes and bone: advantages and limitations of radiological, radionuclide and hybrid techniques in the assessment of diabetic foot. Minerva Endocrinol. 2009;34(3):237–54.

77. Donovan A, Schweitzer ME. Current concepts in imaging diabetic pedal osteomyelitis. Radiol Clin North Am. 2008;46(6):1105–24.

78. Russell JM, Peterson JJ, Bancroft LW. MR imaging of the diabetic foot. Magn Reson Imaging Clin N Am. 2008;16(1):59–70.

79. Ahmadi ME, Morrison WB, Carrino JA, Schweitzer ME, Raikin SM, Ledermann HP. Neuropathic arthropathy of the foot with and without superimposed osteomyelitis: MR imaging characteristics. Radiology. 2006;238(2):622–31.

80. Meyr AJ, Singh S, Zhang X, Khilko N, Mukherjee A, Sheridan MJ, Khurana JS. Statistical reliability of bone biopsy for the diagnosis of diabetic foot osteomyelitis. J Foot Ankle Surg. 2011;50(6): 663–7.

81. Petrosillo N. Epidemiology of infections in the new century. In: Signore A, Quintero AM, editors. Diagnostic imaging of infections and inflammatory disease: a multidisciplinary approach. 1st ed. Hoboken: Wiley; 2014.

82. Lipsky BA. Osteomyelitis of the foot in diabetic patients. Clin Infect Dis. 1997;25(6):1318–26.

83. Kaleta JL, Fleischli JW, Reilly CH. The diagnosis of osteomyelitis in diabetes using erythrocyte sedimentation rate:a pilot study. J Am Podiatr Med Assoc. 2001;91(9):445–50.

84. Upchurch Jr GR, Keagy BA, Johnson Jr G. An acute phase reaction in diabetic patients with foot ulcers. Cardiovasc Surg. 1997;5(1):32–6.

85. Bencardino JT, Restrepo-Velez Z, Bujan R, Jaramillo D. Radiological Imaging of osteomyelitis. In: Signore A, Quintero AM, editors. Diagnostic imaging of infections and inflammatory disease: a multidisciplinary approach. 1st ed. New Jersey: Wiley & Sons; 2014. p. 29–53.

86. Lesens O, Desbiez F, Vidal M, Robin F, Descamps S, Beytout J, et al. Culture of per-wound bone specimen: a simplified approach for the medical management of diabetic foot osteomyelitis. Clin Microbiol Infect. 2011;17(2):1469–691.

87. Senneville E, Melliez H, Beltrand E, Legout L, Valette M, Cazaubiel M, et al. Culture of percutaneous bone biopsy specimens for diagnosis of diabetic foot osteomyelitis: concordance with ulcer swab cultures. Clin Infect Dis. 2006;42(1): 57–62.

88. Centers for Disease Control and Prevention. National diabetes fact sheet: national estimates and general information on diabetes and prediabetes in the United States, 2011. Atlanta, GA: U.S. Department of Health and Human Services, Centers for Disease Control and Prevention; 2011.

89. Berendt AR, Peters EJ, Bakker PK, Embil JM, Eneroth M, Hinchliffe RJ, et al. Diabetic foot osteomyelitis: a progress report on diagnosis and a systematic review of treatment. Diabetes Metab Res Rev. 2008;24 Suppl 1:S145–61.

90. Lazaro-Martinez JL, Aragon-Sanchez J, Garcia-Morales E. Antibiotics versus conservative surgery for treating diabetic foot osteomyelitis: a randomized comparative trial. Diabetes Care. 2014;37:789–95.

91. Mouzopoulos G, Kanakaris NK, Kontakis G, Obakponovwe O, Townsend R, Giannoudis PV. Management of bone infections in adults: the surgeon's and microbiologist's perspectives. Injury. 2011;42 Suppl 5:S18–23.

92. Zaoutis T, Localio AR, Leckerman K, Saddlemire S, Bertoch D, Keren R. Prolonged intravenous therapy versus oral antimicrobial therapy for acute osteomyelitis in children. Pediatrics. 2009;123(2):636–42.

93. Conterno LO, Turchi MD. Antibiotics for treating chronic osteomyelitis in adults. Cochrane Database Syst Rev [Internet]. 2013 Sep [cited 2014 Aug 7]. http://onlinelibrary.wiley.com.libproxy. temple. edu/doi/10.1002/14651858.CD004439.pub3/abstract.

94. Carek PJ, Dickerson LM, Sack JL. Diagnosis and management of osteomyelitis. Am Fam Physician. 2001;63(12):2413–20.

95. Henke PK, Blackburn SA, Wainess RW, Cowan J, Terando A, Proctor M, et al. Osteomyelitis of the foot and toe in adults is a surgical disease. Ann Surg. 2005;241(6):885–94.

96. Simpson AH, Deakin M, Latham JM. Chronic osteomyelitis. The effect of the extent of surgical resection on infection-free survival. J Bone Joint Surg Br. 2001;83(3):403–7.

97. Eckardt JJ, Wirganowicz PZ, Mar T. An aggressive surgical approach to the management of chronic osteomyelitis. Clin Orthop Relat Res. 1994;298:229–39.

98. Melamed EA, Peled E. Antibiotic impregnated cement spacer for salvage of diabetic osteomyelitis. Foot Ankle Int. 2012;33(3):213–9.

99. Roukis TS, Landsman AS. Salvage of the first ray in a diabetic patient with osteomyelitis. J Am Podiatr Med Assoc. 2004;94(5): 492–8.

100. Schweinberger MH, Roukis TS. Salvage of the first ray with external fixation in the high-risk patient. Foot Ankle Spec. 2008;1(4):210–3.

101. Londahl M. Hyperbaric oxygen therapy as adjunctive treatment for diabetic foot ulcers. Int J Low Extrem Wounds. 2013;12(2):152–7.

102. Londahl M, Katzman P, Nilsson A, Hammarlund C. Hyperbaric oxygen therapy facilitates healing of chronic foot ulcers in patients with diabetes. Diabetes Care. 2010;33(5):998–1003.

103. Davis JC, Heckman JD, DeLee JC, Buckwold FJ. Chronic non-hematogenous osteomyelitis treated with adjunctive hyperbaric oxygen therapy. J Bone Joint Surg Am. 1986;68(8):1210–7.

104. Estherhai Jr JL, Pisarello J, Brighton CT, Heppenstall RB, Gellman H, Goldstein G. Adjunctive hyperbaric oxygen therapy in the treatment of chronic refractory osteomyelitis. J Trauma. 1987;27(7):763–8.

105. Fang RC, Galiano RD. Adjunctive therapies in the treatment of osteomyelitis. Semin Plast Surg. 2009;23(2):141–7.

106. Margolis DJ, Gupta J, Hoffstad O, Papdopoulos M, Glick HA, Thom SR, et al. Lack of effectiveness of hyperbaric oxygen therapy for the treatment of diabetic foot ulcer and the prevention of amputation: a cohort study. Diabetes Care. 2013;36(7):1961–6.

107. Kranke P, Bennett MH, Martyn-St James M, Schnabel A, Debus SE. Hyperbaric oxygen therapy for chronic wounds. Cochrane Database Syst Rev. 2012;18(4), CD004123.

108. Gentry LO, Rodriguez-Gomez G. Ofloxacin versus parenteral therapy for chronic osteomyelitis. Antimicrob Agents Chemother. 1991;35(3):538–41.

109. Stengel D, Bauwens K, Sehouli J, Ekkernkamp A, Porzsolt F. Systematic review and meta-analysis of antibiotic therapy for bone and joint infections. Lancet Infect Dis. 2001;1(3):175–88.

110. Snyder RJ, Cohen MM, Sun C, Livingston J. Osteomyelitis in the diabetic patient: diagnosis and treatment. Part 2: medical, surgical, and alternative treatments. Ostomy Wound Manage. 2001;47(3):24–30. 3.

111. Widatalla AH, Mahadi SEI, Shawer MA, Mahmoud SM, Abdelmageed AE, Ahmed ME. Diabetic foot infections with osteomyelitis: efficacy of combined surgical and medical treatment. Diabet Foot Ankle. 2012;3:18809–15. http://diabeticfootandankle.net/index. php/dfa/article/view/18809.

112. Akarsus S, Tekin L, Safaz I, Goktepe AS, Yazicioglu K. Quality of life and functionality after lower limb amputations: comparison between uni- vs bilateral amputee patients. Prosthet Orthot Int. 2013;37(1):9–13.

113. Boutoille D, Feraille A, Maulaz D, Krempf M. Quality of life with diabetes-associated foot complications: comparison between lower-limb amputation and chronic foot ulceration. Foot Ankle Int. 2008;29(11):1074–8.

114. Deans SA, McFadyen AK, Rowe PJ. Physical activity and quality of like: a study of a lower-limb amputee population. Prosthet Orthot Int. 2008;32(2):186–200.

115. Asano M, Rushton P, Miller WC, Deathe BA. Predictors of quality of life among individuals who have a lower limb amputation. Prosthet Orthot Int. 2008;32(2):231–43.

116. Horgan O, MacLachlan M. Psychosocial adjustment to lower-limb amputation: a review. Disabil Rehabil. 2004;26(14–15):837–50.

117. Toursarkissian B, Shireman PK, Harrison A, D'Ayala M, SchoolField J, Sykes MT. Major lower-extremity amputation: contemporary experience in a single Veterans Affairs institution. Am Surg. 2002;68(7):606–10.

118. Evans KK, Attinger CE, Al-Attar A, Salgado C, Chu CK, Mardini S, Neville R. The importance of limb preservation in the diabetic population. J Diabetes Complications. 2011;25(4):227–31.

119. Tice AD, Hoaglund PA, Shoultz DA. Outcomes of osteomyelitis among patients treated with outpatient parenteral antimicrobial therapy. Am J Med. 2003;114(9):723–8.

120. Mader JT, Calhoun JH, Lazzarini L. Adult long bone osteomyelitis. In: Calhoun JH, Mader JT, editors. Musculoskeletal infections. New York: Marcel Dekker; 2003. p. 133–64.

121. Buckholtz JM. The surgical management of osteomyelitis: with special reference to a surgical classification. J Foot Surg. 1987;26 Suppl 1:s17–24.

Emily A. Cook and Jill F. Ashcraft

Overview

By generic definition, osteomyelitis is an infectious usually painful inflammatory disease of bone often of bacterial origin that may result in the death of bone tissue [1]. Unlike superficial soft-tissue infections, bacteria associated with osteomyelitis possess a multitude of virulence factors and biofilm forming adhesions, which contribute to the development and characteristic chronicity of the disease. The early and accurate diagnosis of osteomyelitis is imperative to facilitate effective treatment and decrease associated morbidity of affected patients. In the varying stages of osteomyelitis from acute to chronic, the symptomatic identifiers are not consistent, complicating the processes of diagnosis and treatment.

Osteomyelitis Classifications

Osteomyelitis has been categorized as acute, subacute, or chronic, with the presentation of each type based on the time of onset. Acute osteomyelitis develops within 2 weeks after infection, subacute osteomyelitis within 1–2 months, and chronic osteomyelitis after 3 months [2]. These stages challenge the diagnosis of the disease, as each presents with varying identifiers. This nomenclature has thus been argued as nondescript to the true nature of the process. To address this issue, additional terminology is often incorporated alongside osteomyelitis classifications, including residual,

recurrent, refractory, or recalcitrant. Additional classification systems have emerged to include other important characteristics such as extent of bone and bone marrow involvement and important host factors.

The Waldvogel classification system is an early classification system which divides osteomyelitis into the categories of hematogenous, contiguous, and chronic [3]. This classification system is often still considered a primary classification system, but does not assist the physician in surgical or antibiotic therapy. Other classifications have been developed to emphasize different clinical aspects of osteomyelitis. These classifications include those of Ger, Weiland, May, and Cierny-Mader (Table 2.1) [4–8].

Classifications of osteomyelitis are one small part of accurately defining the diagnosis and are lacking any merit in helping physicians determine etiology. It is the complexity of osteomyelitis that makes the initial diagnosis so challenging, and classifications do not completely nor clearly aid in defining the extent of the disease or guide precise treatments. The standard of care for osteomyelitis, by necessity, has therefore advanced beyond classification guided treatment in order to aid in appropriate early recognition and prevention of long-term consequences.

Risk Factors for Osteomyelitis

When considering all of the possible limitations in diagnostic techniques, physician understanding of associated risk factors for osteomyelitis plays a role in how a diagnosis of osteomyelitis may be made. These risk factors may include the patient's age, gender, comorbidities, and exposure history. Exposures can be due to trauma, surgery, presence of tubes or external connectors, drugs, and more.

When considering age, acute osteomyelitis can be diagnosed at any age, but is the most commonly seen within the first to second decades of life. Conversely, chronic osteomyelitis frequency increases with age. Generally, patients under 18 years of age are more likely to have hematogenous

E.A. Cook, DPM, MPH, CPH, FACFAS (✉)
Division of Podiatric Surgery, Department of Surgery,
Mount Auburn Hospital, 330 Mount Auburn Street, Cambridge,
MA 02138, USA
e-mail: ecook@mah.harvard.edu

J.F. Ashcraft, DPM
Harvard Medical School, Mount Auburn Hospital,
330 Mount Auburn Street, Cambridge, MA 02138, USA
e-mail: jashcraf@mah.harvard.edu

© Springer International Publishing Switzerland 2015
T.J. Boffeli (ed.), *Osteomyelitis of the Foot and Ankle*, DOI 10.1007/978-3-319-18926-0_2

Table 2.1 Osteomyelitis classification systems: Ger, Weiland, May, and Modified Cierny-Mader [2, 5–8]

	Classification systems			
Cierny-Mader staging system for osteomyelitis	Stage 1: Medullary osteomyelitis	A Host: healthy		
	Stage 2: superficial osteomyelitis	B Host:		
		Bs: Systemic compromise		
		Bl: Local compromise		
		Bls: Local and systemic compromise		
	Stage 3: localized osteomyelitis	C Host: Treatment worse than the disease		
	Stage 4: diffuse osteomyelitis			
	• Factors affecting immune surveillance, metabolism, and local vascularity			
	• Systemic factors (Bs): malnutrition, renal or hepatic failure, diabetes mellitus, chronic hypoxia, immune disease, extremes of age, immunosuppression, or immune deficiency			
	• Local factors (Bl): chronic lymphedema, venous stasis, major vessel compromise, arteritis, extensive scarring, radiation fibrosis, small-vessel disease, neuropathy, tobacco abuse			
Ger	Simple sinus	Chronic superficial ulcer	Multiple sinuses	Multiple skin lined sinuses
Weiland	Type I			Open with exposed bone without evidence of osseous infection but with soft-tissue infection
	Type II			Circumferential, cortical, and endosteal infection. X-ray with diffuse inflammation and increased bone density, and spindle-shaped sclerotic thickening of cortex. Bone resorption and sequestrum with involucrum
	Type III			Cortical and endosteal infection with segmental bone defect
	• Chronic OM with wound with exposed bone, positive bone cultures, and drainage for 6 months. Soft tissue and location of bone involved			
May	Type I	Intact tibia and fibula capable of withstanding functional loads	Rehabilitation time, 6–12 weeks	
	Type II	Intact tibia with bone graft needed only for structural support	Rehabilitation time, 3–6 months	
	Type III	Tibial defect <6 cm long with an intact fibula	Rehabilitation time, 6–12 months	
	Type IV	Tibial defect >6 cm and an intact fibula	Rehabilitation time, 12–18 months	
	Type V	Tibial defect >6 cm long without a usable intact fibula	Rehabilitation time, >18 months	
	• Focused on the status of the tibia after soft-tissue and skeletal debridement			

osteomyelitis unless otherwise indicated [9]. On the contrary, bacteremia in adults rarely results in osteomyelitis, and secondary spread from a contiguous focus of infection, such as from surgical wounds or ulcerations, are more common. No studies have shown that age is itself a risk factor; however, patients who are over the age of 60 are more likely to suffer extreme complications from the disease, such as lower extremity amputations [10].

In regard to gender, no studies are conclusive of the most affected population. In one study, of 100 patients, there was found a 1:1 male to female ratio [10]. Another study, by Lavery et al., showed that of over 151 patients with lower extremity infections, the ratio was nearly equal, at 52 % male [11]. However, fungal osteomyelitis has been reported to have a statistically significant male dominance [12]. Gender should not be considered an independent risk factor and osteomyelitis can affect anyone. Overall, both age and gender cannot be used as a sole predictor of osteomyelitis; however, those with multiple comorbidities and increased age are at risk for a worse prognosis.

Specific comorbidities that weaken the host's immune system increase the risk for a worse prognosis in the setting of osteomyelitis. A patient with diabetes has an increased risk for osteomyelitis, especially when there is poor glycemic control and presence of neuropathy. A retrospective cohort study of 8,905 patients found that 15 % of those with diabetes and a foot ulcer developed osteomyelitis at or after diagnosis [13]. Other medical conditions resulting in immunosuppression, organ transplants, or any condition that alters neutrophil defense, humoral immunity or cell-mediated immunity, can increase susceptibility to infection and increase the risk of undiagnosed osteomyelitis. Additionally, those with chronic immunosuppression are more likely to be diagnosed with fungal originated osteomyelitis [12].

Circulation disorders are another risk factor that may decrease host immune response and increase the potential of a deep infection. Secondarily, these conditions decrease laboratory markers of infection and increase the difficulty of diagnosis and treatment effectiveness. Peripheral vascular disease can be seen in patients with poorly controlled diabetes, smokers, sickle cell disease, and more. All of these conditions increase the risk for peripheral vascular disease, which in turn can greatly increase the risk of osteomyelitis and reduce the effectiveness of therapy [14, 15].

Obvious exposures, such as a previous history of osteomyelitis or open wounds, elevate the risk for osteomyelitis. Recent trauma or osseous surgery in any population is also a risk factor for osteomyelitis. A severe bone fracture or a deep puncture wound provides organisms a portal of entry into osseous structures or nearby soft tissues. In particular, surgical correction following open trauma involving osseous or articular surfaces increases patient risk in developing osteomyelitis [9].

Infected hardware is a devastating complication, especially with joint replacement procedures, carrying with it a poor prognosis for salvage of the implant. Specific factors related to poor prognosis in the setting of infected hardware include symptoms of inflammation, swelling, and pain to the site of the implant. The patients may also present with a history of a previous infection, upper respiratory tract infection, or bacteremia [16, 17]. Given the scope and severity of this topic, a later chapter is dedicated towards hardware and joint infections.

Patients who are on long-term external connections, external fixation, external tubing, or catheters and drains are also at greater risk for osteomyelitis. This includes patients associated with dialysis machines, urinary catheters, PICC lines or central lines, digital Kirchner wires, and external fixation devices for lower limb procedures (Fig. 2.1).

Patients who are exposed to injectable illicit drugs are also more likely to develop osteomyelitis. Illicit drug abusers typically use nonsterile techniques and have decreased immune systems due to prolonged abuse, making them not only susceptible to osteomyelitis, but to more resistant strains of bacteria. These potentially resistant but often polymicrobial infections can be found in up to 46 % of IV drug abuse cases [18].

Certain prescription medications may make a patient more susceptible to infection and simultaneously decrease inflammatory markers used in diagnosis of osteomyelitis. Immunosuppressive medications and medications that can mask symptoms of acute osteomyelitis include corticosteroids, tumor necrosis factor (TNF) inhibitors, antibiotics, chemotherapy agents, and more [12].

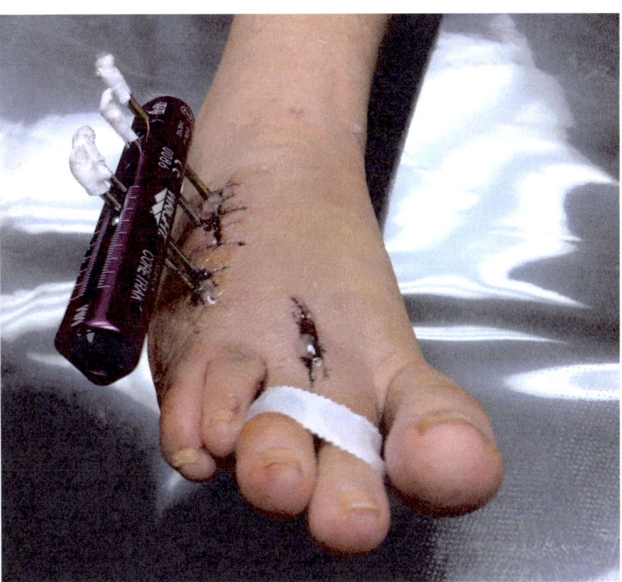

Fig. 2.1 Clinically infected monorail for the treatment of brachymetatarsalgia with portal of entry to the fourth metatarsal diaphysis

Different environmental settings are associated with a greater prevalence of osteomyelitis in certain patient subsets. Populations of hospitalized patients with a history of previous ulceration and infection have a higher prevalence of osteomyelitis than nondiabetic patients with open wounds seen in an outpatient ambulatory care clinic. In one study, 87.3 % of all hospitalized patients diagnosed with osteomyelitis had a previous history of trauma or skin infection [9]. But with all this considered, risk factors although helpful in gaining clinical suspicion, cannot be utilized as the sole diagnostic tool for lower extremity osteomyelitis.

Vital Signs

Initial evaluation of a patient with concerns for osteomyelitis should include assessment of vital signs. Vital signs should include temperature, blood pressure, heart rate, and respiratory rate. These markers are essential in evaluating the stability of a patient at risk for an acute infection. Infectious Disease Society of America (IDSA) guidelines specify that fever is defined as: (1) A single oral temperature >100 °F (>37.8 °C); or (2) repeated oral temperatures >99 °F (>37.2 °C) or rectal temperatures >99.5 °F (>37.5 °C); or (3) an increase in temperature of >2 °F (>1.1 °C) over the baseline temperature [19].

Fever or elevated temperature is a poor indicator of osteomyelitis due to its inconsistency and lack of specificity and sensitivity. Furthermore, the presence or absence of a fever should be interpreted depending on the specific population. Immunocompromised patients may have a normal temperature reading in the presence of severe infection as they may lack the systemic inflammatory response that a non-compromised patient would have. For similar reasons, patients with diabetes may have no fever present in the setting of acute and/or chronic osteomyelitis. Studies have found that up to 82 % of patients with diabetes have a normal oral temperature of <100.5 °F in the face of acute osteomyelitis. Sensitivity for fever and acute osteomyelitis was only 19 % and specificity could not be calculated as patients without osteomyelitis were not included [20].

Conversely, a pediatric patient may have a higher rise in temperature with a less serious medical condition. Yet, not all pediatric patients with osteomyelitis will have an elevated temperature. In one study, only 32 % of the pediatric patients presented with oral temperatures greater than 37.5 °C. All had confirmed cultured osteomyelitis of the lower extremity, but not all had elevated temperatures [21]. The type of organism may also influence body temperature. Ju et al. demonstrated that temperature appeared to be more elevated in those infected with MRSA vs MSSA, the difference being 38.8 °C and 37.2 °C, respectively [22]. When considering the pediatric and hematogenous group, the incidence of fever is also not an appropriate sole predictor for osteomyelitis.

Although fever is not a specific indicator of osteomyelitis, IDSA guidelines state that a temperature of >38 °C demonstrates a serious lower extremity infection with associate systemic inflammatory response and requires appropriate efficient treatment [19]. In the circumstance of an elevated temperature, the patient may have concomitant osteomyelitis, but this could be determined only in the appropriate clinical setting with adjuvant diagnostic criteria matching.

Clinical Signs and Symptoms

When considering clinical signs, the presence of inflammation, erythema, edema, and purulence does not independently determine the diagnosis of osteomyelitis. IDSA guidelines, however, do provide the clinician with a validated method for grading the severity of a general infection (Table 2.2) [19]. Despite this validated instrument, classic signs and symptoms of infection may be absent or masked by the coexistence of previously discussed comorbidities including vascular disease, diabetes, and neuropathy. Other conditions such as Charcot neuroarthropathy and gout may appear clinically similar to a patient with osteomyelitis.

Hematogenous osteomyelitis occurs predominantly in prepubertal children. Patients usually present within several days to 1 week after the onset of symptoms, and therefore most often present in the acute phase. Patients often present with local signs of infection, including erythema, edema, tenderness to the involved bone, decreased range of motion, and warmth to the specific area. In addition, patients often have signs of systemic illness, including fever, chills, pain, irritability, and lethargy. Common locations affected by hematogenous osteomyelitis include the metaphysis of long bones, particularly the tibia and femur. In adults, hematogenous osteomyelitis is rare; however, the most common site is the vertebral bodies, followed by long bones, pelvis, and clavicle [2, 12].

Acute, subacute, and chronic forms of contiguous osteomyelitis more commonly occur in adults. Acute osteomyelitis is usually more representative of what is considered

Table 2.2 Infectious disease society of America (IDSA) guidelines on clinical appearance of infection [19]

IDSA Guidelines on clinical appearance of infection	Grade	IDSA infection severity
No signs of symptoms of infection	1	Uninfected
Infection involving the skin and the subcutaneous tissue	2	Mild
At least two of the following items are present		
1. Local swelling or induration		
2. Erythema >0.5–2 cm around the ulcer		
3. Local tenderness or pain		
4. Local warmth		
5. Purulent discharge (thick, opaque to white, or sanguineous secretion)		
Other causes of an inflammatory response of the skin are excluded (e.g., trauma, gout, acute Charcot neuro-osteoarthropathy, fracture, thrombosis, venous stasis)		
Erythema >2 cm plus 1 of the items described above (swelling, tenderness, warmth, discharge) or infection involving structures deeper than the skin and subcutaneous tissues such as abscess, osteomyelitis, septic arthritis, fasciitis	3	Moderate
No systematic inflammatory response signs, as described below		
Any foot infection with the following signs of a systemic inflammatory response syndrome	4	Severe
Two or more of the following conditions:		
1. Temperature >38 or <36 °C		
2. Heart rate >90 beats/min		
3. Respiratory rate >20 breaths/min or Pa CO_2 <32 mmHG		
White blood cell count >12,000 or <4,000/mm^3 or 10 % immature band forms		

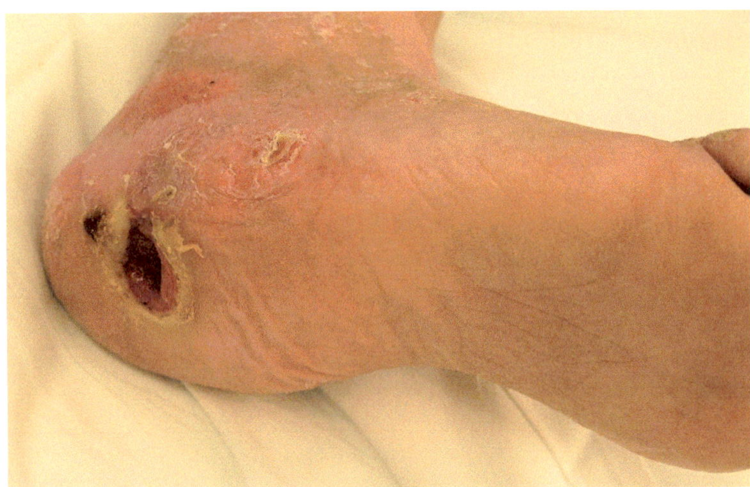

Fig. 2.2 Chronic nonhealing neuropathic diabetic heel wound with mild localized erythema and edema. Further evaluation revealed a sinus tract which probed to the calcaneus and radiographic changes consistent with osteomyelitis. Pathologic and microbiologic bone examination further confirmed the diagnosis of chronic osteomyelitis

cardinal signs of infection: erythema, edema, tenderness to the bone involved (in the absences of neuropathy), decreased range of motion in the affected limb, drainage, and malodor. Chronic osteomyelitis may lack clinical signs and symptoms but is more likely in the presence of a chronic draining sinus tract, an open wound not responding to standard therapies, compound fractures, and wounds that have been present for a long period of time (Fig. 2.2). Contiguous osteomyelitis in patients without diabetes, usually do present with some signs and symptoms from a traumatic or surgical wound [23].

In the diabetic foot, these infections almost always occur by contiguous spread, usually from a chronic ulcer. Osteomyelitis occurs in up to 15 % of patients with a diabetic foot ulcer and up to 20 % in those with infected foot ulcerations [13, 24, 25]. Osteomyelitis should be considered in patients with diabetes with a nonhealing foot wound, despite adequate perfusion and optimization of wound care and offloading [26]. In the setting of diabetes and peripheral neuropathy, infection occurs most often in the prominent bones of the feet, most frequently metatarsals. This is often due to biomechanical deformity, ill-fitting shoe gear, or an incident of trauma combined with peripheral neuropathy. Physical exam usually reveals some type of foot deformity alongside evidence of peripheral neuropathy (Fig. 2.3). The contiguous site of infection is typically a neuropathic ulcer, though paronychia from a toenail deformity, cellulitis or puncture wound are possible other sources.

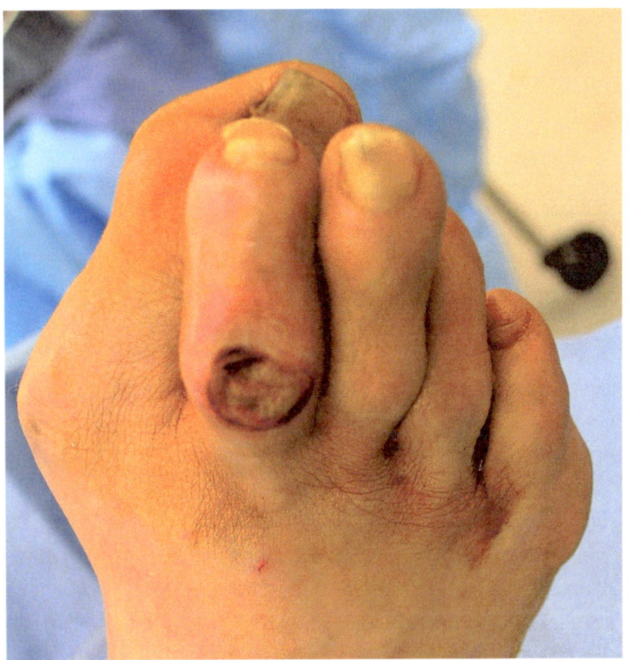

Fig. 2.3 The combination of forefoot pathology with peripheral neuropathy in a patient with diabetes is one of the most common pathways for the development of diabetic foot ulcers and eventual osteomyelitis

Wound Characteristics

Whenever there is an open wound, wound duration, size and depth should be assessed to aid in the diagnosis of osteomyelitis. Available evidence, however, does not justify using any one or combination of these wound characteristics as the sole criterion for diagnosing osteomyelitis.

Duration

A long-standing ulcer overlying a bony prominence, especially in the presence of adequate vascular supply, should raise the suspicion of underlying osteomyelitis if the wound is nonhealing and adequately offloaded. Calcaneal fractures, for example, are less likely to develop osteomyelitis if either traumatic and/or surgical wounds are able to heal within three months following initial injury [27].

Size

The association between the presence of osteomyelitis and the cross-sectional area of a wound has also been studied. The assumption has been that size of the ulcer has been considered predictive of osteomyelitis, however, the evidence to support this is limited and with conflicting evidence.

The diagnosis of underlying osteomyelitis on the basis of an ulcer area of ≥ 2 cm^2 may have a sensitivity of 56 % and a specificity as high as 92 % [25, 26, 28]. However, another found that the wound area was ≥ 2 cm^2 in 76.9 % of the patients with osteomyelitis and 69.2 % of the patients without osteomyelitis [29]. Another study found that increasing ulcer area had a protective effect with increasing ulcer size [30]. Measurement error is also a major concern with all studies assessing wound size. Most studies utilize measurements of the longest and widest diameters of a wound which do not reflect irregular shapes and depth [13].

These findings demonstrate that wound size is an unreliable guide to the presence of bone infection in a lower extremity ulcer. It can, however, be utilized as an adjuvant to the diagnosis for osteomyelitis.

Depth

It is thought that bone that is visible at the base of a wound is likely to be infected, especially when the clinical setting is appropriate. In a study where the prevalence of osteomyelitis was 68 %, the presence of exposed bone at the base of an ulcer had a sensitivity of only 32 % but a specificity of 100 % [25, 26]. Other studies have found that a wound depth greater than 3 mm was in 65–89.7 % of the patients with osteomyelitis but also in 80.8 % without osteomyelitis [29, 30]. Once again, it should be noted that accurate measurement of wound depth is difficult due to inconsistent measuring methods and irregular wound surfaces.

Depth via the Probe to Bone Test

In the absence of bone exposure, the probe-to-bone (PTB) test may be a useful diagnostic aid for osteomyelitis. While the PTB test is technically simple to execute, it is one of the most widely disputed clinical test for diagnosis of osteomyelitis. This is due to the challenges in properly interpreting existing clinical data on the PTB test.

To properly perform a PTB test, an examiner uses a sterile metallic blunt probe to gently probe the depth of a wound. If the probe touches bone, the finding is positive, whereas the inability to probe the base of a wound to periosteum, joint space, or bone is a negative result (Fig. 2.4).

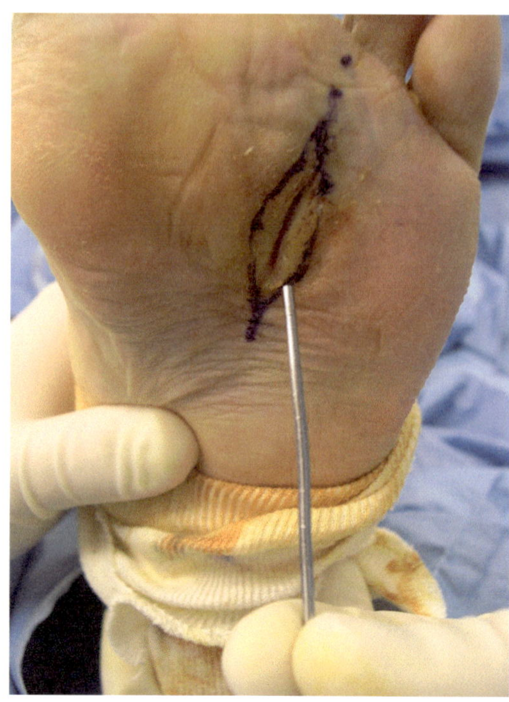

Fig. 2.4 To properly perform a probe-to-bone test, a metallic blunt probe is utilized to gently probe the wound base to ascertain whether or not a hard or gritty end point is felt indicating that a wound extends to bone, periosteum, or joint space

The first study to assess the PTB test was by Grayson and colleagues who examined a series of 76 hospitalized patients with limb-threatening infected diabetic foot ulcers on intravenous antibiotics. This was a nested retrospective cohort study from a previously performed randomized clinical trial. Diagnosis of osteomyelitis was based on histopathologic cultures and/or radiographic findings in combination with clinical criteria. The presumed prevalence of osteomyelitis in this population was 68 %. This study found that a positive PTB test had a sensitivity of 66 % and specificity of 87 %, giving a positive predictive value (PPV) of 89 % and a negative predictive value (NPV) of 56 % for the diagnosis of osteomyelitis [31]. The primary concern of this study is that because all wounds were from in-patient limb-threatening diabetic foot ulcers, the pre-test probability for osteomyelitis is much higher than wounds seen in the general population.

Another study with a high prevalence of osteomyelitis (72.5 %) evaluated the PTB test in 338 patients with 356 episodes of foot infection. Diagnosis of osteomyelitis was based on both bone histology and culture. Almost all patients required surgical debridement of osteomyelitis and therefore biopsies were taken at the time of surgery. The sensitivity, specificity, and positive and negative predictive values for a positive PTB test for the diagnosis of osteomyelitis were 95 %, 93 %, 97 %, and 83 %, respectively [32].

Conversely, two studies evaluated the PTB test in a patient population with a lower prevalence of osteomyelitis. Shone and colleagues examined the PTB test in 81 consecutive patients with 101 ft ulcers presenting to an out-patient multidisciplinary clinic. Inclusion criteria included both clinically infected and noninfected ulcers, and the prevalence of osteomyelitis was estimated to be 23.5 %. The diagnosis of osteomyelitis was determined from a blinded clinical examiner in combination with radiographs and MRI when indicated. Microbiologic bone specimens were collected in a small subset of patients. Researchers reported a sensitivity of 38 %, specificity of 91 %, negative predictive value of 85 %, and positive predictive value of only 53 % for positive probe-to-bone tests to diagnose osteomyelitis [33].

A prospective longitudinal cohort study evaluated the PTB test in 247 consecutive patients. Baseline prevalence of osteomyelitis was estimated to be 12 %, and all patients were seen in an out-patient-based specialty clinic. All infected ulcers had plain radiographs taken and additional imaging if deemed necessary. If osteomyelitis was suspected based on clinical exam and imaging modalities, histopathologic and microbiologic bone specimens were taken via aseptic technique to confirm the diagnosis of osteomyelitis. Patients with acute infections were not yet on antibiotics at the time of the PTB test examination. In this series, a positive PTB test had a sensitivity of 87 %, specificity of 91 %, negative predictive value of 96 %, and positive predictive value of only 57 %. The likelihood ratio for a positive test result was 9.40; the likelihood ratio for a negative test result was 0.14. This study emphasized that the probability of osteomyelitis among patients who had negative PTB test in this out-patient setting was very low [34].

To summarize, in order to properly interpret the PTB test, one must consider the population it is being performed within. The studies with the highest prevalence of osteomyelitis were referral centers (i.e., in-patient setting) with a population of ulcers that were infected and not responding to standard therapies. It was found that in a population with a high baseline prevalence for osteomyelitis, a positive PTB test had a high positive predictive value but a lower negative predictive value (Fig. 2.5) [31–33]. However, in studies examining the PTB test in a patient population with a lower pre-test probability of osteomyelitis (i.e., out-patient or clinic setting that included noninfected wounds), the PPV was much lower. Conversely, a negative PTB test had a high negative predictive value in these out-patient settings (Fig. 2.6) [33, 34]. In other words, the combined evidence of these studies suggest that the PTB test helps a clinician rule out osteomyelitis in an out-patient-based setting and rule-in osteomyelitis in populations with a high prevalence of osteomyelitis. These results confirm the importance of considering disease prevalence in assessing the PPV and NPV in diagnostic tests.

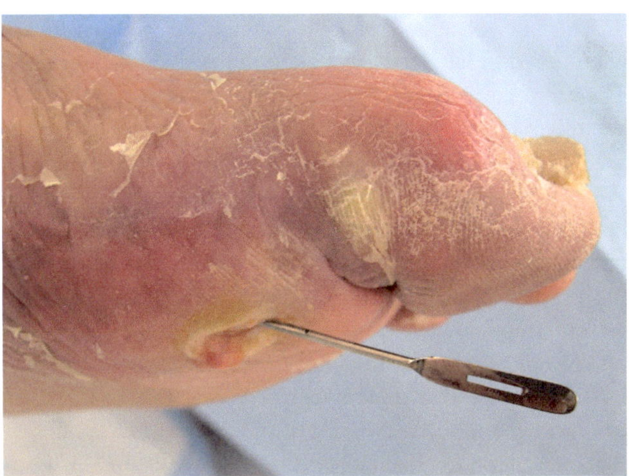

Fig. 2.5 Probe-to-bone test in an in-patient setting (high pre-test probability), making the positive predictive value of the PTB test very high

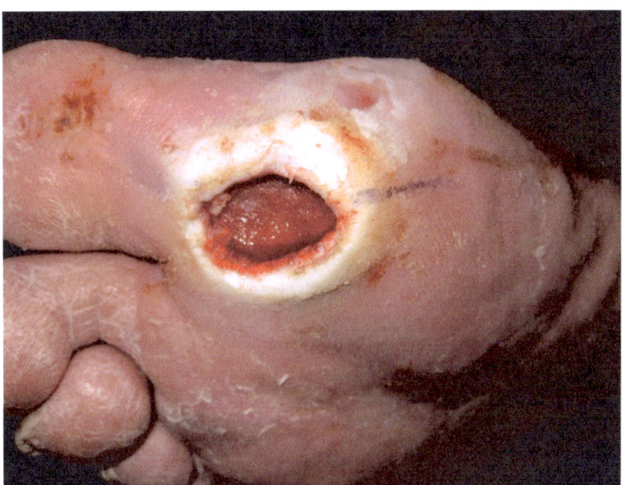

Fig. 2.6 This wound has a lower positive predictive value and higher negative predictive value with the PTB test as it is a noninfected contiguous foot ulcer in an out-patient setting

Questions of the accuracy of osteomyelitis diagnosis, reliability, and reproducibility of the PTB test have all been discussed in the literature. Not all wounds underwent osseous histologic and/or pathologic evaluation to confirm the diagnosis of osteomyelitis. Many patients, especially those with severely infected limbs, were already on intravenous antibiotics. But because researchers cannot ethically obtain bone biopsies in noninfected wounds and withhold antibiotics in patients with severe infections, it still calls into question which wounds truly had osteomyelitis and which ones did not. The extremes of pre-test probability also make little difference to post-test probability. When the pre-test probability is approximately 50 %, however, then a positive or negative probe-to-bone test could possibly improve the post-test probability [35].

The inter-observer reliability of the PTB test has also been found to have only moderate to fair concordance [36]. Therefore, even though the PTB test appears simple, it should only be considered properly performed and interpreted by an appropriate specialist or experienced examiner. Wound location may also influence to reliability of the PTB test. In a study of only forefoot diabetic foot ulcers, greater inter-observer agreement was found within wounds involving the central metatarsals and hallux as opposed to plantar lesser digital wounds [36].

Overall, when considering clinical assessment of diagnostic measures for osteomyelitis, a combination approach has been found to be more effective. Some studies suggest that clinicians might be more proficient at detecting the presence of osteomyelitis rather than detecting its absence based on clinical examination alone [24, 25]. But when a clinician suspects osteomyelitis, further investigation and/or referral is warranted.

Bone Biopsy

The gold standard for the diagnosis of osteomyelitis is a microbiologic and histologic bone culture. However, this procedure is not always practical in noncompliant neuropathic patients, especially if the biopsy requires a plantar incision. Biopsy may also be contraindicated in patients with severe peripheral vascular disease. Proper bone biopsy technique is critical and will be discussed in a future chapter. There is no standardized definition of a "bone biopsy" to diagnose osteomyelitis and one should keep in mind that the microbiologic and histopathologic specimens provide two separate pieces of information. Regardless of technique and definition, bone biopsy has come under scrutiny due to the capriciousness of several studies.

The microbiological aspect of bone biopsy helps physicians gauge antibiotic treatment. Once a specimen is collected, the specimen is analyzed for infectious organisms to help hone antibiotic treatment. In the ideal world, the specimen would be collected from an area infected with live organisms and identification would equate to appropriate treatment. With this being considered, studies have shown that there are underlying flaws with biopsy techniques and outcomes. Weiner and colleagues assessed 44 bone biopsy specimens and found that a positive microbiologic and negative histologic result was just as likely as a negative microbiologic and positive histologic result ($P>0.05$) [37]. False positives are possible via contamination from contiguous tissue. Additionally, overlying soft-tissue infection does not correlate with the bony involvement. A study by Senneville et al. demonstrated that the results of bone and swab cultures were identical in only 17.4 % of patients [38]. False negative results

are also possible if there is a low level of microorganisms or if the biopsy technique missed the infected site [39]. Additionally, prior or concomitant antibiotic use can affect the sample. IDSA guidelines recommend obtaining a culture prior to the initiation of antibiotics if possible. Ideally, antibiotics should be discontinued 48 h to as long as two weeks prior to biopsy [19]. Finally, unusual microorganism can affect the test if incorrect tests were ordered, such as fungal osteomyelitis, which may not be included in a typical analysis.

Histopathologic analysis of bone specimens has been used as the referent standard for many studies in the diagnosis of osteomyelitis [30–32, 34, 40–42]. However, the reliability of histopathologic analysis has come into question in more recent years. One study examined the reliability of diagnosing osteomyelitis from 39 consecutive histopathologic bone specimens from four board certified, experienced surgical pathologists. This study found that there was only complete agreement of osteomyelitis in 13/39 specimens (33 %). There was a clinically significant disagreement of whether or not osteomyelitis was present in 16/39 specimens (41 %). Finally, only 50 % of pathologist agreed between acute vs chronic osteomyelitis. Given these results, the authors of this study recommended that histopathologic bone biopsy should not be the "reference standard" for diagnosis of diabetic osteomyelitis given poor inter-rater reliability [43]. The more concerning concept is that higher quality studies evaluating diagnosis of osteomyelitis, utilized bone biopsy as the reference to determine results. Given that the gold standard has come into question, it is likely that we do not know the true reliability or validity of any test used to diagnose osteomyelitis. The reliability of histopathologic interpretation of bone specimens warrants additional study in order to determine methods in improving its reliability.

Laboratory Evaluation

It is an appealing idea that blood tests and serology can more accurately and less subjectively give a quick and reliable diagnosis for osteomyelitis. Unfortunately, there is no blood test that can independently diagnose osteomyelitis. Local inflammatory signs and symptoms may be blunted due to the presence of diabetes, vascular insufficiency, peripheral neuropathy, and leukocyte dysfunction. Published reports of the sensitivity, specificity, and predictive value of various diagnostic methods is complicated by inconsistent operational definitions and outcome measures, as well as the variability in the prevalence of osteomyelitis in the populations studied. It has been found, however, that laboratory makers can be used in combination to help diagnose, and more importantly, monitor treatment of osteomyelitis.

Blood Cultures

Blood cultures are often obtained when osteomyelitis is suspected, though often negative, except in cases of hematogenous osteomyelitis. In a study by Goergens et al., only 22 % of the patients diagnosed with hematogenous osteomyelitis had positive blood cultures [21]. Most scenarios dictate that blood cultures will be only be positive in the setting of acute bacteremia which may or may not have an associated incident of osteomyelitis.

Leukocytosis

IDSA guidelines indicate that an elevated white blood cell count (WBC) can be indicative of a serious inflammatory reaction in the setting of an acute infection [19]. However, the sensitivity and specificity of leukocytosis in osteomyelitis has been found to be rather imprecise. An elevated white cell count was shown in one retrospective study to be absent in approximately half of patients presenting with bone infection. Sensitivity for diagnosis of osteomyelitis of an elevated white blood cell count has been found to be as low as 14 % [20]. Furthermore, WBC and neutrophil counts have been shown to be of little value in diagnosing mild infection in diabetic foot ulcers, as there was no significant difference between grade 2 and grade 1 ulcer patients [44]. Despite severity of the infection, WBC counts are often normal even in the setting of acute osteomyelitis. Patients who do not have a significant inflammatory reaction, especially those with underlying immunosuppression or anemia may even have decreased white counts in the setting of acute infection. However, some authors have found that WBC counts higher than 11.0×10^9/L and a neutrophil percentage greater than 70 % were useful laboratory markers for osteomyelitis when combining this data with additional patient and wound characteristics [30].

Acute Phase Reactants

Acute phase reactants are defined as those proteins whose serum concentrations increase or decrease by at least 25 % during inflammatory states. Contrary to its name, acute phase reactant (APR) changes can be seen in both acute and chronic inflammatory conditions. Changes in APRs are not specific to infection and actually nonspecifically reflect physiologic responses to inflammatory processes or any type of tissue injury. Most APRs are produced by hepatocytes and therefore liver function can influence certain APRs. Conditions influenced by APRs include but are not limited to infection (both soft tissue and osteomyelitis), trauma, certain malignancies, inflammatory arthritides, any other chronic inflammatory condition, anemia, age, recent surgery, obesity, and renal disease [45, 46]. APRs may either increase or decrease as a result of an influential condition and are termed positive or negative APRs, respectively. Examples of positive APRs include C-reactive protein (CRP), fibrinogen, ceruloplasmin, interleukin-1, hepcidin, haptoglobin, and procalcitonin. Examples of negative APRs include albumin and transferrin [45, 47–49]. Some APRs are believed to respond more to infection and therefore are the best studied when considering the diagnosis of osteomyelitis. These APRs include erythrocyte sedimentation rate (ESR), CRP, and procalcitonin [45, 46, 49, 50].

Erythrocyte Sedimentation Rate

An elevated erythrocyte sedimentation rate (ESR) is often used to aid in the diagnosis and monitoring a patient with osteomyelitis. ESR is a not an actual protein but instead indirectly measures acute phase reactants that reflects plasma viscosity, primarily fibrinogen. The ESR is defined as the rate (mm/h) at which erythrocytes suspended in plasma settle when placed in a vertical tube.

ESR on average will elevate in the presence of both soft-tissue and bone infection. Some studies have found an elevated ESR in 96 % of cases in which bone was involved [20]. The ability of ESR to differentiate between cellulitis and osteomyelitis has been studied but is considered controversial and inconsistent. An early cohort study retrospectively examined 29 diabetic foot ulcers with either osteomyelitis or cellulitis. The study found that the ulcers with osteomyelitis demonstrated a mean erythrocyte sedimentation rate of 104 mm/h while the cellulitis group had a mean erythrocyte sedimentation rate of 44 mm/h [42]. Subsequent studies have found that on average, ESR tends to be higher in patients with osteomyelitis than those with only soft-tissue infection [41, 51–53].

However, there have been wide reports of the sensitivity and specificity of ESR and the optimal cut-off value is unknown. When considering patients with an ESR >70 mm/h, some studies have found a specificity of 100 %, but sensitivity ranged from only 28 to 50 % [25, 26, 54]. Other studies found less optimal sensitivities and specificities in patients with an ESR >70 mm/h and proposed different optimal cut-off levels. Michail and colleagues found that an ESR >70 mm/h had 0.61 sensitivity and 0.79 specificity, whereas the optimal cut-off level in their study was ≥67 mm/h with 0.84 sensitivity, 0.75 specificity, 0.71 positive predictive value, and 0.86 negative predictive value [52]. Other studies found that the optimal ESR cut-off was >65 mm/h and when combined with a wound size of >2 cm², sensitivity was 83 %, specificity 77 %, PPV 80 %, and NPV 81 % in the ability to diagnosis osteomyelitis [41] Peters and colleagues agree that ESR is the best studied laboratory value for diagnosing osteomyelitis, with a pooled analysis demonstrating an ESR >70 mm/h has a pooled positive likelihood ratio of 11 and a pooled negative likelihood ratio of 0.34 [24, 42, 55].

Overall, ESR alone is not an adequate predictor of an osteomyelitic infection. This is in part due to other variables that influence the ESR. Anemia and other erythrocyte-related diseases greatly influence ESR as the shape, size, and number of erythrocytes will influence the sedimentation rate. Anemia, age, and obesity can all increase ESR [56–60] Markedly elevated ESR levels defined as ESR values >100 mm/h can be seen in other conditions besides infection including renal disease and other inflammatory disorders [61] Many patients with osteomyelitis from a contiguous diabetic foot wound may also have concomitant renal disease. And ESR levels are often elevated in patients with renal insufficiency with over 60 % of patients with end-stage renal disease or nephrotic syndrome having ESR levels >60 mm/h [61–64].

Although ESR is familiar, well studied and simple to order, one must consider its significant disadvantages and low specificity in order to properly interpret its value. If ordered, ESR must be paired with other findings specific for osteomyelitis to improve the sensitivity and specificity. ESR can therefore be coupled with other modalities to aid in the diagnosis of osteomyelitis, and more importantly to help trend treatment effectiveness.

When utilizing ESR to monitor treatment effectiveness, it is important to note that it does not trend quickly. More importantly, when evaluating treatment effectiveness, ESR takes up to 3 months to normalize and elevated values within the first few weeks do not necessarily mean failure of treatment (Table 2.3).

C-Reactive Protein

C-reactive protein is a protein acute phase reactant synthesized by hepatocytes and thought to influence different stages of inflammation [65–67]. Similar to ESR, CRP levels are often elevated but lack specificity to diagnose osteomyelitis.

C-reactive protein concentrations tend to be higher in reported cases of osteomyelitis, but like ESR this sign is also inconsistent. Michail and colleagues found that in general, all inflammatory markers including CRP were significantly higher in patients with osteomyelitis compared to those with soft-tissue infection. However, there were 58.8 % of patients with soft-tissue infection only and 14.8 % with osteomyelitis that had a CRP <10 mg/L [52]. In a study of 265 children, ages 3 months to 15 years with culture-positive osteoarticular infection, the CRP values exceeded 20 mg/L in 95 % of the cases [68].

Determining the optimal CRP cut-off has been assessed and is still undetermined. Jeandrot analyzed CRP as an indicator in the diabetic population and found that CRP was the most informative single parameter. The study found that for a cut-off value of 17 mg/L, sensitivity was 0.727, specificity 1.000, positive predictive value 1.000, and negative predictive value 0.793 [44]. Fleischer et al. found that patients with OM had higher CRP levels compared with those without (OM 10.3 mg/dL versus 4.6 mg/dL, respectively). These researchers as well as others found that a CRP greater than 3.2 mg/dL provided the best sensitivity and specificity. Sensitivity has ranged from 75 to 85 % and specificity of only 67 % when attempting to diagnose cases of osteomyelitis in the reported literature [30, 41].

Questions have been raised about the effectiveness of CRP in special populations. In one study of severe diabetic foot infections, both the neutrophil count and the C-reactive protein level were higher in those with exclusively soft-tissue infection (CRP=68.8 mg/dL) than in those with osteomyelitis (CRP=51.4 mg/dL). This difference was not statistically significant [29]. Peri-prosthetic joint infections have also been found to have elevated CRP levels. The optimal threshold for a CRP level associated with prosthetic joint infection was 15 mg/L for patients with non-inflammatory arthritis and 17 mg/L for those with inflammatory arthritis [69].

CRP therefore lacks specificity in the absence of other radiologic, clinical, and microbiologic data. CRP may also vary in different patient populations. Like ESR, markedly elevated levels (CRP >10 mg/dL) are often seen in more severe infections. However, other conditions may increase CRP such as other inflammatory conditions, viral infections, age, obesity, smoking, diabetes mellitus, hypertension, chronic fatigue, depression, and oral hormone replacement therapy [70–78].

CRP is an APR that trends more quickly than ESR, and can be monitored more frequently when utilized to assess response to osteomyelitis treatment or relapse. Unlike ESR, CRP can be drawn every 48 h if needed and shows significant variations in the level measured. The CRP level should normalize within 1 week of treatment (Table 2.3).

Procalcitonin

Procalcitonin (PCT) is an amino acid protein precursor of the hormone calcitonin and is an APR whose site of origin is uncertain. PCT has been linked with the ability to assess inflammation associated with osteomyelitis and has gained acceptance by some as a marker for diagnosing infection [44]. Some authors claim that its accuracy as a predictor of bacterial infection is higher than that of C-reactive protein [75]. However, similar to other APRs, procalcitonin has been found to lack specificity and sensitivity when left up to its own merits.

Studies have shown that PCT levels are higher in patients with osteomyelitis then those with soft tissue or septic arthritis [79]. An elevated PCT at 0.4 ng/mL was 85.2 %

Table 2.3 Published values of acute phase reactants (APRs) reported to be associated with osteomyelitis and may be helpful in monitoring successful treatment in complex cases [24, 25, 29, 30, 41, 42, 44, 54, 55, 69, 80–82]

APR levels associated with osteomyelitis			
	Published levels	Peak time (days)	Normalizes with treatment
ESR	>65–70 mm/h	3–5	Gradual, by month 3
CRP	>15–3.2 mg/dL	2	Rapid, by day 7
PCT	>0.30–0.5 ng/mL	2	Rapid, by day 7

sensitive and 87.3 % specific in diagnosing septic arthritis and acute osteomyelitis. In comparison, PCT at its conventional cut-off of 0.5 ng/mL is 66.7 % sensitive and 91 % specific [80]. In another study with a baseline prevalence of 54 % osteomyelitis, PCT levels were 66.7 pg/mL in patients with osteomyelitis and 58.6 pg/mL in patients without osteomyelitis. The difference did not reach statistical significance ($P=0.627$) [29]. Uzun et al. had suggested that measurement of PCT levels might be an important diagnostic marker in diabetic foot infections. The authors determined 0.08 ng/mL as cut-off value for PCT with 77 % sensitivity and 100 % specificity in their study. Thus, PCT was deemed to be more specific, and equally sensitive in diabetic foot infection when compared to ESR and WBC [81]. Altay et al. determined higher values than former studies for PCT (0.6 ± 2.1) in diabetic foot infections. They also observed that PCT levels would decline, and range within normal limits (0.05 ± 0.02) after treatment [82].

PCT levels in most studies, especially those in patients who are diabetic with lower extremity ulcerations, are similar for deep soft-tissue diabetic foot infections as compared to osteomyelitis. The broad ranges reported in the literature make PCT less reliable then other values studied. However, a PCT value of >0.30–0.5 ng/mL may be indicative of osteomyelitis. Similar to CRP, PCT trends quickly, and peak values can be seen at 2 days from onset of symptoms, and normalizes with treatment quickly, usually within 1 week (Table 2.3).

Combining Clinical Findings and Laboratory Markers

Acute phase reactants do not appear reliable when studied individually. There are many factors that can increase or decrease the values of these laboratory markers. However, there is a select group of studies that identified the usefulness of combining several ARPs to help assess the clinical presence of osteomyelitis. In one study, 50 % of the patients with soft-tissue infection had normal WBC value ($<10\times109$/L); 6.3 % had ESR <30 mm/h; and 43.8 % had ESR <50 mm/h; 58.8 % had CRP <10 mg/L; and 85.3 % had PCT <0.5 ng/mL.

At baseline, 25.9 % of the patients with osteomyelitis had normal WBC values; 7.7 % had ESR <30 mm/h and 11.5 % had ESR <50 mm/h; 14.8 % had CRP <10 mg/L and 14.8 % had PCT <0.5 ng/mL. The values of all inflammatory markers at baseline were significantly higher in the patients with osteomyelitis than in the patients with soft-tissue infection [52]. Jeandrot et al. found that combining CRP and PCT provided the most relevant formula for distinguishing between grade 1 and grade 2 ulcers. The combination of CRP and PCT was significantly greater than that of CRP or PCT alone ($P<0.05$) [44].

If laboratory tests are ordered, studies suggest that the sensitivity and specificity of diagnosing osteomyelitis increases when combining results with examination findings. Ertugrul et al. found that ESR ≥65 mm/h together with a wound size ≥2 cm^2 had a sensitivity of 83 %, specificity of 77 %, positive predictive value of 80 %, and negative predictive value of 81 % in the diagnosis of osteomyelitis [41]. A recent prospective cohort was reviewed by Game et al. and evaluated combining ulcer depth and CRP or ESR in a cohort of 54 patients with histology-confirmed osteomyelitis. Combining the clinical and laboratory findings (ulcer depth >3 mm or CRP >30 mmol/L, ulcer depth >3 mm or ESR >60 mm/h) improved the sensitivity of the diagnosis of osteomyelitis to 100 % with a specificity of 55 % [26]. Fleischer and colleagues found that strategies which combined ulcer depth with serum inflammatory markers appeared most useful in differentiating ulcerated patients with concomitant bone infections. Wounds that had exposed bone or >3 mm depth alongside a CRP >3.2 mg/dL increased the probability of diagnosing osteomyelitis from 63 to 79 % [30].

Usefulness of laboratory markers may help non-specialty fields identify problematic foot ulcers sooner and consult specialists at an earlier stage of osteomyelitis due to suspiciously elevated values. These labs will also give primary care physicians a heightened awareness of the possibility of osteomyelitis due to the CRP or ESR, when they would have potentially underappreciated the extent/depth of a wound. However, it is up to the specialist to properly interpret laboratory tests and determine the next best course of action. Other factors must be taken into consideration as serologic markers alone cannot diagnose osteomyelitis. With that being said, no clinical picture, or clinical examination can solely diagnose osteomyelitis either. There is no single test that exists that can absolutely diagnose osteomyelitis.

Put simply, a single "reference standard" might not exist for the diagnosis of lower extremity osteomyelitis [83]. The clinician needs to rely on combination of factors including a thorough clinical exam, past medical history, vital signs, serologic and other laboratory markers (only when appropriate and deemed necessary), as well as imaging tools to aid in the diagnosis of this complex disease.

References

1. Merriam W. *Osteomyelitis*. http://www.merriamwebster.com/dictionary/osteomyelitis (2014). Accessed 10 Aug 2014.
2. Carek PJ, Dickerson LM, Sack JL. Diagnosis and management of osteomyelitis. Am Fam Physician. 2001;63(12):2413–20.
3. Waldvogel FA, Papageorgiou PS. Osteomyelitis: the past decade. N Engl J Med. 1980;303(7):360–70.
4. Cierny 3rd G, Mader JT, Penninck JJ. A clinical staging system for adult osteomyelitis. Clin Orthop Relat Res. 2003;414:7–24.
5. May Jr JW, Jupiter JB, Weiland AJ, Byrd HS. Clinical classification of post-traumatic tibial osteomyelitis. J Bone Joint Surg Am. 1989;71(9):1422–8.
6. Ger R. Muscle transposition for treatment and prevention of chronic post-traumatic osteomyelitis of the tibia. J Bone Joint Surg Am. 1977;59(6):784–91.
7. Mader JT, Shirtliff M, Calhoun JH. Staging and staging application in osteomyelitis. Clin Infect Dis. 1997;25(6):1303–9.
8. Weiland AJ, Moore JR, Daniel RK. The efficacy of free tissue transfer in the treatment of osteomyelitis. J Bone Joint Surg Am. 1984;66(2):181–93.
9. Prieto-Perez L, Perez-Tanoira R, Petkova-Saiz E, Perez-Jorge C, Lopez-Rodriguez C, Alvarez-Alvarez B, et al. Osteomyelitis: a descriptive study. Clin Orthop Surg. 2014;6(1):20–5.
10. Aziz Z, Lin WK, Nather A, Huak CY. Predictive factors for lower extremity amputations in diabetic foot infections. Diabet Foot Ankle 2011;2. 10.3402/dfa.v2i0.7463. Epub 2011 Sep 20.
11. Lavery LA, Armstrong DG, Wunderlich RP, Mohler MJ, Wendel CS, Lipsky BA. Risk factors for foot infections in individuals with diabetes. Diabetes Care. 2006;29(6):1288–93.
12. Gamaletsou MN, Kontoyiannis DP, Sipsas NV, Moriyama B, Alexander E, Roilides E, et al. Candida osteomyelitis: analysis of 207 pediatric and adult cases (1970-2011). Clin Infect Dis. 2012;55(10):1338–51.
13. Ramsey SD, Newton K, Blough D, McCulloch DK, Sandhu N, Reiber GE, et al. Incidence, outcomes, and cost of foot ulcers in patients with diabetes. Diabetes Care. 1999;22(3):382–7.
14. Schirmer S, Ritter RG, Fansa H. Vascular surgery, microsurgery and supramicrosurgery for treatment of chronic diabetic foot ulcers to prevent amputations. PLoS One. 2013;8(9), e74704.
15. Vuorisalo S, Venermo M, Lepantalo M. Treatment of diabetic foot ulcers. J Cardiovasc Surg (Torino). 2009;50(3):275–91.
16. Stone PA, Barnes ES, Savage T, Paden M. Late hematogenous infection of first metatarsophalangeal joint replacement: a case presentation. J Foot Ankle Surg. 2010;49(5):489; e1–e4.
17. Stinchfield FE, Bigliani LU, Neu HC, Goss TP, Foster CR. Late hematogenous infection of total joint replacement. J Bone Joint Surg Am. 1980;62(8):1345–50.
18. Allison DC, Holtom PD, Patzakis MJ, Zalavras CG. Microbiology of bone and joint infections in injecting drug abusers. Clin Orthop Relat Res. 2010;468(8):2107–12.
19. Lipsky BA, Berendt AR, Cornia PB, Pile JC, Peters EJ, Armstrong DG, et al. Infectious diseases society of America clinical practice guideline for the diagnosis and treatment of diabetic foot infections. Clin Infect Dis. 2012;54(12):e132–73.
20. Armstrong DG, Lavery LA, Sariaya M, Ashry H. Leukocytosis is a poor indicator of acute osteomyelitis of the foot in diabetes mellitus. J Foot Ankle Surg. 1996;35(4):280–3.
21. Goergens ED, McEvoy A, Watson M, Barrett IR. Acute osteomyelitis and septic arthritis in children. J Paediatr Child Health. 2005;41(1-2):59–62.
22. Ju KL, Zurakowski D, Kocher MS. Differentiating between methicillin-resistant and methicillin-sensitive Staphylococcus aureus osteomyelitis in children: an evidence-based clinical prediction algorithm. J Bone Joint Surg Am. 2011;93(18):1693–701.
23. Fritz JM, McDonald JR. Osteomyelitis: approach to diagnosis and treatment. Phys Sportsmed 2008; 36(1):nihpa116823.
24. Peters EJ, Lipsky BA. Diagnosis and management of infection in the diabetic foot. Med Clin North Am. 2013;97(5):911–46.
25. Newman LG, Waller J, Palestro CJ, Schwartz M, Klein MJ, Hermann G, et al. Unsuspected osteomyelitis in diabetic foot ulcers. Diagnosis and monitoring by leukocyte scanning with indium in 111 oxyquinoline. JAMA. 1991;266(9):1246–51.
26. Game FL. Osteomyelitis in the diabetic foot: diagnosis and management. Med Clin North Am. 2013;97(5):947–56.
27. Merlet A, Cazanave C, Dauchy FA, Dutronc H, Casoli V, Chauveaux D, et al. Prognostic factors of calcaneal osteomyelitis. Scand J Infect Dis. 2014;46(8):555–60.
28. Dinh MT, Abad CL, Safdar N. Diagnostic accuracy of the physical examination and imaging tests for osteomyelitis underlying diabetic foot ulcers: meta-analysis. Clin Infect Dis. 2008;47(4):519–27.
29. Mutluoglu M, Uzun G, Sildiroglu O, Turhan V, Mutlu H, Yildiz S. Performance of the probe-to-bone test in a population suspected of having osteomyelitis of the foot in diabetes. J Am Podiatr Med Assoc. 2012;102(5):369–73.
30. Fleischer AE, Didyk AA, Woods JB, Burns SE, Wrobel JS, Armstrong DG. Combined clinical and laboratory testing improves diagnostic accuracy for osteomyelitis in the diabetic foot. J Foot Ankle Surg. 2009;48(1):39–46.
31. Grayson ML, Gibbons GW, Balogh K, Levin E, Karchmer AW. Probing to bone in infected pedal ulcers. A clinical sign of underlying osteomyelitis in diabetic patients. JAMA. 1995;273(9):721–3.
32. Aragon-Sanchez J, Lipsky BA, Lazaro-Martinez JL. Diagnosing diabetic foot osteomyelitis: is the combination of probe-to-bone test and plain radiography sufficient for high-risk inpatients? Diabet Med. 2011;28(2):191–4.
33. Shone A, Burnside J, Chipchase S, Game F, Jeffcoate W. Probing the validity of the probe-to-bone test in the diagnosis of osteomyelitis of the foot in diabetes. Diabetes Care. 2006;29(4):945.
34. Lavery LA, Armstrong DG, Peters EJ, Lipsky BA. Probe-to-bone test for diagnosing diabetic foot osteomyelitis: reliable or relic? Diabetes Care. 2007;30(2):270–4.
35. Wrobel JS, Connolly JE. Making the diagnosis of osteomyelitis. The role of prevalence. J Am Podiatr Med Assoc. 1998;88(7):337–43.
36. Alvaro-Afonso FJ, Lazaro-Martinez JL, Aragon-Sanchez FJ, Garcia-Morales E, Carabantes-Alarcon D, Molines-Barroso RJ. Does the location of the ulcer affect the interpretation of the probe-to-bone test in the diagnosis of osteomyelitis in diabetic foot ulcers? Diabet Med. 2014;31(1):112–3.
37. Weiner RD, Viselli SJ, Fulkert KA, Accetta P. Histology versus microbiology for accuracy in identification of osteomyelitis in the diabetic foot. J Foot Ankle Surg. 2011;50(2):197–200.
38. Senneville E, Melliez H, Beltrand E, Legout L, Valette M, Cazaubiel M, et al. Culture of percutaneous bone biopsy specimens for diagnosis of diabetic foot osteomyelitis: concordance with ulcer swab cultures. Clin Infect Dis. 2006;42(1):57–62.
39. Jeffcoate WJ, Lipsky BA. Controversies in diagnosing and managing osteomyelitis of the foot in diabetes. Clin Infect Dis. 2004;39 Suppl 2:S115–22.
40. Ertugrul MB, Baktiroglu S, Salman S, Unal S, Aksoy M, Berberoglu K. The diagnosis of osteomyelitis of the foot in diabetes: microbiological examination vs magnetic resonance imaging and labelled leucocyte scanning. Diabet Med. 2006;23(6):649–53.
41. Ertugrul BM, Savk O, Ozturk B, Cobanoglu M, Oncu S, Sakarya S. The diagnosis of diabetic foot osteomyelitis: examination findings and laboratory values. Med Sci Monit. 2009;15(6):CR307–12.
42. Kaleta JL, Fleischli JW, Reilly CH. The diagnosis of osteomyelitis in diabetes using erythrocyte sedimentation rate: a pilot study. J Am Podiatr Med Assoc. 2001;91(9):445–50.

43. Meyr AJ, Singh S, Zhang X, Khilko N, Mukherjee A, Sheridan MJ, et al. Statistical reliability of bone biopsy for the diagnosis of diabetic foot osteomyelitis. J Foot Ankle Surg. 2011;50(6):663–7.

44. Jeandrot A, Richard JL, Combescure C, Jourdan N, Finge S, Rodier M, et al. Serum procalcitonin and C-reactive protein concentrations to distinguish mildly infected from non-infected diabetic foot ulcers: a pilot study. Diabetologia. 2008;51(2):347–52.

45. Gabay C, Kushner I. Acute-phase proteins and other systemic responses to inflammation. N Engl J Med. 1999;340(6):448–54.

46. Kushner I. The phenomenon of the acute phase response. Ann N Y Acad Sci. 1982;389:39–48.

47. Gabay C, Smith MF, Eidlen D, Arend WP. Interleukin 1 receptor antagonist (IL-1Ra) is an acute-phase protein. J Clin Invest. 1997;99(12):2930–40.

48. Nemeth E, Valore EV, Territo M, Schiller G, Lichtenstein A, Ganz T. Hepcidin, a putative mediator of anemia of inflammation, is a type II acute-phase protein. Blood. 2003;101(7):2461–3.

49. Nijsten MW, Olinga P, The TH, de Vries EG, Koops HS, Groothuis GM, et al. Procalcitonin behaves as a fast responding acute phase protein in vivo and in vitro. Crit Care Med. 2000;28(2):458–61.

50. Bedell SE, Bush BT. Erythrocyte sedimentation rate. From folklore to facts. Am J Med. 1985;78(6 Pt 1):1001–9.

51. Mutluoglu M, Uzun G, Ipcioglu OM, Sildiroglu O, Ozcan O, Turhan V, et al. Can procalcitonin predict bone infection in people with diabetes with infected foot ulcers? A pilot study. Diabetes Res Clin Pract. 2011;94(1):53–6.

52. Michail M, Jude E, Liaskos C, Karamagiolis S, Makrilakis K, Dimitroulis D, et al. The performance of serum inflammatory markers for the diagnosis and follow-up of patients with osteomyelitis. Int J Low Extrem Wounds. 2013;12(2):94–9.

53. Rabjohn L, Roberts K, Troiano M, Schoenhaus H. Diagnostic and prognostic value of erythrocyte sedimentation rate in contiguous osteomyelitis of the foot and ankle. J Foot Ankle Surg. 2007;46(4):230–7.

54. Eneroth M, Larsson J, Apelqvist J. Deep foot infections in patients with diabetes and foot ulcer: an entity with different characteristics, treatments, and prognosis. J Diabetes Complications. 1999;13(5–6):254–63.

55. Butalia S, Palda VA, Sargeant RJ, Detsky AS, Mourad O. Does this patient with diabetes have osteomyelitis of the lower extremity? JAMA. 2008;299(7):806–13.

56. Yudkin JS, Stehouwer CD, Emeis JJ, Coppack SW. C-reactive protein in healthy subjects: associations with obesity, insulin resistance, and endothelial dysfunction: a potential role for cytokines originating from adipose tissue? Arterioscler Thromb Vasc Biol. 1999;19(4):972–8.

57. Ham TCCF. Sedimentation rate of erythrocytes. Medicine (Baltimore). 1938;17:447.

58. Hayes GS, Stinson IN. Erythrocyte sedimentation rate and age. Arch Ophthalmol. 1976;94(6):939–40.

59. Miller A, Green M, Robinson D. Simple rule for calculating normal erythrocyte sedimentation rate. Br Med J (Clin Res Ed). 1983;286(6361):266.

60. Leff RD, Akre SP. Obesity and the erythrocyte sedimentation rate. Ann Intern Med. 1986;105(1):143.

61. Fincher RM, Page MI. Clinical significance of extreme elevation of the erythrocyte sedimentation rate. Arch Intern Med. 1986;146(8):1581–3.

62. Bathon J, Graves J, Jens P, Hamrick R, Mayes M. The erythrocyte sedimentation rate in end-stage renal failure. Am J Kidney Dis. 1987;10(1):34–40.

63. Shusterman N, Kimmel PL, Kiechle FL, Williams S, Morrison G, Singer I. Factors influencing erythrocyte sedimentation in patients with chronic renal failure. Arch Intern Med. 1985;145(10):1796–9.

64. Arik N, Bedir A, Gunaydin M, Adam B, Halefi I. Do erythrocyte sedimentation rate and C-reactive protein levels have diagnostic usefulness in patients with renal failure? Nephron. 2000;86(2):224.

65. Paakkonen M, Peltola H. Bone and joint infections. Pediatr Clin North Am. 2013;60(2):425–36.

66. Black S, Kushner I, Samols D. C-reactive protein. J Biol Chem. 2004;279(47):48487–90.

67. Marnell L, Mold C, Du Clos TW. C-reactive protein: ligands, receptors and role in inflammation. Clin Immunol. 2005;117(2):104–11.

68. Paakkonen M, Kallio MJ, Kallio PE, Peltola H. Sensitivity of erythrocyte sedimentation rate and C-reactive protein in childhood bone and joint infections. Clin Orthop Relat Res. 2010;468(3):861–6.

69. Cipriano CA, Brown NM, Michael AM, Moric M, Sporer SM, Della Valle CJ. Serum and synovial fluid analysis for diagnosing chronic periprosthetic infection in patients with inflammatory arthritis. J Bone Joint Surg Am. 2012;94(7):594–600.

70. Giles JT, Bartlett SJ, Andersen R, Thompson R, Fontaine KR, Bathon JM. Association of body fat with C-reactive protein in rheumatoid arthritis. Arthritis Rheum. 2008;58(9):2632–41.

71. Kushner I, Rzewnicki D, Samols D. What does minor elevation of C-reactive protein signify? Am J Med. 2006;119(2):166.e17–28.

72. Slade GD, Ghezzi EM, Heiss G, Beck JD, Riche E, Offenbacher S. Relationship between periodontal disease and C-reactive protein among adults in the atherosclerosis risk in communities study. Arch Intern Med. 2003;163(10):1172–9.

73. Ranganath VK, Elashoff DA, Khanna D, Park G, Peter JB, Paulus HE, et al. Age adjustment corrects for apparent differences in erythrocyte sedimentation rate and C-reactive protein values at the onset of seropositive rheumatoid arthritis in younger and older patients. J Rheumatol. 2005;32(6):1040–2.

74. Wener MH, Daum PR, McQuillan GM. The influence of age, sex, and race on the upper reference limit of serum C-reactive protein concentration. J Rheumatol. 2000;27(10):2351–9.

75. Simon L, Gauvin F, Amre DK, Saint-Louis P, Lacroix J. Serum procalcitonin and C-reactive protein levels as markers of bacterial infection: a systematic review and meta-analysis. Clin Infect Dis. 2004;39(2):206–17.

76. Krüger S, Ewig S, Papassotiriou J, et al. Inflammatory parameters predict etiologic patterns but do not allow for individual prediction of etiology in patients with CAP: results from the German competence network CAPNETZ. Respir Res. 2009;10:65.

77. Le Gall C, Desideri-Vaillant C, Nicolas X. Significations of extremely elevated C-reactive protein: about 91 cases in a French hospital center. Pathol Biol (Paris). 2011;59(6):319–20.

78. Vanderschueren S, Deeren D, Knockaert DC, Bobbaers H, Bossuyt X, Peetermans W. Extremely elevated C-reactive protein. Eur J Intern Med. 2006;17(6):430–3.

79. Shen CJ, Wu MS, Lin KH, Lin WL, Chen HC, Wu JY, et al. The use of procalcitonin in the diagnosis of bone and joint infection: a systemic review and meta-analysis. Eur J Clin Microbiol Infect Dis. 2013;32(6):807–14.

80. Maharajan K, Patro DK, Menon J, Hariharan AP, Parija SC, Poduval M, et al. Serum Procalcitonin is a sensitive and specific marker in the diagnosis of septic arthritis and acute osteomyelitis. J Orthop Surg Res. 2013;8:19. doi:10.1186/1749-799X-8-19..

81. Uzun G, Solmazgul E, Curuksulu H, Turhan V, Ardic N, Top C, et al. Procalcitonin as a diagnostic aid in diabetic foot infections. Tohoku J Exp Med. 2007;213(4):305–12.

82. Altay FA, Sencan I, Senturk GC, Altay M, Guvenman S, Unverdi S, et al. Does treatment affect the levels of serum interleukin-6, interleukin-8 and procalcitonin in diabetic foot infection? A pilot study. J Diabetes Complications. 2012;26(3):214–8.

83. Berendt AR, Peters EJ, Bakker K, Embil JM, Eneroth M, Hinchliffe RJ, et al. Diabetic foot osteomyelitis: a progress report on diagnosis and a systematic review of treatment. Diabetes Metab Res Rev. 2008;24 Suppl 1:S145–61.

Diagnostic Imaging of Osteomyelitis of the Foot and Ankle

3

Susan B. Truman

Accurate diagnosis of osteomyelitis of the foot and ankle is important in order to plan treatment for the patient with a foot and ankle ulceration or infection. Prompt initiation of antibiotic therapy in the early stages of infection can cure disease before surgical intervention is needed. Delayed diagnosis can contribute to an increase in rate of complications including bone necrosis and destruction as well as chronic infection and an increased need for surgical intervention. Although osteomyelitis can often be diagnosed clinically, many patients who are diabetic with foot ulcerations do not mount an immune response and thus early physical exam signs of osteomyelitis can be difficult to detect. In addition, in patients with underlying arthropathy or neuropathy, clinical symptoms of these diseases can mimic osteomyelitis. For these reasons imaging is an essential adjunct to clinical evaluation in determining the presence and extent of infection. This chapter will review the advantages and disadvantages of the imaging modalities frequently used for imaging of osteomyelitis and will also review several of the common diagnostic challenges that are confronted in everyday practice.

Radiography

Radiographs are often the first imaging study ordered when a patient presents with suspected osteomyelitis of the foot and ankle. Radiographs are readily available in most clinic and hospital settings and they are inexpensive. Radiographic signs of osteomyelitis include decreased density of bone, lytic changes and cortical erosion, trabecular destruction, bone necrosis, brodie abscess, sclerosis, and periosteal reaction (Fig. 3.1). Radiographs have limited utility in the early diagnosis of osteomyelitis due to low sensitivity in the early stages of osteomyelitis. In one study examining

hematogenous osteomyelitis early radiographs obtained just after the patient presented to the hospital had a sensitivity of only 16 % and a specificity of 96 % [1]. Another study that examined 24 cases of osteomyelitis demonstrated that plain films were negative in 25 % of the patients who had pathologically proven osteomyelitis [2]. Nawaz et al. found sensitivity for diagnosis of osteomyelitis on plain films of 63 % and a specificity of 87 % [3]. An additional meta-analysis found the sensitivity of radiographs is between 28 and 75 % [4]. The low sensitivity on radiographs is due to the fact that radiographically visible changes in the bone can take up to 2–3 weeks to develop after the clinical onset of disease. It is estimated that radiographic changes will not be visible until there has been destruction of between 40 and 60 % of the bone matrix. For this reason radiographs are not a reliable way to diagnose osteomyelitis early in its presentation. That said, a positive X-ray with rarefaction of the bone and cortical erosion is highly suggestive of osteomyelitis, and can often help plan immediate treatment. Since a negative X-ray does not exclude early osteomyelitis, and if there is a high clinical suspicion for osteomyelitis, further imaging should be obtained if the initial X-ray is negative.

There can be false positives when the patient has an underlying arthropathy or neuropathy which can mimic the findings of osteomyelitis on plain films [2]. For this reason at our institution, many patients with positive X-rays still go on to have an magnetic resonance imaging (MRI) in order to delineate the extent of disease and soft tissue findings prior to surgery.

Computed Tomography

Computed Tomography (CT) is not frequently used for diagnosis of early osteomyelitis as it shares several of the deficiencies associated with radiographs. Early osteomyelitis which has not yet progressed to cortical destruction is not well seen and thus CT is not particularly sensitive in early osteomyelitis. In addition, CT has a high radiation dose relative to the

S.B. Truman, M.D. (✉)
St. Paul Radiology and HealthPartners,
767 Linwood Ave, St. Paul, MN 55015, USA
e-mail: struman@stpaulrad.com

T.J. Boffeli (ed.), *Osteomyelitis of the Foot and Ankle*, DOI 10.1007/978-3-319-18926-0_3

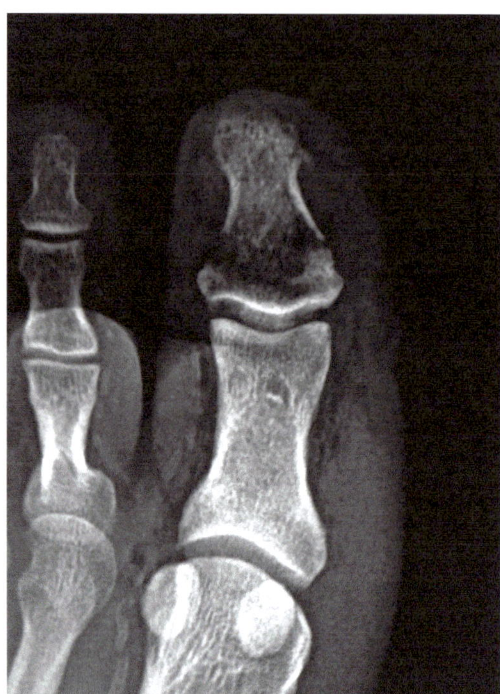

Fig. 3.1 Plain film of the great toe demonstrates typical plain film findings of osteomyelitis including cortical erosion and destruction at the medial tip of the distal phalanx, lytic changes, and destruction of the trabecula in the proximal portion of the bone, soft tissue swelling, and air in the soft tissues

clinical information, which can be obtained, and thus CT is primarily used in patients who have a contraindication to MRI scanning. The findings of osteomyelitis on CT are similar to those seen on radiographs and include trabecular rarefaction, cortical destruction and erosion, and periosteal reaction. These findings are often seen in better detail on CT scan than on X-rays due to the thin slice thickness. In addition, small pockets of gas can be seen and CT can often identify fluid collections when they are not visible by X-ray [5, 6].

Nuclear Medicine Scans

Technetium 99m Phosphate Bone Scans

Bone scintigraphy is a very sensitive test and is usually performed as a three-phase study. The patient is injected with Technetium 99m-labeled diphosphonates, usually methylene diphosphonate (MDP), and images are obtained immediately after injection for a dynamic flow phase. This is followed with static images during an immediate blood pool phase and then delayed imaging 2–4 h later for a bone phase. Focused spot views are very helpful when evaluating the foot and ankle. On a 3-phase bone scan hyperfusion, hyperemia, and focal increased uptake in the bone of interest are seen with a diagnosis of osteomyelitis (Fig. 3.2a–c). The scan will be

positive in early phases of osteomyelitis within 24–48 h of initial symptoms. Although the sensitivity of bone scan is reported at 80–90 % in multiple studies [7, 8], the specificity is much lower and is closer to 50 % in multiple studies [9–12]. A meta-analysis by Termaat et al. found a pooled specificity of 25 % for bone scintigraphy [13]. The binding of the 99mTc-MDp to the hydroxyapatite in the bone is responsible for the radiotracer uptake and thus any condition which causes bone turnover with osteoblastic activity will demonstrate increased radiotracer uptake on a bone scan. Disease processes such as neuroarthropathy, fracture, prior surgery, or malignancy can all cause a false positive bone scan in a patient who is being evaluated for osteomyelitis. In addition, the lack of anatomic detail on bone scan can make exact delineation of extent of disease difficult.

Given the known lack of specificity, Jay et al. evaluated whether the results of the bone scan, either positive or negative, affected amputation rates or clinical treatment and found that there was no difference in treatment or in amputation rates based on whether the bone scan was positive or negative. Jay et al. recommend that bone scan not be used in evaluation of foot and ankle osteomyelitis due to its lack of specificity and unlikely effect on treatment decisions [14].

For these reasons, bone scan is not often used as the imaging method of choice following plain films; however, 3 phase Tc99m-MDp scanning remains a reasonable imaging technique in patients who cannot have an MRI particularly if they do not have underlying arthropathy or neuropathy or a recent history of trauma.

Labeled White Blood Cell Scans

Indium-labeled leukocytes have been used extensively for evaluation for osteomyelitis. The radiolabeled white blood cells accumulate at the site of infection and will not accumulate in locations without infection such as fractures, malignancy, or neuropathic joints. This makes labeled white cell scans particularly useful in diagnosing osteomyelitis in patients with underlying neuropathic joints. The sensitivity of the test reported in the literature extends from 72 to 100 % [12, 15, 16]. Despite the high sensitivity the Indium-labeled leukocyte study has disadvantages that include a 24-h waiting period before imaging can begin as well as low resolution of the images which makes it difficult to determine the exact location of the osteomyelitis (Fig. 3.3). Schauwecker et al. used a concurrent bone scan for determining anatomic location and found improved sensitivity and specificity with a sensitivity of 100 % and a specificity of 83 % [17]. There can be false positives as well due to the accumulation of white cells in the infected soft tissues and the fact that low anatomic resolution can make exact location of infection difficult to determine.

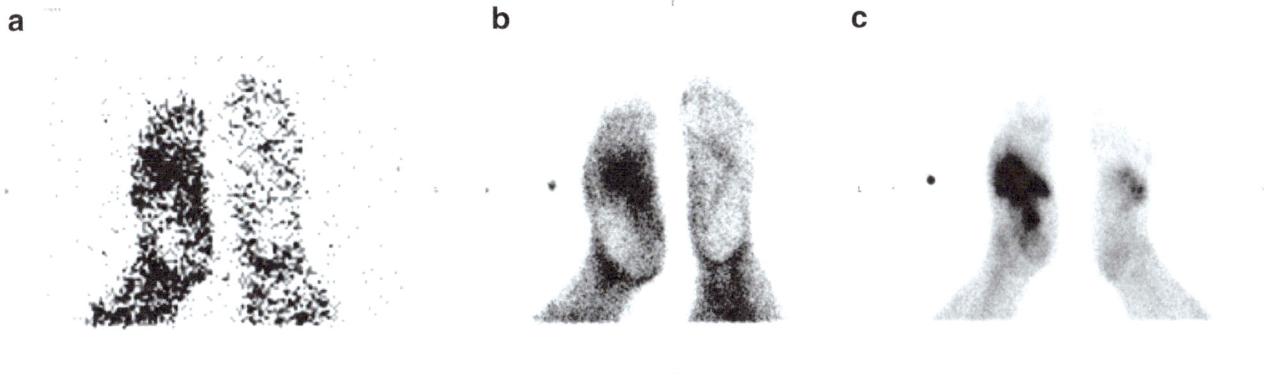

Fig. 3.2 3-Phase bone scan demonstrates typical findings of osteomyelitis. (**a**) Blood flow image, (**b**) blood pool image, and (**c**) delayed image all demonstrate increased uptake of Tc 99m MDP in the region of the base and proximal right fourth metatarsal

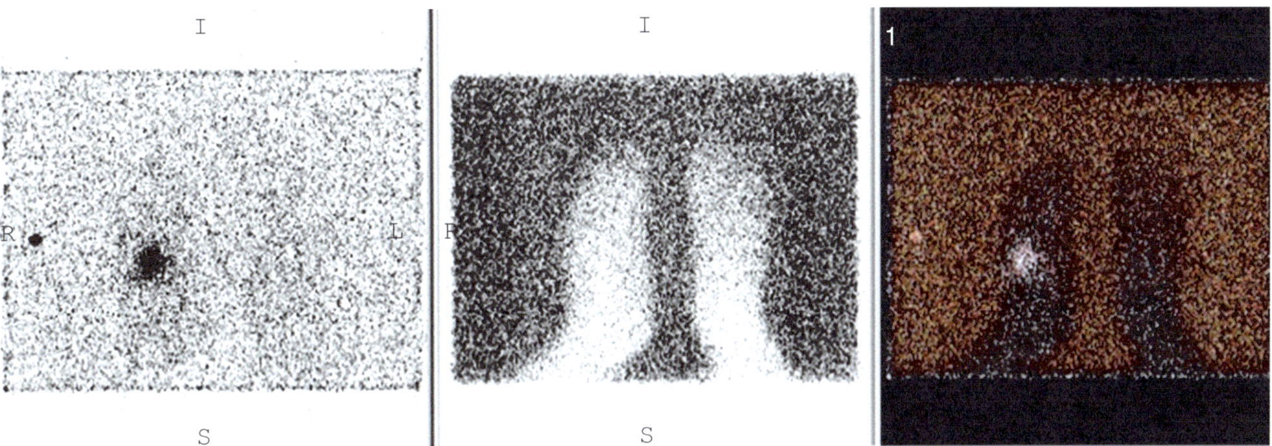

Fig. 3.3 Indium-111-labeled white blood cell scan performed on the patient who had the bone scan in Fig. 3.2. Focal uptake of Indium-labeled white cells seen in the same region of the foot confirms osteo- myelitis. Lack of anatomic detail makes delineation of location of uptake difficult without the bone scan which was performed contemporaneously

Technetium 99m hexamethylpropylamine oxine (HMPAO)-labeled leukocytes are also used and are more cost effective than Indium-labeled cells. Tc-99m HMPAO scanning is also based on the accumulation of white blood cells at sites of infection and thus it shares the advantages of higher specificity due to lack of accumulation in patients with arthropathy, neuropathy, and trauma that Indium scanning has. In addition, it can be performed and completed on the same day, allowing for a more timely diagnosis than Indium white blood cell scanning affords. The sensitivity of the exam is between 85 and 90 % [9, 11]. Despite high sensitivity and specificity of the labeled white cell scans, these are still usually a problem-solving technique used in unusual situations such as patients with extensive hardware which cannot be imaged by MRI or in patients with equivocal findings by other imaging modalities due to underlying neuropathic changes.

Positron Emission Tomography Imaging

Positron emission tomography (PET) has also been studied as an emerging tool for the evaluation of osteomyelitis. PET scans are very expensive and not available in many hospitals on a routine basis and thus PET is unlikely to become a mainstay of imaging for the infected foot and ankle. PET scanning involves injection of fluorodeoxyglucose (FDG). Metabolically active tissues including infected tissues use more glucose and thus accumulate more radiotracer. Data regarding the sensitivity and specificity of PET scans is variable. Nawaz et al. compared PET, MRI, and plain films in patients with diabetic foot ulcers. They found a sensitivity of 81 % and a specificity of 93 % for PET and a sensitivity of 91 % and specificity of 78 % for MRI. They concluded that PET scan is a reasonable alternative in patients who have a contraindication to MRI scanning [3]. Kagna et al. found that PET/CT had a sensitivity of 100 % with a specificity of 93 % for diagnosis of osteomyelitis in the diabetic foot [18]. Basu found that PET was very useful in diagnosing infection in patients with underlying Charcot foot and PET had a sensitivity of 100 % in this setting in comparison to MRI which had a sensitivity of 76.9 % in the setting of Charcot [19]. Although these researchers found high sensitivity for PET, there are conflicting data in the literature. Familiari found only 43 % sensitivity and 67 % specificity for PET/CT [20]. The data are discordant and it is uncertain as to why these scientists have obtained dramatically different results [21]. Given these conflicting data, PET is best used in complex situations in which standard imaging techniques such as MRI and white blood cell scanning cannot be performed easily.

Magnetic Resonance Imaging

MRI is usually the preferred method of imaging for diagnosis of osteomyelitis. MRI is widely available, fairly quick to perform in most centers, and does not use radiation. In addition, scans can be obtained in multiple anatomic planes. MRI images have excellent spatial resolution and are very useful for evaluation of bone marrow as well as of soft tissue structures providing significantly more anatomic detail than nuclear medicine scans. The anatomic detail is helpful in defining the extent of disease which is very important to surgical planning. MRI is also very useful in depicting soft tissue complications in addition to bony involvement. MRI demonstrates abscesses, tendon involvement, and cellulitis with much greater detail than US or CT [22]. Finally MRI has been shown to be cost effective [23].

A standard MRI of the extremity for evaluation of osteomyelitis usually involves a combination of T1 weighted and T2 weighted sequences in multiple anatomic planes as well as imaging after intravenous administration of a gadolinium contrast agent. The exam should be tailored to the site of ulceration and suspected infection. Dedicated smaller field of view imaging of the forefoot or hindfoot is preferable to using a larger field of view in an attempt to include the entire foot and ankle in one exam. Given the size of most feet, the large FOV required to include the entire foot and ankle leads to a decrease in resolution of smaller structures such as the smaller bones of the midfoot and forefoot. This renders the study less useful since less anatomic detail is available. A dedicated extremity coil designed for the foot and ankle should be utilized.

At our institution the exam includes sagital short tau inversion recovery (STIR) images and sagital T1 weighted images, coronal T1 weighted images, and coronal FSE T2 weighted images with fat saturation, axial T1 weighted images, and axial FSE T2 weighted images with fat saturation.

The coronal images are helpful for visualization of ulcerations along the plantar aspect of the forefoot. The relationship of the ulcer to the underlying bone is well seen on coronal imaging. The coronal images are also useful for evaluation of the marrow. Sagital imaging often demonstrates calcaneal ulcerations better than the coronal or axial imaging. Use of fat saturation is important on the T2 weighted exams so that marrow edema can be adequately visualized. Frequently in the distal toes the fat saturation is uneven and thus the bone marrow appears high signal on the T2 weighted images which renders diagnosis of marrow edema impossible. During scanning if the fat saturation in the toes is not adequate, STIR imaging can be substituted for the fat suppressed T2 weighted images. STIR imaging often is lower in resolution but it does not rely on chemical fat saturation and thus can be very useful for visualization of marrow edema particularly in the distal phalanges.

The majority of cases of osteomyelitis in the foot result from direct spread of infection from an ulcer in the skin down into the soft tissues and to the bone. These ulcerations typically occur in patients with diabetes who have developed peripheral neuropathy due to microvascular disease. The vascular disease both causes the neuropathy and also causes impairment in wound healing which predisposes the patient to ongoing infection at the site of the open ulcer. The distribution of foot ulcers depends to some degree on gait and activity and will vary from patient to patient; however, the vast majority of ulcers in the forefoot occur at the fifth metatarsal, first metatarsal, and at the distal phalanx of the great toe. In the hindfoot, the calcaneus is the bone which is most frequently affected. Ledermann et al. demonstrated in a study of 161 ft in 158 patients there were 130 cases of osteomyelitis. Of these 130 cases of osteomyelitis, all but one spread from a skin ulcer or defect down to the subjacent bone [24].

Callus formation is often a precursor to ulceration and calluses are seen frequently in diabetic patients. The distribution of callous is similar to the sites of maximal skin pressure. Thus, calluses are seen in the feet under the metatarsal heads, adjacent to the first metatarsal base, and in patients with a neuropathic foot adjacent to the cuboid. Calluses appear on MRI as soft tissue prominences which are focal and low signal on T1 weighted scans with variable signal on T2 weighted scans. The variability of the signal on T2 weighted scans is due to the variable amount of granulation tissue and inflammation in the callus. The callous will often enhance and care must be taken not to confuse the enhancing callous with focal infection. Repeated micro-trauma to the callus can result in an ulceration in the callus which as described above is often slow to heal in diabetics with vascular disease [25].

Ulcerations on MRI appear as a skin defect often with heaped up margins due to the presence of an underlying callus. The ulcerations are often high signal on T2 weighted scans due to surrounding infection and cellulitis and they will often enhance avidly as well. The ulceration can extend down to the surface of the bone or alternatively a sinus tract may be present extending from the ulceration to the surface of the bone. The presence of an ulcer and the contiguous abnormal signal extending from the ulcer to the bone is a hallmark finding in the diagnosis of osteomyelitis by MRI [26, 27] (Fig. 3.4). The presence or absence of an ulceration can help differentiate marrow edema related to osteomyelitis from reactive marrow edema or marrow edema related to other causes such as stress reaction or trauma. In patients without an ulcer, marrow edema in the bone is less likely to represent osteomyelitis [26, 27].

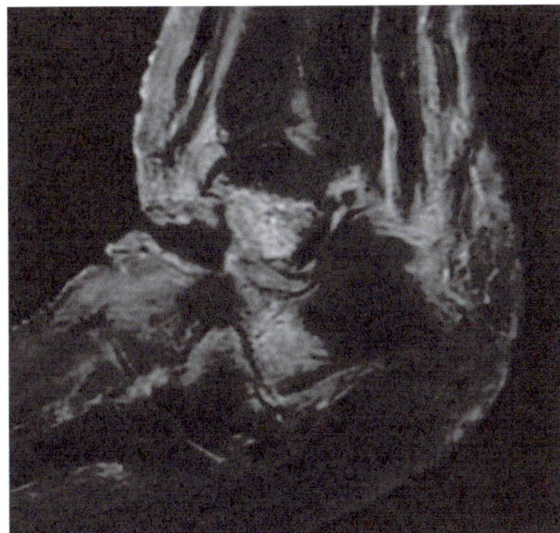

Fig. 3.4 Soft tissue ulceration over the dorsum of the foot extending down to the talus. Erosion of the talus with cortical destruction and marrow enhancement. Extensor tendons are also disrupted

Diagnosis of osteomyelitis by MRI is made by identifying abnormal marrow in the bone that is typically signified by low signal replacing the marrow on T1 weighted scans and high signal in the same location of T2 weighted scans. Enhancement of the bone on fat suppressed T1 weighted images can also be useful in making the diagnosis. Marrow signal changes are always present in osteomyelitis but can also be present due to other disease processes such as reactive edema secondary to inflammation, trauma, stress reaction, or tumor. There are several factors that can help differentiate marrow edema secondary to osteomyelitis from marrow edema related to one of these other causes. These factors include presence of an ulcer with extension to the bone as well as the relative signal intensity of the edema, confluence of the abnormal signal, and presence of the abnormal signal on more than one type of sequence [27, 28] (Fig. 3.5a–c).

On T1 weighted imaging, the signal in cases of osteomyelitis is lower than the normal marrow and typically isointense or hypointense to the musculature [28]. The marrow changes on the T1 weighted images are due to infiltration of the marrow by infection with replacement of the normal marrow with pus and necrosis. Features of the abnormal T1 weighted signal that are highly correlated with true positive cases of osteomyelitis include a geographic medullary distribution of the abnormal signal as well as a confluent pattern of the abnormal marrow signal [29] (Fig. 3.6a,b). Collins et al. found that in 100 % of their study cases with surgically proven osteomyelitis there was decreased signal in the marrow on T1 weighted scans in a geographic distribution and a confluent pattern with T2 marrow signal intensity in the same location [29]. Johnson et al. confirmed these findings and found that in 19/20 cases of confirmed osteomyelitis,

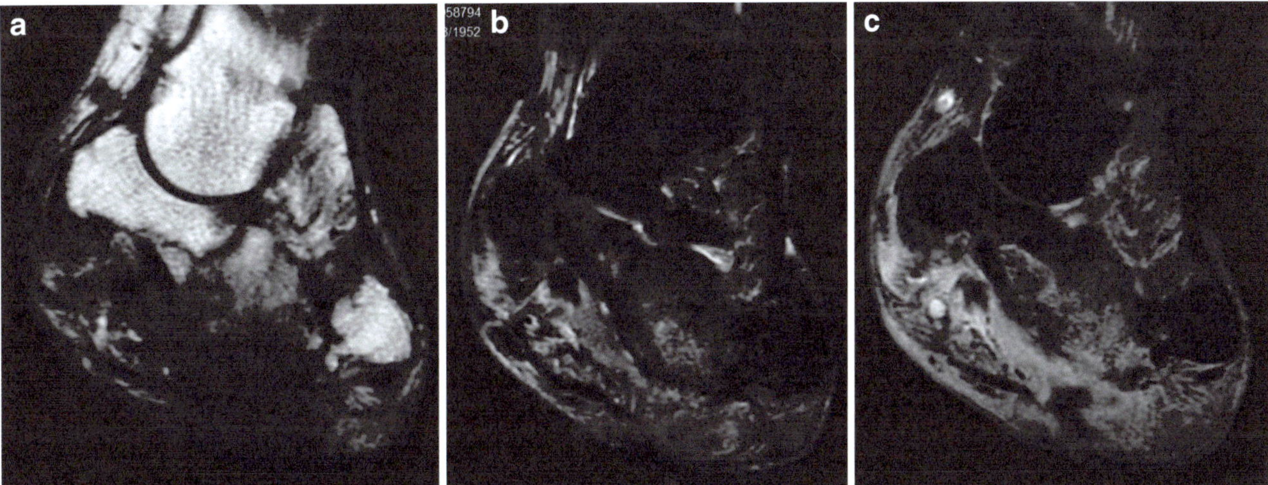

Fig. 3.5 Diabetic patient with foot infection and an ulceration deep to the cuboid. (**a**) On the T1 weighted image, there is abnormal signal within the marrow and cortical destruction. On the T2 weighted image, (**b**) there is marrow edema in the cuboid. (**c**) A sinus tract extends down to the bone and the bone enhances post gadolinium administration. Diagnosis is aided by the presence of the ulceration as well as of abnormal signal on multiple sequences

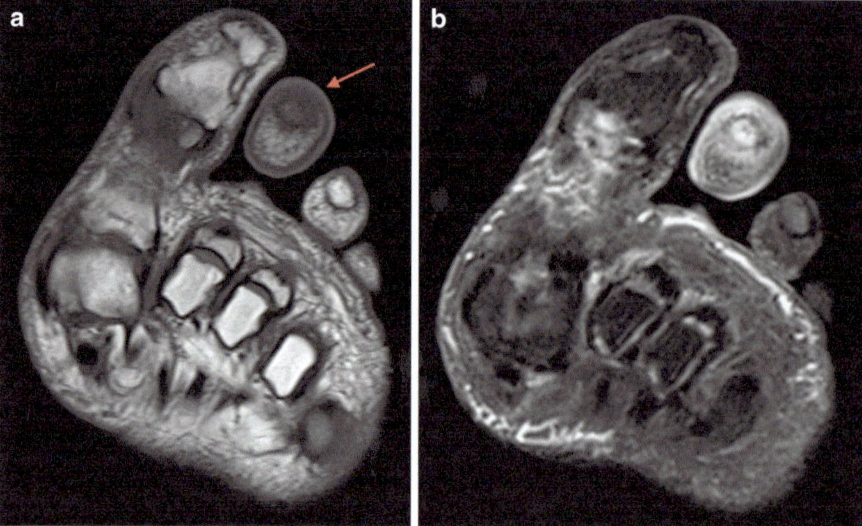

Fig. 3.6 T1 weighted axial image (**a**) of the toes in a patient with osteomyelitis demonstrates low signal in the marrow of the second distal phalanx completely replacing the normal bright fatty signal (*arrow*). Normal marrow signal can be seen for comparison in the distal phalanges of the first and third toes. Coronal T2 weighted image (**b**) of the toes demonstrating concordant increased T2 signal in the second distal phalanx

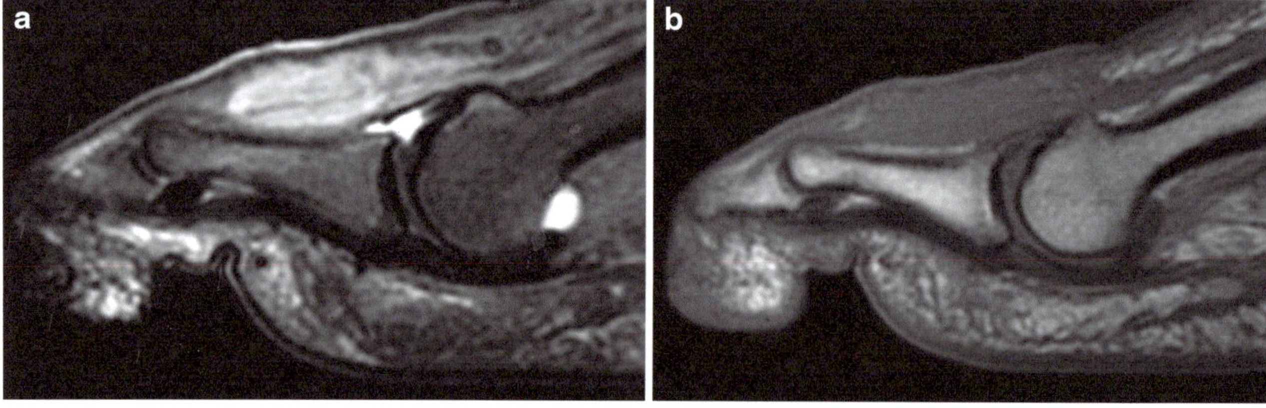

Fig. 3.7 T2 weighted image (**a**) demonstrates edema in the bone deep to a focal abscess; (**b**) however, on the T1 weighted scan the marrow signal remains normal. Normal signal on T1 weighted scans in conjunction with increased signal on T2 weighted scans is a pattern seen in reactive marrow edema and should not be mistaken for osteomyelitis

decreased marrow signal on T1 weighted images was present with a geographic distribution and confluent pattern. None of the cases of confirmed osteomyelitis in this study had hazy reticulated abnormal signal on the T1 weighted scans. The sensitivity of the combination of the findings of geographic distribution of abnormal signal and confluent pattern of abnormal signal was 95 % and the specificity was 91 % in this study using T1 weighted imaging features alone [28]. Morrison et al. also found that using the abnormal signal on T1 weighted scans yielded an average sensitivity of 92 % and a specificity of 86 % [26].

In several studies the presence of abnormal signal in the marrow on T1 weighted scans which has a hazy or reticulated pattern is more suggestive of reactive marrow edema than of osteomyelitis [26, 27, 29, 30]. On T2 weighted scans osteomyelitis is visualized as increased signal due to marrow edema at the site of infection. Marrow edema on the T2 weighted scans is a nonspecific finding as there are many conditions beside osteomyelitis which can also cause increased signal on the T2 weighted scans [27]. Frequently in patients with soft tissue ulceration there will be reactive marrow edema in the adjacent bone. This will typically be reticulated in appearance and less confluent that marrow edema secondary to osteomyelitis. It is helpful to review the T2 weighted scans in conjunction with the T1 weighted scans. When patients have normal signal on the T1 weighted scans and edema on the T2 weighted scans, osteomyelitis is less likely to be present than if the marrow is abnormal on both T1 weighted scans and T2 weighted scans [29] (Fig. 3.7a,b). The T2 weighted scans are also particularly useful when they are normal as normal marrow signal on T2 weighted imaging excludes the diagnosis of osteomyelitis [27].

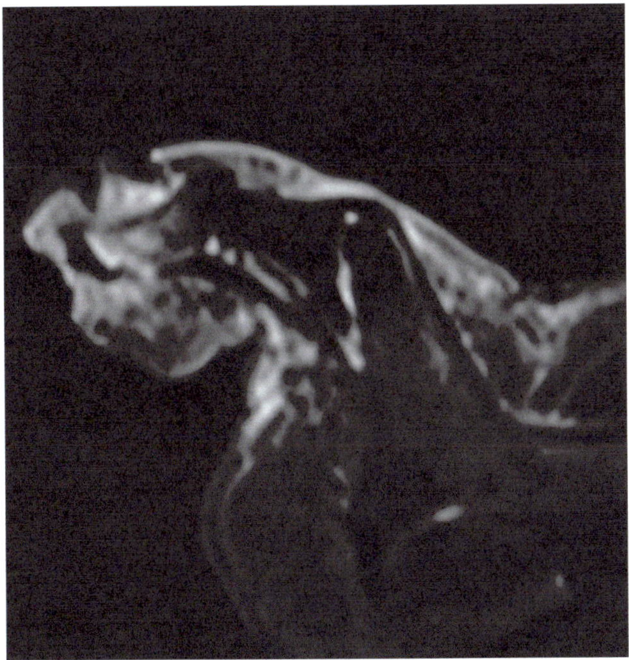

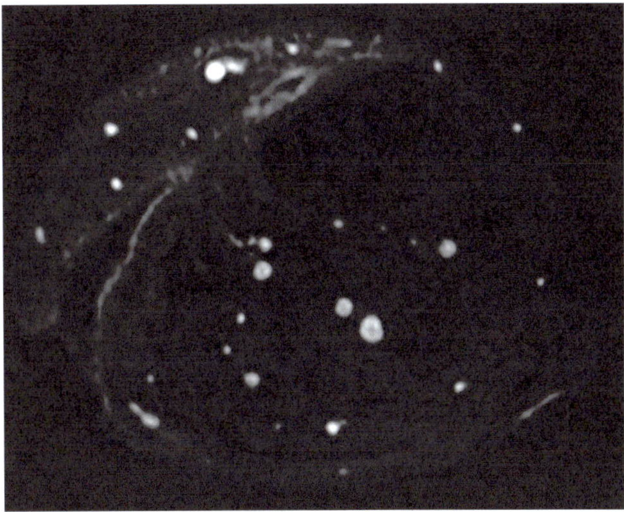

Fig. 3.9 T1 weighted fat suppressed image obtained after administration of intravenous gadolinium demonstrates a draining abscess in the posterior medial soft tissues. This has an enhancing rim and is draining via a sinus tract and ulcer. There is no underling osteomyelitis in this patient

Fig. 3.8 Sagital T1 weighted fat suppressed image obtained after intravenous administration of gadolinium contrast demonstrates a skin ulceration at the tip of the toe with enhancement of the subjacent distal phalanx consistent with osteomyelitis

Gadolinium contrast enhanced imaging is also useful during MRI imaging of osteomyelitis (Fig. 3.8). Scans are typically performed in two anatomic planes after gadolinium contrast administration. Morrison et al. demonstrated a high sensitivity and specificity for MRI diagnosis of osteomyelitis with fat suppressed post gadolinium contrast imaging with a sensitivity of 88 % and specificity of 93 %. With nonenhanced MR imaging alone in this study, the sensitivity for detecting osteomyelitis was 79 % and the specificity was 53 %. The low specificity with routine unenhanced imaging is due to the fact that marrow edema can be present for multiple reasons unrelated to osteomyelitis. Morrison also found that gadolinium enhancement improved the conspicuity of soft tissue abscesses and bone abscesses as well as of sinus tracts [26, 31]. Schmid also found similar sensitivity and specificity of gadolinium enhanced imaging in diagnosis of osteomyelitis in comparison to the STIR images [32]. The STIR images are very useful when contrast cannot be administered but additional data regarding soft tissue abnormalities such as abscesses and tendon involvement is less well visualized with STIR imaging than on post contrast imaging.

Of note, patients need to be screened for renal disease prior to the administration of gadolinium contrast. Patients with poor renal function do not clear the gadolinium chelates and there is a risk of developing nephrogenic systemic fibrosis after gadolinium contrast injection in these patients. In patients without adequate renal function, gadolinium contrast imaging cannot be performed [33, 34].

MRI is also helpful in delineating the extent of disease when osteomyelitis is present. Osteomyelitis can spread to adjacent joints and septic arthritis is a common concurrent diagnosis in patients with osteomyelitis. Typically septic arthritis in a diabetic patient is due to an associated soft tissue infection or ulceration [35]. Findings in septic arthritis include joint effusion, synovial thickening and enhancement, perisynovial enhancement, marrow edema on T1 weighted and T2 weighted scans. Synovial outpouchings are also frequently seen. Occasionally the joint will communicate with a sinus tract leading to an ulceration. Of the visualized markers of septic joint on MRI synovial enhancement and joint effusion are the two diagnostic features that are most closely correlated with the diagnosis of a septic joint [30].

In addition to septic joint, MRI can also delineate abscesses in patients with cellulitis and skin ulceration (Fig. 3.9). These abscesses can be soft tissue abscesses as well as bony abscesses. Diagnosis of an abscess requires incision and drainage and thus early identification is crucial for appropriate intervention. Lederman et al. examined 161 ft of 158 patients with foot infections and suspected osteomyelitis and found abscesses in 18 % of the patients. More than half of these abscesses were in the forefoot and the majority were in the plantar muscle compartment. All of the forefoot abscesses were related to contiguous ulcers. Abscesses were more commonly found in patients who had had prior surgery. More than one third of patients had abscesses in this study in the midfoot and hindfoot, and in these patients the abscesses were several centimeters from the ulceration and up to 9 cm away in some cases [36].

Abscesses are often small in size in the foot and ankle and they are high signal on T2 weighted scans. Abscesses are also well seen on post contrast fat saturated imaging as rim enhancing fluid-filled structures. In patients with cellulitis and soft tissue edema who have significantly increased single on T2 weighted scans throughout the soft tissues of the foot due to edema, small abscesses can be difficult to detect on T2 weighted images against the background hyperintensity. Post gadolinium imaging is very helpful in the visualization of abscesses in these patients, as the diffuse edema will not enhance. The non-enhancement of the surrounding edematous tissues allows the rim enhancing abscess to stand out from the background soft tissues.

Tendon involvement is also common in patients with osteomyelitis and foot and ankle infection. Lederman et al. demonstrated that approximately half the patients who require surgery for foot and ankle infections have evidence of tendon infection on MRI. The most commonly affected tendons were the tendons of the first and 5th toes and the Achilles tendon. Peroneal tendons are also often involved when there is an ulceration over the lateral malleoli. This pattern reflects the common sites of ulceration. In the forefoot, the majority of the tendon disease involved the flexor tendons, again mirroring the usual location of the ulcerations seen in the forefoot. An area of peritendinous enhancement that runs though a region of infected soft tissues in proximity to an ulceration is suspicious for septic tenosynovitis (Fig. 3.10). High signal in the tendon on T-2 weighted scans and peritendinous edema can be seen with infection, however, these signs can also be seen due to mechanical injuries and thus are nonspecific [37].

Defining the scope of osteomyelitis including complications such as septic arthritis, tendon involvement, and abscess formation when present is important because knowledge of

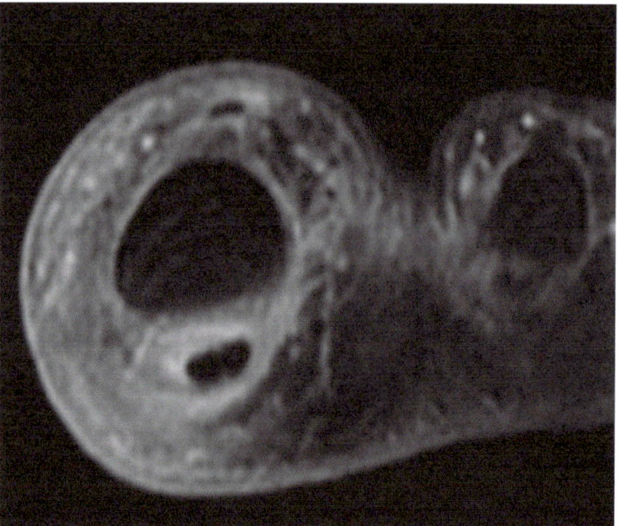

Fig. 3.10 T1 weighted fat suppressed image obtained after intravenous gadolinium contrast administration demonstrates enhancement around the flexor hallucis tendon. The tendon tracks through a region of soft tissue infection adjacent to an ulceration and findings are consistent with infected tenosynovitis

the extent of the diseases translates into more appropriate surgery with preservation of as much of the foot as possible. Morrison et al. demonstrated that in patients who had MRI for diagnosis and went onto a foot sparing limited surgical resection, none of the patients developed recurrence at the site of resection within 1 month of resection. This suggests that MRI is helpful in describing the extent of disease such that surgeons can appropriately plan surgeries which are effective and preserve the foot [23.]

MRI has repeatedly been shown to be overall highly sensitive and specific for the diagnosis of osteomyelitis. The sensitivity ranges form 77 to 100 % and the specificity ranges from 79 to 100 % [23, 24, 38, 39]. A meta-analysis of the data by Dinh et al. demonstrated a pooled sensitivity of 90 % and a pooled specificity of 79 % [4]. Another meta-analysis performed by Kapoor et al. also found that MRI imaging is significantly better than technetium 99m bone scan, plain films, and white blood cell studies for the diagnosis of osteomyelitis [40]. Please note that many of the primary studies that have been conducted were conducted between 1990 and 2000 and there have been significant advances in MRI technology since that time with better resolution imaging obtained on the newer magnets. Given improved equipment, these statistics may underrepresent the current sensitivity and specificity of MRI for detection of osteomyelitis.

Diagnostic Challenges in Diagnosing Osteomyelitis in the Presence of Neuroarthropathy

Although the sensitivity and specificity of MR imaging for diagnosis of osteomyelitis is high, neuropathic osteoarthropathy or Charcot foot presents additional diagnostic challenges when osteomyelitis is suspected. In the early phases of neuroarthropathy, the foot will present as warm, swollen, and inflamed. On MRI, there is often high signal on T2 weighted imaging and low signal on T1 weighted imaging within the bones which are also the usual findings in osteomyelitis [41]. In patients with neuropathic arthropathy however, there is usually no evidence of skin ulceration of subcutaneous soft tissue signal abnormality which are typically seen in osteomyelitis. The findings in neuropathy often involve multiple joints and are seen on both sides of the joints and this constellation is less commonly seen in osteomyelitis. In the chronic phases of neuropathy, edema and enhancement are less prominent; however there is development of significant disorganization and deformity secondary to resorbtion, repeated fractures, and dislocations. Disease at the Lisfranc joint results in dislocation of the metatarsals and results in the classic "rocker bottom" deformity. This deformity causes increased pressure on the cuboid and ulceration and infection in this location can occur [42].

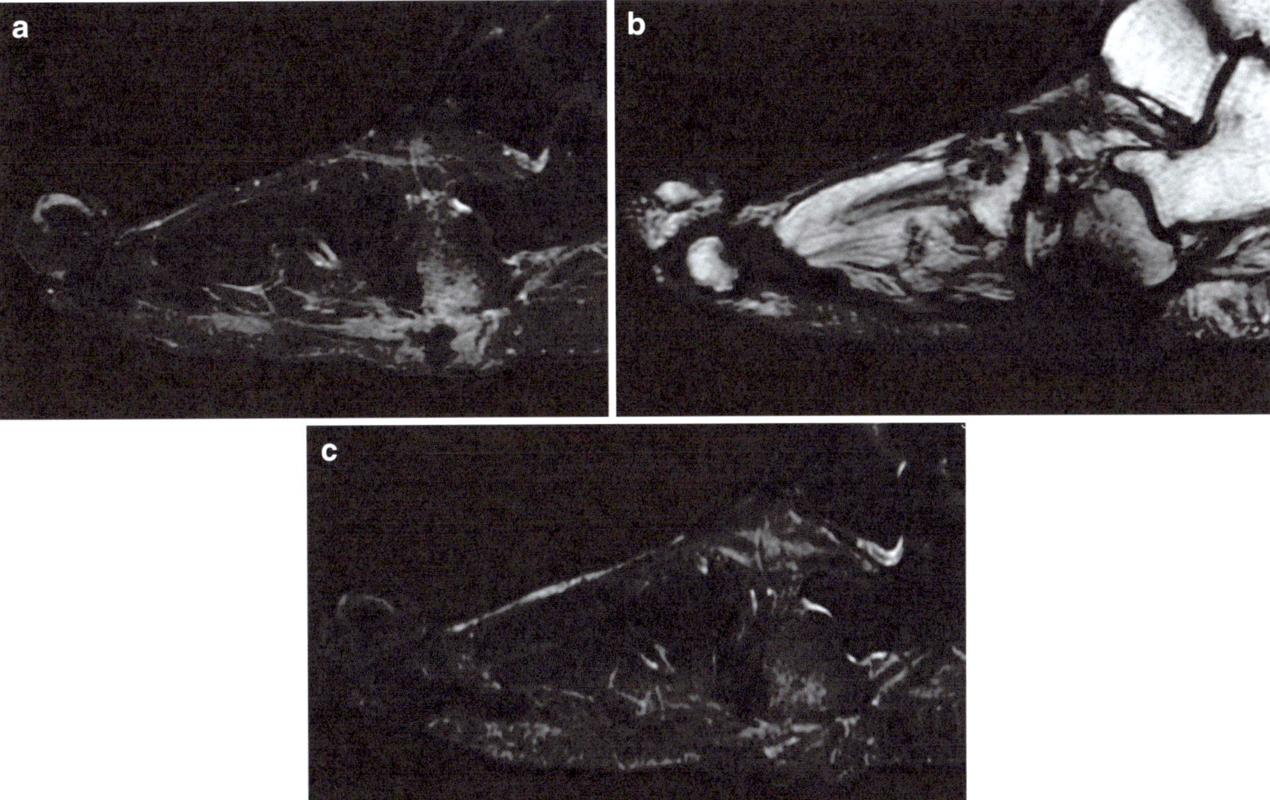

Fig. 3.11 Patient has underlying neuroarthropathy with foot infection and an ulceration deep to the cuboid. (**a**) A sinus tract extends down to the bone which is enhancing. (**b**) On the T1 weighted image, there is confluent abnormal signal within the marrow and cortical destruction. On the T2 weighted image (**c**), there is marrow edema in the cuboid. In this patient with underlying Charcot neuroarthropathy, the deep ulceration and sinus tract are definitive evidence of osteomyelitis

Diagnosing osteomyelitis in patients with underlying neuropathic osteoarthropathy is a diagnostic dilemma. It can be very difficult to definitively diagnose on MRI. Ahmadi et al. studied 128 neuropathic joints in 63 patients and analyzed multiple separate signs on MR imaging in order to define their relative utility for diagnosis of osteomyelitis in patients with underlying neuroarthropathy. They found that presence of a sinus tract, replacement of soft tissue fat, diffuse marrow signal changes, joint erosion, thick rim enhancement of a joint effusion, or diffuse joint enhancement are the best indicators of superimposed osteomyelitis in this setting (Fig. 3.11a–c). They found that the preservation of subcutaneous fat, absence of fluid collections, presence of subchondral cysts, and presence of intraarticular bodies all suggest uninfected neuroarthropathy [43]. Lederman et al. suggest several principles which can help guide the radiologist in making this distinction. First of all, the majority of infections are due to ulceration and contiguous spread of infection. Neuropathy on the other hand is primarily an articular disease and thus if the patient has marrow signal changes in subarticular location without ulceration, simple neuropathy is more likely. In addition, neuropathy is usually polyarticular where as infection spreads locally and thus is usually seen in a focal area. Finally, neuropathic arthropathy is most commonly seen in the midfoot where as infection and osteomyelitis usually occur at the common sites of ulceration which are the metatarsal heads and calcaneus [44].

Nuclear medicine scans can also be helpful in diagnosing osteomyelitis in patients with underlying neuroarthropathy. Tagged white blood cell scans can be performed as the white cells will accumulate at the site of infection and should not accumulate if the patient has uninfected neuroarthropathy. The tagged white cell scan can also be combined with a three-phase bone scan or a sulfur colloid scan in order to improve sensitivity and specificity [45, 46]. Basu et al. demonstrated that FDG-PET imaging could reliably differentiate neuroarthropathy from neuroarthropathy with superimposed infection with a sensitivity of 100 % and a specificity of 94 % [19].

Conclusion

Imaging diagnosis of osteomyelitis usually begins with X-rays. X rays provide an inexpensive widely available tool for initial evaluation. If a patient has no signs of osteomyelitis, the diagnosis is not excluded or confirmed and if there is high clinical suspicion the patient will need additional imaging if the study is negative. In most situations, MRI is the imaging test of choice due to its high sensitivity and specificity, good anatomic detail for evaluation of both bone and soft tissue structures, and its relative availability. In certain situations, nuclear medicine studies may be useful when MRI cannot be performed due to contraindications. In addition, nuclear medicine studies can also be useful in helping diagnose neuroarthropathy with superimposed osteomyelitis from uninfected neuroarthropathy.

References

1. Malcius D, Jonkus M, Kuprionis G, Maleckas A, Monastyreckiene E, Uktveris R, Rinkevicius S, Barauskas V. The accuracy of different imaging techniques in diagnosis of acute hematogenous osteomyelitis. Medicina (Kaunas). 2009;45(8):624–31.
2. Yuh WT, Corson JD, Baraniewski HM, Rezai K, Shamma AR, Kathol MH, Sato Y, el-Khoury GY, Hawes DR, Platz CE, et al. Osteomyelitis of the foot in diabetic patients: evaluation with plain film, 99mTc-MDP bone scintigraphy, and MR imaging. AJR Am J Roentgenol. 1989;152(4):795–800.
3. Nawaz A, Torigian DA, Siegelman ES, Basu S, Chryssikos T, Alavi A. Diagnostic performance of FDG-PET, MRI, and plain film radiography (PFR) for the diagnosis of osteomyelitis in the diabetic foot. Mol Imaging Biol. 2010;12(3):335–42.
4. Dinh MT, Abad CL, Safdar N. Diagnostic accuracy of the physical examination and imaging tests for osteomyelitis underlying diabetic foot ulcers: meta-analysis. Clin Infect Dis. 2008;47:519–27.
5. Gold RH, Hawkins RA, Katz RD. Bacterial osteomyelitis: findings on plain radiography, CT, MR and scintigraphy. AJR Am J Roentgenol. 1991;157:365–70.
6. Chandnani VP, Beltran J, Morris CS, et al. Acute experimental osteomyelitis and abscesses: detection with MR imaging versus CT. Radiology. 1990;175:233–6.
7. Capriotti G, Chianelli M, Signore A. Nuclear medicine imaging of diabetic foot infection: results of meta-analysis. Nucl Med Commun. 2006;27(10):757–64.
8. Eckman MH, Greenfield S, Mackey WC, Wong JB, Kaplan S, Sullivan L, et al. Foot infections in diabetic patients: decision and cost-effectiveness analyses. JAMA. 1995;273(9):712–20.
9. Harvey J, Cohen MM. Technecium-99 labeled leukocytes in diagnosing diabetic osteomyelitis in the foot. J Foot Ankle Surg. 1997;36:120–6.
10. Devillers A, Moissan A, Hennion F, et al. Contribution of technetium 99m hexamethylpropylene amine oxime labeled leucocyte scintigraphy to the diagnosis of diabetic foot infection. Eur J Nucl Med. 1998;25:132–8.
11. Blume PA, Dey HM, Dailey LJ, et al. Diagnosis of pedal osteomyelitis with Tc-99m HMPAO labeled leucocytes. J Foot Ankle Surg. 1997;36:120–6.
12. Palestro CJ, Caprioli R, Love C, et al. Rapid Diagnosis of pedal osteomyelitis in diabetics with a technetium 99m labeled monoclonal antigranulocyte antibody. J Foot Ankle Surg. 2003;42:2–8.
13. Termaat MF, Raijmakers PG, Scholten HJ, Bakker FC, Patka P, Haarman HJ. The accuracy of diagnostic imaging for the assessment of chronic osteomyelitis: a systematic review and meta-analysis. J Bone Joint Surg Am. 2005;87(11):2464–71.
14. Jay PR, Michelson JD, Mizel MS, Magid D, Le T. Efficacy of three-phase bone scans in evaluating diabetic foot ulcers. Foot Ankle Int. 1999;20(6):347–55.
15. Newman LG, Waller J, Palestro CJ, et al. Unsuspected osteomyelitis in diabetic foot ulcers: diagnosis and monitoring by leukocyte scanning with indium In111 oxyquinolone. JAMA. 1991;266:1246–51.
16. Johnson JE, Kennedy EJ, Shereff MJ, et al. Prospective study of bone, indium-111-labeled whit blood cell, and gallium-67 scanning for the evaluation of osteomyelitis in the diabetic foot. Foot Ankle Int. 1996;17:10–6.
17. Schauwecker DS, Park HM, Burt RW, et al. Combined bone scintigraphy and indium-111 leukocyte scans in neuropathic foot disease. J Nucl Med. 1988;29:1651–5.
18. Kagna O, Srour S, Melamed E, Militianu D, Zohar K. FDG PET/CT imaging in the diagnosis f osteomyelitis in the diabetic foot. Eur J Nucl Med Mol Imaging. 2012;39:1545–50.
19. Basu S, Chryssikos T, Houseni M, Scot Malay D, Shah J, Zhuang H, Alavi A. Potential role of FDG PET in the setting of diabetic neuro-osteoarthropathy: can it differentiate uncomplicated Charcot's neuroarthropathy from osteomyelitis and soft-tissue infection? Nucl Med Commun. 2007;28(6):465–72.
20. Familiari D, Glaudemans AW, Vitale V, Prosperi D, Bagni O, Lenza A, Cavallini M, Scopinaro F, Signore A. Can sequential 18F-FDG PET/CT replace WBC imaging in the diabetic foot? J Nucl Med. 2011;52(7):1012–9.
21. Palestro CJ. 18F-FDG and diabetic foot infections: the verdict is. J Nucl Med. 2011;52(7):1009–11.
22. Donovan A, Schweitzer ME. Current concepts in imaging diabetic pedal osteomyelitis. Radiol Clin North Am. 2008;46(960):1105–24.
23. Morrison WB, Schweitzer ME, Wapner KL, Hecht PJ, Gannon FH, Behm WR. Osteomyelitis in feet of diabetics: clinical accuracy, surgical utility, and cost-effectiveness of MR imaging. Radiology. 1995;196(2):557–64.
24. Ledermann HP, Morrison WB, Schweitzer ME. MR image analysis of pedal osteomyelitis: distribution, patterns of spread, and frequency of associated ulceration and septic arthritis. Radiology. 2002;223(3):747–55.
25. Chatha DS, Cunnningham PM, Schweitzer ME. MR imaging of the diabetic foot: diagnostic challenges. Radiol Clin North Am. 2005;43(4):747–59.
26. Morrison WB, Schweitzer ME, Batte WG, et al. Osteomyelitis of the foot: relative importance of primary and secondary MR imaging signs. Radiology. 1998;207:625–32.
27. Craig JG, Amin MB, Wu KW, et al. Osteomyelitis of the diabetic foot: MR imaging-pathologic correlation. Radiology. 1997;203(3):849–55.
28. Johnson PW, Collins MS, Wenger DE. Diagnostic utility of T1 weighted MRI characteristics in evaluation of osteomyelitis of the foot. AJR Am J Roentgenol. 2009;1929(1):96–100.
29. Collins MS, Schaar MM, Wenger DE, Madrekar JN. T1 weighted MRI characteristics of pedal osteomyelitis. AJR Am J Roentgenol. 2005;185:386–93.
30. Karchensky M, Schweitzer ME, Morrison WB, et al. MRI Findings of septic arthritis and associated osteomyelitis in adults. AJR Am J Roentgenol. 2004;182:119–22.
31. Morrison WB, Schweitzer ME, Bock GW, Mitchell DG, Hume EL, Pathria MN, Resnick D. Diagnosis of osteomyelitis: utility of fat-suppressed contrast-enhanced MR imaging. Radiology. 1993;189(1):251–7.
32. Schmid MR, Hodler J, Vienne P, Binkert CA, Zanetti M. Bone marrow abnormalities of foot and ankle: STIR versus T1-weighted contrast-enhanced fat-suppressed spin-echo MR imaging. Radiology. 2002;224(2):463–9.
33. ACR Manual on Contrast Media Version 9, 2013. ACR Committee on Drugs and Contrast Media.

34. Sadowski EA, Bennett LK, Chan MR, et al. Nephrogenic systemic fibrosis: risk factors and incidence estimation. Radiology. 2007;243:148–57.
35. Lipsky BA, Berendt AR, Deery HG, Embil JM, Joseph WS, Karchmer AW, LeFrock JL, Lew DP, Mader JT, Norden C, Tan JS. Diagnosis and treatment of diabetic foot infections. Clin Infect Dis. 2004;39(7):885–910.
36. Ledermann HP, Morrison WB, Schweitzer ME. Pedal abscesses in patients suspected of having pedal osteomyelitis: analysis with MR imaging. Radiology. 2002;224(3):649–55.
37. Ledermann HP, Morrison WB, Schweitzer ME, Raikin SM. Tendon involvement in pedal infection: MR analysis of frequency, distribution, and spread of infection. AJR Am J Roentgenol. 2002;179(4): 939–47.
38. Croll SD, Nicholas GGG, Osborne MA, et al. Role of magnetic resonance imaging in the diagnosis of osteomyelitis in diabetic foot infections. J Vasc Surg. 1996;24:266–70.
39. Levine SE, Neagle CE, Esterhai JL, et al. Magnetic resonance imaging for the diagnosis of osteomyelitis in the diabetic patient with a foot ulcer. Foot Ankle Int. 1994;15:151–6.
40. Kapoor A, Page S, Lavalley M, Gale DR, Felson DT. Magnetic resonance imaging for diagnosing foot osteomyelitis: a meta-analysis. Arch Intern Med. 2007;167:125–32.
41. Marcus CD, Ladam-Marcus VJ, Leone J, Malgrange D, Bonnet-Gausserand FM, Menanteau BP. MR imaging of osteomyelitis and neuropathic osteoarthropathy in the feet of diabetics. Radiographics. 1996;16(6):1337–48.
42. Morrison WB, Ledermann HP, Schweitzer ME. MR imaging of the diabetic foot. Magn Reson Imaging Clin N Am. 2001;9(3): 603–13.
43. Ahmadi ME, Morrison WB, Carrino JA, Schweitzer ME, Raikin SM, Ledermann HP. Neuropathic arthropathy of the foot with and without superimposed osteomyelitis: MR imaging characteristics. Radiology. 2006;238(2):622–31.
44. Ledermann HP, Morrison WB. Differential diagnosis of pedal osteomyelitis and diabetic neuroarthropathy: MR imaging. Semin Musculoskelet Radiol. 2005;9(3):272–83.
45. Palestro CJ, Harendra HM, Mahendra P, et al. Marrow versus infection in the Charcot joint: indium-111 leukocyte an dtechnetium-99m sulfur colloid scintigraphy. J Nucl Med. 1998;39: 346–50.
46. Seabold JE, Flickinger FW, Kao SC, Gleason TJ, Kahn D, Nepola JV, Marsh JL. Indium-111-leukocyte/technetium-99m-MDP bone and magnetic resonance imaging: difficulty of diagnosing osteomyelitis in patients with neuropathic osteoarthropathy. J Nucl Med. 1990;31(5):549–56.

Bone Biopsy Techniques

4

Ryan R. Pfannenstein, Shelby B. Hyllengren, and Troy J. Boffeli

Introduction

The key to effective management of osteomyelitis in the foot or ankle is early and accurate diagnosis which allows for prompt treatment typically involving a tailored combination of antibiotic therapy and surgical intervention. Antibiotic treatment is ideally culture-directed, yet wound cultures do not always accurately reflect the causative organisms [1]. Open surgical treatment of infection readily allows for bone biopsy, but percutaneous biopsy may also be performed as part of the preoperative planning process or in cases where isolated medical treatment is appropriate. A timely diagnosis is especially critical in diabetes-related osteomyelitis since limb or life-threatening infection can develop rapidly [2]. The foot and ankle are particularly prone to osteomyelitis due to contiguous spread of infection from adjacent ulcers or direct inoculation of bone associated with deep puncture wounds due to the relatively subcutaneous nature of the underlying bone and joint structures [3]. Less commonly, the mechanism of infection is hematogenous, whereby osteomyelitis can be mistaken for other disorders such as gout, cellulitis, or septic arthritis since there is no overlying wound.

Unfortunately, osteomyelitis can be difficult to diagnose and the initial clinical symptoms may be sparse [4, 5]. Berendt recommended a high suspicion for osteomyelitis in wounds that do not improve despite 4–6 weeks of appropriate conservative treatment [6]. Failure to heal in 4–6 weeks unfortunately describes most neuropathic, ischemic, decubi-

tus, and venous wounds on the foot or ankle. Larson identified a sensitivity and specificity of 33 % and 60 %, respectively, when diagnosing osteomyelitis based on clinical findings alone [7]. Clinical signs of infection persisting longer than 10 days have been associated with the development of necrotic bone and osteomyelitis [8]. The probe-to-bone (PTB) test is a useful aid in the diagnosis of osteomyelitis and should be a routine part of the physical exam in patients with foot or ankle wounds. Negative PTB may be more useful to exclude the diagnosis of osteomyelitis while positive PTB raises suspicion for, but is not diagnostic of osteomyelitis [9, 10].

Despite the widely held "gold standard" status of bone biopsy, the degree to which biopsy is definitive is highly dependent on the technique used to obtain the biopsy, pre-biopsy antibiotics that may affect culture yield, and diagnostic criteria used by the pathologist. A poorly obtained specimen is of little clinical utility and evidence-based guidelines are deficient regarding the optimal biopsy technique. Lack of consistent diagnostic criteria used to establish a pathologic diagnosis also raises questions about the accuracy of bone biopsy [11]. The clinician should evaluate the entire clinical picture including clinical exam findings, laboratory assessment, radiographic workup, pathologic biopsy, and bone culture in order to accurately diagnose osteomyelitis.

The invasive nature of biopsy suggests that the procedure is not without inherent risks, especially in patients with proven history of compromised wound healing. The goal of bone biopsy is to obtain a representative sample of bone without contamination of the specimen and without causing harm to the patient. The variables that need to be considered to accomplish these goals are the focus of this chapter. Selection of the ideal biopsy technique is largely based on which bone is being biopsied, the size and location of ulceration, the quality of the surrounding soft tissue, presence of active cellulitis, and need for wide resection including partial foot amputation. Biopsy is often part of larger bone resection procedure such as digital amputation, metatarsal head resection, or partial calcanectomy where the same technical pearls are important in order to enhance the accuracy of the biopsy specimen [12].

R.R. Pfannenstein, D.P.M., F.A.C.F.A.S. (✉)
T.J. Boffeli, D.P.M., F.A.C.F.A.S.
Institute for Education and Research, Regions Hospital/
HealthPartners, 640 Jackson St, St. Paul, MN 55101, USA
e-mail: ryan.r.pfannenstein@healthpartners.com;
troy.j.boffeli@healthpartners.com

S.B. Hyllengren, D.P.M.
Allina Health Cambridge Medical Center,
701 South Dellwood St, Cambridge, MN 55008, USA
e-mail: Shelby.b.hyllengren@gmail.com

© Springer International Publishing Switzerland 2015
T.J. Boffeli (ed.), *Osteomyelitis of the Foot and Ankle*, DOI 10.1007/978-3-319-18926-0_4

Case examples are included to demonstrate our patient selection criteria and surgical pearls for percutaneous trephine biopsy, open wound excision with corticotomy, joint arthroplasty with bone biopsy, and bone biopsy associated with partial foot amputation.

Is Bone Biopsy the "Gold Standard"?

A variety of diagnostic modalities exist for the identification of osteomyelitis, but the current standard remains a bone biopsy including histopathologic evaluation and culture. Recent controversy has challenged bone biopsy as the "reference standard." The reality is that no standardized definition exists for "bone biopsy," thus making it a target for review. In 2011, Meyr examined the statistical reliability of bone biopsy in diagnosing diabetes-related osteomyelitis of the foot by comparing the interpretation of bone specimens by four different board certified pathologists. The study found complete agreement among all pathologists in only 33 % (13/39) of the specimens. The researchers concluded that bone biopsy has a limited reliability in diagnosing diabetic foot osteomyelitis based on the histopathologic analysis of bone. They recommended that a combination of diagnostic information be used to guide definitive treatment decisions, rather than bone biopsy alone [11].

The overall clinical picture should always be considered when determining the appropriate treatment course including patient symptoms, physical exam findings, inflammatory marker labs, leukocytosis, and imaging results. For any disease, the ideal diagnostic test is 100 % sensitive (no false negatives) and 100 % specific (no false positives). Despite the significant medical and surgical advances that have been made in the evaluation and management of ulcers and osteomyelitis, bone biopsy, remains the most accurate method to make a diagnosis of osteomyelitis [7].

Laboratory tests including c-reactive protein (CRP), erythrocyte sedimentation rate (ESR), and white blood cell (WBC) count can be normal or near normal at initial clinical presentation of osteomyelitis. Lab tests primarily monitor disease progression and treatment rather than determining the diagnosis of osteomyelitis [13]. ESR and CRP are acute phase reactants (APR) that can increase in both acute and chronic inflammatory conditions and changes are not specific to infection. WBC values are often normal in diabetic patients despite the severity of infection and the sensitivity for diagnosis of osteomyelitis on an elevated WBC count is very low (14 %) [14]. When these labs are obtained in the early stages of treatment before suspicion for osteomyelitis arises, they can serve as a baseline value that should be compared to labs obtained when concern for infection increases. However, keep in mind these laboratory values lack specificity for

osteomyelitis. More information can be found in Chap. 2 on the clinical and laboratory diagnosis of osteomyelitis.

It is also important to remember that radiographs and MRI can be misleading and cannot necessarily distinguish between an inflammatory or infectious process. Also, imaging studies may lag behind initial onset of osteomyelitis, especially plain radiographs which can appear normal in the early stages of bone infection. Previous studies have shown that plain films have a sensitivity of 88 % in identifying osteomyelitis; however, the literature has mostly focused on the larger bones of the body, such as the pelvis or femur. A recent study that focused on the small bones of the foot found that plain films only have a diagnostic sensitivity and specificity of 50 % and 80 %, respectively, with a high risk of obtaining a false-negative result [7]. The amount of time that osteomyelitis has been present is also an important determinant of the reliability and sensitivity of radiographs. It is estimated that radiographic changes will not be visible until destruction of 40–60 % of the bone matrix has occurred, a process which can take 2–3 weeks. Therefore, plain films are highly unreliable when diagnosing osteomyelitis in its early presentation. Bone scintigraphy or bone scans using radiolabeled leukocytes have a documented 100 % sensitivity, but a low specificity (50 %) as they accumulate in sites of both infection and inflammation. There has also been a significant problem with false-positive results in radionuclide bone scanning [15]. Chapter 3 provides further discussion regarding diagnostic imaging of osteomyelitis. In summary, bone biopsy remains a useful component in the workup and diagnosis of osteomyelitis.

What Constitutes a Bone Biopsy?

Bone biopsy for suspected osteomyelitis typically refers to both microbiologic bone culture and histologic analysis. The microbiological portion identifies the causative organism(s) and helps guide antibiotic treatment, while the histological aspect determines the diagnosis of osteomyelitis. Our standard protocol includes aerobic and anaerobic culture as diabetic foot infections are commonly polymicrobial. A fungal or acid-fast culture can be added depending on the clinical situation. Fungal or mixed fungal-bacterial ulcer infections have a relatively low incidence (less than 5 %) and there is no indication for routine mycologic ulcer testing. However, this possibility should be considered in cases where the ulcer infection continues to progress despite standard antibacterial therapy and wound care, and in the chronically infected ulcer [16].

Bone biopsy can be performed using open or minimally invasive percutaneous techniques. Fluoroscopy may be used to guide the trephine position for minimally invasive biopsy procedures. An open biopsy requires a larger incision and can be done as an isolated procedure or as part of an open incision and drainage, joint arthroplasty, or amputation procedure [17].

Should Antibiotics be Held Prior to Bone Biopsy?

Under ideal circumstances, antibiotics should be discontinued a minimum of 48 h prior to bone biopsy [1, 18, 19]. However, holding antibiotics for several days is not always practical from a clinical standpoint. It is often counterproductive to withhold antimicrobial treatment in hospitalized patients with acute infection or in patients with escalating clinical symptoms despite current medical treatment. Biopsy is commonly part of a larger open procedure like amputation; therefore, it is desirable to maintain optimal condition of the surrounding soft tissues. Chronic infection or suspected infection without an open wound makes holding antibiotics more practical.

Kim retrospectively reviewed culture results in patients with vertebral osteomyelitis and found that prior antibiotic exposure of greater than 4 days duration was associated with negative culture results. Antibiotic use 1–3 days prior to culture was not statistically significant [20]. Similar results have been recreated with an overall negative culture rate from 40 to 60 % with biopsies performed after initiation of antibiotics [21]. Conversely, Wu studied 75 patients who underwent image-guided core biopsies for suspected osteomyelitis. Of the 41 patients with histologically confirmed osteomyelitis, 17 (41 %) had received antibiotics within 24 h before biopsy. They found that this factor did not have any significant association with positive or negative culture results ($p=0.23$). Although this difference was not statistically significant, they did detect a lower culture positivity rate in patients on antimicrobial therapy prior to biopsy versus patients off therapy. Therefore, they recommend discontinuing antibiotics at least 24 h before biopsy. They also concluded that other clinical factors including fever, elevated WBC count, elevated ESR, and histologic type of osteomyelitis (i.e., acute or chronic) did not have a significant correlation with obtaining positive or negative cultures [13].

How to Interpret Bone Biopsy Results

The degree to which bone biopsy provides a "definitive diagnosis" is debatable since clinical judgment is required when interpreting histopathologic findings and culture results. Many factors influence these results including potential contamination at the time of biopsy or laboratory handling, pre-biopsy antibiotic therapy, diagnostic criteria used by the pathologist, past infection in the area and location from where the biopsy was taken. For example, a negative biopsy of the first metatarsal head does not rule out infection in the proximal phalanx. Table 4.1 provides a guide to assist with diagnosis of osteomyelitis based on biopsy results and consideration of the entire clinical picture.

Bone Biopsy Techniques

Bone biopsy ranges from procurement of a bone specimen as part of an open incision and drainage or amputation procedure to an isolated percutaneous trephine technique. Needle biopsy has been shown to be a highly accurate method of diagnosing osteomyelitis, providing valid qualitative results with sensitivity and specificity rates above 70 % and 95 %, respectively [22, 23]. The trephine biopsy technique also has the advantage of being relatively noninvasive and inexpensive and can be performed at bedside or in the outpatient clinical setting. The larger bones of the rearfoot and ankle are more easily identifiable without the need for intraoperative imaging making bedside needle biopsy more practical.

Table 4.1 Interpreting bone biopsy results

	(+) Culture	(-) Culture
(+) Pathology	Osteomyelitis is present with coordinating positive culture results to identify causative organism.	This scenario may indicate chronic osteomyelitis without heavy bacterial load or may occur when antibiotics are not held prior to biopsy.
(-) Pathology	Contamination may have occurred from an adjacent open wound or when handling the specimen. If strong suspicion of osteomyelitis based on clinical and radiographic picture, consider repeat biopsy of adjacent bone or discuss diagnostic criteria with pathologist.	Reconsider clinical picture as non-infectious conditions mimic osteomyelitis including Charcot arthropathy, gout, fracture, etc.

Bone biopsy typically involves histopathologic evaluation and microbiologic culture. This two-tiered biopsy approach improves accuracy; however, the results are subjected to variable interpretation leading to clinical uncertainty. Diagnostic accuracy is improved by considering the entire clinical picture including exam findings, intraoperative observations, radiographic workup, bone culture, and histopathologic assessment

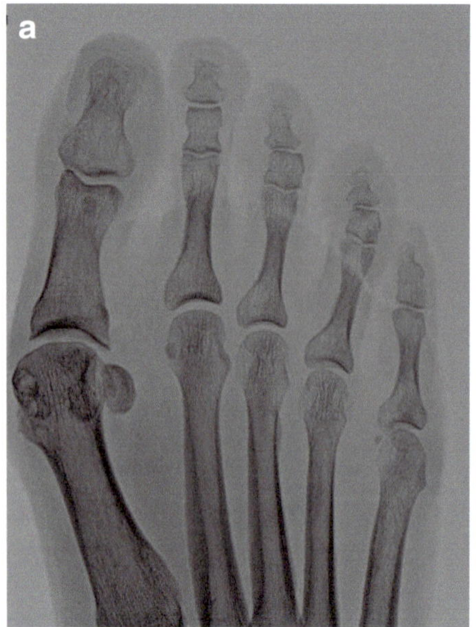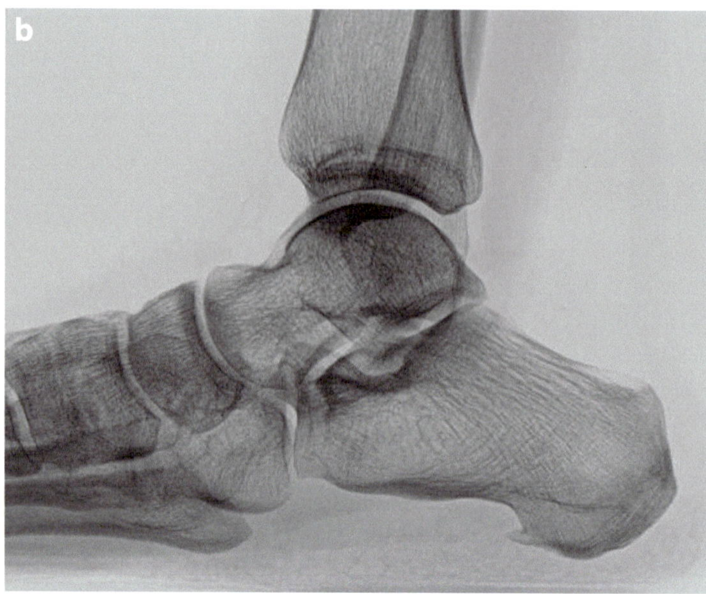

Fig. 4.1 Selection of the ideal bone biopsy technique. (**a**) The small bones of the forefoot are less amenable to percutaneous trephine biopsy and more amenable to open biopsy or wide resection. (**b**) The larger bones of the midfoot and rearfoot are less amenable to wide resection due to concerns about loss of structural integrity of the foot and more amenable to trephine techniques. Open biopsy is frequently the most practical approach for osteomyelitis associated with contiguous spread of infection from an adjacent wound since incision and drainage procedures are typically needed for wound-related infection. There is greater risk of cross contamination with open biopsy yet the location from where the specimen is extracted is more accurate with regard to the bone most likely to be infected

The smaller bones of the forefoot are less amenable to closed needle or trephine biopsy in part because it is difficult to obtain the biopsy without causing significant damage to the structure of the lesser (2–5) digital phalanges or even metatarsals. Ultimately, any bone in the foot could be accessed for a needle biopsy, but fluoroscopic guidance may be helpful to ensure correct bone identification (Fig. 4.1). There are risks associated with needle or trephine bone biopsy including pathologic fracture, joint damage, spreading or seeding bone infection, soft tissue damage, pain, bleeding, and nerve injury.

Open bone biopsy is typically performed in the operating room but clinic-based open biopsy is possible under certain circumstances such as digital infection and ulceration. Open biopsy may involve joint arthroplasty, cortical debridement of exposed bone after wound excision, or wide resection including partial foot amputation or partial calcanectomy. Biopsy is commonly performed at the time of the incision and drainage procedure and is often repeated for staged surgery. Repeat cultures are not necessary at revision surgery unless infection is not responding to current antibiotic therapy. The bone specimen is frequently taken from bone that would otherwise be discarded, as in the case of amputation or digital arthroplasty.

Trephine Bone Biopsy of the Small Bones of the Forefoot

While less practical for digits 2–5, trephine biopsy of the hallux and first metatarsal is common due to large bone structure with less likelihood of joint injury or pathologic fracture. An office or bedside protocol is demonstrated in Fig. 4.2. A medial midline approach is most practical to avoid the plantar weight bearing surface, the dorsal and plantar tendons, the nail or nail matrix, and neurovascular structures. Dorsal and plantar amputation flaps are also unaffected by this biopsy location.

Wound Excision and Open Corticotomy with Bone Biopsy

Wound infection with secondary contiguous spread of osteomyelitis to the prominent underlying bone is commonly treated with wound excision, decortication, bone biopsy, and remodeling of bone irregularity. A staged approach is common and flap surgery may be used to provide coverage of the exposed cancellous bone. This surgical protocol is detailed in Fig. 4.3.

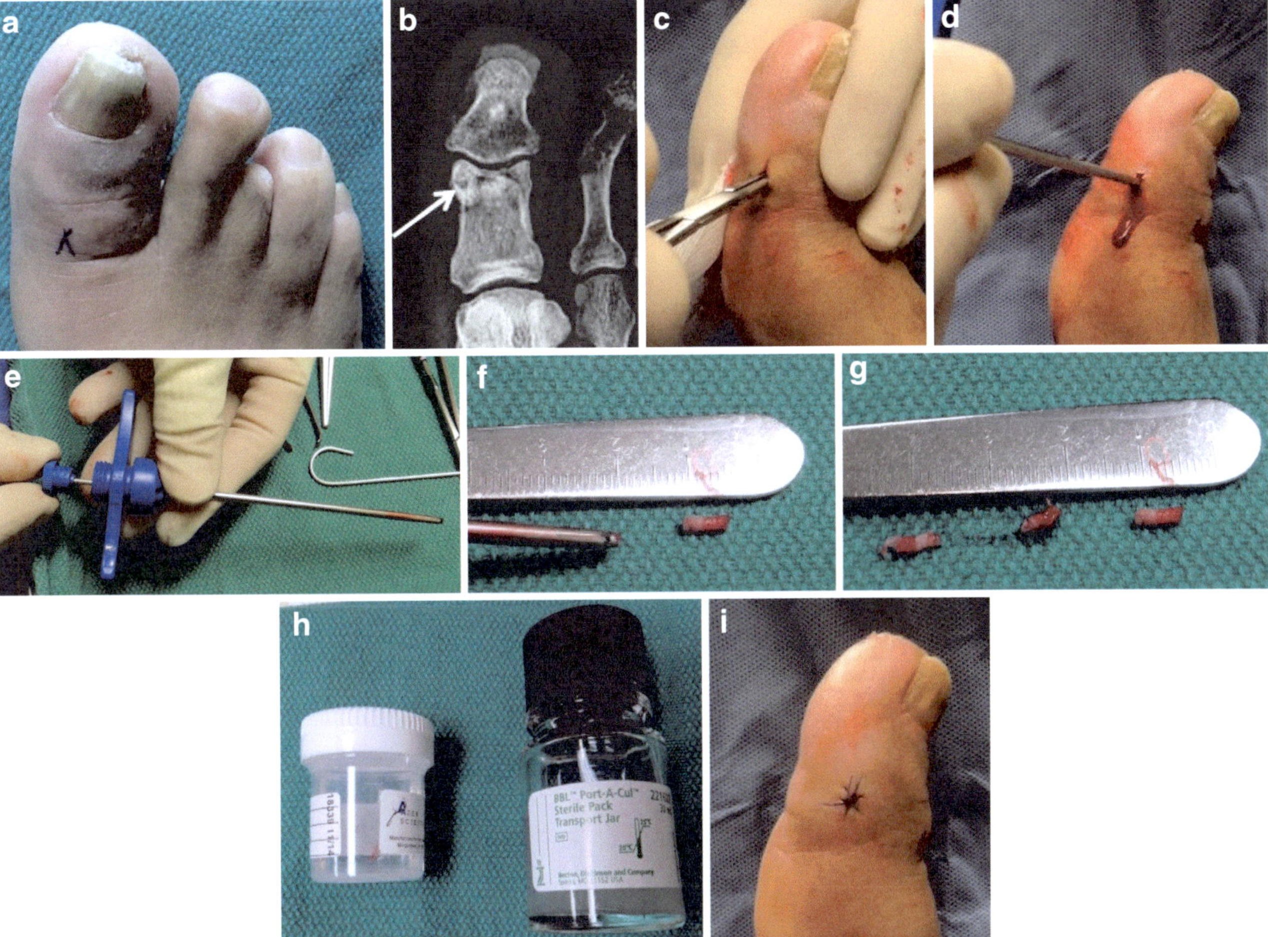

Fig. 4.2 Trephine bone biopsy of the hallux. (**a**, **b**) Bone biopsy was performed for clinical appearance of first toe infection with correlating suspicious radiographic changes (*arrow*). The phalanges of the first toe are large enough for small trephine biopsy although there is risk of pathologic fracture or joint damage with this technique. Bedside or office-based biopsy is possible and requires minimal instrumentation. A small stab incision was made directly over the desired area of biopsy. (**c**) Care was taken to avoid neurovascular structures along the medial side of the toe and midline incision is helpful from this regard. Blunt dissection down to the bone level was performed with a mosquito hemostat. (**d**) The trephine or biopsy needle was positioned against the medial cortex of the proximal phalanx. The trephine was then carefully advanced through the cortex and into the medullary canal. A slight "wobble" technique disengages the biopsy specimen from the surrounding bone and minimizes chance for pathologic fracture. (**e**, **f**) The plunger was then used to extract the bone graft from the trephine. (**g**) Several small specimens can be obtained through one cortical puncture. Direct inspection of the biopsy specimen confirmed a relatively normal bone appearance without intraosseous pus or necrosis. (**h**) A small specimen was placed in the culture jar and the remainder was placed in formalin for histopathologic evaluation. (**i**) A simple suture can be placed which minimizes bleeding and risk of postprocedure contamination

Joint Arthroplasty with Bone Biopsy

Inter-phalangeal and metatarsal phalangeal joint wounds complicated by osteomyelitis are typically associated with deformity including hammertoe contracture, bone spurs, and hallux valgus. Deformity is largely responsible for the non-healing wound and a biopsy is obtained through an open procedure. This approach, which is outlined in Fig. 4.4, allows for wound excision, drainage of joint infection, joint arthroplasty, deformity correction, bone biopsy, and possible wound closure. Digital procedures can be performed in the clinic and staged surgery is common with subsequent conversion to ray amputation depending on biopsy results and clinical response.

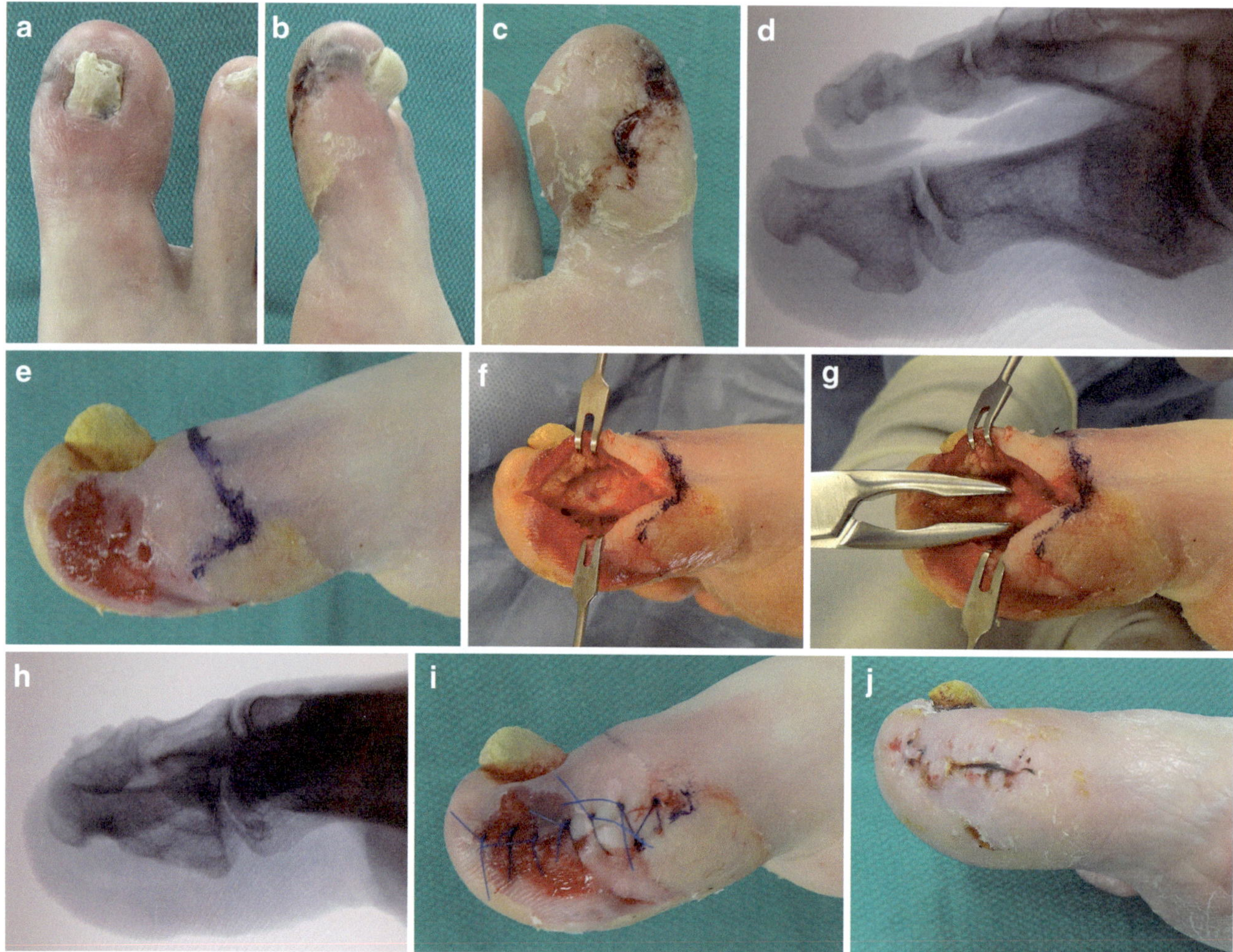

Fig. 4.3 Open resection biopsy of the hallux distal phalanx.(**a–d**) Local infection at the tip of the first toe combined with radiographic evidence of bone erosion within the distal phalanx raised concern for osteomyelitis. (**e, f**) Medial incision directly through the wound is not ideal for biopsy but allowed direct access for bone resection and biopsy. Note how the distal symes incision is drawn, which is the planned procedure if osteomyelitis is not resolved with biopsy and medical treatment. (**g**) A rongeur is used to take a nip of bone from the medial aspect of the distal phalanx. Prominent bone is oftentimes the nidus for recurrent ulceration which is also the bone most likely to develop osteomyelitis. (**h**) Bone biopsy that removes the source of the ulcer is ideal to allow wound healing and avoid wound recurrence. (**i, j**) Primary closure allows delayed revision surgery depending on clinical response and biopsy results

Partial Foot Amputation with Bone Biopsy

Partial foot amputation provides specimen for biopsy with the opportunity to attempt to achieve a clean margin. Procurement of bone from the area of infection is commonly performed on the back table away from the clean surgical site to avoid cross contamination. Additionally, clean margin biopsy is commonly taken. The surgical protocol is demonstrated in Fig. 4.5.

Trephine Bone Biopsy of the Large Bones of the Rearfoot or Ankle

The calcaneus is easily amenable to trephine biopsy with the lateral approach being most common to avoid the medial neurovascular structures. An in-office setup of this technique is shown in Fig. 4.6. The lateral approach also avoids biopsy through a plantar or posterior wound. Care is taken to biopsy close to the wound, yet avoid cross contamination. Trephine

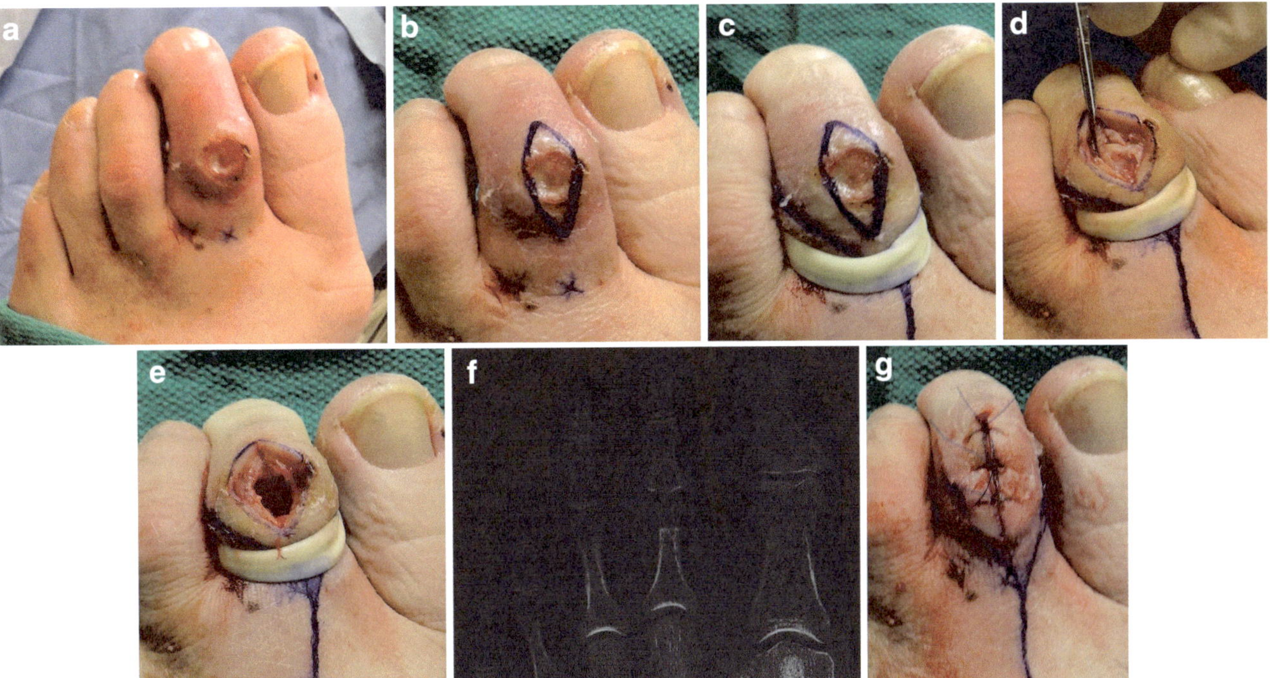

Fig. 4.4 Open biopsy of the second proximal interphalangeal joint. (**a**) Dorsal proximal interphalangeal joint (PIPJ) ulceration associated with hammertoe deformity commonly leads to osteomyelitis and joint infection. Trephine biopsy does not resolve the bone prominence and does not allow incision and drainage of the infection. (**b**) Open biopsy allows excision of the ulcer and access to the involved bone and joint. (**c**) An elastic drain tourniquet is used for office-based biopsy. Incisions are drawn here for planned toe amputation which may be required depending on clinical response and biopsy results. (**d**) Full depth excision of the wound and disarticulation of the PIPJ allows direct access for biopsy. (**e**, **f**) Resection of the head of the proximal phalanx allows biopsy as well as reduction of bone prominence and relaxation of contracture deformity. (**g**) Primary closure can be performed depending on the quality of the surrounding tissue and size of the wound defect

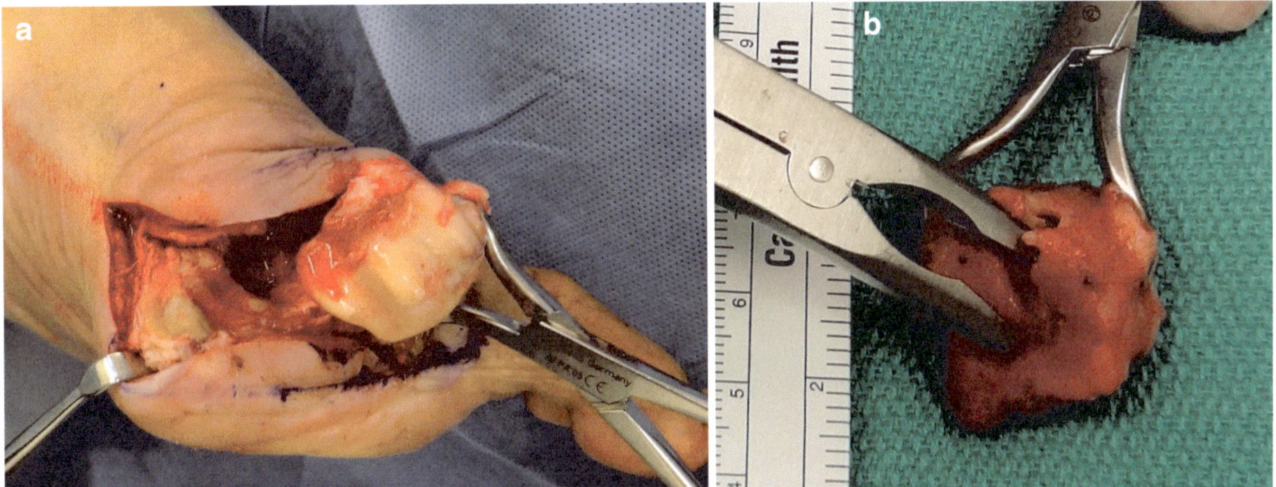

Fig. 4.5 Open resection biopsy of the first metatarsal head. (**a**) Resection of the first metatarsal head was performed as part of a first ray amputation procedure. Deep bone biopsy was taken on the back table to avoid cross contamination with the surgical wound. (**b**) A sterile rongeur was used to remove a section of bone for culture. The remainder of the first metatarsal head was placed in formalin for pathologic biopsy. The internal medullary canal of the residual first metatarsal shaft can also be biopsied with a curette for proximal margin biopsy

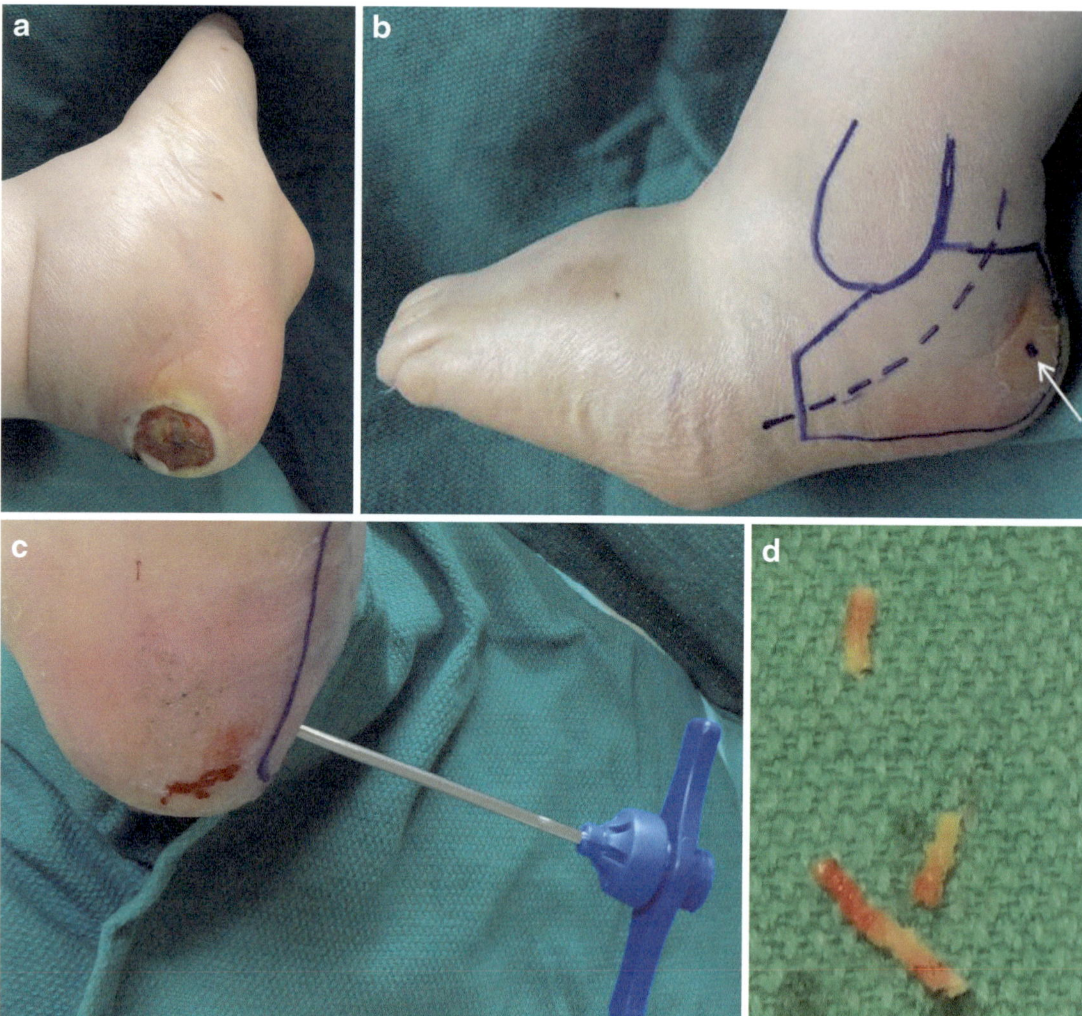

Fig. 4.6 Trephine biopsy of the calcaneus. (**a**) Posterior heel wound with suspected calcaneal osteomyelitis. Office-based trephine biopsy was taken through intact adjacent soft tissues lateral to the wound using a no-touch technique to avoid cross contamination from the chronic wound. (**b**) The outline of the calcaneus and distal fibula was drawn and the sural nerve is represented by the *dashed line*. The dot marks the biopsy site (*arrow*). (**c**) The trephine or biopsy needle was advanced through the cortex and into the cancellous bone after stab incision. Note that the biopsy was being taken deep to the wound in the area most likely to be infected. (**d**) The biopsy specimen was sectioned and processed for culture and pathologic examination

biopsy minimally impacts the structural integrity of the calcaneus and immediate weight bearing would rarely result in pathologic fracture. Post-biopsy radiographs are helpful to monitor healing progress. A bone biopsy can also be readily obtained after hardware removal if there is concern for infection utilizing a curette as shown in Fig. 4.7.

A similar approach is used for the fibula, distal tibia, and cuboid. The navicular, talus, and cuneiforms are smaller and less easily palpable making image-guided trephine biopsy more useful.

Conclusion

The diagnosis of osteomyelitis of the foot and ankle is ideally made by evaluating the entire clinical picture including local exam findings, relevant labs, imaging studies, and most importantly bone biopsy results. The diagnostic utility of bone biopsy is highly dependent on timing of biopsy in relation to antibiotic treatment, proper biopsy technique to avoid contamination from adjacent open wounds, and location of the biopsy

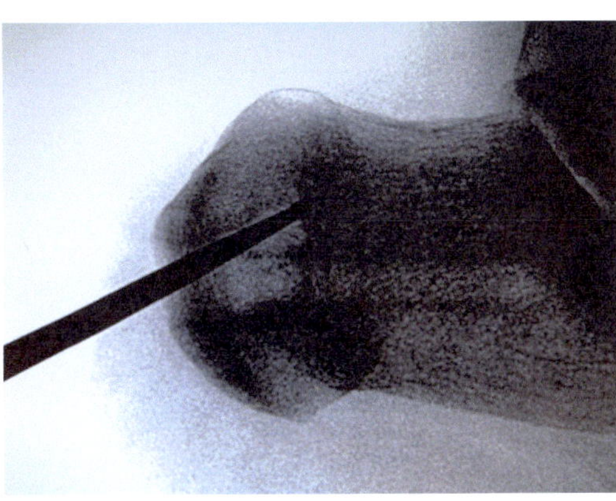

Fig. 4.7 Image-guided curettement of osteomyelitis. Osteomyelitis associated with hardware complication after calcaneal osteotomy. Debridement with a curette after screw removal allowed bone biopsy and resection of the nidus of infection

to ensure that a representative sample is obtained. A variety of biopsy techniques are available depending on location of infection in the foot or ankle, extent of local wounds, and need for amputation. Careful attention to established biopsy protocols helps to minimize the risk of harm to the patient using minimally invasive techniques where appropriate.

References

1. Senneville E, Melliez H, et al. Culture of percutaneous bone biopsy speciemens for diagnosis of diabetic foot osteomyelitis: concordance with ulcer swab cultures. Clin Infect Dis. 2006;42:57–62.
2. Brem H, Sheehan P, Rosenberg HJ, Schneider JS, Boulton AJM. Evidence-based protocol for diabetic foot ulcers. Plast Reconstr Surg. 2006;117:193s–209.
3. Lavery LA, Peters EJ, Armstrong DG, Wendel CS, Murdoch DP, Lipsky BA. Risk factors for developing osteomyelitis in patients with diabetic foot wounds. Diabetes Res Clin Pract. 2009;54: e132–66.
4. Kaldau NC, Brorson S, Jensen PE, Schultz C, Arpi M. Bilateral polymicrobial osteomyelitis with *Candida tropicalis* and *Candida krusei*: a case report and an updated literature review. Int J Infect Dis. 2012;16:e16–22.
5. Butalia S, Palda VA, Sargeant RJ, Detsky AS, Mourad O. Does this patient with diabetes have osteomyelitis of the lower extremity? JAMA. 2008;299:806–13.
6. Berendt AR, Peters EJG, et al. Diabetic foot osteomyelitis: a progress report on diagnosis and a systematic review of treatment. Diabetes Metab Res Rev. 2008;24:S145–61.
7. Larson DL, Gilstrap J, Simonelic K, Carrera GF. Is there a simple, definitive, and cost-effective Way to diagnose osteomyelitis in the pressure ulcer patient? Plast Reconstr Surg. 2011;126:670–6.
8. Prieto-Perez L, Perez-Tanoira R, Petkova-Saiz E, Perez-Jorge C, Lopez-Rodriquez C, Alvarez-Alvarez B, Polo-Sabau J, Esteban J. Osteomyelitis: a descriptive study. Clin Orthop Surg. 2014; 6:20–5.
9. Lavery LA, Armostrong D, Peter EJG, Lipsky BA. Probe-to-bone test for diagnosing diabetic foot osteomyelitis. Diabetes Care. 2007;30(2):270–4.
10. Grayson ML, Gibbons GW, Balogh K, Levin E, Karchmer AW. Probing to bone in infected pedal ulcers: a clinical sign of underlying osteomyelitis in diabetic patients. JAMA. 1995;273:721–3.
11. Meyr AJ, Singh S, Zhang X, Khilko N, Mukherjee A, Sheridan MJ, Khurana JS. Statistical reliability of bone biopsy for the diagnosis of diabetic foot osteomyelitis. J Foot Ankle Surg. 2011;50(6):663–7.
12. Atway S, Nerone VS, Springer KD, Woodruff DM. Rate of residual osteomyelitis after partial foot amputation in diabetic patients: a standardized method for evaluating bone margins with intraoperative culture. J Foot Ankle Surg. 2012;51:749–52.
13. Wu JS, Gorbachova T, Morrison WB, Haims AH. Imaging-guided bone biopsy for osteomyelitis: are there factors associated with positive or negative cultures? AJR Am J Roentgenol. 2007;188(6):1529–34.
14. Armstrong DG, Lvery LA, Sariaya M, Ashry H. Leukocytosis is a poor indicator of acute osteomyelitis of the foot in diabetes mellitus. J Foot Ankle Surg. 1996;35:280–3.
15. Lewis VL, Bailey MH, Pulawski G, Kind G, Bashioum RW, Hendrix RW. The diagnosis of osteomyelitis in patients with pressure sores. Plast Reconstr Surg. 1988;81:229–32.
16. Mlinaric-Missoni E, Kalenic S, Vukelic M, de Syo D, Belicza M, Vazic-Babic V. Candida infection of diabetic foot ulcers. Diabetol Croat. 2005;34:29–35.
17. Simon MA, Biermann JS. Biopsy of bone and soft-tissue lesions. J Bone Joint Surg. 1993;75:616–21.
18. Lipsky BA, Berendt AR, Cornia PB, Pile JC, Peters EJ, Armostrong DG, et al. Infectious diseases society of America clinical practice guideline for the diagnosis and treatment of diabetic foot infections. Clin Infect Dis. 2013;54:e132–73.
19. Witso E, Persen L, Loseth K, Bergh K. Adsorption and release of antibiotics from morselized cancellous bone. In vitro studies of 8 antibiotics. Acta Orthop Scand. 1999;70:298–304.
20. Kim CJ, Song SH, Park WB, Kim ES, Park SW, Kim HB, Oh MD, Kim NJ. Microbiologically and clinically diagnosed vertebral osteomyelitis: impact of prior antibiotic exposure. J Antimicrob Chemother. 2012;56:2122–4.
21. Marschall J, Bhavan KP, Olsen MA, Fraser VJ, Wright NM, Warren DK. The impact of prebiopsy antibiotics on pathogen recovery in hematogenous vertebral osteomyelitis. Clin Infect Dis. 2011;52: 867–72.
22. Fugere MC, Malluche HH. Comparison of different bone-biopsy techniques for qualitative and quantitative diagnosis of metabolic bone diseases. J Bone Joint Surg. 1983;65:1314–8.
23. Han H, Lewis VL, Wiedrich TA, Patel PK. The value of jamshidi core needle bone biopsy in predicting postoperative osteomyelitis in grade IV pressure ulcer patients. Plast Reconstr Surg. 2002;110:118–22.

Pathologic Diagnosis of Osteomyelitis

5

Suzanne B. Keel

As at other anatomic sites, the foot has four primary routes of contamination leading to osteomyelitis: (1) hematogenous, (2) contiguous spread, (3) direct implantation, and (4) post-operative infection [2]. Infections are common in diabetic patients. Uncontrolled diabetes leads to hyperglycemia, an impaired inflammatory response to pathogens, and tissue ischemia [8]. In the diabetic patient, contiguous spread from an infected chronic skin ulcer is the most common route of bone infection. The inflammatory process manifests itself as cellulitis of the soft tissues before reaching the periosteum and causing periostitis, or penetrating a joint capsule leading to septic arthritis. Involvement of the periosteum may damage the periosteal blood supply to the bone leading to cortical necrosis. Any irritation and lifting of the periosteum can cause reactive periosteal new bone formation. Once the inflammation breaches the periosteum to involve the underlying cortical bone, osteitis is present. Only when the medullary portion of the bone is involved by the inflammatory process is the term osteomyelitis appropriate.

Even in the days of Hippocrates (460–370 BC) bone infection was recognized. However it was not until much later when Pasteur pointed to microbes as responsible for causing "a boil of the bone marrow" [9]. By the mid-nineteenth century, the quality of the microscope was good enough to be useful in diagnosing disease [6]. The discovery of penicillin broadened the treatment options for osteomyelitis from just surgery alone. In this modern era, therapy for osteomyelitis is tailored to the individual patient. Antibiotic courses will differ and, fortunately, amputation is no longer a certain outcome. But regardless of therapy, successful treatment of osteomyelitis relies on early diagnosis.

Although clinical examination, probe to bone test, laboratory studies, and imaging studies are helpful in diagnosing osteomyelitis, the gold standard for a definitive diagnosis is a bone biopsy demonstrating the characteristic histologic features of osteomyelitis, coupled with a positive culture of the infected bone [3–5, 7, 10, 12, 13]. The biopsy should be taken from an abnormal area, either radiographically abnormal if there is no overlying skin abnormality, or an area deemed abnormal at the base of an ulcer. Bone biopsy samples obtained adjacent to the infected portion of bone may only demonstrate reactive changes, a clinically unhelpful pathologic diagnosis. Samples should be taken for culture as well as microscopic examination. In a single institution review of 39 cases of osteomyelitis by four pathologists, there was complete agreement on the histopathologic diagnosis of osteomyelitis by all four pathologists in only 33 % of cases, indicating microscopic examination alone may not be a reliable method to accurately diagnose osteomyelitis [15]. Culture of the bone increases the diagnostic accuracy of osteomyelitis and directs antibiotic therapy but may yield false negative results in the setting of prior antibiotic treatment [2, 11, 17, 18, 20].

In the patient with a chronic foot wound, the inflammation reaches the bone by direct extension from the ulcer. The inflammatory response to bacterial infection is predominantly neutrophilic and the cells gain access to the bone either by penetration of the periosteum or joint capsule [19] (Fig. 5.1). In their quest to eradicate the infecting pathogens, neutrophils produce cytokines, including interleukins and tissue necrosis factor, which damage the tissue and cause necrosis and edema [16]. The cellular response to infection is diminished when the vascular supply is damaged, as in the diabetic patient. Penetration of the periosteum by inflammation also compromises the blood supply to the bone, diminishing the cellular response to infection even more.

Bone is a dynamic organ. Normal, healthy bone is composed primarily of lamellar bone (Fig. 5.2). Osteoblasts lay down unmineralized osteoid in layers, or lamellae. Osteoblasts surrounded by bone are called osteocytes, and they reside within spaces called lacunae. The osteocytes communicate with each other via cytoplasmic processes called canaliculi. Osteoclasts are responsible for breaking

S.B. Keel, M.D. (✉)
Department of Pathology, Regions Hospital,
640 Jackson Street, St. Paul, MN 55101, USA
e-mail: Suzanne.b.keel@healthpartners.com

T.J. Boffeli (ed.), *Osteomyelitis of the Foot and Ankle*, DOI 10.1007/978-3-319-18926-0_5

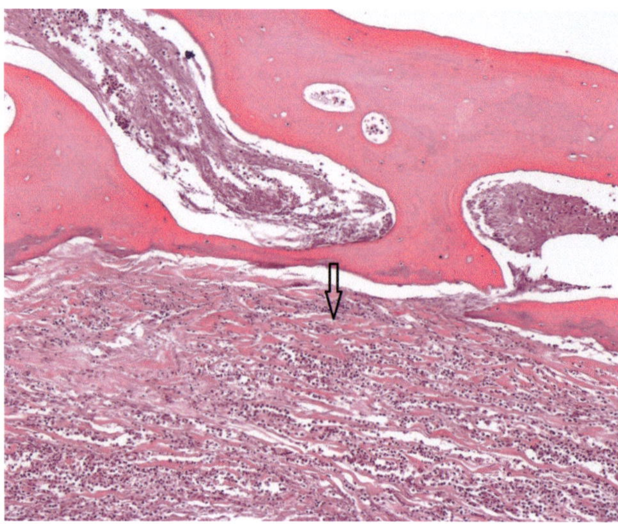

Fig. 5.1 Acute osteomyelitis: Neutrophils infiltrate through the fibrous periosteum (*arrow* on periosteum) and into the cortical bone

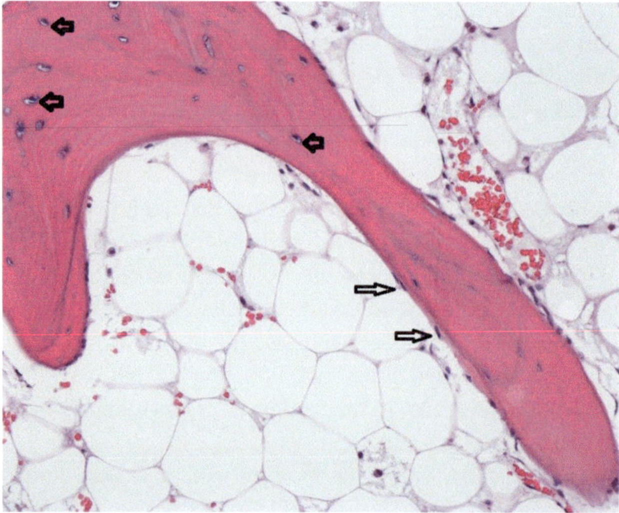

Fig. 5.2 Normal bone: Mature lamellar cancellous bone composed of layers of mineralized osteoid matrix. Inactive osteoblasts on the surface of the bone trabeculae (*long arrows*). Osteocytes within the bone matrix reside within lacunae (*short arrows*). The marrow space is filled with mature fat

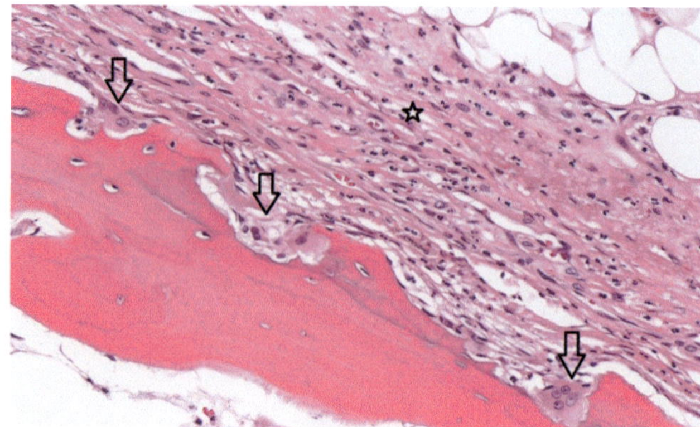

Fig. 5.3 Subperiosteal scalloping of cortex by activated osteoclasts (*arrow* osteoclasts). Neutrophils infiltrate the fibrous periosteum (*star*)

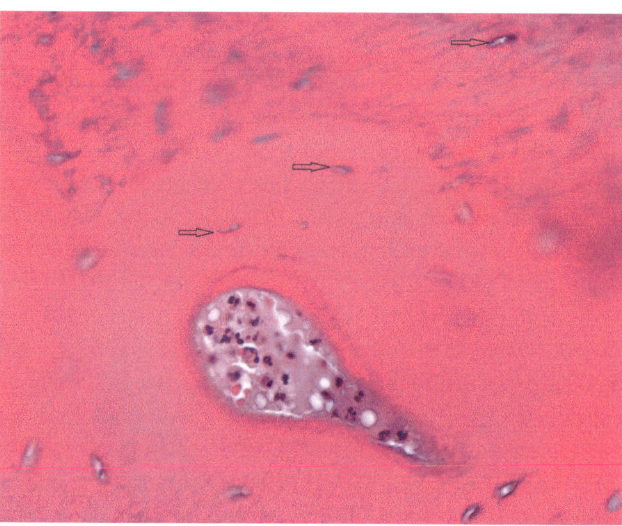

Fig. 5.4 Acute osteomyelitis: Neutrophils within a Haversian system of cortical lamellar bone. The bone is necrotic so most of the lacunae are void of osteocyte nuclei (*arrows*)

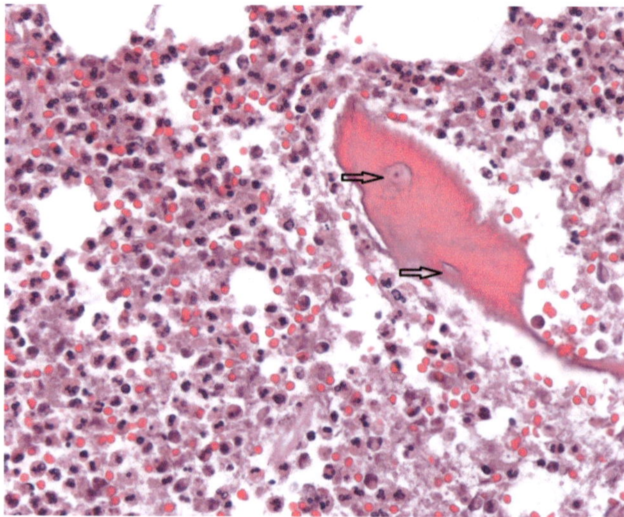

Fig. 5.5 Acute osteomyelitis: Necrotic trabecular bone surrounded by neutrophils. Note the absence of viable osteocyte nuclei within lacunae due to bone necrosis (*arrows*)

down the bone by a process of resorption. Together the osteocytes, osteoblasts, and osteoclasts remodel the bone in response to mechanical forces, calcium and phosphate levels, as well as other hormones and cytokines.

When an infection breeches the periosteum and reaches cortical bone, osteoclastic resorption occurs causing scalloping of the cortical surface (Fig. 5.3). Pathogens and neutrophils gain access to the medullary canal via Haversian systems in the cortical bone (Fig. 5.4) and the host response of osteoclastic bone resorption continues. Because a bone is virtually a closed system, the edema from the inflammatory response increases the intramedullary pressure, impairing the blood supply further. Microscopic bone necrosis is evident after approximately 48 h (Fig. 5.5) [19]. Left untreated or

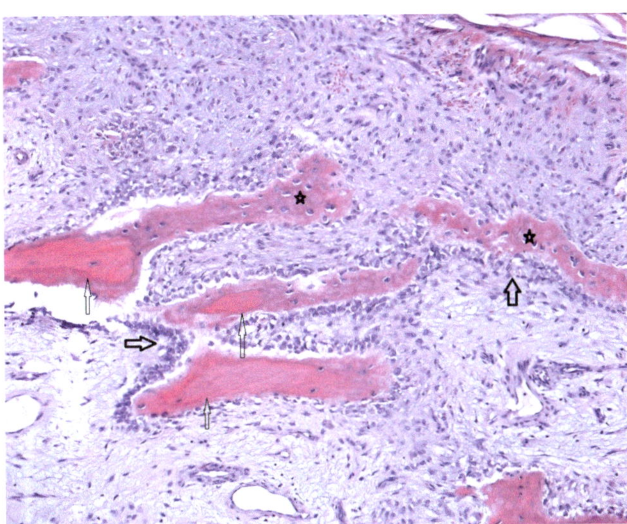

Fig. 5.6 Subperiosteal new woven bone with osteoblastic rimming may be produced in osteomyelitis and other conditions (*dark arrows* on activated osteoblasts). The woven bone (*stars*) is haphazardly arranged and lacks the lamellae, or lines, present in mature lamellar bone (*thin arrows* on lamellar bone)

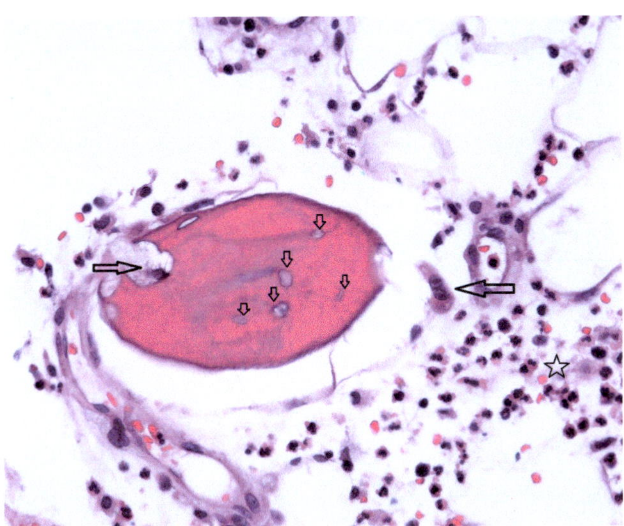

Fig. 5.7 Acute osteomyelitis: Necrotic bone with osteoclastic resorption (*long arrows*). The lacunae are devoid of osteocyte nuclei (*short arrows*). The marrow space contains abundant neutrophils (*star*)

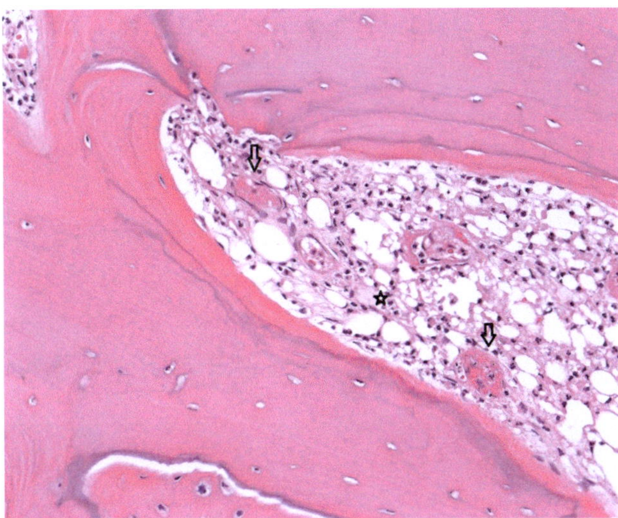

Fig. 5.8 Acute osteomyelitis: Intravascular thrombi within the marrow space composed of pink, granular fibrin (*arrows*). Abundant neutrophils fill the marrow space (*star*)

partially treated, the process becomes chronic and gross necrosis may become evident. The term sequestrum refers to an area of segmental osteonecrosis which has become separate from the adjacent viable bone and may be identifiable in imaging studies [16]. As bone necrosis continues, the inflammatory activity stimulates the production of osteoblastic new woven bone formation between the periosteum and cortex (Fig. 5.6), termed the involucrum, which encases the sequestrum and strengthens the bone in the damaged area, much like a fracture callus.

The key histologic features of acute osteomyelitis are neutrophils in close association with necrotic bone, and osteoclastic activity with bone scalloping. Bone necrosis is recognized by the absence of osteocytes within lacunae (Fig. 5.7). Other histologic features may also be present such as marrow edema, marrow necrosis, and intravascular thrombi (Fig. 5.8). As the inflammatory process continues, osteoblasts produce woven bone to rebutress trabeculae of necrotic lamellar bone in a reparative process referred to as creeping substitution. Septic arthritis is characterized by acute inflammation involving the joint capsule, synovium, or damaging the articular cartilage (Figs. 5.9 and 5.10).

Without effective therapy, between 5 and 25 % of acute osteomyelitis patients will develop chronic osteomyelitis [16]. Histologically, chronic osteomyelitis is characterized by necrotic bone as seen in acute osteomyelitis, with scalloping and creeping substitution, as well as marrow fibrosis and a plasma cell infiltrate (Figs. 5.11 and 5.12).

The pathologic findings of acute and chronic osteomyelitis are fairly straight forward and the diagnosis should be manageable with a good biopsy. One setting in which the diagnosis of acute osteomyelitis may be problematic is a patient who had a recent procedure at the same site. Postsurgical changes include trabecular disruption with bone necrosis and fibrinopurulent cellular response, similar to osteomyelitis (Fig. 5.13). The difference is that the postsurgical changes will be localized to the area adjacent to where the bone had been previously manipulated. Heterotopic ossification may enter the differential diagnosis of osteomyelitis clinically and/or radiographically. Histologically, heterotopic ossification may be woven bone early on, and after time may be indistinguishable from mature cortical and cancellous bone. Acute and chronic osteomyelitis may also involve heterotopic bone.

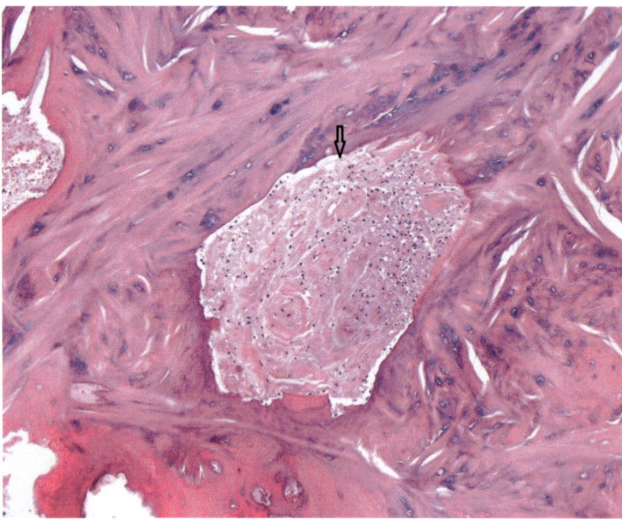

Fig. 5.9 Acute inflammation involving fibrocartilage of a tendon insertion site (*arrow neutrophils*)

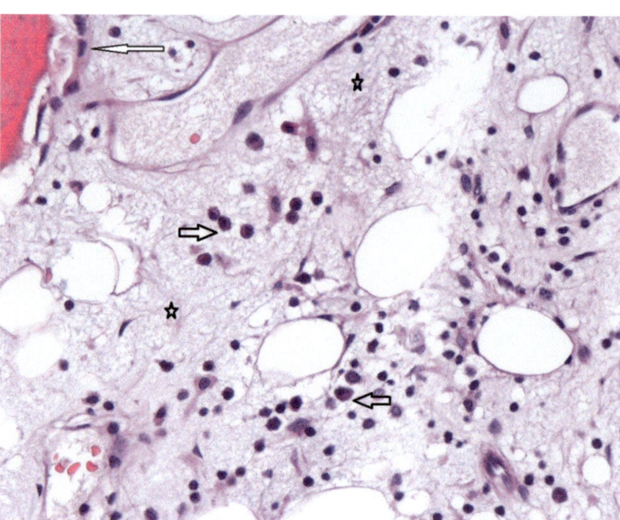

Fig. 5.12 Chronic osteomyelitis: The marrow space contains frothy appearing edema (*stars*) and plasma cells with eccentric nuclei (*fat arrows*). Activated osteoblasts produce new bone (*thin arrow*)

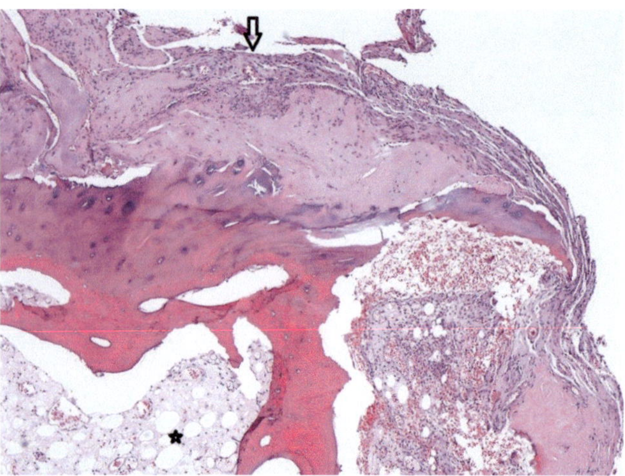

Fig. 5.10 Septic arthritis: Neutrophils destroy the articular hyaline cartilage in septic arthritis (*arrow* articular cartilage) (star marrow space)

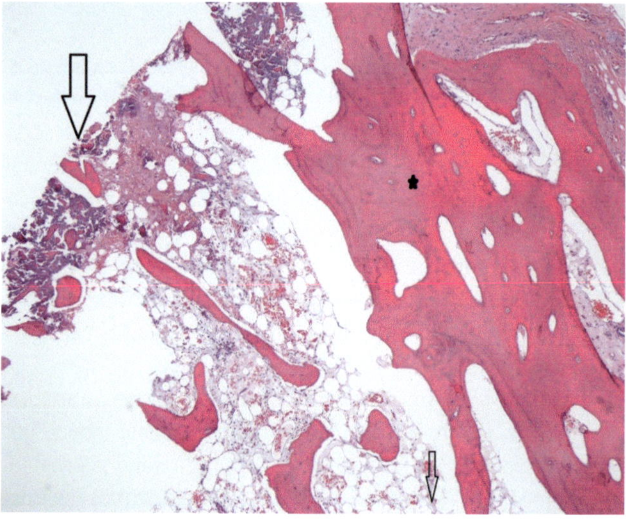

Fig. 5.13 Postsurgical site change with trabecular bone disruption, bone necrosis and fibrin and neutrophils combined at the margin (*large arrow*). Normal fatty marrow away from surgical margin (*small arrow*). The lamellar cortical bone appears healthy and not involved by inflammation or osteoclastic activity (*star*)

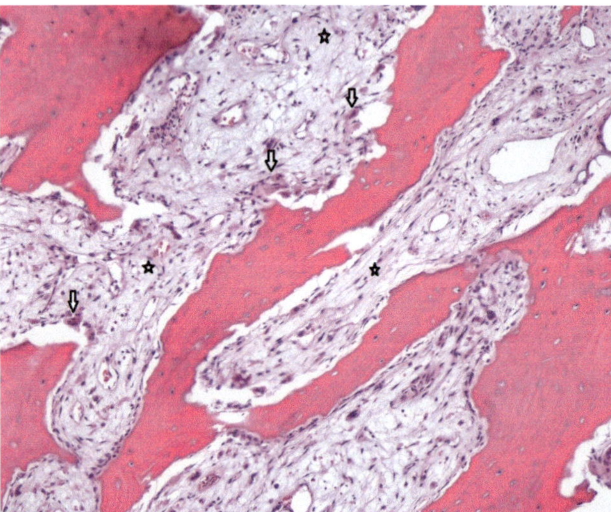

Fig. 5.11 Chronic osteomyelitis: Abundant osteoclastic activity (*arrows*), loss of osteocyte nuclei within lacunae, and the normal fatty marrow is replaced by fibrosis (*stars*)

Long-term complications of chronic osteomyelitis include sinus tract formation, pathologic fracture, and neoplasia [16]. Malignancy arising in chronic osteomyelitis of the foot is rare [1]. Squamous cell carcinoma is the most common malignancy associated with chronic osteomyelitis, but fibrosarcoma, myeloma, and lymphoma have all been reported [14]. Amputation is the treatment of choice for local control of malignancy.

References

1. Altay M, Arikan M, Yildiz Y, Saglik Y. Squamous cell carcinoma arising in chronic osteomyelitis in foot and ankle. Foot Ankle Int. 2004;25:805–9.
2. Calhoun JH, Manring MM. Adult osteomyelitis. Infect Dis Clin North Am. 2005;19:765–86.
3. Dinh T, Snyder G, Veves A. Current techniques to detect foot infection in diabetic patient. Int J Low Extrem Wounds. 2010;9:24–30.
4. Ertugrul MB, Baktiroglu S, Salman S, Unal S, Aksoy S, Berberoglu K, et al. The diagnosis of osteomyelitis of the foot in diabetes: microbiological examination vs. magnetic resonance imaging and labelled leucocyte scanning. Diabet Med. 2006;23:649–53.
5. Ertugrul BM, Savik O, Ozturk B, Cobanoglu M, Oncu S, Sakarya S. The diagnosis of diabetic foot osteomyelitis: examination findings and laboratory values. Med Sci Monit. 2009;15:CR307–12.
6. Fechner RE. The birth and evolution of American surgical pathology. In: Rosai J, editor. Guiding the surgeon's hand, the history of American surgical pathology. Washington, DC: American Registry of Pathology, Armed Forces Institute of Pathology; 1997. p. 7–21.
7. Fleischer AE, Didyk AA, Woods JB, Burns SE, Wrobel JS, Armstrong DG. Combined clinical and laboratory testing improves diagnostic accuracy for osteomyelitis in the diabetic foot. J Foot Ankle Surg. 2009;48:39–46.
8. Frykberg RG, Zgonis T, Armstrong DG, Driver VR, Giurini JM, Kravitz SR, et al. Diabetic foot disorders: a clinical practice guideline. J Foot Ankle Surg. 2006;45:S1–66.
9. Klenerman L. A history of osteomyelitis from the Journal of Bone and Joint Surgery: 1948–2006. J Bone Joint Surg Br. 2007;89(5):667–70.
10. Lavery L, Armstrong DG, Peters EJG, Lipsky BA. Probe-to-bone test for diagnosing diabetic foot osteomyelitis. Diabetes Care. 2007;30:270–4.
11. Lipsky BA. Osteomyelitis of the foot in diabetic patients. Clin Infect Dis. 1997;25:1318–26.
12. Lipsky BA, Berendt AR, Deery HG, Embil JM, Joseph WS, Karchmer AW, et al. Diagnosis and treatment of diabetic foot infections. Clin Infect Dis. 2004;39:885–910.
13. Lozano RM, Fernandez ML, Hernandez DM, Montesinos JV, Jimenez SG, et al. Validating the probe-to-bone test and other tests for diagnosing chronic osteomyelitis in the diabetic foot. Diabetes Care. 2010;33:2140–5.
14. McGrory JE, Pritchard DJ, Unni KK, Ilstrup D, Rowland CM. Malignant lesions arising in chronic osteomyelitis. Clin Orthop Relat Res. 1999;362:181–9.
15. Meyer AJ, Singh S, Zhang X, Khilko N, Mukherjee A, Sheridan MJ, et al. Statistical reliability of bone biopsy for the diagnosis of diabetic foot osteomyelitis. J Foot Ankle Surg. 2011;50:663–7.
16. Rosenberg AR. Bones, joints, and soft tissue tumors. In: Kumar V, Abbas AK, Fausto N, Aster JC, editors. Robbins and cotran pathologic basis of disease. Philadelphia: Saunders Elsevier; 2010. p. 1221–3.
17. Senneville E, Melieze H, Beltrand E, Legout L, Valette M, Cazaubiel M, et al. Culture of percutaneous bone biopsy specimens for diagnosis of diabetic foot osteomyelitis: concordance with ulcer swab cultures. Clin Infect Dis. 2005;42:57–62.
18. Shank CF, Feibel JB. Osteomyelitis in the diabetic foot: diagnosis and management. Foot Ankle Clin North Am. 2006;11:775–89.
19. Vigorita VJ. Osteomyelitis and septic arthritis. In: Vigorita VJ, editor. Orthopaedic pathology. Philadelphia: Lippincott Williams & Wilkins; 2008. p. 220–64.
20. Weiner RD, Viselli SJ, Fulkert KA, Accetta P. Histology versus microbiology for accuracy in identification of osteomyelitis in the diabetic foot. J Foot Ankle Surg. 2011;50:197–200.

Chris A. Manu, David B. Banach, Peter A. Blume,
Baver E. Sumpio, and Michael E. Edmonds

The underlying principle behind medical treatment is to administer antibiotics while providing a local environment that enhances antibiotic efficacy [1]. This approach requires an accurate and prompt diagnosis and optimization of host defences, which should be carried out within a multidisciplinary team approach. Bone infection in the foot and ankle most commonly arises from contiguous soft tissue infection via a skin wound and rarely from direct inoculation of offending pathogen into bone. Patients with diabetes form a significant proportion of the cohort with foot and ankle osteomyelitis. Peripheral arterial disease, neuropathy, and nephropathy are major comorbidities associated with diabetes, and all increase the risk of foot ulceration and osteomyelitis. It is estimated that 15 % of patients with diabetes will develop an ulcer in their lifetime due to neuropathy [2]. Patients with diabetes are at an 80 % increased risk of cellulitis, a fourfold increased risk of osteomyelitis, and a twofold risk of both sepsis and death caused by infection [3]. The prevalence of diabetes is estimated to increase by 165 % between 2001 and 2050 [4]. Osteomyelitis is present in approximately 20 % of cases of diabetic foot infection [5, 6]. Osteomyelitis of the foot and ankle is therefore a significant concern in patients with diabetes, and greatly increases the likelihood that the patient will require a lower-extremity amputation [7, 8]. Medical management can therefore be discussed in three main parts: indications for medical management, antibiotic therapy, and adjunctive therapies.

Indications for Medical Management

It is important to have a clear awareness of the role of medical management of osteomyelitis of the foot and ankle. Advantages and disadvantages are shown in Table 6.1. The decision is ideally reached through a multidisciplinary team approach [9]. Recent studies have shown that antibiotics alone may apparently eliminate bone infection in many cases [10]. There is also evidence that early amputation of infected digits may be non-curative in that remnants of infected bone may be left after surgical treatment [11]. To assist with the dilemma over the choice of medical or surgical treatment, the Infectious Disease Society of America (IDSA) in its 2012 guidelines of the management of diabetic foot infections [12] proposed four situations in which nonsurgical management of osteomyelitis might be considered:

1. When infection is confined to the forefoot, and there is minimal soft tissue loss.
2. When the patient has limb ischemia caused by unreconstructable vascular disease but wishes to avoid amputation.
3. When there is no acceptable surgical target (i.e., radical cure of the infection would cause unacceptable loss of function).
4. When the patient and healthcare professional agree that surgical management carries excessive risk or is otherwise not appropriate or desirable.

Classification of osteomyelitis may be of some value in determining the indication for medical treatment as well as its

C.A. Manu, M.B.B.S., B.Sc., M.R.C.P.
Diabetic Foot Clinic, Department of Diabetics,
Kings College Hospital, London, SE59RS, UK
e-mail: chris.manu@nhs.net

D.B. Banach, M.D., M.P.H., M.S.
Section of Infectious Diseases, Yale School of Medicine,
8 Twinbrook Dr, Woodbridge, CT 06525, USA

P.A. Blume, D.P.M., F.A.C.F.A.S.
Professor of Surgery, Surgery Orthopedics and Rehabilitation
Anesthesia, Yale New Haven Hospital,
508 Blake St, New Haven, CT 06545, USA
e-mail: peterib@snet.net

B.E. Sumpio, M.D. • M.E. Edmonds, M.D. (⊠)
Diabetic Foot Clinic, Department of Diabetics, Kings College
Hospital, London, SE59RS, UK

Professor of Surgery, Surgery Orthopedics and Rehabilitation
Anesthesia, Yale New Haven Hospital, 508 Blake St.,
New Haven, CT 06545, USA
e-mail: baver.sumpio@yale.edu; michael.edmonds@nhs.net

© Springer International Publishing Switzerland 2015
T.J. Boffeli (ed.), *Osteomyelitis of the Foot and Ankle*, DOI 10.1007/978-3-319-18926-0_6

Table 6.1 Advantages and disadvantages of medical management of osteomyelitis

Advantages	Disadvantages
Avoids surgical procedure	Increases risk of infection recurrence
Potentially avoids hospitalization	Risk of re-ulceration if uncorrected foot deformity
Preserves more of foot	Antibiotic-related toxicities
May shorten duration of hospitalization	Risk of developing antibiotic resistance
	Risk of *Clostridium difficile* disease

Antibiotic treatment for osteomyelitis is associated with moderate or severe adverse events in 4.8 % of patients treated with oral antibiotics and 15.5 % patients treated with parenteral antibiotics [12, 46]

possible prognosis. Although several classifications of osteomyelitis have been advocated, none is universally accepted. With regard to the foot and ankle, the Cierny-Mader staging and classification system categorizes the disease according to the extent of anatomical involvement and host physiological factors [13]. The Waldvogel classification system incorporates the mechanism of infection (hematogenous or contiguous) and the presence of vascular insufficiency [14]. However, a classification system, according to the duration of disease seems more relevant with regard to clinical management of foot and ankle osteomyelitis. This allows division of osteomyelitis into acute or chronic and is generally distinguished according to the duration of the symptoms of infection (i.e., < or >2 weeks, respectively) although this definition is arbitrary [15].

Acute osteomyelitis develops within 2 weeks and is characterized by infection presenting with small vessel thrombosis, vascular congestion, and oedema. In the diabetic foot, this occurs with rapid onset and is accompanied by severe soft tissue infection leading to an acute osteomyelitis, needing immediate antibiotic treatment and urgent surgical debridement.

Chronic osteomyelitis is an infection of bone which usually occurs by contiguous spread and has been present for several weeks [16]. There may be associated soft tissue infection. Occasionally, it may take months or possibly years to develop and is often characterized by the presence of necrosis on bone histology, new bone formation, and drainage or sinus tracts [16]. Since this finding may be present early during the natural history of the disease, its role in the classification into acute versus chronic by duration of disease is uncertain. Indeed, many reported studies do not use an osteomyelitis classification system. In others, the most commonly used classification was simply "acute" versus "chronic." Unfortunately, most authors do not provide definitions of acute and chronic osteomyelitis and when given, the threshold between acute and chronic ranges from 20 days to 6 months making interpretation of published literature difficult.

One specific entity of osteomyelitis is bone infection in the foot and ankle associated with a prosthesis. Some bacteria associated with prosthesis infections such as *S. epidermidis*, adhere to a biofilm that protects the organism from phagocytosis and impedes delivery of the antibiotic.

Antibiotic Therapy

Introduction

The mainstay of medical management of osteomyelitis is prompt and appropriate antibiotic therapy. Studies have shown that antibiotics alone may eliminate bone infection in many cases [9]. Antibiotic therapy should ideally target the pathogen(s) with a narrow spectrum when feasible, utilizing bone culture results when possible [17].

The initial antibiotic regimen should treat the likely causative pathogen, with few adverse effects. Treatment may be modified once the organism is identified. Parenteral and oral antibiotics may be used alone or in combination depending on microorganism sensitivity and patient compliance. There are many factors that affect treatment choices, such as antibiotic bone penetration, method of administration, and duration of therapy. Systematic reviews have demonstrated the lack of evidence supporting specific antibiotics for diabetic foot osteomyelitis [18], and no antibiotic has shown superiority in the eradication of osteomyelitis. The clinical outcome was better for acute than chronic osteomyelitis in 8 of the 12 studies which allowed comparison and few statistically significant differences were observed between the tested treatments [19].

Choice of Antibiotics

There are many factors that may affect treatment choices, such as spectrum of antimicrobial activity, antibiotic bone penetration, method of administration, and duration of therapy. The choice of antimicrobial therapy is now complicated by the increasing prevalence of antibiotic-resistant organisms, including methicillin-resistant *Staphylococcus aureus* (MRSA) and multidrug-resistant gram-negative pathogens. Systematic reviews have demonstrated the poor evidence base for making any specific recommendation on antibiotic therapy for diabetic foot osteomyelitis [20–22].

Overall, antibiotic treatment of acute and chronic osteomyelitis should be considered as two distinct entities with regard to the choice of the most appropriate antibiotics and the need for surgery. Antibiotic treatment can be further divided into empirical and targeted treatment. Empirical therapy is necessary when initially treating an infection and when it is not possible to isolate causative organisms from the infection site. Targeted therapy is making an antibiotic choice which is tailored to the organisms isolated from cultures preferably obtained from infected bone. Empirical and targeted therapy will be considered for both acute and chronic osteomyelitis.

Acute Osteomyelitis: Empirical Therapy

Empirical antibiotic therapy should treat the pathogens that are expected according to the severity of infection and the patient's medical history. In acute infection, it is essential to start antibiotic treatment immediately, and as early as possible in the infectious process, and in this setting empirical antibiotic therapy should be prescribed while waiting for the culture results [23]. In acute osteomyelitis, *S. aureus* and β-hemolytic streptococci are the leading organisms, but enterobacteriaceae can also be involved. In acute osteomyelitis, infections should be assumed to be polymicrobial, and include mixtures of aerobic and anaerobic organisms [24, 25]. Antibiotics with activity predominantly against gram-positive organisms (staphylococci and streptococci) [24] and broad-spectrum antibiotics with increased activity against gram-negative organisms and obligate anaerobes [26] appear equally effective. Initial empiric regimens may need to include multiple antibiotics with activity against different classes of pathogens [24]. It is still not clear if antibiotic therapy should be selected based on the sensitivities of all isolated organisms or only those judged most likely to be pathogenic.

There is controversy regarding the choice of specific antibiotics. A recent systematic review demonstrated the poor evidence base for making any recommendation on antibiotic therapy for diabetic foot osteomyelitis [18]. There is no specific evidence for superiority of any specific antibiotic agent or treatment strategy, route, or duration of therapy. Some authorities advise broad-spectrum antibiotic therapy to treat as many as possible of the likely organisms that can cause osteomyelitis including gram-positive, gram-negative, and anaerobic organisms. Use of broad-spectrum agents such as ampicillin-sulbactam, piperacillin-tazobactam, or a carbapenem will provide empiric activity against most potential aerobic and anaerobic pathogens. β-lactams are the best-suited agents for the treatment of acute bacterial osteomyelitis given their intense bactericidal activity and bone concentration β-Lactam antibiotics (penicillins, cephalosporins, and carbapenems) penetrate bone at levels ranging from ~5 to 20 % of those in serum [19]. However, because serum levels of parenterally delivered β-lactam antibiotics are so high, absolute bone levels are likely to exceed target minimum inhibitory concentrations of causative bacteria in most cases. β-lactam penetration is higher in infected than in uninfected bone [25]. The main limitation of antibiotic therapy in these situations is the size of the infecting inoculum that may reduce its efficacy and may favor the selection of resistance. A rapid decrease in the size of the inoculum is essential to prevent development toward a chronic stage of osteomyelitis. Surgical debridement is the most effective way to rapidly and efficiently reduce the inoculum especially in cases of abscesses and wet gangrene which contain very large infecting inoculums [23].

Table 6.2 Summary of factors influencing the choice of antibiotics

Scenarios	Antibiotic choice
Empirical treatment	Need to treat gram-positive organisms, including *S. aureus*
Known isolate	Guided by sensitivities from cultures
Polymicrobial or non-hospital acquired	Consider need to treat gram-negative organisms, including pseudomonas, and anaerobes
Hospital acquired infections	Consider the need to treat multidrug-resistant organisms, including methicillin-resistant *Staphylocccus aureus*
Previous treatment with antibiotics	Consider need to treat multi-resistant organisms
Foot or ankle with prosthesis	Consider inclusion of rifampicin when appropriate

The choice of antimicrobial therapy is complicated by the increasing prevalence of antibiotic-resistant organisms, especially MRSA, and vancomycin may be included as initial empiric therapy. Among the most recently available antibiotics, ertapenem and daptomycin are promising agents for the outpatient treatment of osteomyelitis due to antibiotic-resistant organisms. Addition of adjunctive rifampicin to other antibiotics may improve cure rates. Examples of scenarios influencing antibiotic choice are given in Table 6.2.

Empirical Antibiotics for Acute Osteomyelitis

Dosages are suggested but may need adjustment according to clinical state
- Piperacillin-tazobactam 3.375 g IV q6h
- Ampicillin-sulbactam 3 g IV q6h
- Ticarcillin-clavulanate 3.1 g IV q6h
- If multidrug-resistant gram-negative enterobacteriaceae is suspected:
  - Ertapenem 1 g IV q24h
- Patients with penicillin allergy and osteomyelitis
  - Clindamycin 600 mg IV q6h or 450 mg PO q6h or metronidazole 500 mg IV q8h or 400 mg PO q8h plus ciprofloxacin 750 mg PO or 400 mg IV q12h or levofloxacin 750 mg IV/PO daily, or moxifoxacin 400 mg IV/PO daily
- If MRSA is suspected and if MRSA screen positive
  - Add vancomycin 15 mg/kg IV q12h
  - If a contraindication exists to the use of vancomycin, an alternative anti-MRSA agent such as linezolid, daptomycin, or ceftaroline may be used

Acute Osteomyelitis: Targeted Therapy

After empirical parenteral therapy, targeted therapy, dependent on culture results, should be initiated intravenously, with eventual transfer to oral therapy. The recent IDSA guidelines recommend a short duration (2–5 days) when a radical resection leaves no remaining infected tissue, and a prolonged treatment (>4 weeks) when there is persistent infected and/or necrotic bone [12]. If there is a need to continue intravenous antibiotics, ceftriaxone and ertapenem are useful for prolonged courses of outpatient antibiotic therapy based on convenient once daily dosing.

Oral Therapy Following Intravenous Treatment for Patients with Acute Osteomyelitis

- Ciprofloxacin 750 mg PO q12h plus clindamycin 300–450 mg PO q6h or
- Levofloxacin 750 mg PO daily plus clindamycin 300–450 mg PO q6h or
- Moxifloxacin 400 mg PO daily

Chronic Osteomyelitis: Empirical Therapy

In nonrandomized studies of adults with chronic osteomyelitis, 4–6 weeks of parenteral β-lactam antibiotic therapy cures 60–90 % of cases. The varying cure rates may be related to variable diagnostic criteria, use of concomitant surgical debridement notably reported in only two studies [26, 27], or duration of follow-up. In multiple studies, the cure rates of infections caused by Pseudomonas were lower than those for other pathogens [28, 29]. Vancomycin achieves low cure rates for chronic osteomyelitis [30]. In patients receiving outpatient parenteral antibiotic therapy of osteomyelitis, treatment of *S. aureus* infection with vancomycin (compared with β-lactam agents) had an odds ratio (OR) for recurrence of 2.5 by multivariate analysis [31, 32]. Other independent risk factors for recurrence were diabetes mellitus (OR, 1.9), peripheral arterial disease (OR, 7.9), and infection with Pseudomonas (OR, 2.2). Antibiotics with high propensity to select resistance within the infecting population (e.g., rifampicin, fluoroquinolones, fusidic acid, fosfomycin) should not be used empirically in monotherapy, especially at the start of treatment as the inoculum size is the largest [23].

In most cases, the antibiotic therapy of chronic osteomyelitis is less urgent compared with acute osteomyelitis. The aim of the antibiotic therapy of chronic osteomyelitis is to complete the microbial eradication that depends, for the most part, on the efficacy of surgical debridement. Antibiotics with activity on stationary phase growth, intracellular and biofilm diffusion may play a major role in the eradication of the latent bacteria responsible for chronic osteomyelitis. Thus, despite the limitations of clinical and experimental studies, rifampicin may have a role in the treatment of staphylococcal chronic osteomyelitis as has ciprofloxacin in the treatment of gram-negative chronic osteomyelitis and levofloxacin for staphylococcal osteomyelitis.

A retrospective cohort study over 6 years treated diabetic forefoot ulcers with underlying osteomyelitis with empirical antibiotic therapy targeting *S. aureus* and β-haemolytic streptococci, the most common organisms involved [33]. Co-amoxiclav was chosen as the first-line treatment because of its good oral bioavailability and bone penetration. Treatment was monitored with MRI and if there was no change in the associated bone signal on MRI, the antibiotics were continued for a further 3-month cycle with repeat MRI. This treatment achieved high rates of healing and low rates of amputation.

Chronic Osteomyelitis: Targeted Therapy

After starting initial empiric therapy, good microbiologic data are critical in developing a further antibiotic treatment plan in chronic osteomyelitis. Antibiotic therapy directed by culture of bone (as compared with empiric therapy) was associated with a significantly higher rate of resolution of the bone infection without surgery after a mean of 12 months' follow-up [34]. It is still not clear if antibiotic therapy should be based on the sensitivities of all isolated organisms or against those judged, most likely to be pathogenic. Antibiotics may be less effective in treating areas of necrotic bone. Also antibiotic delivery is limited where biofilm formation reduces penetration of antibiotics to the infective focus. Thus the standard surgical practice has been to remove infected and necrotic bone in chronic osteomyelitis. However, in some cases, successful treatment of diabetic foot osteomyelitis can be achieved with antibiotic therapy alone [35].

Oral Therapy in Targeted Treatment of Chronic Osteomyelitis

Penetration of antibiotics into bone has been extensively assessed using different methods for sample preparation, drug analysis, and data handling. The published data show substantial variability in the reported mean bone penetration between drugs and between different studies of the same drug. Landersdorfer et al. conducted a systematic literature research of published articles on bone penetration of antibiotics [36]. Mean bone to serum concentration ratios range from 0.3 to 1.2 for quinolones, macrolides, and linezolid, from 0.15 to 0.3 for cephalosporins and glycopeptides, and from 0.1 to 0.3 for penicillins. For the majority of antibiotics studied, the ratios were higher for cancellous bone than for cortical bone and for lipophilic versus hydrophilic antibiotics [36]. Satisfactory bone concentrations of a given antibiotic, and low minimal inhibitory concentrations (MICs) against the offending pathogens routinely assessed at the microbiology laboratory, do not guarantee a satisfactory result in chronic osteomyelitis [23]. A subpopulation of bacteria in a slow-growth phase (the so-called small colony variants) is capable of penetrating cells and surviving intracellularly [37]. These bacteria are insensitive to those antibiotics which are only active on replicating microorganisms (e.g., β-lactams and glycopeptides) and those without intracellular diffusion. After antibiotic treatment, bacteria in latency can return to a logarithmic growth phase, which may partially explain why chronic osteomyelitis may relapse. Bacteria identified in these relapsing infections retain the same antibiotic susceptibility profile as the original strains [38]. Other orally available agents to which many community-associated strains of methicillin-resistant *Staphylococcus aureus* (MRSA) are usually susceptible are doxycycline and clindamycin. Doxycycline penetrates, and discolors, teeth and bone, but concentrations range from as low as 2 % in axial skeletal bone [39] to as high as 86 % in mandibular bone [40]. Clindamycin penetrates bone at levels of approximately 40–70 % of serum, and its bone levels should exceed the MICs of susceptible MRSA isolates. Fluoroquinolones, linezolid, and trimethoprim have been found to achieve bone concentrations at ~50 % of serum [41]. Although the sulfamethoxazole component of trimethoprim-sulfamethoxazole (TMP-SMX) has inferior penetration (10–20 %), its serum concentrations are 20-fold higher than those of trimethoprim. Thus its bone concentrations generally exceed the MICs of susceptible organisms. Because TMP-SMX exhibits concentration-dependent killing, higher doses (i.e., 7–10 mg/kg trimethoprim, or two double-strength tablets twice per day) (one double strength tablet is trimethoprim–sulfamethoxazole 160 mg–800 mg) may result in greater efficacy when treating chronic osteomyelitis. The lack of a fixed 1:5 ratio of concentrations of trimethoprim and sulfamethoxazole at the site of infection does not impair their synergy [42].

An oral antibiotic option for treatment of anaerobic osteomyelitis is metronidazole, which penetrates bone at concentrations approximating those in serum. Rifampicin also achieves concentrations in bone near, or exceeding, those in serum. Because serum concentrations of rifampicin increase markedly at doses >450 mg/day [43], prescribing 600 mg once daily should be sufficient. Adjunctive rifampicin therapy has been studied in two randomized clinical trials of patients with chronic osteomyelitis caused by *S. aureus* [44, 45]. More patients who received rifampicin in addition to other antibiotics were cured compared with those who did not (17 of 20 [85 %] vs. 12 of 21 [57 %]; *P* = .05 by Fisher's exact test), and no patient terminated therapy due to rifampicin-related adverse effects. Finally, both fusidic acid and fosfomycin penetrate bone extremely well, at concentrations in excess of target MICs.

In summary, oral options for the treatment of chronic osteomyelitis based on pharmacokinetic considerations include fluoroquinolones, TMP-SMX, or fosfomycin for susceptible gram-negative bacilli, and TMP-SMX, clindamycin, and linezolid for susceptible gram-positive infections. Rifampicin and fusidic acid are reasonable adjunctive agents for combination therapy.

There have been few randomized trials of systemic therapy for osteomyelitis in adults. A systematic review published in 2009 found only eight small trials, with a total of 228 evaluable subjects [46]. A composite analysis of the five trials that compared oral with parenteral treatment did not find a significant difference in remission rate at ≥12 months of follow-up, but the rate of moderate or severe adverse events was significantly higher with parenteral than with oral agents (15.5 % vs 4.8 %, respectively). Conterno and da Silva Filho [46] showed there was no statistically significant difference between patients treated with oral versus parenteral antibiotics, in the remission rate 12 or more months after treatment. Single trials with very few participants have found no statistically significant differences in remission rates or adverse events for the following three comparisons: parenteral plus oral versus parenteral only administration; two oral antibiotic regimens; and two parenteral antibiotic regimens. Limited evidence suggests that the method of antibiotic administration (oral versus parenteral) does not affect the rate of disease remission if the bacteria are sensitive to the antibiotic used. Despite advances in both antibiotics and surgical treatment of chronic osteomyelitis long-term recurrence may be 20–30 % [46].

Treatment of Specific Organisms

Antibiotic choice should be tailored to the organism isolated from infected bone, when and if possible. Below are sample organisms and recommended definitive antibiotic treatment with a summary in Table 6.3.

Staphylococcus Aureus and Methicillin-Resistant *S. Aureus*

S aureus is the predominant pathogen isolated in all forms and stages of osteomyelitis. Strains are increasingly methicillin-resistant due to the continued increase in hospital-associated MRSA and the emergence of community-associated MRSA [47, 48]. When methicillin-sensitive, it can be treated with an anti-staphylococcal penicillin (flucloxacillin, nafcillin, oxacillin) or first generation cephalosporin, but therapy options for MRSA includes vancomycin, daptomycin, linezolid trimethoprim-sulfamethoxazole plus rifampicin, and clindamycin depending on susceptibility testing [49]. In a salvage study of patients with MRSA osteomyelitis, which had failed to respond to previous therapy, all nine patients who were treated with daptomycin had clinical resolution of their infection by the end of therapy, but one patient subsequently relapsed [50]. Larger retrospective studies on the treatment of chronic osteomyelitis with

Table 6.3 Summary of some specific antibiotic choices commonly used in the United States

Organism	Potential antibiotic choice
Methicillin-sensitive staphylococci	Oxacillin, nafcillin, cefazolin, ceftriaxone
Methicillin-resistant staphylococci	Vancomycin, daptomycin, linezolid, trimethoprim-sulfamethoxazole plus rifampicin, clindamycin
Streptococci	Penicillins and cephalosporins, vancomycin (if penicillin-resistant organism or patient has beta-lactam allergy)
Enterococci	Ampicillin (if sensitive), vancomycin, daptomycin, linezolid
Gram-negative organisms	Parenteral options include broad-spectrum penicillins and cephalosporins, oral fluoroquinolones
Polymicrobial	Broad-spectrum e.g., ampicillin-sulbactam, piperacillin-tazobactam, or a carbapenem
Unusual and atypical organisms	Treatment should be pathogen-specific and based on in vitro antibiotic susceptibility testing

daptomycin have reported cure rates of 65–75 % [51]. Rifampicin has an optimal intercellular concentration and is used in combination with cell-wall active antibiotics to achieve synergistic killing and to prevent rapid emergence of resistant strains. Linezolid is active against MRSA, inhibits bacterial protein synthesis, has excellent bone penetration, and is administered intravenously or orally, though concerns have been raised regarding side effects associated with its long-term use. Case reports suggest the potential for quinupristin-dalfopristin and tigecycline to cure chronic osteomyelitis, but clinical data are limited [52]. Tetracyclines, including doxycycline and tigecycline, are not generally first-line treatments for MRSA bone infections.

Coagulase-Negative Staphylococci

Although less virulent than *S. aureus* the coagulase-negative staphylococci (CNS) have become important pathogens, in the foot and ankle, due to frequency of posttraumatic and prosthetic device-associated and implant-associated infections in the foot and ankle. Treatment of methicillin-susceptible CNS is similar to treatment of MSSA, but the majority of CNS strains are methicillin-resistant. Susceptibilities to fluoroquinolones, clindamycin, trimethoprim-sulfamethoxazole, and tetracyclines are more variable. Methicillin-resistant CNS osteomyelitis is usually treated with intravenous vancomycin. Daptomycin and linezolid have also been used, but published experience is limited.

Streptococcus spp.

Most streptococcal osteomyelitis is due to the beta-haemolytic streptococci, especially *Streptococcus agalactiae* (group B) and *Streptococcus pyogenes* (group A). These organisms remain highly susceptible to penicillins and cephalosporins, and intravenous penicillin G remains the drug of choice, though other intravenous penicillins, cephalosporins, and carbapenems are also effective. Intravenous cefazolin and ceftriaxone are probably equivalent to penicillin and allow more convenient dosing. For penicillin allergic patients, clindamycin may be used, though resistance to this agent is increasing. For isolates resistant to penicillin and cephalosporins, treatment decisions should be based on in vitro susceptibility data. Vancomycin or linezolid remains an option for isolates resistant to or patients intolerant of other antibiotics.

Enterococci and Vancomycin-Resistant Enterococci

Enterococcal osteomyelitis was formerly a complication of enterococcal bacteremia and endocarditis, but enterococci and vancomycin-resistant enterococci (VRE) are increasingly important in chronic osteomyelitis of the foot and ankle in diabetic and ischemic ulcers and in device-associated infections. Enterococci are intrinsically resistant to many antibiotics including cephalosporins and clindamycin. Most enterococcal infections are caused by *Enterococcus faecalis*. These organisms are usually susceptible to ampicillin, although this drug is only bacteriostatic, and intravenous ampicillin is the drug of choice. At present, *Enterococcus faecium* causes an increasing proportion of enterococcal infections, and is usually ampicillin and carbapenem-resistant. It is increasingly vancomycin-resistant as well [53]. Most reported experience for treatment of ampicillin-resistant VRE osteomyelitis has been with linezolid [54].

Other agents used include chloramphenicol, tetracyclines, daptomycin, and quinupristin-dalfopristin. Tigecycline is also active against VRE. Linezolid resistance develops more frequently in enterococci than in staphylococci. Combination therapy with aminoglycosides and cell-wall agents for enterococcal osteomyelitis is associated with significant nephrotoxicity [55]. Ampicillin—ceftriaxone can be a reasonable synergistic combination to treat orthopedic infections due to *E. faecalis* though data to support this combination is limited and based on its use in other enterococcal infections.

Gram-Negative Organisms

Treatment of osteomyelitis caused by gram-negative pathogens depends on the infecting organism and in vitro susceptibility data. Oral options for treatment of gram-negative infections are more limited than for gram-positive infections and include fluoroquinolones and trimethoprim-sulfamethoxazole. Tigecycline can also be used for some acinetobacter and klebsiella infections but is not active against pseudomonas. Parenteral options include broad-spectrum penicillins and cephalosporins, aztreonam, carbapenems, and aminoglycosides. Fluoroquinolones have excellent oral bioavailability and may be used in patients who can absorb oral medications in the treatment of susceptible organisms.

Anaerobes

The role of anaerobes in polymicrobial osteomyelitis of the foot and ankle is uncertain. Several antibiotics frequently used in the management of diabetic foot infections including co-amoxiclav, piperacillin-tazobactam, cefamycines (cefoxitin, cefotetan), carbapenems, metronidazole, moxifloxacin, tigecycline, and linezolid have anaerobic activity. Metronidazole is highly bioavailable with excellent tissue diffusion and potent bactericidal activity against anaerobes making it a useful agent for the treatment of osteomyelitis due to obligate anaerobes.

Polymicrobial Infections

Most osteomyelitis in diabetic foot infections and ischemic ulcers is polymicrobial and includes mixtures of aerobic and anaerobic organisms. Microbiologic specimens may identify the most abundant pathogens but may not identify important organisms, and not all isolated organisms are equally virulent. The need to treat an organism in a mixed culture depends in part on its suspected relative virulence and the role in a polymicrobial foot infection. Initial empiric regimens may include several drugs with activity against different classes of pathogens. Use of broad-spectrum agents such as ampicillin-sulbactam, piperacillin-tazobactam, or a carbapenem can provide empiric activity against most potential aerobic and anaerobic pathogens, but even these broad-spectrum agents may be inadequate, especially if MRSA is a concern.

Osteomyelitis Due to Unusual and Atypical Organisms

Bone and joint tuberculosis is a notable presentation of extrapulmonary tuberculosis, comprising 11 % of cases of extrapulmonary disease in the United States. Treatment regimens for tuberculous osteomyelitis are similar to those for pulmonary disease and include initiation of isoniazid, rifampicin ethambutol, and pyrazinamide, with revision of therapy based on susceptibilities. Regimens consisting of two or more drugs continued for at least 6–9 months are recommended by the American Thoracic Society [56]. Atypical mycobacterial organisms that can cause bone infection include *Mycobacterium marinum*, *Mycobacterium kansasii*, and *Mycobacterium avium*. In immunocompromised patients (organ transplant recipients, patients receiving highly immunosuppressive medications) fungal pathogens and other bacterial infections including nocardia may be potential causes of osteomyelitis and should be treated with pathogen-guided antimicrobials based on in vitro susceptibility testing.

Treatment of the Foot and Ankle Infected Prosthesis

Some bacteria, such as staphylococci in prosthesis infections, adhere to a biofilm that protects the organism from phagocytosis and impedes delivery of the antibiotic. Rifampicin is often recommended to be used in combination with other antibiotics for staphylococcal infections because it penetrates the biofilm. When feasible, infected prosthetic material should be removed. Long-term, culture-guided suppressive antibiotic therapy should also be considered when removal of an infected prosthesis cannot be performed. Good bioavailability, low toxicity, and adequate bone penetration are important factors in guiding suppressive treatment. If the infection recurs after 6 months of suppressive antibiotic treatment and infected prosthetic material cannot be removed, a lifelong regimen of suppressive therapy may be considered.

Studies of suppressive therapy with administration of rifampicin, ofloxacin, fusidic acid, and trimethoprim-sulfamethoxazole for 6–9 months have been performed in patients with infected orthopedic implants. Studies have shown that, after discontinuation of antibiotics, infection did not recur in 67 % of patients treated with trimethoprim-sulfamethoxazole, in 55 % of patients treated with rifampicin and fusidic acid, and in 50 % of patients treated with rifampicin and ofloxacin [57]. Relapses usually result in a form of chronic osteomyelitis and may be treated with antibiotics and surgical debridement but can persist for years with frequent therapeutic failure.

In another trial, Zimmerli et al. [58] randomized patients with prosthetic devices infected with Staphylococcus spp. to receive either rifampicin or placebo, plus ciprofloxacin, for 3–6 months. In the per-protocol population, cure rates were 100 % for rifampicin-treated versus 58 % for placebo-treated patients ($P<.02$). Notably, the causative pathogen in four of the five patients whose infection failed to respond to ciprofloxacin monotherapy developed resistance to ciprofloxacin.

Route of Therapy

No particular route, either parenteral or oral, has been shown to be either superior or inferior to the other. Adequate levels of antibiotics can be achieved through intravenous or highly bioavailable oral medications. Oral and parenteral therapies can therefore achieve similar cure rates; Table 6.4 shows a sample of potent oral antibiotics for treatment of osteomyelitis. Furthermore, oral therapy avoids risks associated with intravenous catheters and is generally less expensive, making

Table 6.4 A sample of potent oral antibiotics for treatment of osteomyelitis

Oral agent	Activity
Clindamycin	Gram-positive bacteria, including staphylococci
Linezolid	Methicillin-resistant *Staphylococcus aureus* (MRSA) and vancomycin-resistant enterococcus (VRE)
Quinolones, e.g., ciprofloxacin	Gram-negative organisms
Trimethoprim-sulfamethoxazole	Staphylococci, gram-negative organisms
Rifampicin	*Staphylococcus aureus*, including MRSA, used in combination with other cell-wall active antibiotics

it a reasonable choice for osteomyelitis caused by susceptible organisms. [18] Single trials with very few participants have found no statistically significant differences for remission or adverse events for the following three comparisons [16]:

1. Parenteral plus oral versus parenteral only administration.
2. Two oral antibiotic regimens.
3. Two parenteral antibiotic regimens.

Limited evidence suggests that the method of antibiotic administration (oral versus parenteral) does not affect the rate of disease remission if the bacteria are sensitive to the antibiotic used [18].

Game and Jeffcoate reported on 113 patients who were treated nonsurgically with antibiotic therapy [59]. Oral therapy was chosen for 80 % of patients, while the other 20 % received intravenous followed by oral antibiotics. The mean duration of therapy for oral treatment was 9 weeks, while the intravenous group had a mean duration of 2 weeks. Overall, 93 of 113 (82 %) were in remission at 12 months. The results of this study concur with the results reported in a study by Embil et al., who treated diabetic osteomyelitis with oral therapy in 79 patients [60]. Patients were treated with a mean of 3 oral antibiotics, and duration lasted an average of 40 weeks. With this therapy, 80 % patients achieved remission with a mean relapse free period of 50 weeks. Valabhji et al. also demonstrated that high rates of healing and low rates of amputation were achieved with medical treatment which was guided by MRI and was associated with long courses of antibiotics, but nevertheless, particularly low relapse rate [33].

Oral antibiotics that have been proven to be effective include clindamycin, rifampicin, trimethoprim-sulfamethoxazole, and fluoroquinolones. Clindamycin is given orally after initial intravenous treatment for 1–2 weeks and has excellent bioavailability. It is active against most gram-positive bacteria, including staphylococci. Peters et al. assessed the available evidence for accepted treatments of

diabetic foot osteomyelitis, and found no significant differences in outcome associated with any particular treatment strategy [61].

Duration of Therapy

The most appropriate duration of therapy for any type of foot infection is not well defined, especially in the diabetic foot. It is important to consider the presence and amount of any residual dead or infected bone and the state of the soft tissues. When a radical resection leaves no remaining infected tissue, only a short duration of antibiotic therapy is needed. Alternatively, if infected bone remains despite surgery, the IDSA guidelines advocate for prolonged treatment. Table 6.5 is a summary of the IDSA guidelines for duration of treatment.

Given the potential adverse effects that may occur during the antibiotic therapy, it is essential to ensure appropriate medical follow-up comprising both clinical and biological assessments. A satisfactory assessment for an adequate duration of treatment needs to be a multifactorial approach in the evaluation of the patient and may include a combination of the following three domains:

1. Detailed clinical assessment of the patient and site of infection for signs of residual infection.
2. Biochemical tests to assess and track resolution of the osteomyelitis. A potential testing strategy may include:
   - C-Reactive Protein, ESR, procalcitonin, white blood cell and neutrophil count.
3. Radiological assessment to compare baseline tests at diagnosis.
   - E.g.: X-rays and MRI scans.

Although the length of antibiotic therapy is frequently discussed in the literature, there is no clear evidence to support a specific duration of therapy. Classically, 4–6 weeks of parenteral antibiotics is utilized in conjunction with debridement to eradicate osteomyelitis. More recently, reports have shown it is possible to have a shorter treatment with parenteral and longer treatment with highly bioavailable oral therapy [10].

Acute osteomyelitis can usually respond to short duration of antibiotic treatment alone, but chronic osteomyelitis is associated with avascular necrosis of bone and formation of sequestrum, and usually requires a longer duration of treatment for its medical management. Animal studies and observations show that bone revascularization after debridement takes about 4–6 weeks [62]. The optimal duration of therapy for chronic osteomyelitis remains uncertain. There is no evidence that antibiotic therapy for more than 4–6 weeks

Table 6.5 IDSA guidelines for diabetic foot osteomyelitis

Severity or extent	Route of administration	Duration of therapy
No residual infected tissue (e.g., post amputation)	Parenteral or oral	2–5 days
Residual infected soft tissue (but not bone)	Parenteral or oral	1–3 weeks
Residual infected bone (but viable)	Initial parenteral, then consider oral switch	4–6 weeks
No surgery possible, or residual dead bone postoperatively	Initial parenteral, then consider oral switch	More than 3 months

IDSA 2012 guidelines: suggested route, and duration of antibiotic therapy for bone or joint infection

improves outcomes compared with shorter regimens, and there is no evidence that prolonged parenteral antibiotics will penetrate the necrotic bone [19].

Local Antibiotic Therapy

There is limited evidence supporting the effectiveness of local antibiotics in treating osteomyelitis. The primary benefit achieved with local antibiotic delivery vehicles is the ability to obtain extremely high levels of antibiotic without increasing systemic toxicity. Antibiotic-loaded bone cement represents the current standard as an antibiotic delivery vehicle in orthopedic surgery. Composite biomaterials that simultaneously provide function of antibiotic delivery, and also contribute to the process of bone regeneration represent the most ideal class of local antibiotic delivery vehicles [63].

Local antibiotic delivery with antibiotic-loaded acrylic bone cement has been used extensively in the management of chronic osteomyelitis and implant-related infections. Self-made antibiotic-loaded bone cement beads, which are cheaper and antibiotic specific, have been shown to elute less effectively than commercial antibiotic-loaded cement beads [64]. The commercial formulation of antibiotic cement produces an inhibition zone that is larger and more regular than the manually mixed preparation.

In clinical practice, low-dose antibiotic eluting bone cement is often used. Although all carriers showed a burst release, low-dose antibiotic spacers showed little additional release after the first week, compared to the longer duration of antibiotic elution from commercial high dose antibiotic cement [65]. Moojen et al. cautioned the use of low-dose antibiotic bone cement for spacers because unsuccessful eradication of infection could result. Prospective, randomized trials are needed to evaluate the role of localized antibiotic therapy as adjunctive treatments for osteomyelitis in diabetic foot infections.

Adjunctive Therapies

Splinting or "Off-Loading": Osteomyelitis in the foot and ankle of patients with diabetes and neuropathy may trigger the development of acute Charcot neuroarthropathy or an unstable foot. It is therefore important to consider the need for "off-loading" the foot with devices such as total contact casting or air cast boots. This in turn helps to prevent foot deformity as well as improves pain relief [66].

Hyperbaric Oxygen Therapy: Systematic reviews note that studies are of variable quality [67], and a recent RCT [68] suggests a potential role in wound healing.

Pain Control: Although not always reported in patients with diabetic neuropathy, patients with osteomyelitis of the foot and ankle can present with deep bone pain. Although the emphasis for medical management is usually placed on antimicrobial therapy, the need to provide adequate analgesia should not be overlooked, especially in acute and sub-acute osteomyelitis. Chronic osteomyelitis can also be associated with pain, especially in the presence of an abscess formation [69].

Patient Education: It may not be possible to prevent osteomyelitis but its effect can be limited through increased awareness among patient groups with high risk. Patient education by healthcare providers should promote early recognition and presentation and prompt treatment. Medical management may require prolonged use of antibiotics patients in patients who are systematically well and thus good patient education and understanding is needed to maximize compliance with antibiotic and adjunctive treatment. Table 6.6 is a list of patient groups who may be at high risk of developing osteomyelitis.

Adequate patient education is of particular relevance in patients with diabetes mellitus, who may lack some of the early signs and symptoms of infection due to their concomitant neuropathy.

Summary

There is increasing use of medical management of the foot and ankle osteomyelitis. Specific indications for the initiation of medical therapy are recognized. At this time, there is a lack of high quality clinical studies to guide medical therapy. However it is important to understand the microbiology of diabetic foot infections, including osteomyelitis, and to be aware of available antibiotics used in the treatment of osteomyelitis, routes of administration and considerations that may guide duration of antibiotic therapy.

Table 6.6 Patient groups with high risk of osteomyelitis

Trauma (orthopedic surgery or open fracture)	Diabetes mellitus	Presence of catheter-related bloodstream infection
Prosthetic orthopedic device	Alcoholism	Sickle cell disease
Peripheral arterial disease	Immunosuppression	Tuberculosis
Chronic joint disease	Intravenous drug abuse	HIV and AIDS

These patients need to be aware of their increased risk of developing osteomyelitis and their associated risk of poor healing

References

1. Berendt AR, Peters EJ, Bakker K, et al. Specific guidelines for treatment of diabetic foot osteomyelitis. Diabetes Metab Res Rev. 2008;24 Suppl 1:S190–1.
2. Frykberg RG, Wittmayer B, Zgonis T. Surgical management of diabetic foot infections and osteomyelitis. Clin Podiatr Med Surg. 2007;24(3):469–82.
3. Shank CF, Feibel JB. Osteomyelitis in the diabetic foot: diagnosis and management. Foot Ankle Clin. 2006;11(4):775–89.
4. Wukich DK, Sung W. Charcot arthropathy of the foot and ankle: modern concepts and management review. J Diabetes Complications. 2008;16.
5. Newman LG, Waller J, Palestro CJ, et al. Unsuspected osteomyelitis in diabetic foot ulcers. Diagnosis and monitoring by leukocyte scanning with indium in 111 oxyquinoline. JAMA. 1991;266:1246–51.
6. Grayson ML, Gibbons GW, Habershaw GM, et al. Use of ampicillin/sulbactam versus imipenem/cilastatin in the treatment of limb-threatening foot infections in diabetic patients. Clin Infect Dis. 1994;18:683–93.
7. Lipsky BA. Osteomyelitis of the foot in diabetic patients. Clin Infect Dis. 1997;25:1318–26.
8. Lavery LA, Armstrong DG, Wunderlich RP, Mohler MJ, Wendel CS, Lipsky BA. Risk factors for foot infections in individuals with diabetes. Diabetes Care. 2006;29(6):1288–93.
9. Sumpio BE, Armstrong DG, Lawrence A, Lavery LA, Andros G, SVS/APMA writing group. The role of interdisciplinary team approach in the management of the diabetic foot. A Joint Statement from the Society for Vascular Surgery and the American Podiatric Medical Association. J Vasc Surg. 2010;51(6):1504–6.
10. Jeffcoate WJ, Lipsky BA. Controversies in diagnosing and managing osteomyelitis of the foot in diabetes. Clin Infect Dis. 2004;39 Suppl 2:s115–22.
11. Kowalski TJ, et al. The effect of residual osteomyelitis at the resection margin in patients with surgically treated diabetic foot infection. J Foot Ankle Surg. 2011;50(2):171–5.
12. Lipsky BA, Berendt AR, Cornia PB, et al. 2012 Infectious Diseases Society of America clinical practice guideline for the diagnosis and treatment of diabetic foot infections. Clin Infect Dis. 2012;54: e132–73.
13. Cierny G, Mader JT, Pennick JJ. A clinical staging system for adult osteomyelitis. Contemp Orthop. 1985;10:17–37.
14. Waldvogel FA, Medoff G, Swartz MN. Osteomyelitis: a review of clinical features, therapeutic considerations and unusual aspects (first of three parts). N Engl J Med. 1970;282:198–206.
15. Lew DP, Waldvogel FA. Osteomyelitis. Lancet. 2004;364:369–79.
16. Lazzarini L, Lipsky BA, Mader JT. Antibiotic treatment of osteomyelitis: what have we learned from 30 years of clinical trials? Int J Infect Dis. 2005;9(3):127–38.
17. Lipsky B. Treating diabetic foot osteomyelitis primarily with surgery or antibiotics: have we answered the question? Diabetes Care. 2014;37:593–5.
18. Cochrane Review Conterno LO, Turchi MD. Antibiotics for treating chronic osteomyelitis in adults. Cochrane Database of Syst Rev 2013, 9.
19. Spellberg B, Lipsky BA. Systemic antibiotic therapy for chronic osteomyelitis in adults. Clin Infect Dis. 2012;54:393–407.
20. Berendt AR, Peters EJ, Bakker K, et al. Diabetic foot osteomyelitis: a progress report on diagnosis and a systematic review of treatment. Diabetes Metab Res Rev. 2008;24 Suppl 1:S145–61.
21. Concia E, Prandini N, Massari L, Ghisellini F, Consoli V, Menichetti F. Osteomyelitis: clinical update for practical guidelines. Nucl Med Commun. 2006;27(8):645–60.
22. Lipsky BA, Berendt AR, Deery GH, Infectious Diseases Society of America, et al. IDSA guidelines: diagnosis and treatment of diabetic foot infections. Clin Infect Dis. 2004;39:885–910.
23. Senneville E, Nguyen S. Current pharmacotherapy options for osteomyelitis: convergences, divergences and lessons to be drawn. Expert Opin Pharmacother. 2013;14:723–34.
24. Lipsky BA, Itani K, Norden C. Treating foot infections in diabetic patients: a randomized, multicenter, open-label trial of linezolid versus ampicillin-sulbactam/amoxicillin-clavulanate. Clin Infect Dis. 2004;38(1):17–24.
25. Handa N, Kawakami T, Kitaoka K, et al. The clinical efficacy of imipenem/cilastatin sodium in orthopedic infections and drug levels in the bone tissue. Jpn J Antibiot. 1997;50:622–7.
26. LeFrock JL, Carr BB. Clinical experience with cefotaxime in the treatment of serious bone and joint infections. Rev Infect Dis. 1982;4(Suppl):S465–71.
27. MacGregor RR, Gentry LO. Imipenem/cilastatin in the treatment of osteomyelitis. Am J Med. 1985;78:100–3.
28. Bach MC, Cocchetto DM. Ceftazidime as single-agent therapy for gram-negative aerobic bacillary osteomyelitis. Antimicrob Agents Chemother. 1987;31(10):1605–8.
29. Gomis M, Herranz A, Aparicio P, Filloy JL, Pastor J. Cefotaxime in the treatment of chronic osteomyelitis caused by gram-negative bacilli. J Antimicrob Chemother. 1990;26(Suppl A):45–52.
30. Dombrowski JC, Winston LG. Clinical failures of appropriately-treated methicillin-resistant Staphylococcus aureus infections. J Infect. 2008;57:110–5.
31. Tice AD, Hoaglund PA, Shoultz DA. Outcomes of osteomyelitis among patients treated with outpatient parenteral antimicrobial therapy. Am J Med. 2003;114:723–8.
32. Tice AD, Hoaglund PA, Shoultz DA. Risk factors and treatment outcomes in osteomyelitis. J Antimicrob Chemother. 2003;51: 1261–8.
33. Valabhji J, Oliver N, Samarasinghe D, Mali T, Gibbs RG, Gedroyc WM. Conservative management of diabetic forefoot ulceration complicated by underlying osteomyelitis: the benefits of magnetic resonance imaging. Diabet Med. 2009;26(11):1127–34.
34. Senneville E, Lombart A, Beltrand E, et al. Outcome of diabetic foot osteomyelitis treated nonsurgically: a retrospective cohort study. Diabetes Care. 2008;31(4):637–42.
35. Malhotra R, Claire Shu-Yi Chan, Aziz Nather. Diabet Foot Ankle. 2014; 5: 10.3402/dfa.v5.24445.
36. Landersdorfer CB, Bulitta JB, Kinzig M, et al. Penetration of antibacterials into bone: pharmacokinetic, pharmacodynamic and bioanalytical considerations. Clin Pharmacokinet. 2009;48:89–124.
37. Widmer AF, Frei R, Rajacic Z, Zimmerli W. Correlation between in vivo and in vitro efficacy of antibioticagents against foreign body infections. J Infect Dis. 1990;162:96–102.

38. Patel R. Biofilms and antibiotic resistance. Clin Orthop Relat Res. 2005;437:41–7.

39. Dornbusch K. The detection of doxycycline activity in human bone. Scand J Infect Dis Suppl. 1976;9:47–53.

40. Bystedt H, DAhlbäck A, Dornbusch K, Nord CE. Concentrations of azidocillin, erythromycin, doxycycline and clindamycin in human mandibular bone. Int J Oral Surg. 1978;7:442–9.

41. Wacha H, Wagner D, Schafer V, Knothe H. Concentration of ciprofloxacin in bone tissue after single parenteral administration to patients older than 70 years. Infection. 1990;18:173–6.

42. Burman LG. The antimicrobial activities of trimethoprim and sulfonamides. Scand J Infect Dis. 1986;18:3–13.

43. Peloquin CA, Jaresko GS, Yong CL, Keung AC, Bulpitt AE, Jelliffe RW. Population pharmacokinetic modeling of isoniazid, rifampin, and pyrazinamide. Antimicrob Agents Chemother. 1997;41:2670–9.

44. Van der Auwera P, Klastersky J, Thys JP, Meunier-Carpentier F, Legrand JC. Double-blind, placebo-controlled study of oxacillin combined with rifampin in the treatment of staphylococcal infections. Antimicrob Agents Chemother. 1985;28:467–72.

45. Norden CW, Bryant R, Palmer D, Montgomerie JZ, Wheat J. Chronic osteomyelitis caused by Staphylococcus aureus: controlled clinical trial of nafcillin therapy and nafcillin-rifampin therapy. South Med J. 1986;79:947–51.

46. Conterno LO, da Silva Filho CR. Antibiotics for treating chronic osteomyelitis in adults. Cochrane Database Syst Rev. 2009;3, CD004439.

47. Bocchini CE, Hulten KG, Mason Jr EO, et al. Panton-Valentine leukocidin genes are associated with enhanced inflammatory response and local disease in acute hematogenous Staphylococcus aureus osteomyelitis in children. Pediatrics. 2006;117:433–40.

48. Klevens RM, Morrison MA, Nadle J, et al. Invasive methicillin-resistant Staphylococcus aureus infections in the United States. JAMA. 2007;298:1763–71.

49. Liu C, Bayer A, Cosgrove SE, et al. Clinical practice guidelines by the Infectious Diseases Society of America for the treatment of methicillin-resistant Staphylococcus aureus infections in adults and children. Clin Infect Dis. 2011;52:e18–55.

50. Finney MS, Crank CW, Segreti J. Use of daptomycin to treat drug-resistant gram-positive bone and joint infections. Curr Med Res Opin. 2005;21:1923–6.

51. Holtom PD, Zalavras CG, Lamp KC, Park N, Friedrich LV. Clinical experience with daptomycin treatment of foot or ankle osteomyelitis: a preliminary study. Clin Orthop Relat Res. 2007;461:35–9.

52. Chen PL, Yan JJ, Wu CJ, et al. Salvage therapy with tigecycline for recurrent infection caused by ertapenem-resistant extended-spectrum beta-lactamase-producing Klebsiella pneumoniae. Diagn Microbiol Infect Dis. 2010;68:312–4.

53. Rice LB. Antimicrobial resistance in gram-positive bacteria. Am J Infect Control. 2006;34:S11–9.

54. Graham AC, Mercier RC, Achusim LE, Pai MP. Extended interval aminoglycoside dosing for treatment of enterococcal and staphylococcal osteomyelitis. Ann Pharmacother. 2004;38:936–41.

55. Falagas ME, Siempos II, Papagelopoulos PJ, Vardakas KZ. Linezolid for the treatment of adults with bone and joint infections. Int J Antimicrob Agents. 2007;29:233–9.

56. Blumberg HM, Burman WJ, Chaisson RE, Daley CL, Etkind SC, Friedman LN, Fujiwara P, Grzemska M, Hopewell PC, Iseman MD, Jasmer RM, Koppaka V, Menzies RI, O'Brien RJ, Reves RR, Reichman LB, Simone PM, Starke JR, Vernon AA. American Thoracic Society/Centers for Disease Control and Prevention/Infectious Diseases Society of America: treatment of tuberculosis. Am J Respir Crit Care Med. 2003;167:603–62.

57. Calhoun JH, Manring MM. Adult osteomyelitis. Infect Dis Clin North Am. 2005;19(4):765–86.

58. Zimmerli W, Widmer AF, Blatter M, Frei R, Ochsner PE. Role of rifampin for treatment of orthopedic implant-related staphylococcal infections: a randomized controlled trial. Foreign-Body Infection (FBI) Study Group. JAMA. 1998;279:1537–4.

59. Game FL, Jeffcoate WJ. Primarily non-surgical management of osteomyelitis of the foot in diabetes. Diabetologia. 2008;51(6):962–7.

60. Embil JM, Rose G, Trepman E, et al. Oral antimicrobial therapy for diabetic foot osteomyelitis. Foot Ankle Int. 2006;27(10):771–9.

61. Peters EJ, Lipsky BA, Berendt AR, Embil JM, Lavery LA, Senneville E, et al. A systematic review of the effectiveness of interventions in the management of infection in the diabetic foot. Diabetes Metab Res Rev. 2012;28:142.

62. Lazzarini L, Mader JT. Osteomyelitis in long bones. J Bone Joint Surg Am. 2004;86:2305–18.

63. Hanssen AD. Local antibiotic delivery vehicles in the treatment of musculoskeletal infection. Clin Orthop Relat Res. 2005;437:91–6.

64. Samuel S, Ismavel R, Boopalan PR, Matthai T. Practical considerations in the making and use of high-dose antibiotic loaded bone cement. Acta Orthop Belg. 2010;76:543–5.

65. Moojen DJ, Hentenaar B, Charles Vogely H, Verbout AJ, Castelein RM, Dhert WJ. In vitro release of antibiotics from commercial PMMA beads and articulating hip spacers. J Arthroplasty. 2008;23:1152–6.

66. Donegan R, Sumpio B, Blume PA. Charcot foot and ankle with osteomyelitis. Diabet Foot Ankle. 2013;1:4. doi:10.3402/dfa.v4i0.21361.

67. Goldman RJ. Hyperbaric oxygen therapy for wound healing and limb salvage: a systematic review. PM R. 2009;1(5):471–89.

68. Löndahl M, Katzman P, Nilsson A, Hammarlund C. Hyperbaric oxygen therapy facilitates healing of chronic foot ulcers in patients with diabetes. Diabetes Care. 2010;33(5):998–1003.

69. Yazdi H, Shirazi MR, Eghbali F. An unusual presentation of subacute osteomyelitis: a talus brodie abscess with tendon involvement. Am J Orthop (Belle Mead NJ). 2012;41(3):E36–8.

Acute Hematogenous Osteomyelitis of the Foot and Ankle in Children

Ralph J. Faville, Jr.

Bacteria may invade bones following traumatic injury, contiguous spread from adjacent foci, surgically created wounds or by bacterial dissemination through the blood stream, acute hematogenous osteomyelitis (AHO). Trauma as a cause of osteomyelitis results from puncture wounds or open fractures. Contiguous spread to bone may occur when there is an abutting infected joint (septic arthritis) or muscle (pyomyositis). Osseous infections secondary to surgical procedures occur at a rate of 1–1.5 %. This occurs when a previously clean surgical site becomes contaminated with bacteria [1]. This may also occur when bacteria enter the surgical wound during the surgical procedure with eruption of infection in the days or weeks to follow. Likewise poor skin and soft tissue integrity may lead to a surgical wound dehiscence with subsequent colonization and infection. The most common infecting organism in any form of osteomyelitis is *Staphylococcus aureus*. About 20 % of individuals outside the newborn period are colonized with staph, harboring the organism in the anterior nares, groin and axilla [2].

The frequency of AHO varies with the socioeconomics of the country or location being less than one per ten thousand children per year in affluent countries and two to three times that in economically deprived regions [3]. The differences are likely due to earlier diagnosis and treatment of cutaneous, pyogenic lesions that, when not treated early, may lead to bacteremia and hematogenous spread to a boney nidus. Peak ages for developing AHO are 2–5 years. Except in infancy, boys with AHO outnumber girls by greater than two to one [4].

R.J. Faville, Jr., M.D. (✉)
Department of Pediatric Infectious Disease, Gillette
Childrens Speciality Healthcare, 200 University Avn,
St Paul, MN, 55101, USA
e-mail: Rfaville@gillettechildrens.com

Pathophysiology of AHO

The initial event in the genesis of AHO is a bacterial pathogen entering the circulation generally at a site remote from the subsequent infection. Common sites of entry are infected insect bites, infected eczema, impetigo, and paronychia. Upon circulating in the blood stream, while evading circulating neutrophils and fixed phagocytes in spleen, liver, lymph nodes, the surviving bacteria enter the nutrient artery in the bone metaphysis, toward one end of a long, tubular bone (Fig. 7.1).

Terminal arterioles lead to venous sinusoids where blood flow is slow and there is paucity of fixed phagocytes in the walls of the vessels. This creates an ideal environment for bacterial lodgments and proliferation. The bacteria and their released toxins initiate an inflammatory response, chemotactic recruitment of leukocytes, edema, ischemia, and eventually bone necrosis (Fig. 7.2).

Although bones infected with AHO are predominately large tubular bones, no bone is exempt. The femur and tibia are in the lead at 36 % and 33 % respectively as sites for AHO.

By comparison, the calcaneus accounts for 4 %, the metatarsals 2 %, the talus 1 %, and the combined bones of the pelvis 3 % [1, 2].

Where the capsule of a joint encompasses part of the metaphysis such as in the hip, ankle, elbow, and shoulder, extension through the boney cortex and periosteum may lead to septic arthritis. Additionally, in children less than 18 months of age, there may be a patent transphyseal vessel running from the metaphysis, through the physis (growth plate), through the epiphysis, and into the joint space creating continuity between the metaphysis and the adjacent joint. The appearance of septic arthritis in a young child should therefore arouse suspicion of osteomyelitis in an adjacent long bone (Fig. 7.3).

Bacteremia is not an uncommon event and, alone, does not account for the development of AHO. Simultaneous disruption of bone microarchitecture from minor, often not recalled, trauma and bacteremia from a distant focus set the stage for bacterial lodgment and proliferation.

© Springer International Publishing Switzerland 2015
T.J. Boffeli (ed.), *Osteomyelitis of the Foot and Ankle*, DOI 10.1007/978-3-319-18926-0_7

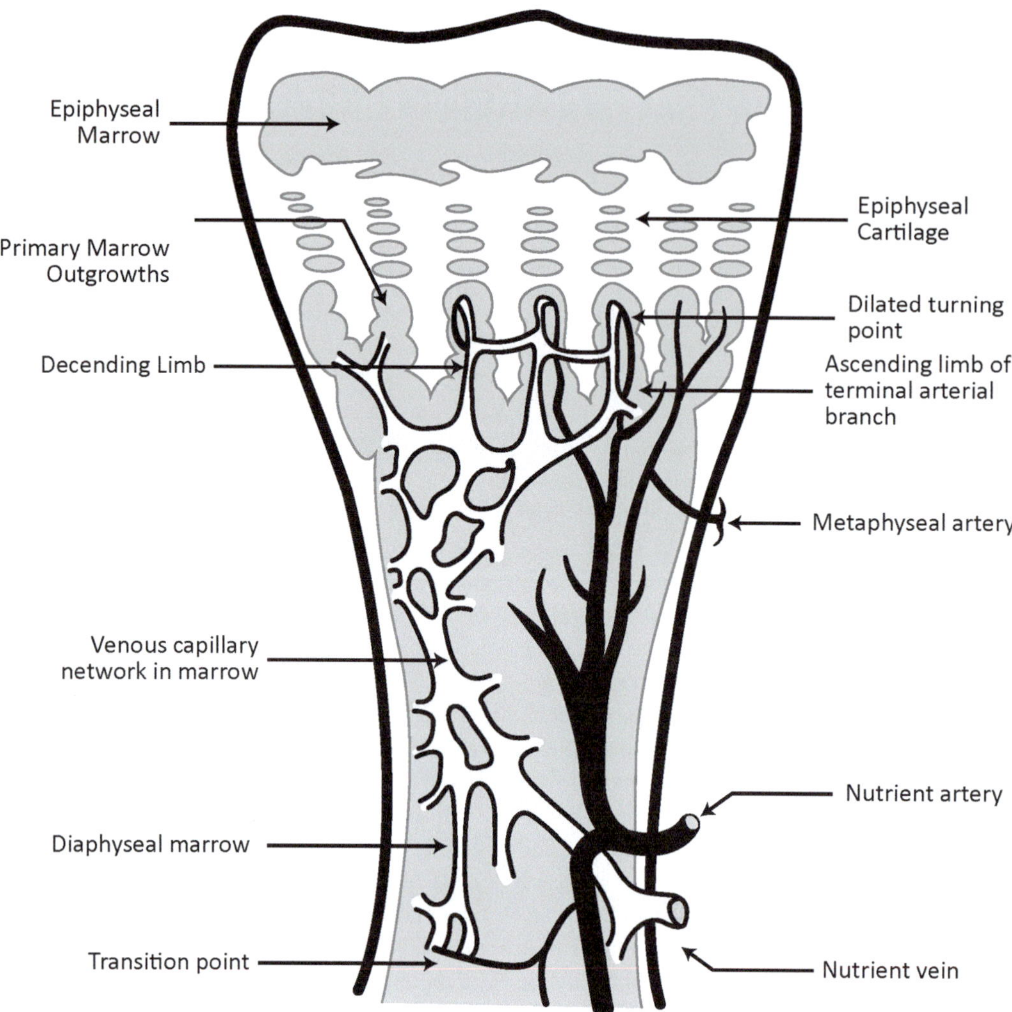

Fig. 7.1 Graphic representation of vascular anatomy of the metaphysis of a tubular bone. Bacteria enter the nutrient artery and lodge into the venous sinusoids

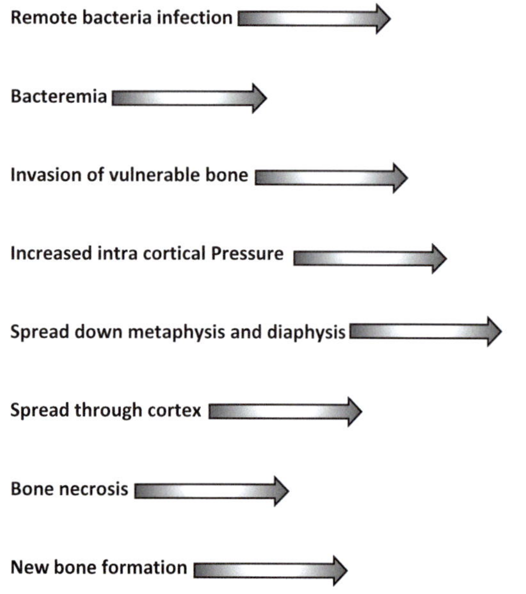

Fig. 7.2 The sequence of events from bacteremia to bone necrosis

This is often referred to as the "bone bruise theory" of skeletal infection.

Making the Diagnosis

Signs and Symptoms

Sustained pain with palpation and pressure over the end of a long bone or directly over a cuboid bone or flat bone along with systemic signs of illness such as fever, malaise, and anorexia justify consideration of osteomyelitis. Additional symptoms may include abnormal gait, with reluctance to bear weight or use an extremity. Other localizing features include localized swelling, warmth, redness, and decreased range of motion. A very late sign occurs when the inflammatory process has penetrated the boney cortex, the periosteum, and soft tissue and forms a fistulous tract to the surface of the skin resulting in purulent drainage.

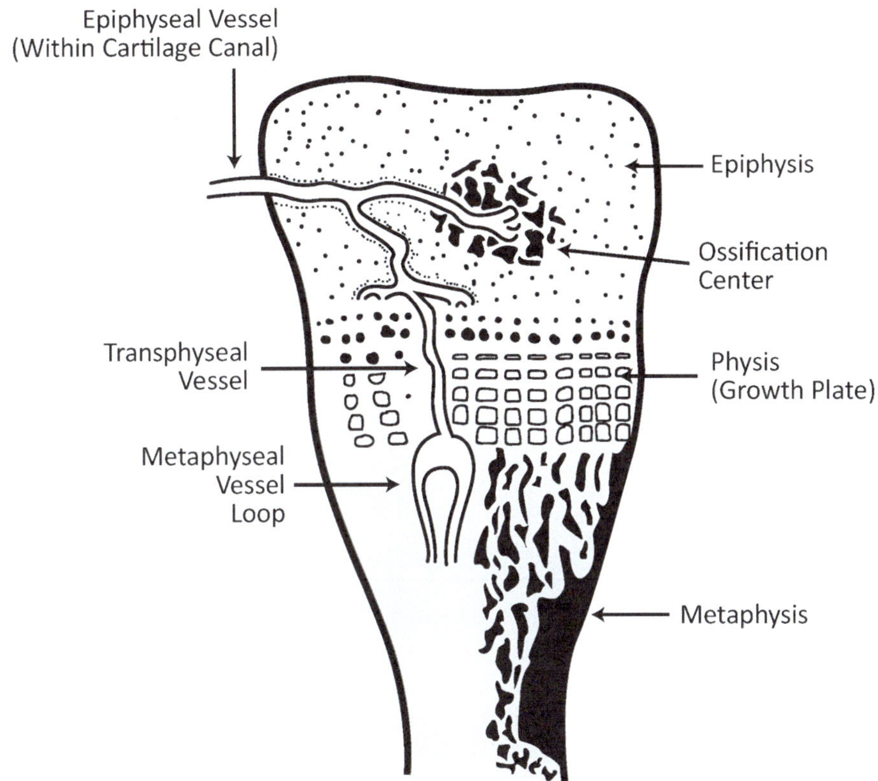

Fig. 7.3 Graphic representation of the metaphysis of a tubular bone of an infant or young child showing the transphyseal vessel

Laboratory Aides

AHO is primarily a clinical diagnosis. Laboratory investigations may help confirm or refute clinical suspicions, but are not absolutes.

Non-specific tests are looking for evidence of inflammatory response. The complete blood count (CBC) usually, but not always, shows a leukocytosis with a predominance of neutrophils (granulocytes). Commonly the total white cell count will be over 12,000 with 60 % or more neutrophils. The c-reactive protein (CRP) is quick to rise with inflammation and quick to fall once appropriate surgical and/or medical treatments are initiated. The erythrocyte sedimentation rate (ESR) rises slowly and may still be rising even after appropriate therapy is initiated. These inflammatory markers should be followed during the course of treatment to assure successful eradication of the infection. These test results are variable depending on the pathogenicity of the organism and the inflammatory response of the host.

Microbiology

The organism responsible for AHO can, more often than not, be found in culture if the cultures are obtained and treated appropriately. Specimens of blood (two independent cultures), joint fluid (if applicable), infected bone and subperiosteal fluid should be obtained. Purulent fluid consists of white blood cells and engulfed bacteria. Optimal cultures are from the bone tissue surrounding the infected fluid.

Scrapings of 1 g of bone tissue (about the size of a pea) and rapid transport to the microbiology laboratory in a transport medium will keep organism alive until agar plates and broth have been inoculated. Generally, aerobic and anarobic cultures are sufficient. Fungal and mycobacteria (TB) cultures may be added in unusual circumstances such as with immunodeficiency and infection not responding to conventional therapy. Successful identification of infecting bacteria should occur in greater than 90 % of cases of AHO. Lack of growth from a culture may occur when antibiotics are given before cultures are obtained, when there are delays in processing the tissue for culture, and when inadequate specimens are submitted to the microbiologist. Direct visualization of the specimen by gram stain may give immediate information of the nature of the infectant such as gram positive cocci or gram negative rod. Once the organism is identified subsequent susceptibility testing will identify optimal antibiotic choices.

At all ages, *Staphylococcus aureus* (coagulase positive staph) is the most prelevent organism. Patients with staph aureus osteomyelitis commonly have this organism as part of their own flora, colonizing anterior nares and skin. Other notable bacteria causing AHO are group B streptococcus in infants, coagulase negative staphylococcus (staph epidermidis), gram negative bacteria such as *Kingella kingae*, and enteric bacteria including *Pseudomonas aeruginosa*. Gonoccal joint infection should be considered in sexually active teens and young adults.

Imaging

Conventional radiography is of limited value in the early detection of AHO because boney changes may take 10–14 days to appear. X-rays are, however, useful to rule out other conditions such as fractures, cysts, or malignancy. The first signs to appear are soft tissue swelling adjacent to the infected metaphysis. The swelling may be accompanied by the displacement of radiolucent muscle and fat planes. The bone cortex is porous. With increasing edema within the metaphysis, infected tissue spreads down the shaft of the metaphysis and diaphysis and outward through the cortex, elevating the periosteum. The periosteum is a tough fibrous sheet that has its own blood supply and remains viable despite the infection all round it. Periosteal reaction and boney rarefaction in the metaphysis are the first osseous changes reflecting bone necrosis and resorption. Dead bone, the sequestrum, becomes surrounded with periosteal new bone, the involucrum. This can be seen on plain X-rays at 2–3 weeks of the onset of symptoms (Fig. 7.4).

Skeletal scintigraphy, or bone scanning, can detect boney changes of osteomyelitis in the first 24–36 h of symptomatic infection [5]. A radioactive marker, technetium methylene diphosphate, is injected intravenously and flows to all tis-

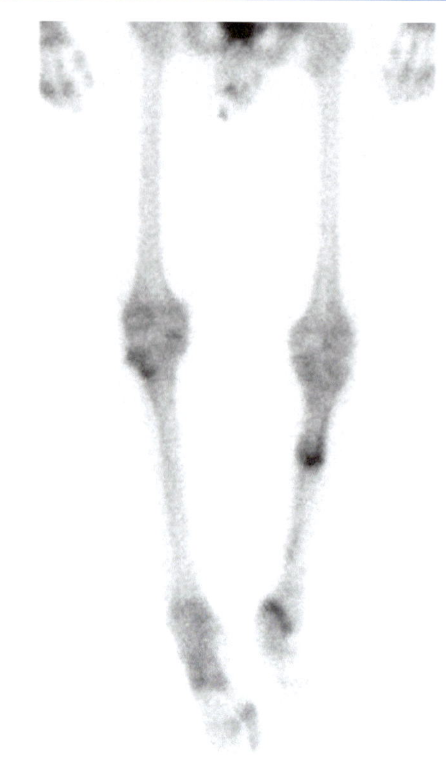

Fig. 7.5 Bone scans showing radioactive hot spots of tibia and calcaneus

sues. It will be more densely concentrated in areas of hyperemia. The compound is taken up by osseous tissue and attaches to the boney matrix. The body is scanned at intervals. The marker will remain longer in bone and especially so in inflamed bone where there is greater osseous blood flow. The resulting scanned image, if positive, will show a defined increased uptake or "hot spot" (Figs. 7.5 and 7.6). When a bone scan is performed late in the course of infection, perhaps 10–15 days into the disease, there may be a "cold spot" indicating that the bone is necrotic and without blood supply. All hot spots are not osteomyelitis. Similar appearing scans may be encountered with tumors, such as Ewings sarcoma, or a skeletal presentation of acute lymphoblastic leukemia.

Magnetic resonance imaging (MRI) is the most specific and, sensitive modality for diagnosing osteomyelitis in its early stages [6]. The T2-weighted signal detects bone marrow edema (Fig. 7.7).

MRI gives optimal anatomic detail of bone and soft tissue inflammation. MRI serves to identify when bone infection has ruptured through the cortex and entered into soft tissue spaces. Most importantly it gives the precise location of infection to the surgeon who may need to aspirate, evacuate, or debride and irrigate the lesion (Figs. 7.8 and 7.9).

The quality of an MRI scan may be compromised if there are any metallic implants in the field of investigation. MRI is

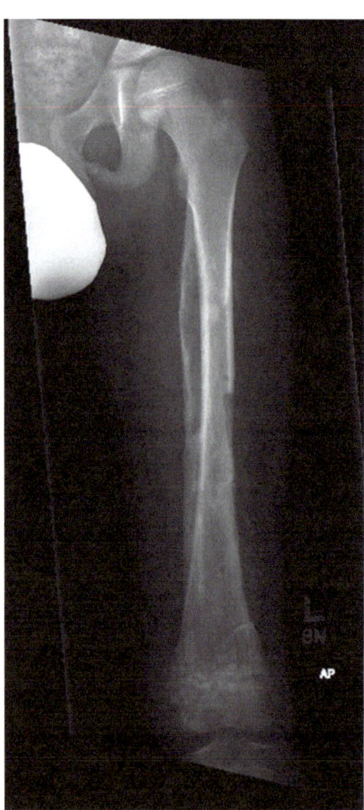

Fig. 7.4 X-ray of femur with advanced osteomyelitis. This depicts necrotic bone distally, lytic lesions of the diaphysis and metaphysis, periosteal reaction and beginning new bone Formation

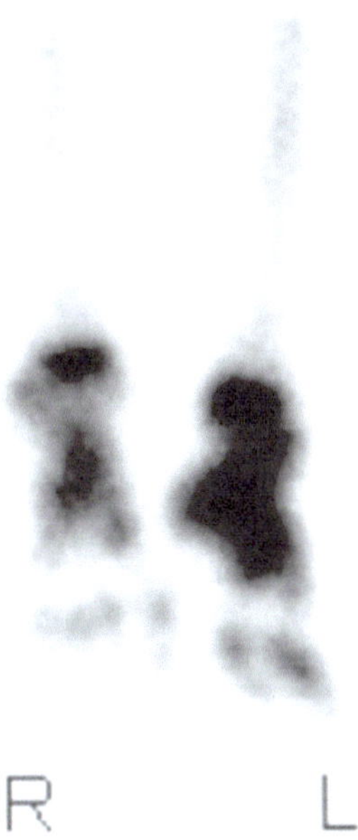

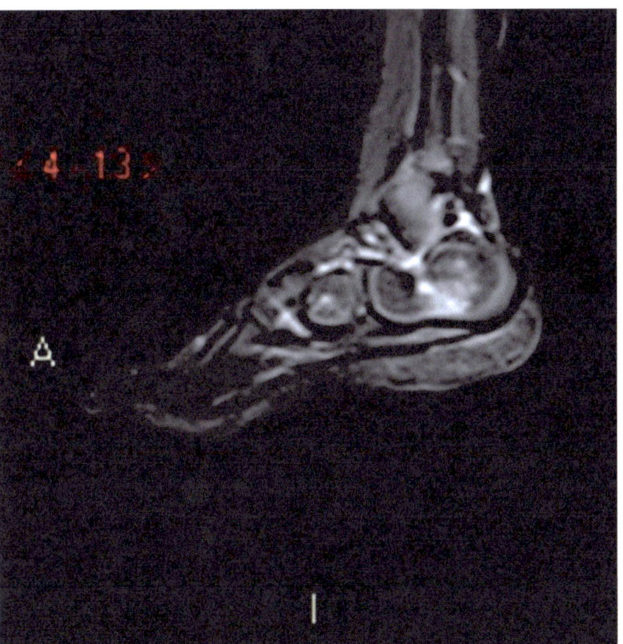

Fig. 7.8 MRI of hindfoot localizing site of inflammation

Fig. 7.6 Respectively in acute hematogenous osteomyelitis

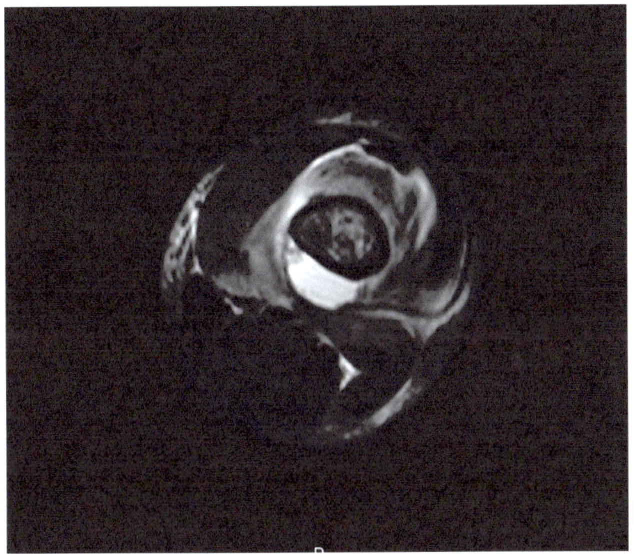

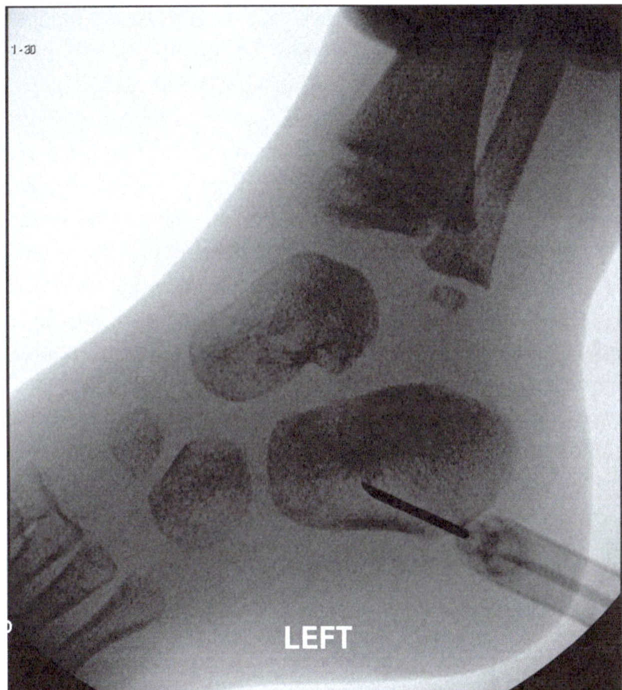

Fig. 7.7 Axial MRI image showing subperiosteal abbess on the T_2 signal

Fig. 7.9 C-arm fluoroscopy showing needle aspiration and/or biopsy of the area of inflammation detected by MRI

costly and, in young children may need to be performed under general anesthesia which adds another significant expense. An MRI scan even over a limited anatomic area can take 45–60 min.

All imaging techniques are limited in their ability to confirm a diagnosis of AHO. They provide the clinician with answers to what is likely and where to biopsy for culture and, if a non-infectious diagnosis is being considered, for histology.

AHO of the Foot

Hematogenous osteomyelitis of the foot is uncommon, accounting for 5–8 % of all AHO in children. Fifty-one percent of these infections are of the calcaneus, 23 % are of the metatarsals, 9 % are of the talus, and 7 % of the phalanges [5]. AHO of the foot, especially the calcaneus, presents more subtly than long bone infections. A history of blunt, nonpenetrating trauma to the affected bone is noted in about 50 % of cases of foot AHO. The injury may be mild and not recalled.

Systemic symptoms of AHO of the foot include fever (often low grade), malaise, and anorexia. Focal symptoms are persistent point tenderness, refusal to bear weight, limping, toe walking, swelling, and redness. The symptoms may be misdiagnosed as inflammation of the growth plate of the calcaneus (apophysitis), inflammation of the tendenous attachments (enthesitis), or plantar fasciitis. Delayed diagnosis may lead to chronic osteomyelitis with bone necrosis, reabsorption, and fusion of the bones of the ankle and foot.

The calcaneus is the foot bone most often affected with AHO [7]. More common is the non-hematogenous infection from a heel prick or the nail through the tennis shoe where organisms such as *Staphylococcus aureus* and *Pseudomonas aeruginosa* are directly innoculated into the bone. As with other sites of AHO, *Staphylococcus aureus* is the bacteria most commonly responsible for infecting the calcaneus. Heel pain out of proportion to any injury should raise suspicion of AHO. X-ray imaging may show lytic lesions and new bone formation if the duration of the infection is 7 days or more. At that point a bone abscess (Brodies abscess) has likely formed and surgical management will be required. Repeated trips to the operating room for debridements and irrigation may be necessary. Recalcitrant cases may require vacuum-assisted wound closure and placement of antibiotic impregnated beads in addition to intravenous antibiotics. AHO of the calcaneus of shorter duration can be identified using MRI. A trephine needle biopsy of a suspected site of infection will allow identification of the organism and its antibiotic susceptibilities. A properly diagnosed and treated case of early osteomyelitis should show considerable improvement of clinical symptoms as well as a decrease in inflammatory laboratory parameters within 48–72 h after starting antibiotic therapy.

AHO has been reported in most of the other bones of the foot. AHO of the metatarsals most commonly affects the first [8]. This presents with limping, focal pain and inability to bear weight. Pathologic fractures, growth arrest, and metatarsal deformity are unpredictable complications. As with other sites of AHO, identification of the bacteria from needle biopsy or surgical decompression, and prolonged antibiotic therapy are required for successful eradication of the infection. Remodeling of the shaft of the metatarsal and valgus deformity may develop despite optimal surgical and antibiotic interventions.

AHO of the talus accounts for less than 1 % of AHO in children [1]. The diagnosis should be considered when a child presents with ankle swelling and limping with antalgic gait. The talus is a flat bone but with a rich blood supply like that of tubular bones. Signs and symptoms of AHO of the talus are subtle and the condition may be misdiagnosed as a result of trauma or cellulitis. Consequently the diagnosis is often delayed resulting in subacute or chronic osteomyelitis with bone necrosis, reabsorption, and pathologic fracture. Ankle instability and restricted dorsiflexion of the ankle are possible sequelae [9].

Treatment of AHO

There are lingering debates about treatment of AHO with antibiotics alone, without needle biopsy or surgery. There are several reports of successful treatment with no surgical intervention. Consideration of the "antibiotics alone" option requires the infection be treated in the first 2–3 days of symptoms. This would be before conventional X-ray imaging would show evidence of boney changes. The clinical course (fever, redness, swelling, and pain) would need to be closely monitored. Blood cultures should be obtained as they may be the only cultures that may allow identification of the organism. With this option, the diagnosis of AHO is not certain, infecting agents are not recovered, and antibiotic susceptibility testing is lacking.

Needle aspiration at the site of maximal tenderness on palpation or a site identified by MRI may confirm or refute the clinical diagnosis, capture the organism, and allow identification and susceptibility testing. More advanced infections will require open debridement and irrigation. Specific antibiotic therapy decisions rest on the results of cultures. Cultures should be obtained of blood, joint fluid (when relevant) and aspirated fluid or tissue from the site of inflammation.

Intravenous antibiotics are given initially for 10–14 days. If there is a suitable oral antibiotic for the offending bacteria, a switch from parenteral to enteral therapy may be made at that time. Generally, oral therapy would continue for another 2 weeks. Changing to oral therapy would require that the patient had made marked clinical improvement and a return to normal or near normal of laboratory inflammatory markers.

Typically a child with AHO would be hospitalized 2–4 days by which time the bacteria would be identified from blood and tissue cultures obtained on day one. Parenteral antibiotic selection is based on gram stain and subsequently modified as directed by susceptibility testing. A peripheral intravenous central catheter (PICC line) is placed if and when the blood culture shows no growth for 48 h. A 2-week course of parenteral antibiotics is completed at home. The patient is seen as an outpatient in 10–14 days for clinical evaluation and repeat of laboratory studies. If all is going well, the PICC line is removed and oral antibiotics, when available, are started and continued for another 2 or 3 weeks with periodic monitoring of temperature, wound appearance, white blood count, and CRP.

Chosing the optimal antibiotic is based on gram stain, culture results, and susceptibility testing. Initial selection may need to be modified as this information becomes available.

If the gram stain shows gram positive cocci (GPC) such as Staphylococcus or Strep pyogenes:

Vancomycin

- Treats all GPCs causing osteomyelitis
- Requires serum through levels to be obtained at least weekly

Nafcillin and other semisynthetic penicillin

- Will not cover MRSA

Clindamycin

- Covers most GPC and some but not all MRSA

Cephalosporin, e.g., cefazolin

- Will not cover MRSA

Linezolid

- Achieves identical blood and tissue levels given intravenously or orally
- Is bacteria static, not cidal
- Very expensive

Because of the increasing frequency of community acquired MRSA, initial treatment of a GPC, infection should include vancomycin with the intent of switching to semisynthetic penicillin, clindamycin, or a cephalosporin if MRSA does not grow.

If the gram stain shows gram negative Rods (GNR) such as *Haemophilus influenza*, or Kingella Kingae, or Pseudomonas:

Piperacillin/tazobactam (*Zosyn*)

- Very broad GNR coverage including pseudomonas

Ceftazidime (*Fortaz*)

- Also has very broad GNR Coverage including Pseudomonas

Pseudomonas is difficult to eradicate. When this organism is identified, two complimentary agents such as piperacillin/tazobactam and tobramycin are commonly ordered.

A perplexing presentation occurs when the gram stain shows many neutrophils but no organisms. When this occurs, an antibiotic regimine is chosen with several factors in mind.

- What is the age of the child? Younger children have a greater propensity to have a broader spectrum of pathogens such as *Kingella Kingae* or *Haemophilus influenza* in addition to Staph.
- How ill is the child? A patient with high fever, malaise, anorexia as well as significantly elevated WBC and CRP would warrant initial broad coverage as there would be little room for error.
- Are there any extenuating factors such as malnutrition, immunodeficiency, or anatomic abnormalities such as congenital heart disease or renal failure?

Any of these scenarios would justify initial antibiotic treatment with a very broad regime covering both gram positive and gram negative bacteria. Alternatively, an older patient perhaps greater than 5 years with recent onset of mild symptoms, low-grade fever, and minimal elevation of inflammatory parameters may be started on single drug coverage such as vancomycin.

More often than not the organism will ultimately grow in cultures. Staph aureus and Strep pyogenes tend to grow out faster 24–48 h, even if they are not seen on gram stain. Other bacteria tend to grow very slowly in culture with no growth appreciated for 4–6 days. These would include Staph coagulase negative (Staph epidermidis) and Kingella Kingae.

Identification of the bacteria and the assoicated susceptibility profile allows the clinician to modify and usually simplify antibiotic regimen. For example, when a gram positive coccus is seen, the initial treatment with vancomycin can be switched to cefazolin if it proves to be sensitive to cephalosporins such as cefazolin or to a semisynthetic penicillin such as nafcillin.

AHO of the bones of the foot as well as the rest of the skeleton are serious but are rarely fatal infections. There may be lifelong sequellae including pathologic fractures, growth plate disruptions with bone angulation deformity and joint destruction due to septic arthritis.

Early detection and identifications of the infecting bacteria coordinated with timely surgical and/or antibiotic treatment achieves the optimal outcome.

References

1. The Red Book. Report of the committee on infectious diseases. Am Acad Pediatr. 2012;2012:873–6.
2. Gorwitz RJ, Krogzon-Moran D, Mc Allister SK, et al. Changes in the prevelance of nasal colonization with Staphylococcus aureus in the United States, 2001–2004. J Infect Dis. 2008;197(9):1226–34.

3. Peltola H, Paakkonen M. Acute osteomyelitis in children. N Engl J Med. 2014;370(4):352–8.
4. Dich VQ, Nelson JD, Haltalin KC. Osteomyelitis in infants and children. Am J Dis Child. 1975;129:1273–8.
5. Treves S. Skeletal scintigraphy in the diagnosis of acute osteomyelitis. Hosp Pract. 1979;14(8):66–72.
6. Lew DP, Valdvogel FA. Osteomyelitis. Lancet. 2004;24(364):369–71.
7. Fox IM, Aponte JM. Hematogenous osteomyelitis of the calcaneus. J Am Pod Med A. 1993;83(12):681–4.
8. Robb JE. Primary acute haematogenous osteomyelitis of an isolated metatarsal in children. Acta Orthop Scand. 1984;55:334–8.
9. Narang S. Pseudomonas osteomyelitis of the talus: review of the pathophysiology and report of a rare case. J Foot Ankle Surg. 2009;48(6):672–6.

Infected Nonunions and Infected Hardware

Jeremy J. Cook and Michael Sganga

Introduction

There are few disease states that challenge a musculoskeletal surgeon like an infected implant. When this infection occurs in the setting of incompletely healed or ununited osseous segments, successful resolution can defy even the most competent of practitioners. Owing to the complexity of this dual diagnosis related to anatomic and functional diversity, few comprehensive guidelines have been delineated that apply throughout the body. Despite a paucity of high-level evidence, consensus has been reached regarding the importance of culture-derived diagnosis, infection control, and osseous stabilization. This chapter will present an overview of this difficult clinical entity and merge the best available evidence with leading practices across specialties. Integration of organizational guidelines, expert opinions, and established foundations of surgical management have resulted in multiple treatment protocols that may serve as decision support tools across the continuum of clinical presentations, particularly for surgeons of foot and ankle pathology.

Pathogenesis of Implant Surgery

Infection is a common risk associated with any surgical intervention, but the presence of an implant substantially elevates the risk of infection during recovery as well as a lifelong risk of seeding infection due to inherent vulnerabilities of their use [1, 2]. As early as 1982, research has shown that the amount of bacterial inoculum required to form infection is 100,000 times less in the presence of an implant [1, 3, 4]. This vulnerability is multifaceted and can be minimized or exacerbated by implant selection. The nature of most biomaterial-associated infections is rooted in colonization by microorganisms and the formation of biofilms [1]. Starting with colonization, this is attributed to the in vivo location of an avascular implant which potentially provides a static site for bacterial colonization that exists outside direct vascular supply. This is relevant because the implant is essentially removed from the influence of the host's immune system meaning spontaneous cure cannot result [1]. Immediately following surgical implantation, the device becomes engulfed in immune-incompetent fibroinflammatory tissue [2]. Surface contaminants introduced perioperatively have an opportunity to colonize the implant during this time which is why antibiotic prophylaxis combined with good sterile technique are important barriers to colonization. This is relevant because once an infection has occurred; antimicrobial agents can only access the implant by diffusion from the surrounding tissues regardless if the medication is delivered orally (PO) or intravenously (IV) [2]. Where standard antibiotic therapy often eradicates planktonic bacteria in a typical infection, the presence of an implant reduces the ability of the medication to adequately penetrate the tissue encapsulating the colonized implants.

Beyond implants serving as colonization sites, the interaction between implant and organism also contributes to the resistance of this disease state. One of the more important interactions is adherence of microorganisms to the implant which can be mediated by specific factors called adhesins and nonspecific factors such as surface tension, hydrophobicity, and electrostatic forces [4]. This can lead to accumulation of the organisms that are interconnected by an extracellular matrix which serves as an isolating barrier against host defenses. This aggregation of organisms and matrix is known as a biofilm [5]. It is important to recognize that bacterial phenotype can vary. Single cells can act independently as with the planktonic state or they can act collectively as is observed within the aggregates of a biofilm growth phenotype [6].

J.J. Cook, DPM, MPH, CPH, FACFAS (✉)
Division of Podiatric Surgery, Department of Surgery,
Mount Auburn Hospital, 330 Mount Auburn Street, Cambridge,
MA 02138, USA
e-mail: jeremycook@post.harvard.edu

M. Sganga, DPM
Mount Auburn Hospital, 330 Mount Auburn Street, Cambridge,
MA 02138, USA

© Springer International Publishing Switzerland 2015
T.J. Boffeli (ed.), *Osteomyelitis of the Foot and Ankle*, DOI 10.1007/978-3-319-18926-0_8

In a typical nonimplant infection, biofilm formation takes time to develop and is associated with chronic infections. Conversely, the presence of an implant permits rapid colonization and biofilm formation [1]. Once a stable aggregation has formed, the bacteria produce extracellular polymeric substance (EPS) forming an antibiotic and host defense-resistant barrier [7].

In addition to functioning as a physical barrier against the host immune response, the microenvironment of the biofilm itself enables resistance mechanisms that make the infection more recalcitrant than a typical infection. One such mechanism is quorum sensing, where cells within a biofilm communicate with each other to change gene expression throughout the aggregate. Similarly, the close proximity of the bacterial cells permits rapid exchange of genes via plasmids. Another consequence of biofilm formation is as metabolites diminish and waste accumulates, the bacteria enter a quiescent state in order to promote long-term survival [5]. This quiescence contributes to the frequently observed indolent nature of this infection and certainly supports the chronicity of this disease.

Even though biofilm formation is a feature commonly observed in infected nonunions; the organisms creating the biofilm and the setting they predominate is varied. Studies have shown that some pathogens are more commonly associated with joint replacements while others are more frequently seen in fracture management. These pathogens are coagulase negative staphylococcus for joint replacements and *Staphylococcus aureus* for fractures [1, 4, 5]. Table 8.1 summarizes the epidemiology of infecting organisms observed both in prosthetic joint and traumatic implants. The prevalence of one organism over another suggests that procedure-specific factors may enhance or inhibit the infective process. Bioimplant characteristics are one such factor that have been extensively studied and continue to evolve with medicine.

Implant Infection and Epidemiology

Fixation methods have evolved in the past century to provide surgeons with a variety of methods to stabilize a fracture. As our understanding of bone healing has become more

Table 8.1 Microbial prevalence varies with the setting of the surgical implants. [1, 4, 5]

	Joint replacement (%)	All fractures (%)
Staphylococcus aureus	12–23	30
Coagulase Negative Staphylococcus	30–43	22
Gram Negative Bacilli	3–6	10
Anaerobes	2–4	5
Enterococci	3–7	3
Streptococci	9–10	1
Polymicrobial	10–12	27
Unknown	10–11	2

sophisticated, so too has our implant selection process become more elaborate. Just as implant design influences bone healing, these same characteristics impart a susceptibility to complications [2]. Copious amounts of literature have explored the effects of implant architecture, surface interaction, and material constitution on infection resistance; but adequate discussion of that topic is a chapter unto itself. In this chapter we will briefly discuss some relevant implant features encountered on a routine basis.

Several studies have demonstrated that surface nanotopography influences susceptibility to infection. In one bench top study, a porous coated cobalt chromium implant required 40 times lower inoculum of bacteria to generate osteomyelitis than its smooth polished control. Yet another study reported greater infection resistance in textured titanium implants as compared to a smooth polished stainless steel control [8]. While surface topography is an important feature, it appears that implant material, which confers biocompatibility, is a more significant consideration.

The most common materials used in fixation or joint replacements are electropolished stainless steel (EPSS) or titanium. Titanium implants have the potential of direct anchorage to bone via a process called osseointegration. Implants that undergo osseointegration connect directly to living bone and have enhanced structural stability. This is in contrast to EPSS implants, where evidence suggests that a thin fibrous tissue is interposed between the device and bone. The presence of any barrier further inhibits circulation and penetration of immunocompetent elements into an already isolated space. This is more common among EPSS materials than titanium [7, 9, 10]. Some authors have concluded that titanium is less susceptible to infection and colonization because its biocompatibility profile also reduces tissue reaction and has less corrosion than traditional stainless steel fixation [11].

Implant architecture is another feature that influences infection potential. Cannulated devices have an intrinsic dead space that is susceptible to colonization and growth. Studies of intramedullary nails found that solid devices were less likely to develop an infection compared to the cannulated designs. Subsequent investigations found that reamed intramedullary devices nails were more likely to become infected than unreamed implants. The authors concluded that unreamed nails better preserve the medullary blood supply and minimize the deadspace [1]. Continuing with the theme of preservation of native tissue, consider the role of plate fixation. Dynamic compression plates (DCP) compress tightly to bone which often leads to necrosis of adjacent periosteum. In a preclinical comparison study conducted by the AO foundation, investigators found that a locking plate design imparts less pressure on the underlying tissue and was ten times more resistant to infection than the DCP [7].

In addition to design characteristics and technique, the function of the implant also impacts the epidemiology of infection. For example, reports indicate that prosthetic joint implants are more prone to infection by gram-positive cocci than gram-negative rods [1]. Even within the domain of prosthetic implants variation exists; where larger weight bearing joints have higher infection rates than smaller and non-weight bearing implants, referring to those of the hand and shoulder versus ankle and knee [1].

The setting of implantation is very important and has a significant impact on the risk of infection. Few studies truly examine the long-term outcomes of overall surgical site infection (SSI) with fixation, however studies indicate that elective surgery carries a lower risk of infection than trauma-related surgery. Roughly 5 % of all inserted internal fixation will become infected including all types [4], and that is of great concern to any surgeon. A large, single center retrospective analysis of all patients undergoing "clean" elective podiatric surgery over a 7-year period found a surgical site infection (SSI) rate of 3.1 %. They reported that 71 % of the cultured pathogens were coagulase positive or negative staphylococcus and an alarming 87 % were resistant to penicillin or ampicillin [12]. Their analysis found that cases that included internal fixation had a statistically significant higher risk for developing post-op infection. A large case–control trial used a multiple logistic regression model to determine that the odds of prosthetic joint infection were 36 times greater in the setting of a SSI [OR: 35.9; 95 % confidence interval 8.3–154.6] [13]. Recent years have seen an increased interest in foot and ankle joint replacements. Technological advancements, particularly in total ankle replacements (TAR), have increased the relevance of periprosthetic joint infection (PJI) to foot and ankle surgeons. PJI is considered to be among the most devastating of prosthetic complications because the majority of infected implants will go on to failure [5, 14]. A 2012 case–control study evaluated the risk factors for periprosthetic ankle joint infection in 130 cases. Risk factors such as any prior surgery in the joint, procedure duration, and low preoperative functional ability were all statistically significant. Among the most significant risk factors for PJI they identified persistent wound dehiscence (OR: 15.38) and wound drainage (OR: 7.0). Conclusions of that study were that prior surgery at the site increased infection by greater than 4.5 times, dehiscence increased chances of wound infection by 15 times, and infection was 7 times more likely with a draining wound [15].

It is contextually important to distinguish between the "clean" elective procedures discussed above and the less controlled environment of trauma. In the setting of traumatic injury, preventing SSI or implant associated infection becomes much more complicated and is heavily dependent on whether it is an open versus closed fracture pattern. Research suggests that trauma cases are 2.5 times more likely to develop SSIs than elective cases [16]. Severity of trauma is strongly related to implant infection risk with closed fractures reported as having an incidence of 1–2 % infection versus infection rates as high as 30 % in open fractures [17].

Focusing on ankle trauma, a database study of 57,183 patients reported that open injuries posed a four times greater risk of developing post-op infection as compared to closed fractures following ORIF [18]. To further elaborate the effect of soft tissue integrity, consider the following outcomes. Internal fixation of tibial fractures via an intramedullary nail has demonstrated infection rates of 2–3 % in closed fractures. In the presence of an open fracture the incidence jumps to 21 %, and in the setting of severe soft tissue damage the incidence of SSI has been as high as 50 % [7].

When dealing with open injuries it is always prudent to focus on the amount of soft tissue destruction and potential coverage. A further complicating issue is the necrosis, perfusion limitations, and lack of immune system ability to reach edematous or severely disrupted soft tissue envelopes [7].

Tenants of Treatment

The previous sections of this chapter have presented the epidemiology, pathogenesis, and risk factors of infected implants. The remaining sections will focus on treatment principles and protocols that enhance outcomes. Because other chapters provide in-depth discussion of imaging and laboratory-based diagnosis/monitoring of bone infections, this chapter will minimize those features. Similarly, specific antibiotic agents and surgical excision extensively covered elsewhere in this book will be limited to their role in the overall treatment paradigm of infected implants.

Much of current treatment practices are an amalgam of traditional teaching, anecdotal evidence, and medicolegal considerations. Just as individual variation exists, so too is there significant variety of treatment protocols between institutions and countries [5]. Despite a diversity of settings and patient factors, the primary management objectives are: elimination of the infection, promote osseous stability, and optimize patient function in the context of the intended original procedure. Management of infected implants and nonunions require a multidisciplinary collaboration that integrates local and systemic antimicrobial therapy with adequate debridement, wound, and dead space management while anticipating the need for osseous stabilization in the setting of ununited bone segments and large deficits with bone graft.

Before discussing specific management protocols we need to consider factors that alter treatment. The importance of timing from the implantation, vector of infection, and host risk factors have been established by countless publications and often direct decision making.

Although there is overlap with treatment approach in a variety of situations, there are other areas where divergence is significant. Merging current practices into a cogent protocol that encompasses every clinical scenario is an impossible task. Instead we've consolidated the treatment protocols by the surgical setting and implant's functional objective, specifically relative to the purpose of the implant within the body. We refer to this as the *Intended Original Procedure*. For instance, when dealing with osteotomies, fractures, and fusions, the therapeutic goals are fundamentally similar. In these settings the implants are intended to promote osteosynthesis, maintain appropriate alignment of osseous segments and rigid stability in an effort to restore or optimize function. Beyond similar therapeutic goals, bone healing in fractures and osteotomies can be treated as equivalent since the process of vascularization and bone formation are analogous despite variations in the details of healing [19, 20].

The other implant setting we will discuss is that of prosthetic joints. Like the previous example, these implants seek to provide good alignment but desired stability is related to the periarticular-implant interface which preserves function of the joint. Prosthetic joints don't require osteosynthesis to achieve their objectives, but compromise of the interface leads to instability and diminished function. The management tenants of these two broad groups not only have several areas of overlap but also significant differences. We will highlight similarity and diversity of treatments later in the formal protocols.

Timing and vector of colonization are innately connected, therefore they are presented here in concert to add to the overall context. Much of the knowledge base regarding these two factors is derived from the prosthetic joint literature and the following discussion will reflect that fact.

The method of infection dissemination aids in identifying the pathologic organism. All surgical implants are vulnerable to two methods of implant colonization: exogenous and hematogenous. Exogenous refers to an inoculation from outside of the body that can occur during the implantation procedure itself or during a subsequent procedure and it usually arises within 2 years postoperatively [1, 21]. An example is postoperative arthrocentesis of the joint. An infection is classified as acute when it arises within just days and is usually due to *Staphylococcus aureus*; or subacute that occurs within weeks and is likely due to Coagulase Negative Staphylococcus [1]. The hematogenous vector occurs when the implant is seeded from another source in the body via the blood stream at any point after surgery [1]. As noted earlier in the chapter, prosthetic implants are at a lifelong risk of colonization and many reports have concluded that any presentation of infection more than two years post-implantation is likely due to hematogenous spread [5, 13, 21–23]. The risk of hematogenous colonization increases in the setting of bacteremia; studies report the rate of PJI as 34–39 % while all other nonarticular implants were shown to have a 7 % chance of seeding [1, 5, 23, 24].

For PJI, the classes are defined as early, delayed, and late [1, 5, 21, 23]. In the early phase, within 1–3 months of joint replacement, the origin is exogenous and it is likely that infection was seeded during implantation. The delayed phase is any time from 3 months up until 2 years postoperative. Clinical presentation typically includes vague symptoms of chronic pain in the absence of systemic signs of infection [22]. It is important to note that any painful prosthetic could represent a PJI or aseptic loosening, and therefore diagnosing and treating this is heavily relied on clinical judgment [21]. Seeding of delayed infection is thought to be through an exogenous source that was acquired during implantation. The late phase of PJI is characterized by onset of greater than 1–2 years postoperatively. The two main causes of late infection are described as hematogenous spread or a late manifestation of infection acquired during insertion. This will present with a more acute and abrupt onset of pain and symptoms and can be accompanied by a concomitant infection at another site in the body [21]. Statistics for elective surgery show that rates of hematogenous spread of infection for total knee or hip are around 1–2 %[21] while elbow or ankle arthroplasty are >5 % with primary implant surgery [1]. In support of that data, a study by Kessler of 26 infected ankle replacements found that 4 (15 %) were seeded by hematogenous origin and the remaining 22 (85 %) were through exogenous means [15]. The overall risk of hematogenous spread to a prosthetic joint is estimated to be 0.25–0.5 % per year, per prosthesis [1]. This points out the lower likelihood of hematogenous spread, however it is a real entity that cannot be overlooked.

The timing of infection in nonarticular fixation is similar to but also differs from that of prosthetic joints. The familiar early, delayed, and late presentations remain, however the time periods of onset are very different as are the most common organisms involved [25]. The early period represents less than two weeks and is described as acquired preoperatively during the trauma or during the implant surgery. These are often high virulence organisms, most commonly *Staphylococcus aureus* and Gram-Negative Bacilli such as *E. coli* [26, 27]. The delayed time frame is between 2 and 10 weeks, delayed and late manifestations are similar in presentation, course, and outcome and therefore grouped together in this discussion [28]. The late presentation is represented by greater than ten weeks and can be acquired during the trauma, implant surgery, or postoperative wound-healing period. This is described as being caused by an organism of low virulence such as Coagulase Negative Staphylococcus or Propionibacterium Acnes. In comparison to prosthetic joint replacements, infection of fracture fixation is rarely caused by hematogenous spread as described above at 7 % versus nearly 40 % of prostheses [24]. The type of pathogen involved in these infections also differs by type of fixation as discussed earlier. A large consecutive study of 132 internal-fixation device-associated infections found that the most common infectious agent was *Staphylococcus aureus* accounting for 30 % of the infections. *Staphylococcus aureus* is most commonly introduced during the preoperative initial trauma or when placing percutaneous fixation [4]. Coagulase negative *Staphylococcus* represented 22 % and Gram-negative Bacilli 10 % of the total isolated pathogens with greater than one pathogen isolated in 27 % of the cases [4].

Foundations of Treatment

Every protocol presented in this chapter will start with the same basic step: incision and drainage with adequate debridement. This stage which we will refer to as the *initial debridement* and is the foundation of our care. The data obtained during this phase will direct all aspects of the comprehensive treatment plan. The initial debridement will: (1) Identify the infectious organism, (2) Excise nonviable tissue and abscess, (3) Stabilize osseous segments, (4) Control infection via culture-directed antimicrobials, (5) Determine the necessity of soft tissue and dead space management.

The decision to perform the initial debridement is dependent on several factors, one of the most important is overall status of the patient. An example is a case where a patient treated with a foot or ankle implant has been hospitalized for sepsis. Infectious disease and the critical care team are unable to identify the source of the infection but suspect that the retained implant may be the nidus. The patient is immunosuppressed and therefore the absence of local signs of infection is unreliable. The medical team believes that the implant must be excluded as the source and determine that the patient is stable enough for incision and drainage with debridement and removal of the implant. This is a clinical scenario that you've either encountered or will encounter at some point in your career. In these instances it is advisable to perform the initial debridement because of the life-threatening consequences. Even if the implant is not the source, the procedure is not wasted effort. The likelihood of a patient with documented sepsis seeding an implant is quite high at just under a 40 % and removal may prevent a future occurrence [1]. Aside from this scenario, the decision to perform the initial debridement is unclear.

Once the decision is made to proceed with initial debridement, performance of the five foundations is critical to an optimal outcome. Other authors have discussed the importance of intraoperative cultures so our focus will be on optimal collection practices as they relate to infected implants and nonunions. During the course of debridement, tissue samples should be collected for aerobic and anaerobic cultures and pathology. Specimens should be collected from deep sources and sinus tracts are notoriously an unreliable culture source when present. If there is a communicating sinus tract or long-standing chronic ulceration then that specimen should be sent to pathology separately to evaluate if malignant transformation has occurred [17]. If circumstances dictate that the implant should be removed, then it should be submitted for microbiologic culture as well. But sensitivity of implant derived cultures can be imprecise. One emerging method of enhancing sensitivity is implant sonication. This technique can dislodge bacteria from the implant and is requested when submitting the implant for cultures. One study of hip and knee infections found that sonication had a sensitivity of 78.5 % while traditional culture only had a sensitivity of 60.8 % in the same patients [21].

Identification of the organism is so important that current recommendations are to withhold antibiotics for 2 weeks prior to debridement in order to increase organism yield from intraoperative samples if medically possible. Many resources advise that intraoperative cultures should be taken from multiple sites to improve accuracy, but the anatomic restrictions of the foot and ankle may restrict this methodology. Finally, in situations where the diagnosis of infection or aseptic loosening is unclear, it is possible to send specimens for frozen section to determine a rapid assessment [21]. This is easily accomplished at most institutions and can have significant repercussions on the treatment plan. Regardless, some organisms do take longer than others to grow in culture so it may be prudent to wait 14 days prior to finalizing plans with the patient.

Debridement has already been discussed in other chapters but will be briefly discussed in the context of this chapter. Aggressive and thorough debridement is an important part of the process since it reduces bioburden, eliminates the nidus of infection and eliminates nonviable tissue in the local environment [15, 29]. Inadequate debridement can lead to spread of the infection and additional tissue loss. It also predisposes the patient to chronic infection and its attendant sequelae. Multiple debridements may be necessary; in fact, a study by Patzak has reported that 26 % of cultures remained positive after the initial debridement [30]. Our experience has been that the more extensive the infection, particularly with gross purulence, that multiple debridements are necessary. This should not be viewed as poor or indecisive care; rather it reflects the difficulty in achieving balance between adequate debridement and tissue preservation.

Where appropriate, early debridement can disrupt biofilm formation or eliminate it completely when performed early and extensively [15]. This specifically involves opening the area, debriding infected soft tissue and washing out the implant only [22]. Occasionally debridement is so extensive that even with stable osseous segments, the potential of iatrogenic fracture becomes a concern. Several studies have concluded that even in the setting of gross stability, if debridement reduces cortical volume to less than 70 %, structural integrity is compromised and must be augmented [31–33]. Several options are available in this situation. Cast immobilization is simple but imprecise. It lacks compression, and can hamper wound care. The latter limitation can be ameliorated by bivalving the cast but at the cost of stability. A more physiologic stabilization is external fixation which imparts stability

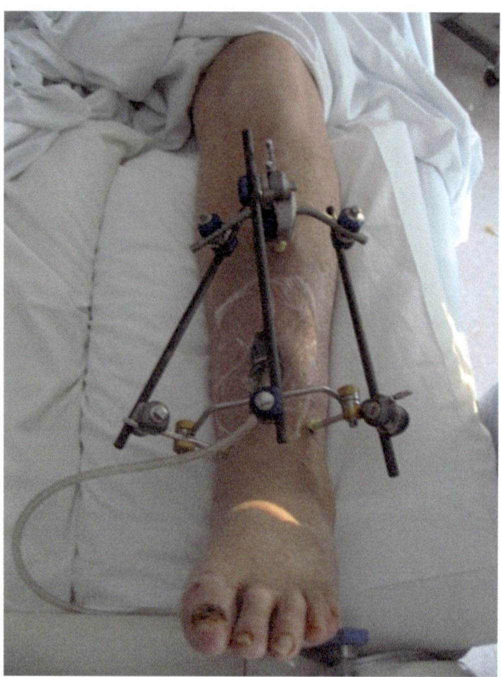

Fig. 8.1 Large segmental bone loss can lead to instability which threatens successful outcomes. External fixation provides excellent stability in a variety of settings and permits inspection of the soft tissue envelope

via wires and pins remote to the infected area (Fig. 8.1). It is superior to cast immobilization in that it provides precise stabilization with the ability for compression and permits wound care. The primary disadvantages are that it is costly, technically demanding, and is frequently poorly tolerated by patients. These same stabilization options are also appropriate in the setting of unstable bone segments. Although stability is obviously important in terms of preserving function; what may be less evident is that stability is beneficial for control of infection.

Preclinical research demonstrated that even with direct inoculation of a fracture site following surgery, unstable fractures were more likely to develop infections. Investigators concluded that fixated fractures were less likely to develop osteomyelitis than unfixated fractures [34, 35]. Worlock expanded on this work and used *Staphylococcus aureus* contaminated implants to determine the effect of rigid versus unstable fixation. He reported that less stable unlocked intramedullary pins had double the risk of developing osteomyelitis than the rigid plate fixation [36]. Earlier work by Friedrich et al., reported that severity of instability impacted infection rate and further stated that there was no observed difference in time to union between infected and uninfected fractures stabilized with rigid fixation [37]. The previous studies highlighted the importance of stability in preventing infection and the Friedrich study evinces that bone healing can occur in the setting of infection given adequate stability. This is particularly pertinent in the early postoperative phase of an osteotomy, fracture or fusion where fixation is critical to stabilization. Currently available evidence generally indicates that as long as a device provides rigid fixation, its role as a nidus and impediment to immunologic response is superseded by the stability it imparts [17, 38]. The consequences of stability on decision making are a good segue into actual treatment protocols.

Protocols

Regardless of any subsequent facts, the first step is adequate initial debridement of infected or nonviable tissue and collection of cultures and pathology specimens (Fig. 8.2). Next, assess osseous stability. Depending on the timing we typically encounter one of three scenarios: (1) the debridement leads to a large defect and the bone segment and implant become unstable; (2) the bone is healed and even after debridement the segment remains stable; (3) the bone is not healed [1, 17, 39, 40]. A preoperative computed tomography (CT) scan can aid in analysis of union as well, although fixation artifact may limit utility. Ultimately, evaluation of bone healing and segmental stability is an intraoperative assessment post-debridement. The first scenario occurs when the debridement leads to a large defect and the bone segment or implant become unstable. In this setting the evidence supports removal of the implant and temporary stabilization and progression through the management protocol. In the second scenario, where following debridement the bone segment is healed and remains stable, then current recommendations are to simply remove the implant and maintain culture-directed systemic therapy for four to six weeks. Removal of the implant in this scenario is simple because the fixation has served its purpose and no longer is necessary. The clarity of this choice becomes less obvious when infectious onset is early in the postoperative period and the bone is unhealed (scenario 3), the titular infected nonunion. For example, if infection occurs less than 4 weeks following fixation of a fracture, there is little chance that the construct will be stable. However, if the infection occurs after that fourth week then it is necessary to determine if fixation is still the primary stabilizing force. This again refers to basics of AO principles and load sharing by implanted fixation which typically remain stable during the first 6 weeks of healing [38]. A study by Sarmiento et al. in 1995 reported that early stability is related to formation of soft callus in fracture healing and begins at 2–3 weeks post-injury. They highlighted that this process provides enough inherent stability to prevent shortening, but may remain vulnerable to angulation [41]. Their observations support the perspective that intrinsic stability can occur early in the healing process. This does not mean to imply the implant should always be removed without subsequent stabilization. As our protocol discusses the use of an

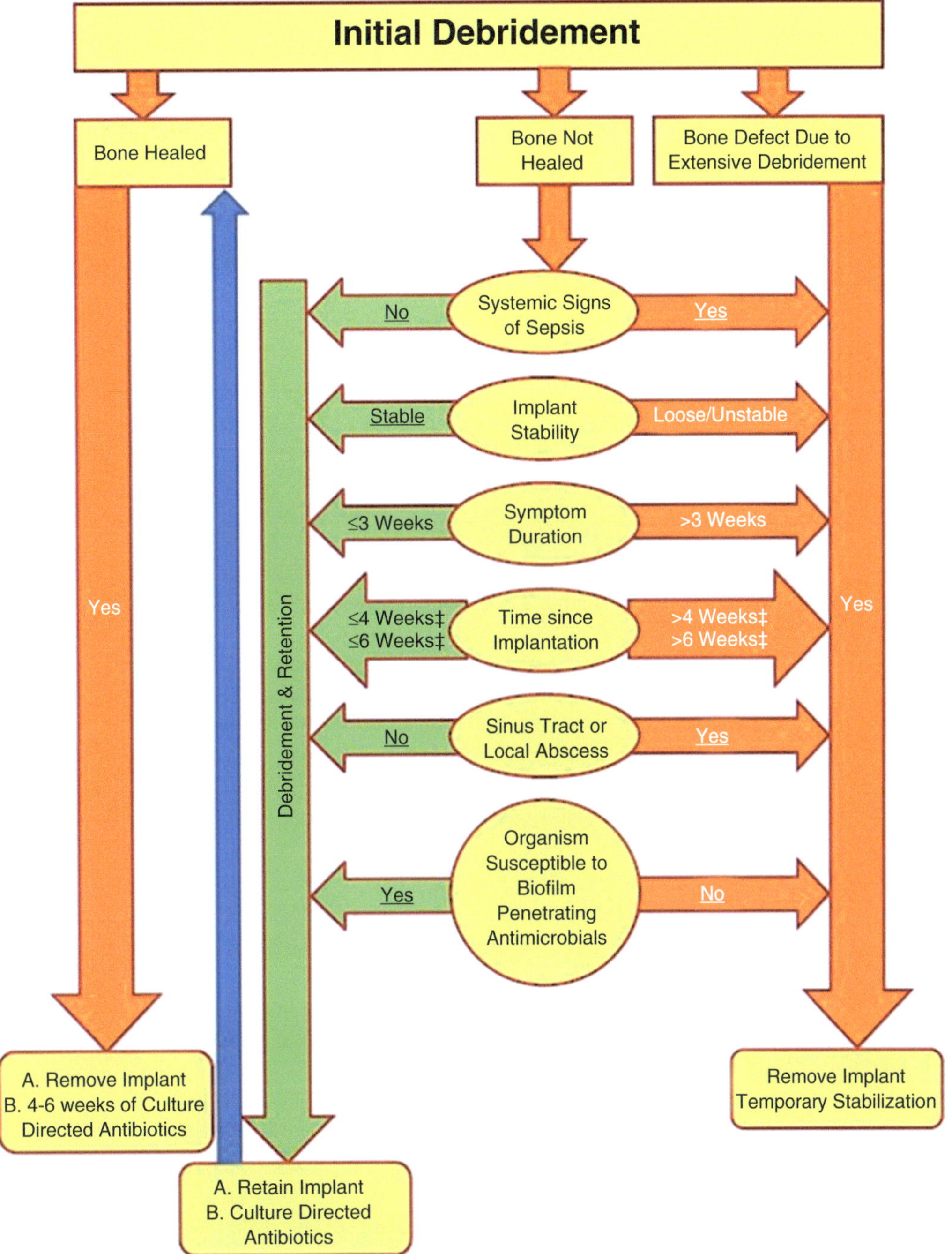

Fig. 8.2 Following the initial debridement, the decision to remove or retain implants must be made. Risk factors have been identified that enhance the likelihood of treatment success. †=Prosthetic joint infection; ‡=Osteotomies, fractures, and fusions. Adapted from Trampuz and Zimmerli [4], Mouzopoulos [17], IDSA [21]

external fixator or cast should be applied in certain situations and limiting weight bearing is certainly advisable as well [31].

Whether to remove or retain hardware in the face of infection is a long-standing topic that remains hotly debated, and like much of medicine requires further investigation. Absolute directives do not exist, but luminaries in biomaterial infection such as Werner Zimmerli, M.D., Andrej Trampuz, M.D., and Peter Ochsner, M.D. have identified risk factors which increase the likelihood of poor outcomes if an implant is retained in the setting of infection. This strategy is referred to as, *debridement with retention*, and has a success rate of greater than 80 % if cases meet the following criteria: the implant is stable, the duration of infection is less than 3 weeks, no sinus tract or abscess are present, and the pathogen is susceptible to antimicrobial therapy [1, 21–23, 42]. Published results demonstrate that if these criteria are not met, successful eradication is between 14 and 68 %, although this is primarily derived from studies of hip and knee prosthetic infections [4, 21, 22, 39, 42, 43]. A brief discussion of the criteria is warranted. Implant stability has been discussed extensively throughout this chapter; the relevance within the prosthetic joint setting is that once instability occurs, revision becomes necessary for consequences independent of the infection such as subsidence. Infections that are less than 3 weeks in duration are generally not as extensive and may not have compromised the implant beyond salvage. Similarly, implants and union sites that are contiguous with an abscess or a sinus tract are more likely to be infected. The virulence and resistance of the organism is also a major factor and the presence of high-risk organisms increase the risk of relapse [23]. Studies demonstrate that in the presence of methicillin-resistant *Staphylococcus aureus* (MRSA) a failure rate of greater than 80 % is seen when attempting the debridement and retention strategy [22, 44]. Zimmerli and Trampuz have consistently identified those difficult-to-treat or resistant organisms which they believe warrant removal of the implant rather retention. These include Rifampin- or Methicillin-resistant *Staphylococcus aureus*, small-colony variants of staphylococci, enterococci, quinolone-resistant *Pseudomonas aeruginosa* or *Candida* [4, 21, 23].

The debridement and retention approach varies somewhat with osteotomies, fractures, and fusions (OFF). Complete eradication of infection is not the primary goal when the site is unhealed or unstable; rather consolidation and preventing chronic osteomyelitis are the primary objectives [1, 39]. In this setting, retention of hardware is appropriate if: the implant is stable and removal would lead to union site instability, infection is less than four (PJI) to six (OFF implant) weeks post-implantation, duration of symptoms less than three weeks, absence of systemic infection, and the culture definitively identifies a low-risk organism susceptible to appropriate antibiotics [4, 21, 23]. Clinical investigations report a 68–86 % success rate when these criteria are met. As noted in the prior section regarding stability, effective rigid internal fixation is beneficial in osteomyelitis control. Utilizing this approach Rightmire found 68 % of patients achieved successful union with the original hardware in place. Likewise, Berkes treated 121 cases complicated by contiguous wound infection and reported 71 % union. Trampuz reported an 86 % success rate in 132 cases of infected fracture fixation. These studies also identified case risk factors which increased the likelihood of failure: heavy smokers, initially open fractures, use of an intramedullary fixation device, or a persistent sinus tract. While the implant is retained, antibiotics are considered suppressive. Once consolidation has occurred, the implant can be removed but appropriate antibiotic therapy should be continued for an additional 4–6 weeks post removal [4]. One must keep in mind that eventual hardware removal after initial retention while awaiting consolidation is not a failure. This is described well in the article by Berkes et al. who state, "Treating an infection at the site of a union is preferable to treating an infection at the site of a nonunion" [39].

Removal of Implants

The rest of the management strategies require removal of the implant (Fig. 8.3). The factors that contribute to this decision are at least partially derived from the risk factors previously discussed. The union site is not healed and the implant is unstable either due to the infection itself or as a result of excessive debridement. The infection onset is delayed to late meaning greater than 4 weeks. Culture results were inconclusive or the organism was high risk. Finally, the presence of a persistent draining sinus tract associated with the implant increases the likelihood that the implant is contaminated.

The main protocols to be discussed are staged exchanges, permanent resection, amputation, and medical therapy. Staged techniques allow for a reimplantation of hardware or restabilization of bone segments following adequate debridement with copious irrigation in a single or multiple surgeries and have improved outcomes [15].

The 1-stage exchange, also referred to as a direct exchange, involves removal of all implant components and cement. The procedure continues with complete debridement of devitalized bone and soft tissue and lastly reimplantation of new clean hardware followed by 4–6 weeks of culture-directed IV or highly bioavailable oral antimicrobial therapy for a total of 12 weeks of antimicrobial therapy. A 1-stage approach most commonly occurs in two scenarios. The diagnosis of aseptic nonunion or implant subsidence is assumed and multiple postoperative cultures yield the same organism consistently. In the second scenario, the pathogenic organism has been identified preinitial debridement via arthrocentesis or cultures and the surgeon decides to perform the procedure in a single stage. In the first scenario, the judicious use of frozen section is useful for determination of aseptic process, and can be combined with intraoperative cultures to rule out infection. The common indications in this setting are that the patient is medically unable or unwilling to undergo a multiple staged procedure. The majority of clinical evidence regarding this approach is derived from total hip replacements where successful outcomes have occurred between 80 and 100 %. The success of the direct exchange has been attributed to extensive debridement and incorporation of antibiotic impregnated cement that secures the new implant [21, 23, 42, 45]. The latter factor limits direct exchange in other prosthetic joints and implants that don't

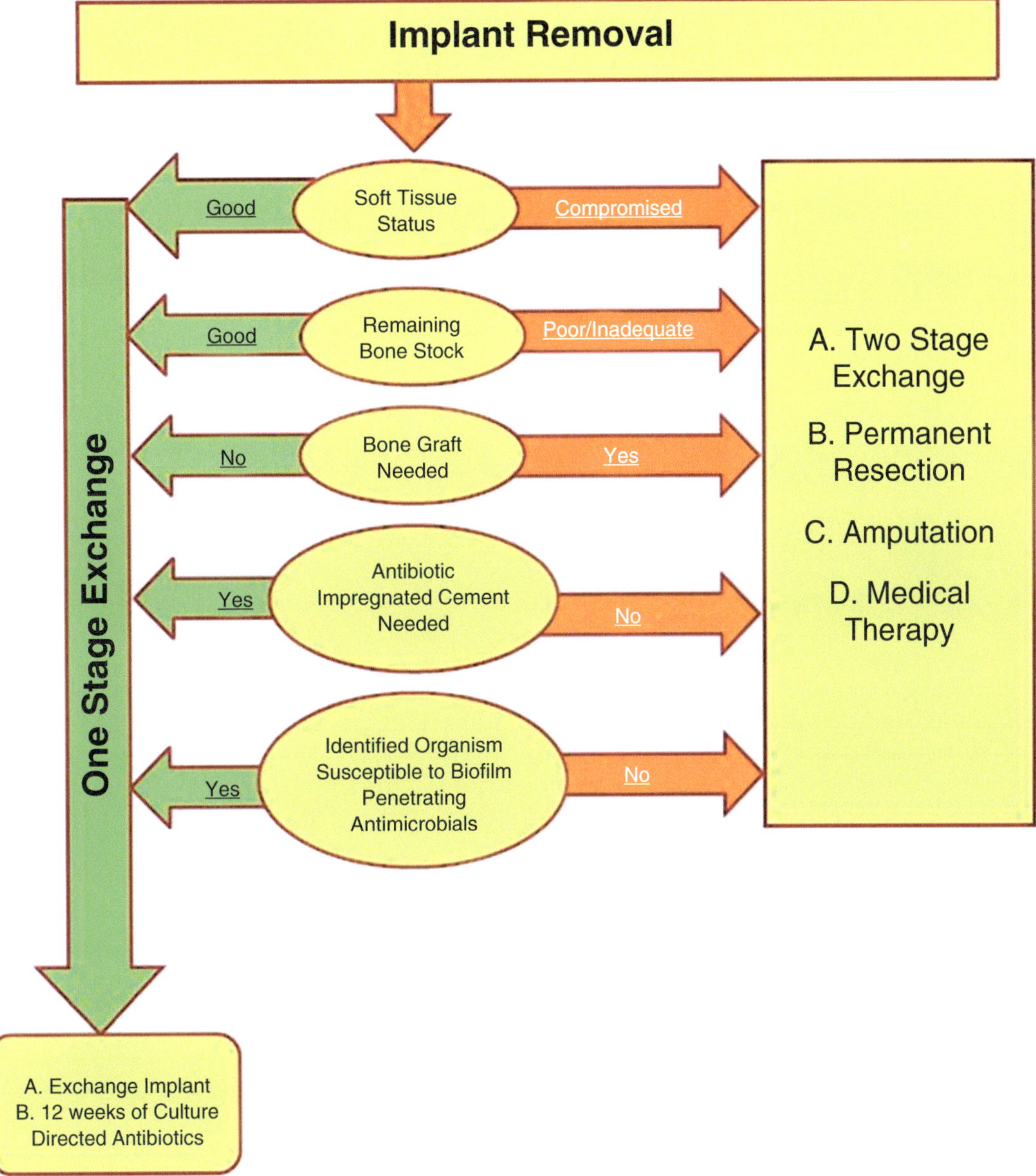

Fig. 8.3 Major considerations for One Stage Exchange. Adapted from Trampuz and Zimmerli [4], Mouzopoulos [17], IDSA [21]

use antibiotic cement or those cases that require bone graft. Advantages of a single-stage exchange are the need for only one procedure, reduced hospitalization and reduced associated cost, and relatively improved patient satisfaction [45]. As noted in the debridement and retention strategy, the presence or absence of certain parameters will optimize the likelihood of success in these cases.

Patients treated with this approach should be relatively healthy with good bone stock capable of supporting the goals of the originally intended procedure and a viable soft tissue envelope. This strategy is not indicated in patients where other attempts have failed at single-stage exchange, infection has involved the neurovascular bundle, or in the setting of active sinus tract [45]. Recommendations differ slightly based on anatomic considerations. For example, based on contemporary Infectious Disease Society of America recommendations total treatment with intravenous or highly bioavailable oral antibiotics with good biofilm penetration should last 6 months for knee replacements and 3 months for hip and ankle replacements [21]. Thus far, the common link between our retention and single-stage exchange strategies has been the persistence of an implant during the antibiotic therapy phase. Prerequisites for this approach are that the pathologic organism is susceptible to antimicrobials with adequate biofilm penetration. The remaining methods will remove the implant during the antimicrobial therapy.

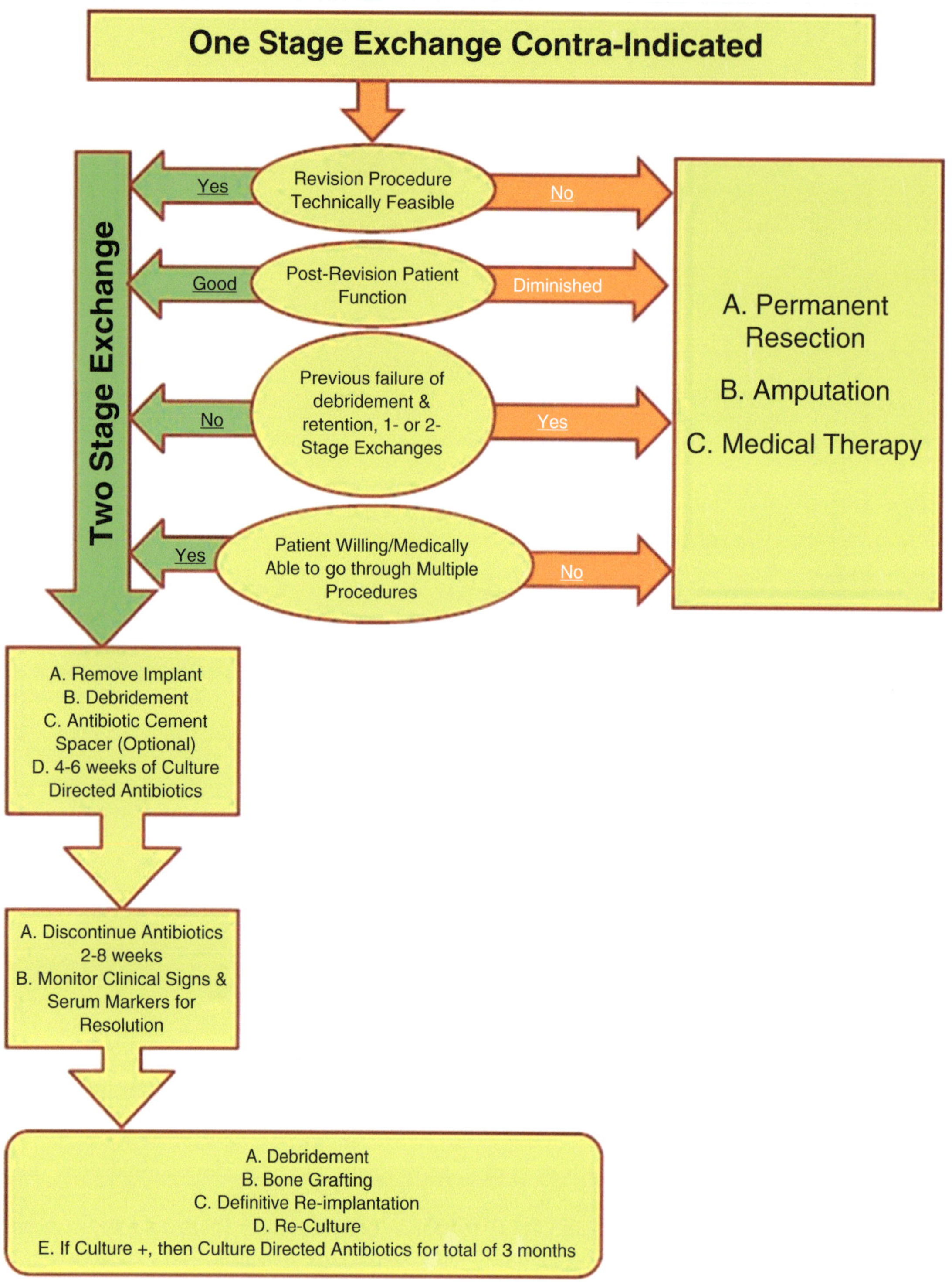

Fig. 8.4 The two-stage (multi-stage) exchange strategy is highly versatile and tolerates comprised soft tissue and poor bone stock. Differences of opinion exist related to the duration of the interval before performing the definitive stage. Adapted from Trampuz and Zimmerli [4], Mouzopoulos [17], IDSA [21]

If circumstances prohibit a direct exchange, then a 2-stage exchange is the next logical step (Fig. 8.4). This approach is the preferred method for management of chronic infections, particularly in unstable or loosening prosthesis. Recent literature points to a success rate of greater than 87 % when implementing a proper 2-stage exchange [21, 23]. It is widely accepted in the literature that treatment of late or chronic infections be treated by two or multiple staged procedures, however, there is no clear evidence that more stages have an improved success rate over single-stage procedures [45]. Regardless of the previously detailed risk factors, surgeon clinical judgment regarding the appropriateness of multiple staged procedures is paramount. Much like the direct exchange, this technique involves removal of all infected prosthetic components and cement followed by debridement of infected and nonviable periprosthetic tissue. Within this same procedure, antibiotic impregnated cement is fashioned into beads or a spacer and used to manage the dead space and eradicate local infection until a permanent implant is inserted. After the initial debridement and implant removal, systemic culture-directed systemic therapy is given for 4–6 weeks followed by an interval of 2–8 weeks without antibiotics in order to monitor serum markers of infection resolution [4, 21, 23]. The minimum duration of 4–6 weeks of systemic antibiotics prior to reimplantation is not arbitrary, but based upon observations related to the time it takes for revascularization of debrided bone [17, 21, 23].

The duration of the latency period for reimplantation is an area that requires further investigation. Currently available evidence recommends delaying the definitive procedure from 2 weeks to several months. Older studies have reported that reimplantation within three weeks of initial debridement has a higher failure rate. Later European studies show acceptable outcomes of reimplantation 2–6 weeks following the initial debridement while simultaneously receiving systemic antibiotics. This shorter latency period has only been successful when the pathologic organism is not MRSA, enterococci, or a multidrug resistant gram-negative organism. If during the planned definitive reimplantation, intraoperative findings suggest persistent infection, then a debridement and reimplantation of antibiotic impregnated cement is indicated followed by another latency period prior to reimplantation of hardware. Regardless of antibiotic latency interval length, new cultures and specimens should be collected during definitive reimplantation. If these are positive for persistent infection, then culture-specific antibiotics should be continued for a total treatment time of 3 months [21, 23]. Although discussed in detail in other chapters, the use of antibiotic impregnated cement is not universally recommended. Some experts discourage their use in infection due to small-colony variants of staphylococci, MRSA, or fungi citing diminished effectiveness. Randomized control trials that assess effectiveness in these difficult-to-treat infections have yet to be performed [21].

The 2-stage exchange is a versatile treatment strategy that is highly effective in most cases because it eliminates the implant as foreign nidus of infection during antimicrobial therapy. It also provides time to resolve concomitant limitations such as severe soft tissue deficits and severe bone loss. Management of large segmental osseous defects is a complicated matter that has been addressed in several ways. One of

the more common techniques used worldwide for long bone defects or infected fracture hardware is the Masquelet technique consisting of two main stages. First, aggressive debridement and resection, with insertion of antibiotic impregnated bone spacer, and application of an external fixator [31]. The second stage occurs approximately 6–8 weeks later where bone cement is removed revealing an induced membrane surrounding the spacer that will be filled with bone graft and fixated by a surgeon preferred method [46–49]. Several modifications to this protocol exist and in long bones include intramedullary nailing with antibiotic cement surrounding the nail [47–49]. McNally et al. described the Belfast technique which is a 2-stage procedure including radical debridement with soft tissue coverage followed by autogenous bone grafting. They report a recurrence rate of only 13 % and a success rate overall of 91 % [17, 50]. The Papineau technique was described in 2005, and includes radical debridement, cancellous bone grafting over granulation tissue, and associate soft tissue closure that has yielded a success rate of 90 % [17, 51]. Patients with risk factors that increased the likelihood of failure such as sinus tracts and difficult-to-treat organisms (MRSA, enterococci, and *Candida*) have also demonstrated better outcomes than the previously described strategies. It is worth mentioning that the presented strategies don't occur in a vacuum. Some recent literature indicates that the effectiveness of a 2-stage exchange is diminished following either, a failed initial debridement and retention, or failed direct exchange approach [21]. Reports of reinfection rates among 2-stage procedures for hip and knee prosthesis range from 9 to 20 % with some reports as high as 28 % in smaller groups with various comorbidities such as diabetes [40, 45]. A prerequisite for a multi-staged exchange is that the patient must be physically willing and able to withstand surgery more than once. Similarly, this strategy mandates a critical and honest assessment of the ultimate outcome. Despite the innate desire to restore the patient to an outcome consistent with the intended original procedure, the infectious process may make this goal unfeasible. In those situations where revision of the IOP is either not possible or the patient's post-revision functional capacity is diminished, then the imperative changes from revision to salvage strategies.

Salvage Strategies

The salvage strategies require acceptance that initial indications are compromised and the new priority is optimization of the overall patient outcome (Fig. 8.5). This may mean conceding or completely rejecting the objectives of the original procedure. One of the accepted methods is via permanent resection. Permanent resection involves debridement of infected/nonviable tissue and implant constructs without

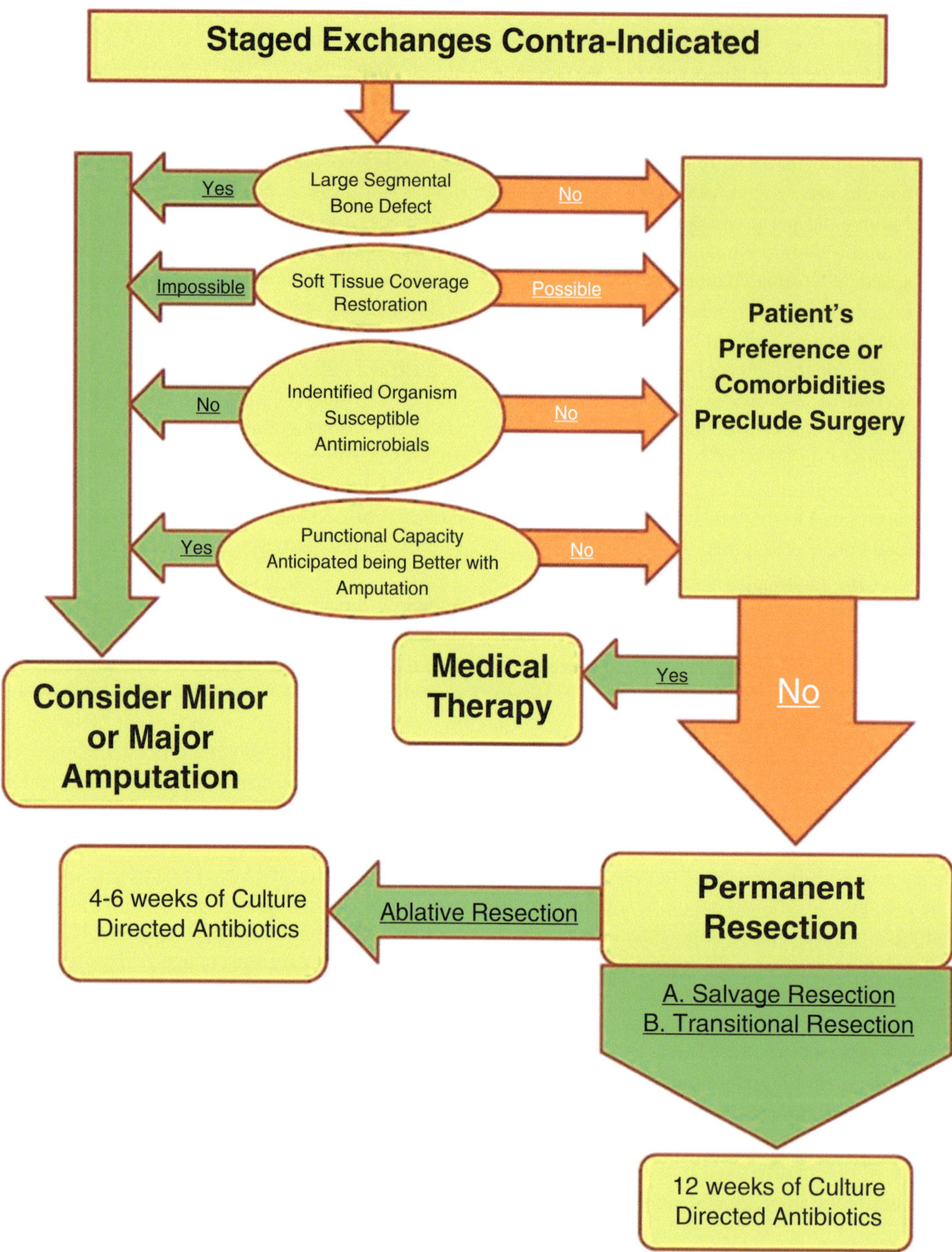

Fig. 8.5 The remaining strategies require compromise of the site-specific objectives in favor of the patient's overall objectives. This ranges from chronic suppressive antimicrobial therapy to amputation, when functional status and overall health are anticipated to be better than less drastic options. Adapted from Trampuz and Zimmerli [4], Mouzopoulos [17], IDSA [21]

revision reimplantation. Following resection these patients are treated with appropriate systemic antibiotics for 4–6 weeks [21, 23]. Within the orthopedic literature this has been most frequently applied in the setting of failed joint replacement and attempted salvage via primary arthrodesis. The permanent resection technique has been successfully utilized in even patients with significant barriers to recovery. Reported success rates range between 60 and 100 % for eradication of infection [21, 23]. The indications are significantly compromised soft tissue envelope, moderate-to-severe bone deficit, and restoration of the original procedure is no longer feasible.

In our experience we have determined that the permanent resection strategy exists on a spectrum that can be divided into subclasses that prioritize overall or site-specific function. These strategies have varying objectives that closely resemble or significantly differ from those of the intended original procedure. We present three variations of permanent resection that allow for retaining as much function as possible while eliminating infection. They are ablative resection, salvage resection, and transitional resection. For ease of understanding, the variants are presented in the context of an infected hemiarthroplasty of the first metatarsophalangeal joint (MTPJ). An ablative resection is a definitive removal of implant, compromised bone and soft tissue. In the infected hemi-arthroplasty example, this could be represented by a Keller procedure. The site-specific function is most compromised but this approach may result in acceptable overall patient function given patient profile. It can be single-staged and therefore absorbable antibiotic impregnated beads can be utilized to augment infection eradication. In nonambulatory and sedentary patients, where function is not crucial or bone loss is excessive following debridement an ablative resection type can be performed. Continuing with our example, arthrodesis of the first MTPJ would be classified as salvage resection of the articulation. The salvage procedure does not salvage the joint; rather it preserves overall function for active patients with better long-term stability than a Keller arthroplasty type resection but at the expense of the site-specific function. We advocate that the definitive arthrodesis be performed in a multi-stage fashion to allow for adequate clearing of infection. The interval placement of antibiotic impregnated spacer can aid in dead space management and reduce the risk of residual pathogens in a site that may require bone grafting. The final subclass is transitional resection where a different type of implant is used to replace the entire joint such as a silastic with grommets. In this example the removal of hemi-implant is performed and exchanged for a total joint replacement. This procedure more closely mimics the original intended procedure and preserves the most site-specific function. For the transitional approach in our example of infection in the setting of hemiarthroplasty the first metatarsal head is assumed infected and cartilage is no longer viable. The benefit of inserting a total silastic joint implant is that it can accommodate a great deal of bone resection while preserving some length and having better stability and function than a Keller arthroplasty. Similar to the salvage resection, we prefer a multi-stage strategy for transitional resections to ensure adequate soft tissue envelope, appropriate resection of bone, and clearance of infection.

When all else fails, the surgeon must weigh the risks of continued debridement surgery and chronic infection against those of amputation. In these cases a consultation to the appropriate service for higher-level amputation such as below-the-knee or above-the-knee is a good choice. In the setting of severe bone loss, nonviable or poor soft tissue coverage, or chronic multidrug resistant infection with persistent draining sinus this may be the best option. Any amputation to be performed should include either a minor or major resection of all infected and nonviable bone and soft tissue. This may be a better long-term option for some patients to eradicate infection, preserve some function and mobility, and allow the patient to move on from infection and the toll a course of multiple surgeries can have on their life. Duration of post-amputation antibiotics is dependent on the thoroughness of surgical eradication. If the surgeon is confident that the amputation has successfully removed all infected and nonviable tissues in the absence of septicemia or bacteremia, then systemic antibiotics can be terminated after 24–48 hours [21]. Conversely, if amputation does not fully excise potentially compromised tissues then systemic antibiotics are recommended for an additional 4–6 weeks [21].

In patients that are unwilling or medically unable to tolerate additional surgical procedures the use of prolonged antimicrobial therapy is feasible. In this setting, the treatment objective is suppression rather than cure. Selection of this strategy requires a susceptible pathogen and collaboration with the infectious disease team to counsel the patient regarding the hazards of therapy and requisite monitoring.

Conclusions

Despite the comprehensive nature of the preceding sections, it is necessary to clarify that there is no universal protocol for all infected implants. The totality of management in cases of infected hardware requires a multispecialty approach, but can lead to successful eradication of infection and functional optimization when executed properly. Adhering to principles of treatment in a logical construct can provide benefits and success rates in the 80–90 % range [1, 2, 4, 21, 23, 40]. This is referencing the current protocols for all orthopedic implants and not exclusively related to foot and ankle pathology. The protocols presented are intended as a decision support tool to optimize outcomes derived from the currently available evidence base. Even with decades of research, expert opinion, and a greater understanding of infectious process than ever before, treatment of this entity is mediated by the surgeon's clinical judgment. This sentiment is expressed well in the most recent IDSA guidelines which explicitly state in recommendation 17 that "the ultimate decision regarding surgical management should be made by the surgeon with appropriate consultation as necessary" [21].

References

1. Zimmerli W, Trampuz A. Biomaterial-associated infection: a perspective from the clinic. In: Moriarty T, Zaat S, Busscher H, editors. Biomaterials associated infection: immunologic aspects and antimicrobial strategies. 1st ed. New York: Springer; 2013. p. 3–25.
2. Ovaska M, Lindahl J, Makinen T, Madanat R, Pulliainen L, Kiljunen V, et al. Postoperative infection—removal of screws and plates? Suomen Ortopedia ja Traumatologia. 2011;34(1):34–6.
3. Zimmerli W, Waldvogel FA, Vaudaux P, Nydegger UE. Pathogenesis of foreign body infection: description and characteristics of an animal model. J Infect Dis. 1982;146(4):487–97.
4. Trampuz A, Zimmerli W. Diagnosis and treatment of infections associated with fracture-fixation devices. Injury. 2006;37 Suppl 2:S59–66.
5. Trampuz A, Zimmerli W. Prosthetic joint infections: update in diagnosis & treatment. Swiss Med Wkly. 2005;135:243–51.
6. Bjarnsholt T. The role of bacterial biofilms in chronic infections. APMIS Suppl. 2013;136:1–51.
7. Schmidmaier G, Gahukamble A, Moriarty T, Richards R. Infection in fracture fixation: device design and antibiotic coatings reduce infection rates. In: Moriarty T, Zaat S, Busscher H, editors. Biomaterials associated infection: immunological aspects and antimicrobial strategies. 1st ed. New York: Springer; 2013. p. 435–54.
8. Calabro L, Lutton C, Seif El Din A, Richards R, Moriarty T. Animal models of orthopedic implant-related infection. In: Moriarty T, Zaat S, Busscher H, editors. Biomaterials associated infection: immunologic aspects and antimicrobial strategies. 1st ed. New York: Springer; 2013. p. 282–3.
9. Hayes JS, Vos DI, Hahn J, Pearce SG, Richards R. An in vivo evaluation of surface polishing of TAN intermedullary nails for ease of removal. Eur Cell Mater. 2009;18:15–26.
10. Hayes JS, Seidenglanz U, Pearce AI, Pearce SG, Archer CW, Richards RG. Surface polishing positively influences ease of plate and screw removal. Eur Cell Mater. 2010;19:117–26.
11. Melcher GA, Hauke C, Metzdorf A, Perren SM, Printzen G, Schlegel U, et al. Infection after intramedullary nailing: an experimental investigation on rabbits. Injury. 1996;27 Suppl 3:SC23–6.
12. Zgonis T, Jolly GP, Garbalosa JC. The efficacy of prophylactic intravenous antibiotics in elective foot and ankle surgery. J Foot Ankle Surg. 2004;43(2):97–103.
13. Berbari EF, Hanssen AD, Duffy MC, Steckelberg JM, Ilstrup DM, Harmsen WS, et al. Risk factors for prosthetic joint infection: case-control study. Clin Infect Dis. 1998;27(5):1247–54.
14. Glazebrook MA, Arsenault K, Dunbar M. Evidence-based classification of complications in total ankle arthroplasty. Foot Ankle Int. 2009;30(10):945–9.
15. Kessler B, Sendi P, Graber P, Knupp M, Zwicky L, Hintermann B, et al. Risk factors for periprosthetic ankle joint infection: a case control study. J Bone Joint Surg Am. 2012;94(20):1871–6.
16. Blam OG, Vaccaro AR, Vanichkachorn JS, Albert TJ, Hillbrand AS, Minnich JM, et al. Risk factors for surgical site infection in the patient with spinal injury. Spine (Phila Pa 1976). 2003;28(13):1475–80.
17. Mouzopoulos G, Kanakaris NK, Kontakis G, Obakponovwe R, Townsend PV, Giannoudis PV. Management of bone infections in adults: the surgeon's and microbiologist's perspectives. Inquiry. 2011;42(5):S18–23.
18. SooHoo NF, Krenek L, Eagan MJ, Gurbani B, Ko CY, Zingmond DS. Complication rates following open reduction and internal fixation of ankle fractures. J Bone Joint Surg Am. 2009;91(5):1042–9.
19. Cruess R, Dumont J, Newton C. Healing of bone. In: Newton N, editor. Textbook of small animal orthopaedics. Philadelphia: J.B. Lippincott; 1985.
20. Cruess RL, Dumont J. Fracture healing. Can J Surg. 1975;18(5):403–13.
21. Osmon D, Berbari EF, Berendt AR, Lew D, Zimmerli WS, Steckelberg JM. Diagnosis and management of prosthetic joint infection: clinical practice guidelines by the Infectious Disease Society of America. Clin Infect Dis. 2013;56(1):1–25.
22. Arnold WV, Shirtlliff ME, Stoodley P. Bacterial biofilms and periprosthetic infections. J Bone Joint Surg Am. 2013;95(24):2223–9.
23. Zimmerli W, Trampuz A, Ochsner PE. Prosthetic-joint infections. N Engl J Med. 2004;351(16):1645–54.
24. Murdoch DR, Roberts SA, Fowler Jr VG, Shah MA, Taylor SL, Morris AJ, et al. Infection of orthopedic prosthesis after Staphylococcus aureus bacteremia. Clin Infect Dis. 2001;32(4):647–9.
25. Leutenegger AF. Acute infection following osteosynthesis. The Umsch. 1990;47(7):593–6.
26. Gustilo RB, Merkow RL, Templeman D. The management of open fractures. J Bone Joint Surg Am. 1990;72(2):299–304.
27. Zych GA, Hutson Jr JJ. Diagnosis and management of infection after tibial intramedullary nailing. Clin Orthop. 1995;315:153–62.
28. Ochsner P, Sirkin M, Trampuz A. Acute infection. In: Ruedi R, Murphy W, editors. AO principles of fracture management. Stuttgart: Thieme; 2006.
29. Giannoudis PV, Faour O, Goff T, Kanakaris N, Dimitriou R. Masquelet technique for the treatment of bone defects: tips-tricks and future directions. Injury. 2011;42(6):591–8.
30. Patzakis MJ, Greene N, Holtom P, Shepherd L, Bravos P, Sherman R. Culture results in open wound treatment with muscle transfer for tibial osteomyelitis. Clin Orthop Relat Res. 1999;360:66–70.
31. Fodor L, Ullmann Y, Soudry M, Calif E, Lerner A. Prophylactic external fixation and extensive bone debridement for chronic osteomyelitis. Acta Orthop Belg. 2006;72(4):448–53.
32. Parsons B, Strauss E. Surgical management of chronic osteomyelitis. Am J Surg. 2004;188(1A Suppl):57–66.
33. Tetsworth K, Cierny 3rd G. Osteomyelitis debridement techniques. Clin Orthop Relat Res. 1999;360:87–96.
34. Merritt K, Dowd JD. Role of internal fixation in infection of open fractures: studies with Staphylococcus aureus and Proteus mirabilis. J Orthop Res. 1987;5(1):23–8.
35. Merritt K. Factors increasing the risk of infection in patients with open fractures. J Trauma. 1988;28(6):823–7.
36. Worlock P, Slack R, Harvey L, Mawhinney R. The prevention of infection in open fractures: an experimental study of the effect of fracture stability. Injury. 1994;25(1):31–8.
37. Friedrich B, Klaue P. Mechanical stability and post-traumatic osteitis: an experimental evaluation of the relation between infection of bone and internal fixation. Injury. 1977;9(1):23–9.
38. Johnson E. Chronic infection and infected non-union. In: Colton C, Dell'Oca A, Holz U, Kellam J, Ochsner PE, editors. AO principles of fracture management. 1st ed. Stuttgart: AO Publisher/Thieme; 2000.
39. Berkes M, Obremskey WT, Scannell B, Ellington JK. Maintenance of hardware after early postoperative infection following fracture internal fixation. J Bone Joint Surg Am. 2010;92(4):823–8.
40. Zalavras CG, Christensen T, Rigopoulos N, Holtom P, Patzakis MJ. Infection following operative treatment of ankle fractures. Clin Orthop Relat Res. 2009;467(7):1715–20.
41. Sarmiento A, Sharpe FE, Ebramzadeh E, Normand P, Shankwiler J. Factors influencing the outcome of closed tibial fractures treated with functional bracing. Clin Orthop Relat Res. 1995;315:8–24.
42. Sherrell JC, Fehring TK, Odum S, Hansen E, Zmistowski B, Dennos A, et al. The Chitranjan Ranawat Award: fate of two-stage

reimplantation after failed irrigation and debridement for periprosthetic knee infection. Clin Orthop Relat Res. 2011;469(1):18–25.

43. Rightmire E, Zurakowski D, Vrahas M. Acute infections after fracture repair: management with hardware in place. Clin Orthop Relat Res. 2008;466(2):466–72.

44. Bradbury T, Fehring TK, Taunton M, Hanssen A, Azzam K, Parvizi J, et al. The fate of acute methicillin-resistant Staphylococcus aureus periprosthetic knee infections treated by open debridement and retention of components. J Arthroplasty. 2009;24(6 Suppl):101–4.

45. Gehrke T, Zahar A, Kendoff D. One-stage exchange: it all began here. Bone Joint J. 2013;95(11 Suppl A):77–83.

46. Masquelet AC, Fitoussi F, Begue T, Muller GP. Reconstruction of the long bones by the induced membrane and spongy autograft. Ann Chir Plast Esthet. 2000;45(3):346–53.

47. Apard T, Bigorre N, Cronier P, Duteille F, Bizot P, Massin P. Two-stage reconstruction of post-traumatic segmental tibia bone loss with nailing. Orthop Traumatol Surg Res. 2010;96(5):549–53.

48. Woon CY, Chong KW, Wong MK. Induced membranes—a staged technique of bone-grafting for segmental bone loss: a report of two cases and a literature review. J Bone Joint Surg Am. 2010;92(1):196–201.

49. Biau DJ, Pannier S, Masquelet AC, Glorion C. Case report: reconstruction of a 16-cm diaphyseal defect after Ewing's resection in a child. Clin Orthop Relat Res. 2009;467(2):572–7.

50. McNally MA, Small JO, Tofighi HG, Mollan RA. Two-stage management of chronic osteomyelitis of the long bones. The Belfast technique. J Bone Joint Surg Br. 1993;75(3):375–80.

51. Beals RK, Bryant RE. The treatment of chronic open osteomyelitis of the tibia in adults. Clin Orthop Relat Res. 2005;433:212–7.

Diagnosis and Management of the Septic Joint

9

Troy J. Boffeli and Jonathan C. Thompson

Introduction

Joint sepsis can present in the ankle or smaller joints of the foot and may arise from hematogenous spread of infection, contiguous bone or wound infection, or direct contamination from trauma. Small joints of the foot, most commonly the digital interphalangeal joints or metatarsophalangeal joints, are often infected by an adjacent ulcer communicating with the joint while less commonly being associated with a hematogenous source. Conversely, isolated joint sepsis from a hematogenous source is more classically observed in the ankle and to a lesser extent the subtalar joint. Due to the hematogenous source and based on the proximal location of the ankle, management of ankle joint sepsis often varies from smaller joints of the foot. Ankle pyarthrosis has been reported to comprise 3.4–15 % of all joint sepsis cases with a mortality rate as high as 11.5 % [1–3]. Concomitant osteomyelitis of the distal tibia or talus is frequently seen in this setting, with a reported incidence of 30 % [4]. The patient is furthermore at high risk for septicemia, subsequent debilitating arthritis, and amputation, so prompt and effective management is of central importance. The majority of this chapter will focus on discussing isolated pyarthrosis from a hematogenous source as opposed to joint sepsis secondary to an adjacent lower extremity infection. The latter is more common in small joints of the foot and can typically be managed with local debridement or amputation options as discussed in the corresponding location-appropriate chapters of this book. Isolated joint sepsis is most commonly appreciated in the ankle and will be the main focus of this chapter.

T.J. Boffeli, DPM, FACFAS
Regions Hospital/HealthPartners Institute for Education and Research, 640 Jackson Street, Saint Paul, MN 55101, USA
e-mail: troy.j.boffeli@healthpartners.com

J.C. Thompson, DPM, MHA, AACFAS (✉)
Orthopedic Center, Mayo Clinic Health System,
1400 Bellinger Street, Eau Claire, WI 54702, USA
e-mail: thompson.jonathan@mayo.edu

Clinical Presentation and Diagnosis

Recognition of ankle pyarthrosis can be difficult due to relatively inconsistent clinical and laboratory findings. The "gold standard" for treatment has been described as the appropriate level of clinical suspicion of an experienced physician [5]. The classical clinical presentation consists of a relatively rapid onset of ankle pain, decreased joint range of motion, swelling, and warmth under 2 weeks in duration (Fig. 9.1) [6–8]. Fever, rigors, and malaise are variably present. The reported sensitivities of joint pain (85 %), edema (78 %), fever (57 %), sweats (27 %), and rigors (19 %) does not provide a clear diagnostic picture [9]. Recent injury to the area may be seen and does not rule out the possibility of joint sepsis. Similarly, polyarticular involvement does not rule out sepsis as a 22 % incidence of multiple joint involvement has been reported [10, 11]. Risk factors raising the index of suspicion for joint sepsis are rheumatoid arthritis, prosthetic joints, low socioeconomic status, intravenous drug use, alcoholism, diabetes, recent corticosteroid injection, and ulceration (Table 9.1) [3, 6, 8, 10–14].

Laboratory studies can aid in establishing the diagnosis of pyarthrosis. Peripheral white blood cell (WBC) count, erythrocyte sedimentation rate (ESR), and C-reactive protein (CRP) have been shown to provide minimal diagnostic value. WBC counts greater than $10,000/\mu L$, ESR over 30 mm/h, and CRP more than 100 mg/L have been shown to exhibit only a mildly increased likelihood of septic arthritis [15, 16]. Dissimilarly, diagnostic arthrocentesis is important in establishing a diagnosis. The technique for performing ankle arthrocentesis is displayed in Fig. 9.2. The synovial fluid white cell count (WCC) has proven to be an effective marker, with the likelihood of joint sepsis increasing markedly as the synovial WCC rises [9]. However, Li and colleagues cite a synovial WCC as low as $17,500/mm^3$ in providing diagnostic sensitivity of 83 % and specificity of 67 % [17]. A synovial WCC of $>50,000/mm^3$ is a threshold above which increases the likelihood of subsequently confirmed cases [3]. Similarly, positive synovial fluid culture has been shown to exhibit a sensitivity of 75–95 % in a

© Springer International Publishing Switzerland 2015
T.J. Boffeli (ed.), *Osteomyelitis of the Foot and Ankle*, DOI 10.1007/978-3-319-18926-0_9

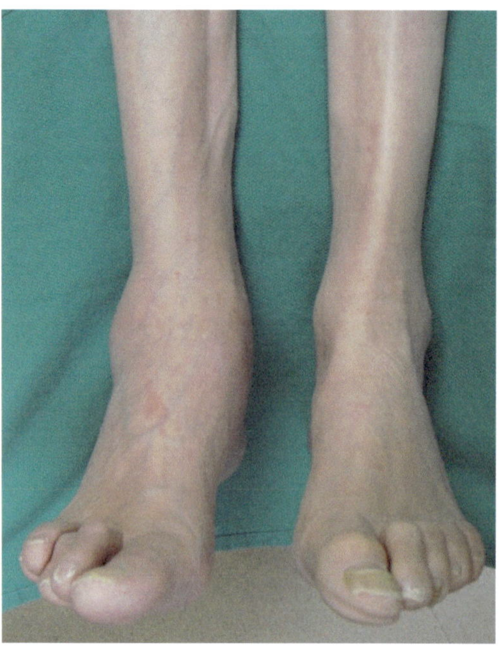

Fig. 9.1 Clinical appearance of ankle joint sepsis The clinical appearance of a septic right ankle and the contralateral unaffected limb are seen. The classical clinical presentation consists of a relatively rapid onset of ankle pain, decreased joint range of motion, swelling, and warmth under 2 weeks in duration. However, presentation can be variable and often does not include all of these features. Thus maintaining a low index of suspicion for joint sepsis is important in a patient presenting with some of these features

Table 9.1 Risk factors for joint sepsis

Rheumatoid arthritis

Prosthetic joints

Low socioeconomic status

Intravenous drug use

Alcoholism

Diabetes

Recent corticosteroid injection

Ulceration

septic joint [18]. Thus the ultimate "gold standard" diagnosis currently rests on the clinical acumen of an experienced physician considering all available clinical and laboratory findings [5].

Differential diagnoses that should be considered with a painful, erythematous ankle are numerous. Klippel developed an extensive list of differentials for acute monoarthritis that can be seen in Table 9.2 [19]. Common differentials that will be encountered in the ankle are trauma, gout, extra-articular infection, hemarthrosis, and post-corticosteroid injection flare. It should be noted that certain differentials are also risk factors for joint sepsis and can be present in tandem with one another. Thus the definitive diagnosis of a differential does not necessarily rule out concomitant infection.

One common example is acute gout; simply establishing the diagnosis of gout does not effectively rule out simultaneous infection. Similarly, patients with rheumatoid arthritis are at higher risk for developing joint sepsis because of the systemic disease process as well as immunosuppressive drug therapy used to manage the disease [20, 21].

In general, joints that exhibit inflammation and arthritis secondary to a number of different entities are at higher risk for sepsis. Robust vascular supply is often appreciated in hypertrophic synovial tissue that forms in an inflamed or arthritic joint. These vessels lack a basement membrane and thus allow blood-borne bacteria easier passage into the joint. Any condition that leads to acute or chronic joint inflammation like arthritis, bone spurs, ankle instability, rheumatoid arthritis or gout may therefore predispose to joint sepsis (Fig. 9.3).

Medical and Surgical Treatment

Prompt and effective treatment of a patient diagnosed with a septic ankle joint serves to lower the potential for morbidity. There have traditionally been few recommendations regarding medical and surgical management. The consensus put forth by the British Society for Rheumatology recommends immediate antibiotic therapy and removal of purulent material from the joint space [14]. This consensus has been consistent with the recommendations put forth by several other studies as well [22–24]. Staphylococci and streptococci have been reported as the most common pathologic organisms in joint sepsis [4, 6, 25–27]. *Staphylococcus aureus* has been reported as the most common pathogen, followed by *Streptococcus* and, rarely, gram-negative rods [4]. While the typical patient without risk factors for gram-negative or resistant bacteria can be treated with the appropriate parenteral penicillin or clindamycin, those considered high-risk for such colonization, such as the diabetic patient, should receive the appropriate empiric therapy. Interdisciplinary management with the involvement of Infectious Disease is often prudent to effectively manage the patient with pyarthrosis.

The means by which the joint is to be evacuated has been a source of debate between the two options of serial joint aspirations versus arthroscopic or open surgical intervention. However, a number of sources recommend immediate arthroscopic irrigation and debridement [1, 28–34]. Given the relatively high mortality rate and potential for morbidity with pyarthrosis, surgical intervention should be performed in an urgent or emergent fashion.

Arthroscopic surgery for pyarthrosis is typically performed under general anesthesia without regional or local anesthetic. External distraction is not used to avoid further disturbance to the edematous soft tissues in the region.

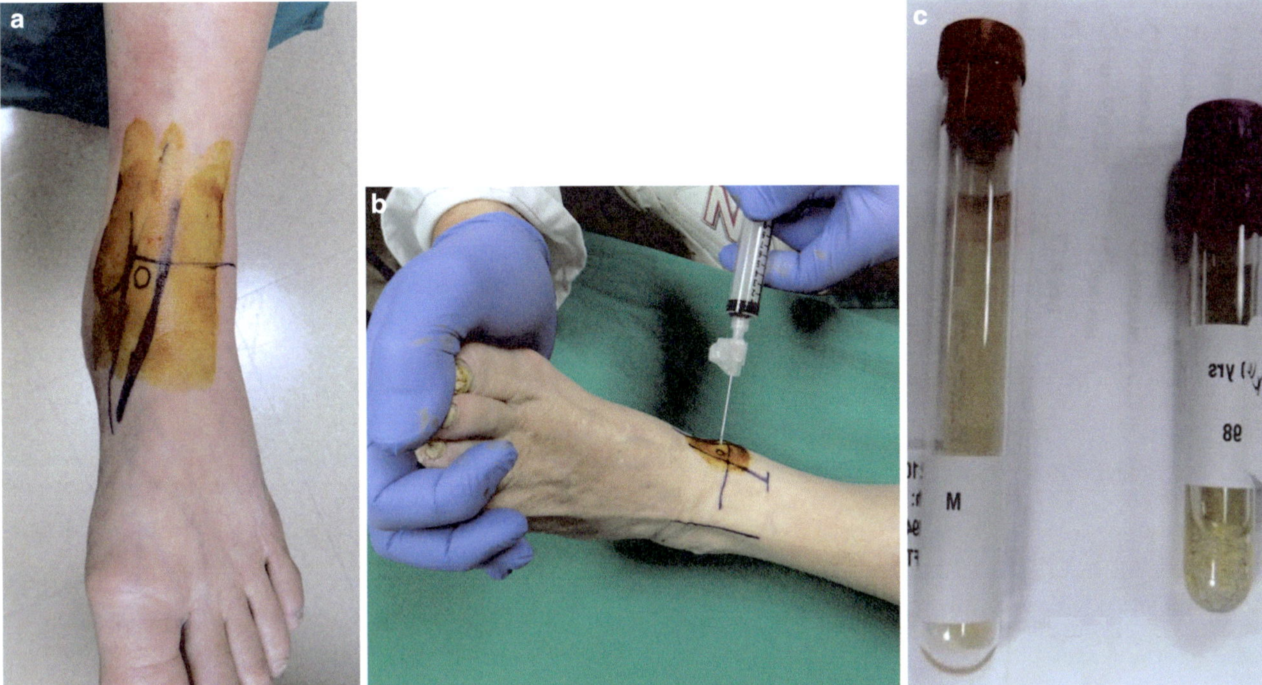

Fig. 9.2 Ankle joint aspiration is typically approached from the anterior medial side of the ankle joint. Site markings similar to an arthroscopic anteromedial portal are used. The joint line is marked by palpation. The anteromedial puncture is made just medial to the tibialis anterior tendon which is lateral to the greater saphenous vein and adjacent saphenous nerve (**a**). The foot is held dorsiflexed at 90° while an 18-gauge needle is introduced into the ankle joint. This technique protects the cartilage on the talar dome from injury during insertion of the large-bore needle (**b**). The needle enters the joint at approximately 45° with the intention of entering the anterior joint capsule recess. Joint distention is oftentimes present with infection making entrance into the joint much easier. Vacuum is then applied through the 12-mL syringe. The tip of the needle frequently becomes obstructed with synovial tissue. A slight pullback or withdrawal technique allows uncorking of the needle at which point several milliliters of yellow, purulent and often watery fluid is aspirated. Normal synovial fluid is typically clear to slightly yellow in appearance while fluid concerning for infection may exhibit a more turbid, discolored, or frankly purulent appearance (**c**). Bloody-appearing fluid with initial aspiration may indicate hemarthrosis; aspirate that becomes increasingly bloody in appearance during aspiration is more likely due to injection-induced hemarthrosis. The specimen for synovial crystal analysis and culture are initially placed in a preservative-free tube (indicated by the red-top tube). One milliliter of aspirate is preferred. An additional milliliter of joint aspirate is then placed into a tube containing ethylenediaminetetraacetic acid (EDTA) (indicated by the lavender-top tube) for synovial white cell count. Less than 1 mL of volume or dilution with saline will compromise the cell count. The synovial white cell count may have to be foregone if a very small quantity of fluid is obtained as the ankle joint does not typically yield a high volume of joint aspirate

Table 9.2 Differential diagnosis for acute monoarthritis

Infection (bacterial, fungal, mycobacterial, viral, spirochete)

Rheumatoid arthritis

Gout

Pseudogout

Apatite-related arthropathy

Reactive arthritis

Systemic lupus erythematosus

Lyme arthritis

Sickle cell disease

Dialysis-related amyloidosis

Transient synovitis of the hip

Plant thorn synovitis

Metastatic carcinoma

Pigmented villonodular synovitis

Hemarthrosis

Neuropathic arthropathy

Osteoarthritis

Intra-articular injury (fracture, soft tissue injury, osteonecrosis)

Adapted from Klippel et al. [19]

Standard anteromedial and anterolateral ankle portals are used as described by Ferkel [35]. The use of lactated Ringer's solution without impregnated antibiotics or antiseptics is well described and is our preference [1]. Use of 3 L unimpregnated lactated Ringer's solution followed by 6 L impregnated with 50,000 units of Bacitracin powder per bag have also been described [34]. Antiseptics are discouraged when healthy cartilage remains due to concerns of chondrotoxicity [1]. A 2.7 mm or 4.0 mm arthroscope is utilized based on surgeon preference. The 4.0 mm arthroscope may allow for more timely debridement and quicker passing of fluid through the joint but may create difficulty in accessing the joint without distraction, particularly in the patient with osteoarthritis-related joint narrowing. When creating the standard portals for joint access, the anteromedial portal is established first followed by the anterolateral portal with the aid of transillumination (Fig. 9.4a). Intraoperative fluoroscopy can be utilized to help determine the appropriate level for portal placement, which is often more challenging in the septic

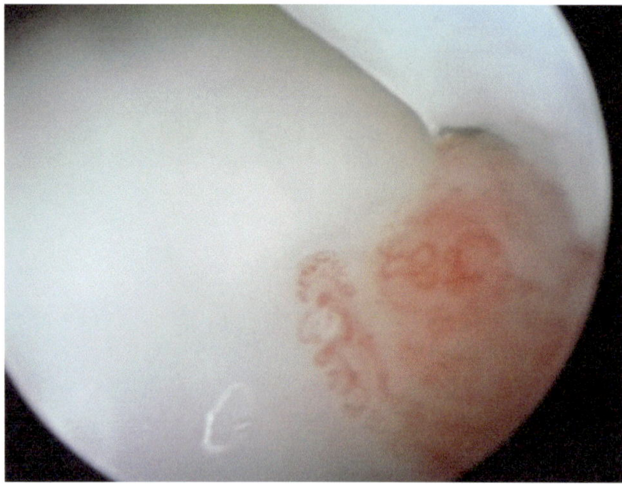

Fig. 9.3 Hypertrophic synovial tissue has robust vascular supply that predisposes to hematogenous joint sepsis. These vessels lack a basement membrane which allows bacteria circulating in the blood to cross into the joint. Any condition that leads to acute or chronic joint inflammation like arthritis, bone spurs, ankle instability, rheumatoid arthritis or gout therefore may predispose to joint sepsis

ankle due to the degree of swelling and extensive internal joint derangement (Fig. 9.4b). When introducing the camera into the joint, difficulty visualizing the articular surface should be anticipated due to a commonly high degree of synovitis with pyarthrosis. The anterolateral portal is then made immediately lateral to the extensor digitorum longus tendon. Care is taken to avoid the intermediate dorsal cutaneous nerve, which can sometimes be visualized with transillumination. An alternate technique involves palpating the nerve on the unaffected limb as the location of this nerve is typically consistent on the contralateral limb [36]. A doppler ultrasound can be used to assess the location of the perforating peroneal artery which is often non-palpable (Fig. 9.4c). After inserting the camera into the medial portal and establishing a lateral portal, a shaver is placed in the anterolateral portal to assist in evacuating fluid for arthroscopic lavage of the joint. In order to maintain continuous egress of fluids, the shaver often needs to remain running as hypertrophied synovial tissue will otherwise obstruct a standard suction tip. High-volume joint lavage allows for arthroscopic inspection

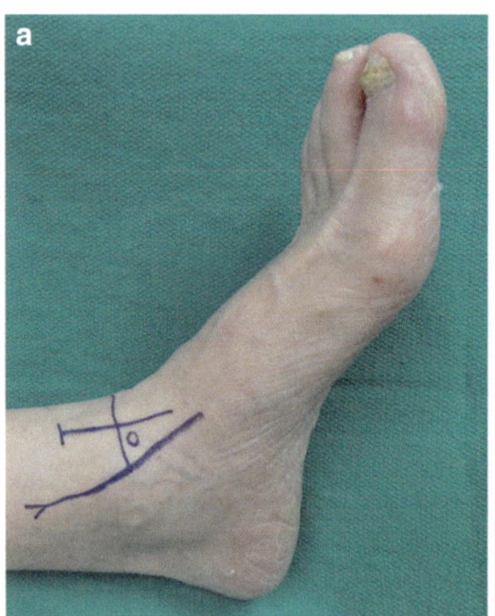
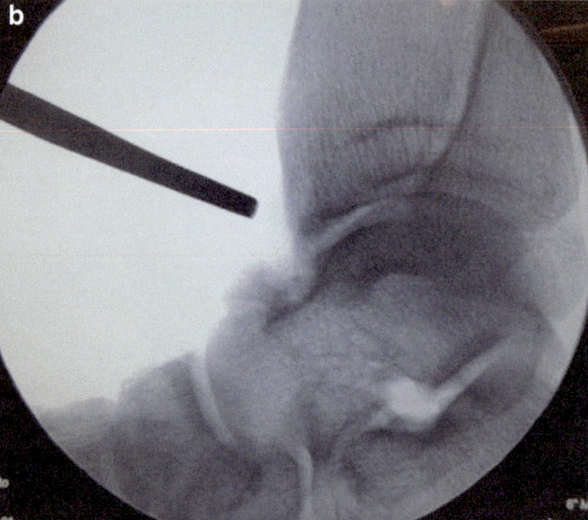
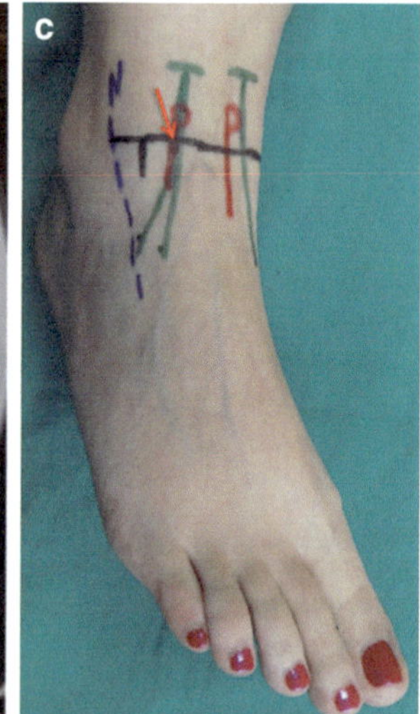

Fig. 9.4 Establishing arthroscopy portals. (**a**) A standard anteromedial portal is created just medial to the tibialis anterior tendon. The portal is lateral to the greater saphenous vein and saphenous nerve. Difficulty is oftentimes encountered with palpating anatomic structures when infection is present. Anterior synovial hypertrophy and localized soft tissue edema largely precludes identification of sensory nerves. Making the portal close to the tibialis anterior is therefore best to avoid the nerve and vein. Identifying the tibialis anterior in pre-op while the patient is awake allows more accurate delineation of tendon location. Making the portal medial to the tibialis anterior also protects the dorsalis pedis artery. (**b**) Determining the joint level can be difficult with an edematous ankle, so fluoroscopy is often valuable in determining the joint line prior to incisious. (**c**) The anterolateral portal is made immediately lateral to the extensor digitorum longus tendon and medial to the intermediate dorsal cutaneous nerve. If not able to be visualized clinically in the superficial tissues, the intermediate dorsal cutaneous nerve can at times be visualized with transillumination. Alternately, the location of this nerve is typically consistent between sides so it is possible to palpate the nerve on the unaffected limb to determine its location in relation to the planned portal on the affected side [36]. A doppler ultrasound can be used to assess the location of the perforating peroneal artery (indicated by *red arrow*), which is not always protected by the overlying tendinous structures

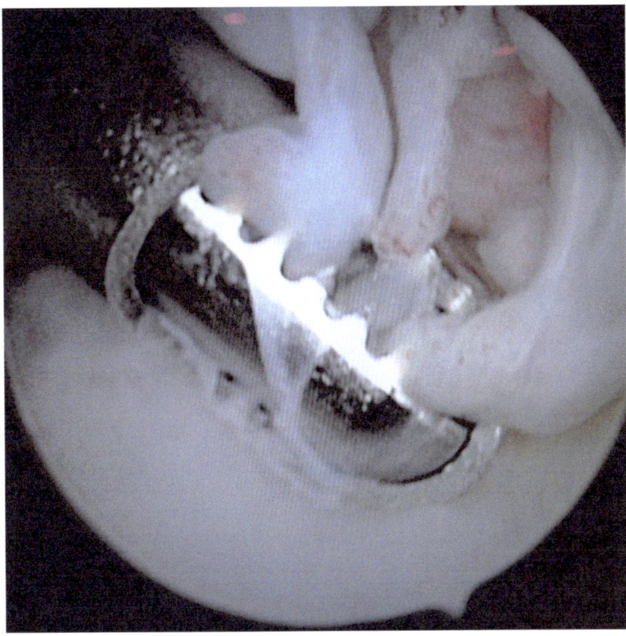

Fig. 9.5 Arthroscopic debridement. Once both portals are established, a shaver is placed in the anterolateral portal, which assists in evacuating fluid upon arthroscopic lavage of the joint. Running the shaver during lavage helps maintain continuous egress of fluids. Hypertrophy of the synovial tissue will otherwise obstruct a standard suction tip. High-volume joint lavage is time consuming but allows the opportunity for arthroscopic inspection and debridement of hypertrophied synovial tissue. The surgeon should expect difficulty finding the shaver and visualizing the joint in advanced cases of joint sepsis. The anterior joint recess is frequently filled with hypertrophied tissue; blind debridement may be necessary, with care being taken to orient the shaver away from the articular surface of the joint

Table 9.3 Septic joint staging and associated surgical treatment

Stage	Intraoperative findings	Surgical treatment
I	Synovitis, turbid fluid, possible petechiae	Single arthroscopic irrigation with minimal debridement
II	Fibrin deposits, purulence, inflammation	Irrigation and debridement with local synovectomy and fibrinectomy, likely to repeat surgery
III	Synovial thickening, formation of multiple pouches caused by adhesions	Multiple irrigation and debridement surgeries, with adhesion resection and partial to subtotal synovectomy
IV	Aggressive synovitis, radiographic changes, subchondral erosions	Consider arthrotomy with multiple irrigations and debridements, removal of loose fragments, and curettage of erosions or cysts

and debridement of hypertrophied synovial tissue while passing fluid through the joint. The surgeon should anticipate difficulty finding the shaver and visualizing the joint in advanced cases of joint sepsis. Because the anterior joint recess is frequently filled with hypertrophied tissue, initial blind debridement may be necessary while being careful to orient the shaver away from the articular surface (Fig. 9.5). At this time a pre-debridement synovial culture and biopsy are obtained.

When assessing the intraoperative appearance of the joint, it is important to have an understanding of the optimal amount of debridement that is likely to be required. Too little debridement can lead to insufficient management of the infection while overly aggressive synovectomy should be avoided as the synovium provides protection against micro-organisms [1, 28]. We routinely correlate the extent of debridement that will be performed with the intraoperative stage of joint sepsis based on criteria put forth by Gaechter [29] (Table 9.3). Stage-based debridement protocols were subsequently described by Stutz and Vispo Seara and later extrapolated for management of ankle joint sepsis by Boffeli [1, 28, 37]. Stage I joint sepsis displays joint fluid opacity and redness of the synovium with minimal synovitis and often requires a single arthroscopic irrigation with minimal

debridement. We recommend joint lavage with at least 9 L of lactated Ringer's solution. Stage II joint sepsis exhibits frank purulence, fibrin clots, and severe inflammation with increased synovitis. Joints falling into this category will typically require irrigation with debridement consisting of local synovectomy and fibrinectomy with a likely need for subsequent irrigation and debridement. In stage III joint sepsis, significant synovial thickening and adhesions.

Staging according to Gaechter [29]: Treatment protocol derived from the typical treatment required to successfully treat patients in previous retrospective studies [1, 28, 34, 37] are encountered, which creates the appearance of intra-articular compartments and leads to limited joint motion. These cases generally require multiple irrigation and debridement procedures consisting of adhesion resection and partial to subtotal synovectomy. Extensive debridement may initially be required in order to simply visualize the joint surface, so care should be taken to verify that the arthroscope is indeed in the intra-articular space during initial debridement. The septic joint exhibiting osseous erosions and radiographic osteolysis are classified as stage IV. These cases require multiple procedures for irrigation and debridement with removal of loose fragments and curettage of cysts. Open arthrotomy should be considered in this setting to provide adequate debridement of the joint. We prefer to avoid arthrotomy if possible as we feel high-volume lavage in a confined joint space via arthroscopy seems to better irrigate a relatively small joint such as the ankle better than an open approach. If intraoperative appearance suggests osseous involvement, magnetic resonance imaging (MRI) should be considered to assess the extent of osteomyelitis in the adjacent structures. The full 9 L of lactated Ringer's solution is passed through the joint, and in some rare instances a greater volume may be required. A post-debridement synovial culture is obtained. The arthroscopy portals are left open to allow drainage of the joint.

While the patient remains hospitalized, repeat surgery may become necessary within two to six days if clinical and laboratory signs of infection persist. Intraoperative staging can provide insight into whether multiple surgeries are likely

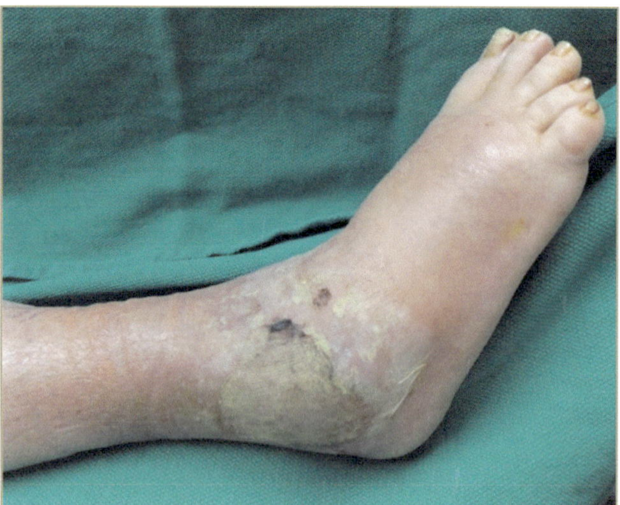

Fig. 9.6 Portal sites at 2 weeks postoperatively which are left open to allow drainage of infection. *Published with permission by the Journal of Foot and Ankle Surgery* [37]

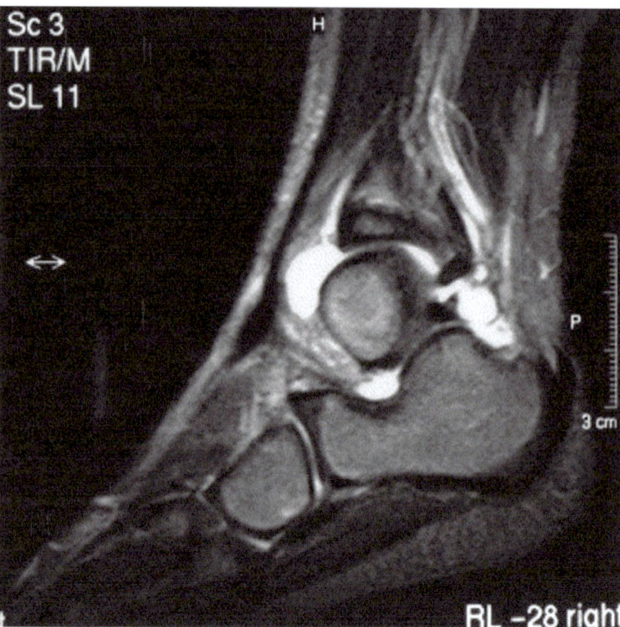

Fig. 9.7 Consider the potential for adjacent osteomyelitis if there is insufficient response to medical and surgical treatment. Adjacent osteomyelitis can be seen in up to 30 % of cases, so MRI should be considered if this is suspected. Communication of infection to the subtalar joint should also be considered when the response to treatment is not as anticipated

to be needed. Our threshold for returning to the operating room is relatively low and contingent on persistent cellulitis, persistent or worsening ankle pain, and inflammatory or WBC lab values remaining significantly elevated. The decision for determining whether repeat surgery is warranted is ultimately based on the clinical suspicion and acumen of the surgeon. Postoperatively, the patient typically requires parenteral antibiotics per Infectious Disease recommendations as available. The patient remains non-weight bearing in a removable boot until the portals have healed, at which time active and passive ankle joint range of motion can be initiated and weight bearing advanced. Physical therapy can be initiated at that time as well to minimize loss of ankle joint range of motion. In our experience, the portals typically heal within 2–3 weeks (Fig. 9.6).

Insufficient Response to Treatment

The stage-guided surgical treatment protocol merely provides insight into the extent and frequency of debridement that is typically anticipated. Thus deviation from these guidelines may be encountered, but significant divergence with an insufficient response to surgical intervention should raise concern for other contributing factors not previously addressed. Adjacent osteomyelitis can occur in up to 30 % of septic ankle joint cases, so an MRI should be considered in these situations [4] (Fig. 9.7). Similarly, communicating subtalar joint sepsis that has not been sufficiently recognized and addressed has been described and should be considered as well [38]. In the rare setting of persistent joint sepsis or adjacent osteomyelitis that is recalcitrant to arthroscopic irrigation and debridement with extended parenteral antibiotic management, arthrodesis of the joint can be considered as a limb-salvage option. This is generally performed in a staged manner, with the initial surgery comprising the resection of infected bone and application of polymethacrylate antibiotic beads or spacers. The spacer serves an antibacterial purpose as well as maintaining length prior to definitive arthrodesis. Alternately, single-stage resection and fusion has been described as well [39]. Joint fusion with bone grafting is performed with either internal fixation, circumferential frame compression arthrodesis, or via a combined internal–external fixation approach [39–41].

Joint Sepsis of the Foot

Isolated joint sepsis secondary to hematogenous inoculation is relatively rare in joints of the foot. On the other hand, the development of joint sepsis through contiguous spread of infection from a neuropathic ulceration or gangrene is much more common. Full-thickness ulcerations at the level of a joint provide a portal for infection. Common areas of ulceration that are at highest risk for joint involvement are the plantar hallux interphalangeal joint (IPJ), the dorsal digital IPJs, ulceration hallux valgus deformities at the medial first

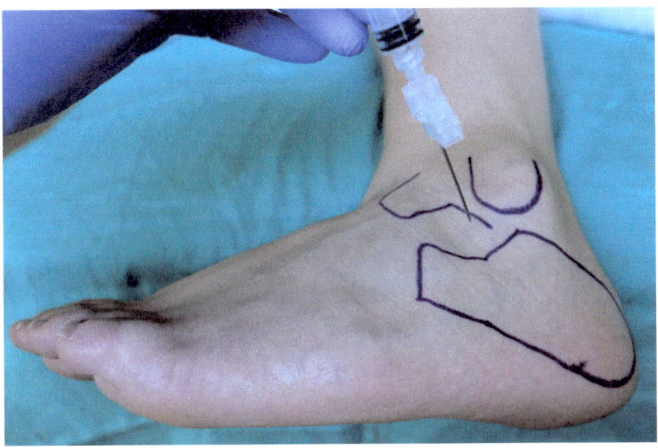

Fig. 9.8 When subtalar joint sepsis is suspected, arthrocentesis is performed at the lateral rearfoot. The sinus tarsi is palpated prior to it being prepped with an antiseptic. An 18-gauge needle is then advanced into the sinus tarsi directed in a posteromedial angle aimed toward the medial malleolus. Joint fluid aspiration may require needle re-direction while maintaining suction on the syringe

metatarsophalangeal joint (MPJ), and plantar MPJ ulcerations. Joint sepsis in these areas with adjacent osseous and soft tissue infection can generally be managed with local debridement or amputation options as discussed in the corresponding location-appropriate chapters of this book.

Subtalar joint sepsis can be encountered in an isolated manner or in communication with ankle joint sepsis. Evaluation and diagnosis of subtalar joint sepsis is similar to that described in the ankle. There should be a low threshold for obtaining imaging such as MRI when subtalar involvement is suspected to determine the extent of infection and rule out other differentials. Initial diagnostic arthrocentesis is performed through the sinus tarsi (Fig. 9.8). Once a septic subtalar joint is identified and the need for surgical intervention determined, irrigation and debridement can either be performed in an arthroscopic or open manner. The arthroscopic approach would generally be reserved for an infectious process that appears low-grade in nature and does not involve extra-articular structures, as may be determined by preoperative MRI. An open approach may be considered if imaging would favor an abscess or adjacent soft tissue involvement. Alternately, an arthroscopic-assisted limited open approach may provide a reasonable option in certain settings.

The first metatarsophalangeal joint may exhibit findings concerning for isolated joint sepsis. Because this joint is commonly affected by gout as well, it is important to distinguish between the two entities. Diagnosis of one is not exclusionary for the other as gout-afflicted joints are predisposed to sepsis. Furthermore, this joint may be predisposed to sepsis due to intra articular inflammation and synovitis created by hallux limitus. Arthrocentesis can be performed through a dorsolateral approach immediately lateral to the extensor

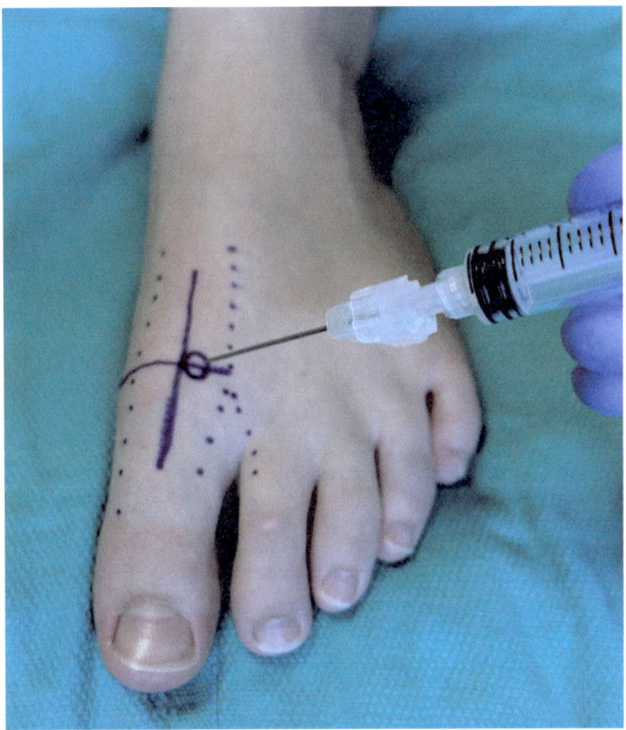

Fig. 9.9 First metatarsophalangeal joint aspiration technique. An inflamed, erythematous first metatarsophalangeal joint can resemble the presentation for either gout or pyarthrosis. Arthrocentesis is often necessary in order to differentiate between the two entities. A confirmed diagnosis of one is not exclusionary for the other as gout-afflicted joints are predisposed to sepsis. Arthrocentesis can be performed through a dorsolateral approach immediately lateral to the extensor hallucis longus tendon. The joint can be distracted for easier access by placing traction on the hallux as tolerated by the patient

hallucis longus tendon (Fig. 9.9). MRI may indicate periarticular involvement that could help differentiate whether to simply pursue open lavage of the joint versus performing a partial first ray resection for osteomyelitis.

While joint sepsis in the foot and ankle is relatively rare, it is important that this diagnosis is considered in the differential of patients exhibiting periarticular erythema, pain, and edema. Despite a history that would not indicate an infectious process, such as a recent injury, such incidents can predispose the patient to developing secondary joint sepsis. Due to the potential for significant morbidity to the patient, joint sepsis should not be overlooked when considering differential diagnoses in the patient with a painful, enflamed joint.

References

1. Vispo Seara JL, Barthel T, Schmitz H, Eulert J. Arthroscopic treatment of septic joints: prognostic factors. Arch Orthop Trauma Surg. 2002;122:204–11.
2. Esterhai Jr JL, Gleb I. Adult septic arthritis. Orthop Clin North Am. 1991;22:503–14.

3. Weston VC, Jones AC, Bradbuy N, Fawthrop F, Doherty M. Clinical features and outcome of septic arthritis in a single UK Health District 1982–1991. Ann Rheum Dis. 1999;58:214–9.

4. Holtom PD, Lawrence B, Zalavras CG. Hematogenous septic ankle arthritis. Clin Orthop Relat Res. 2008;466:1388–91.

5. Mathews CJ, Kingsley G, Field M, et al. Management of septic arthritis: a systematic review. Ann Rheum Dis. 2007;66:440–5.

6. Gupta MN, Sturrock RD, Field M. A prospective 2-year study of 75 patients with adult-onset septic arthritis. Br J Rheumatol. 2001;40: 24–30.

7. Goldenberg DL, Cohen AS. Acute infectious arthritis. A review of patients with nongonococcal joint infections (with emphasis on therapy and prognosis). Am J Med. 1976;60:369–77.

8. Ispahani P, Weston VC, Turner DP, Donald FE. Septic arthritis due to Streptococcus pneumoniae in Nottingham, United Kingdom, 1985–1998. Clin Infect Dis. 1999;29:1450–4.

9. Margaretten ME, Kohlwes J, Moore D. Does this adult patient have septic arthritis? J Am Med Assoc. 2007;297(13):1478–88.

10. Kaandorp CJ, Dinant HJ, van de Laar MA, Moens HJ, Prins AP, Dijkmans BA. Incidence and sources of native and prosthetic joint infection: a community based prospective survey. Ann Rheum Dis. 1997;56:470–5.

11. Dubost JJ, Fis I, Denis P, Lopitaux R, Soubrier M, Ristori JM, et al. Polyarticular septic arthritis. Medicine (Baltimore). 1993;72:296–310.

12. Sharp JT, Lidsky MD, Duffy J, Duncan MW. Infectious arthritis. Arch Intern Med. 1979;139:1125–30.

13. Meijers KA, Dijkmans BA, Hermans J, van den Broek PJ, Cats A. Nongonococcal infectious arthritis: a retrospective study. J Infect. 1987;14:13–20.

14. Coakley G, Mathews CJ, Field M, et al. On behalf of the British Society for Rheumatology Standards, Guidelines, and Audit Working Group. BSR & BHPR, BOA, RCGP, and BSAD guidelines for the management of the hot swollen joint in adults. Rheumatology. 2006;45:1039–41.

15. Söderquist B, Jones I, Fredlund H, Vikerfors T. Bacterial or crystal-associated arthritis? Discriminating ability of serum inflammatory markers. Scand J Infect Dis. 1998;30:591–6.

16. Jeng GW, Wang CR, Liu ST, et al. Measurement of synovial tumor necrosis factor-alpha in diagnosing emergency patients with bacterial arthritis. Am J Emerg Med. 1997;15:626–9.

17. Li SF, Cassidy C, Change C, et al. Diagnostic utility of laboratory tests in septic arthritis. Emerg Med J. 2007;24:75–7.

18. Shmerling RH. Synovial fluid analysis: a critical reappraisal. Rheum Dis Clin North Am. 1994;20:503–12.

19. Klippel JH, Weyand CM, Crofford LJ, Stone JH. Arthritis Foundation: primer on the rheumatic diseases. 12th ed. Atlanta, GA: Arthritis Foundation; 2001.

20. Edwards CJ, Cooper C, Fischer D, et al. The importance of the disease process and disease-modifying antirheumatic drug treatment in the development of septic arthritis in patients with rheumatoid arthritis. Arthritis Rheum. 2007;57:1151–7.

21. Mathews C, Coakley G. Septic arthritis: current diagnostic and therapeutic algorithm. Curr Opin Rheumatol. 2008;20(4):457–62.

22. Shetty AK, Gedalia A. Management of septic arthritis. Indian J Pediatr. 2004;71:819–24.

23. Ferroni A. Epidemiologie et diagnostique bacteriologique des infections osteoarticulairesaigues de l'enfant. Arch Pediatr. 2007;14 suppl 2:S91–6.

24. Lane JE, Moore C, Beckish ML, Stephens JL. Isolated septic arthritis caused by penicillin-resistant Streptococcus pneumonia. South Med J. 2001;94:429–31.

25. Dubost JJ, Soubrier M, De Champs C, Ristori JM, Bussiere JL, Sauvezie B. No changes in the distribution of organisms responsible for septic arthritis over a 20 year period. Ann Rheum Dis. 2002;61:267–9.

26. Eder L, Zisman D, Rosenbaum M, Rosner I. Clinical features and aetiology of septic arthritis in northern Israel. Rheumatology. 2005;44:1559–63.

27. Gupta MN, Sturrock RD, Field M. Prospective comparative study of patients with culture proven and high suspicion of adult onset septic arthritis. Ann Rheum Dis. 2003;62:327–31.

28. Stutz G, Kuster MS, Kleinstruck F, Gaechter A. Arthroscopic management of septic arthritis: stages of infection and results. Knee Surg Sports Traumatol Arthrosc. 2000;8:270–4.

29. Der GA. Gelenkinfekt. Inform Arzt. 1986;6:35–43.

30. Bynum DK, Nunley JA, Goldner JL, Martinez S. Pyogenic arthritis:emphasis on the need for surgical drainage of the infected joint. South Med J. 1982;75:1232–5.

31. Thiery JA. Arthroscopic drainage in septic arthritides of the knee: a multicenter study. Arthroscopy. 1989;5:65–9.

32. Jerosch J, Hoffstetter I, Schroder M, Castro WHM. Septic arthritis: arthroscopic management with local antibiotic treatment. Acta Orthop Belg. 1995;61:126–34.

33. Shadrick D, Mendicinio RW, Catanzariti AR. Ankle joint sepsis with subsequent osteomyelitis in an adult patient. J Foot Ankle Surg. 2011;50:354–60.

34. Mankovecky MR, Roukis TS. Arthroscopic synovectomy, irrigation, and debridement for treatment of septic ankle arthrosis: A systematic review and case series. J Foot Ankle Surg. 2014;53(5): 615–9.

35. Ferkel RD. Arthroscopy of the foot and ankle. New York: Lippincott Williams & Wilkins/Raven Press; 1996.

36. Boffeli TB, Hyllengren SB. The forgotten artery in ankle arthroscopy: is the perforating peroneal artery at risk with Standard Anterolateral Portal Placement? J Foot Ankle Surg 2014.

37. Boffeli TB, Thompson JT. Arthroscopic management of the septic ankle joint: case report of a stage-guided treatment. J Foot Ankle Surg. 2013;52(1):113–7.

38. Wynes J, Harris IV W, Hadfield RA, et al. Subtalar joint septic arthritis in a patient with hypogammaglobulinemia. J Foot Ankle Surg. 2013;52:242–8.

39. Saltzman CL. Salvage of diffuse ankle osteomyelitis by single-stage resection and circumferential frame compression arthrodesis. Iowa Orthop J. 2005;25:47–52.

40. Baumhauer JF, Lu AP, DiGiovanni BF. Arthrodesis of the infected ankle and subtalar joint. Foot Ankle Clin North Am. 2002;7: 175–90.

41. Klouche S, El-Masri F, Graff W, Mamoudy P. Arthrodesis with internal fixation of the infected ankle. J Foot Ankle Surg. 2011;50:25–30.

Surgical Treatment Principles for Diabetic Wounds Complicated by Osteomyelitis

Lindsay Gates, Peter A. Blume, and Bauer E. Sumpio

Introduction

Diabetes is a growing concern worldwide affecting over 250 million people [1]. In the United States alone, the Center for Disease Control estimates that there are 29.1 million people with diabetes and another 1.7 million new cases being diagnosed each year [2]. One of the most frequent and potentially devastating complications affecting about 25 % of diabetic patients during their lifetime is foot ulceration [3]. The progression from foot ulceration to infection and then onto amputation accounts for more than 60 % of all nontraumatic lower extremity amputations annually [2]. Lower extremity amputation can cause significant medical, emotional, and physical stress for patients, with mortality rates following amputation ranging from 13 to 40 % at 1 year, 35–65 % at 3 years, and 39–80 % at 5 years [4]. The mortality rates in these patients are second only to lung cancer mortality rates in the general population, which are estimated to be 86 % at 5 years [5]. For diabetics who do develop foot infections, approximately 20 % have evidence of osteomyelitis; often necessitating immediate treatment and intervention [6, 7]. The optimal treatment for these patients is multifactorial. The anatomical site of infection, vascular supply, extent of soft tissue and bone destruction, presence of necrosis, systemic signs of infection and patient preferences impact management options [8, 9]. The ideal balance between medical and surgical management continues to evolve. Primary surgical intervention, however, is reemerging as the principle treatment choice for diabetic patients with foot wounds complicated by osteomyelitis. The aim of intervention is both limb preservation and reduction of long-term morbidity.

Patients who are diagnosed with diabetic foot osteomyelitis (DFO) are often treated nonsurgically with the use of antimicrobial therapy [10]. The standard recommendation for treating chronic osteomyelitis is 6 weeks of parenteral antibiotic therapy. However, oral antibiotics are available that can achieve adequate levels in bone [11, 12]. Oral and parenteral therapies achieve similar cure rates; however, oral therapy avoids risks associated with intravenous catheters and is generally less expensive [11, 12]. In 2006, a study completed by Embil et al. evaluated 325 consecutive diabetic patients at a specialty wound care center [13]. They found and treated 93 infectious episodes in 79 total patients with oral antimicrobial agents. After a mean follow-up of 40 weeks, 75 (80.5 %) episodes were put into remission. They concluded that oral antimicrobial therapy alone was an effective management strategy in these patients [13]. In a similar study done by Senneville et al. years later, 50 consecutive diabetic patients with nonischemic feet who were diagnosed with osteomyelitis of the toe or metatarsal head and received primary medical treatment were followed [14]. At the conclusion of 12.8 months, results revealed that 63 % of patients were in remission [14]. Many other studies, in turn, have shown similar results, concluding the efficacy of primary nonsurgical treatment in this population [15–17]. However, these studies lacked standardization of diagnostic criteria, showed variability on the choice of outcome measures (readmission vs wound healing vs limb salvage), had heterogeneous populations and small sample sizes, limiting their reliability [10, 18] Based on all of this information, conservative medical therapy alone leaves significant room for improvement in overall patient outcomes. The addition of surgical intervention assists with infection eradication as well as offering the benefit of reconstruction to increase functionality and decrease long-term morbidity in patients with DFO. These principles and techniques will be further discussed throughout this chapter.

L. Gates, M.D. (✉) • P.A. Blume, D.P.M., F.A.C.F.A.S.
Yale New Haven Hospital, 330 Cedar Street, BB 204,
New Haven, CT 06510, USA
e-mail: Lindsay.gates@yale.edu; peter.b@snet.net

B.E. Sumpio, M.D.
Diabetic Foot Clinic, Department of Diabetes, King's College Hospital, London, SE 59RS, UK

Yale New Haven Hospital, 330 Cedar Street, BB 204,
New Haven, CT 06510, USA
e-mail: sumpio@yale.edu

© Springer International Publishing Switzerland 2015
T.J. Boffeli (ed.), *Osteomyelitis of the Foot and Ankle*, DOI 10.1007/978-3-319-18926-0_10

Eradication of Bone and Soft Tissue Infection

The eradication of a bone infection with antimicrobial therapy can be quite challenging due to many factors. Principally, host defenses do not optimally operate in the osseous environment, allowing infecting bacteria to elude inflammatory cells and induce osteolysis [19]. Some bacteria, such as *Staphylococcus aureus*, can produce adhesions for bone matrix proteins becoming incorporated into a relatively impermeable glycocalyx biofilm [19, 20]. The inability of antibiotics to completely eradicate bone infections in patients with DFO leads to recurrence, antibiotic resistance, and increased cost both financially and physically for the patient. The advent of newer broad-spectrum antibiotics which have better bioavailability and penetration and the use of surgical resection of infected and necrotic bone and soft tissue is of critical importance for limb salvage.

The goal for surgical intervention, beyond eradicating infection, is limb sparing; preserving function, and decreasing overall long-term morbidity and mortality. Location of DFO is very important and can be a limiting factor when planning for surgical intervention. In a study by Faglia et al., 350 patients with DFO were evaluated [21]. Osteomyelitis to the forefoot was found in 300 patients (85.7 %), the midfoot in 27 patients (7.7 %) and in the hind foot in 23 patients (6.7 %). In this cohort only one patient with forefoot osteomyelitis (0.33 %) required a transtibial amputation compared to 12 patients with osteomyelitis of the hindfoot/heal. After further analysis with multivariate logistical regression, they found that heel osteomyelitis was an independently significant risk factor for major amputation (OR 15.3; $p<0.001$) [21]. Poor outcomes can be associated with proximal spread of infection as well as delay in proper and complete surgical resection.

Complete resection and reconstruction may or may not be feasible as a single-stage procedure. Pinzur et al. evaluated 73 cases of patients with DFO who underwent a single-staged procedure for treatment [22]. The treatment algorithm included a radical resection of clinically infected bone followed by placement of large smooth percutaneous pins for provisional fixation. Maintenance of the surgically obtained correction was achieved with a three-level preconstructed static circular external fixator that was maintained for a period of 8 weeks in patients with involvement of the foot and a minimum of 12 weeks when the ankle was involved. At 1-year follow-up, Pinzur was able to achieve 95.7 % limb salvage rate with ambulation [22]. In a similar protocol, Paola et al. in 2009 conducted a prospective study of 45 patients with DFO. All patients underwent single-staged debridement and attempted fusion with external fixator. Their results showed that out of 45 patients, 39 were able to heal maintaining the fixation, which stayed in place for an average of 25.7 weeks [23]. In yet another single-stage operative approach to DFOs, Saltzman et al. extensively evaluated 8 patients with diffuse ankle osteomyelitis (5 of which

were diabetic). They attempted fusion of eight ankles and four subtalar joints with all patients receiving concurrent intravenous antibiotics for 6 weeks. At an average of 13.5 weeks, ankle sepsis was eradicated in all patients with 7 of 8 patients having successful ankle fusion. At end of their 3.4-year long-term follow-up, none of the 7 patients required further surgery. Single-stage surgery with aggressive debridement of infected soft tissue and bone, fusion and external fixation can provide an optimal outcome [24].

Patients with extensive infection, bone destruction, and soft tissue involvement, often require multiple staged procedures with aggressive debridement followed by internal fixation alone or in combination with external fixation (Fig. 10.1). Conservation of viable noninfected bone and soft tissue is paramount to a successful outcome. In a study done by Aragon-Sanchez, the investigator's goals were to analyze factors that determined the outcomes of conservative surgical treatment of DFO [25]. A consecutive series of 185 diabetic patients with foot osteomyelitis and histopathological confirmation of bone involvement were followed. All patients underwent early surgical treatment, within 12 h of admission, as an attempt towards foot-sparing interventions. At the conclusion of their study, authors found that 91 patients, 49.2 %, received conservative surgical procedures (no amputation to any part of the foot), 79 patients, 42.7 %, received foot-level/minor amputations, and 15 patients, 8 %, received major amputations. Risk factors for failure of foot conservation in this group included exposed bone, presence of ischemia and necrotizing soft tissue infections. The majority of patients were able to successfully undergo foot conservation. In many of these complicated cases, multiple debridement operations of bone and soft tissue can lead to foot instability and progressive deformity. Reconstruction considerations are especially important in patients who have charcot osteoarthropathy with concurrent osteomyelitis. The goal is eradication of osteomyelitis with antibiotics and surgical resection before final reconstruction. For maintaining deformity correction, Steinmann pins can be used for stabilization with compression from Ilizarov external fixation for midfoot, hindfoot, and/or ankle joints. Other options for surgical reconstruction include internal fixation, external fixation, arthrodesis or exostectomy [11]. A group led by Luca Dalla Paola evaluated a cohort of 45 patients with Charcot arthropathy and osteomyelitis [26]. All patients underwent aggressive surgical debridement with microbiological and histological exams of bone and soft tissue performed to ensure eradication. A hybrid external fixation was placed with the application of a foot plate combined with a unilateral fixator parallel to the tibia. All of these patients were given at least 8 weeks of postoperative antibiotics. At the end of their study, 39 patients healed with a stable ankle fusion and plantar grade foot. There were no reported screw or wire breakage and no pin tract infections. A study by Thordarson et al. mirror these excellent results in a small case series of five patients with

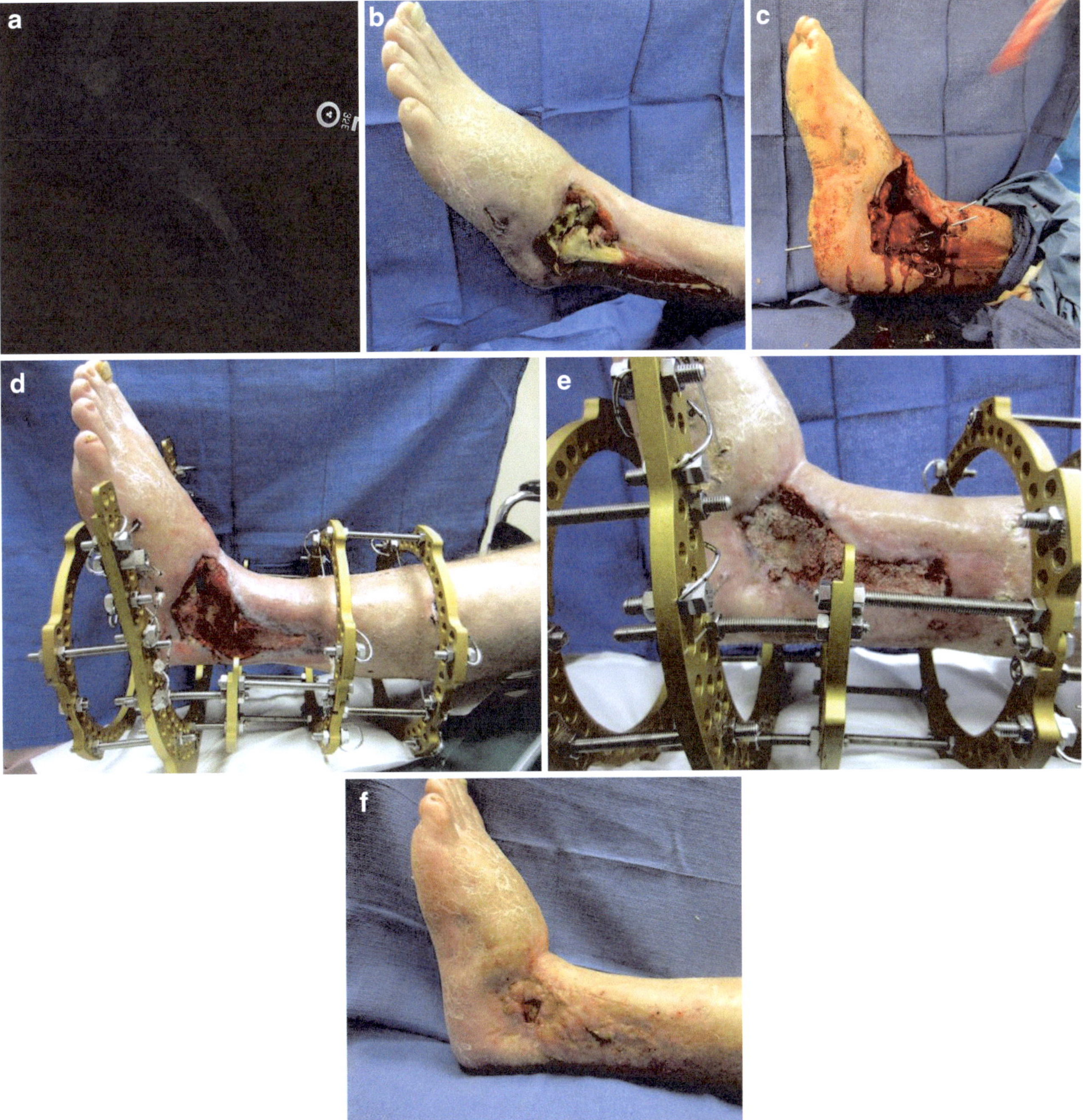

Fig. 10.1 A 70-y/o male with significant peripheral vascular disease with distal ischemia who presented after revascularization with ankle osteomyelitis. (**a**, **b**) X-ray imaging shows diffuse osteopenic changes with nonspecific periosteal reaction in the distal tibia and fibula. (**c**) Patient underwent 3 debridements with talectomy (**d**, **e**). Tibial calca-neal arthrodesis with application of circular frame external fixation. (**f**) Healed tibial calcaneal arthrodesis with healed skin graft after negative pressure wound therapy with wound reconstruction. Patient was able to walk without limitations 5 months after initial procedure

diabetic foot osteomyelitis who underwent radical soft tissue and bone debridement, soft tissue transfers, unilateral external fixation, and antibiotics [27]. All patients had successful fusion and were free of infection at follow-up. Richter et al. also reported on conservative surgery in 45 patients with complicated infections involving the ankle or subtalar joints [28]. Their treatment similarly involved debridement with intraoperative confirmation of infection free-tissue margins.

In this study however, arthrodesis was performed with either two compression screws (29 patients) or two compression screws (16 patients) in combination with additional external fixation for stabilization. In 86.6 % of the patients treated, solid fusion was obtained, 32 of which were able to return to work after an average of 35 weeks. Major amputation was avoided in all but one patient in this study who eventually required a below-knee amputation.

Whether single-stage or multiple-stage surgical procedures are utilized; a key principle to surgical treatment of DFOs is to remove all infected soft tissue and bone. Intraoperative specimens can be sent for histology to ensure free margins at the time of primary intervention or subsequent procedures in the case of delayed results [9, 10, 13, 29]. In a study by Atway et al., 81.8 % of patients with positive bone margins after intervention had poor long-term outcomes. The routine standardized bone margin culture should be obtained in all patients with reinterventions [30]. The evidence reveals that when adequate soft tissue coverage remains after debridement, excellent long-term healing can be achieved. Patients who present with bone involvement can undergo internal and external fixation, separate or in combination for stabilization and simultaneously to allow for eradication of infection and subsequently produce a long-term functional extremity (Fig. 10.2).

Tissue Reconstruction

The surgical approach to osteomyelitis of the diabetic foot and ankle can be dependent upon closure and reconstructive options. Numerous factors impact these complex reconstructive strategies. Surgery still can minimize adverse events with respect to the patient and their outcomes. The reconstructive ladder, a concept familiar to plastic surgeons, provides a framework for this advanced reconstructive decision-making [31]. Several iterations of the reconstructive ladder have been proposed; however one of the most recent versions, created by Janis et al., incorporates the traditional model with new wound healing strategies using negative-pressure wound therapy (NPWT), dermal matrices and increased utilization of local flaps [31]. The base of the ladder is primary closure with the transition to closure by secondary intention, negative pressure wound therapy, skin graft, dermal matrices, local flaps, distant flaps, tissue expansion, and free flaps as a last option. The reconstructive hierarchy created is an obvious simplification of complex decision-making process between the surgeon and patient. The algorithm can guide surgical planning and focus on restoration of limb function [32] (Fig. 10.3).

A successful surgical debridement can lead to complete primary wound closure which is the base of the reconstructive ladder. Garcia Morales et al. looked at 46 patients with DFO who underwent bone and soft tissue debridement and had either primary surgical closure [33] or were allowed to heal by secondary intention [14]. They found that primary

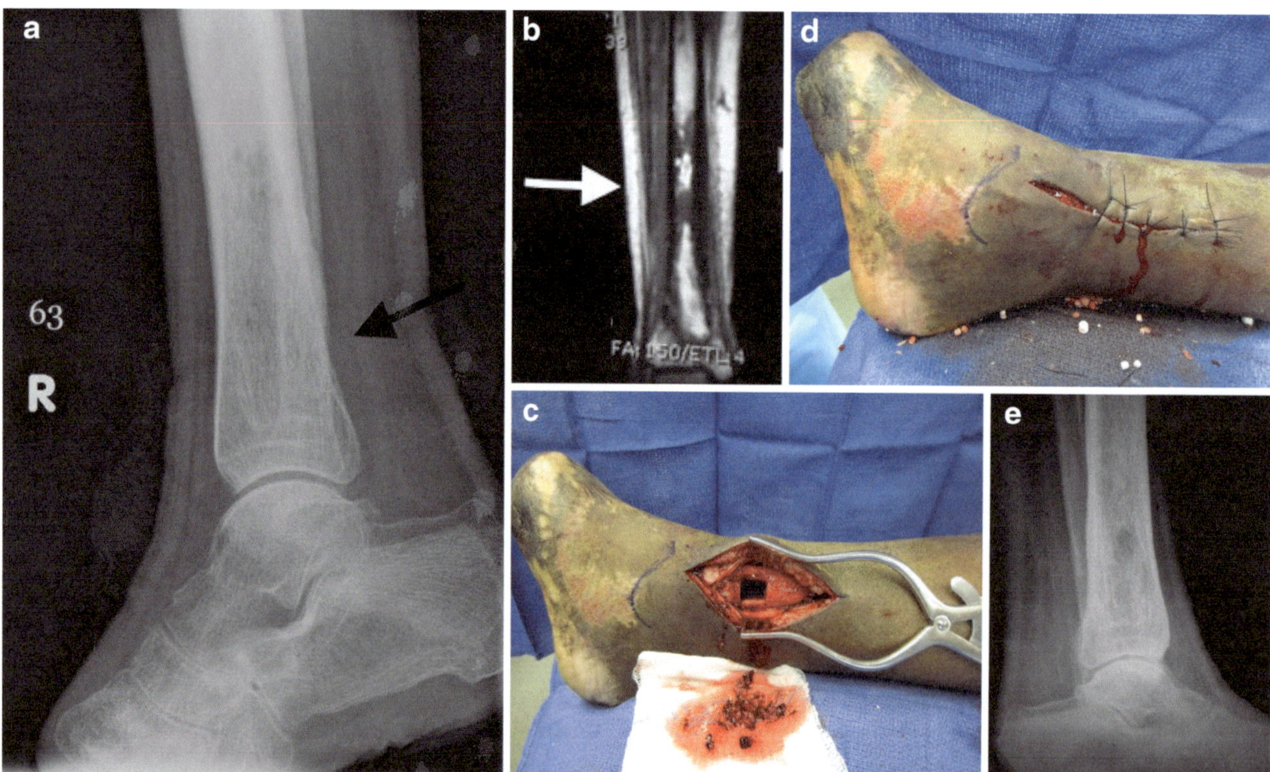

Fig. 10.2 Patient was a 26-year-old female with leukemia who developed hematogenous osteomyelitis after MRSA bacteremia. (**a**) Preoperative X-ray showed a permeative lesion with endosteal scalloping within the distal tibial diaphysis and metaphysis with associated periosteal reaction, suspicious of osteomyelitis. (**b**) MRI confirmed tibial osteomyelitis. (**c**) Underwent single-stage resection of tibial osteomyelitis with window created for packing Stimulan antibiotic beads. (**d**) Primary closure over defect. (**e**) Follow-up X-ray, patient completely healed and able to utilize for walking

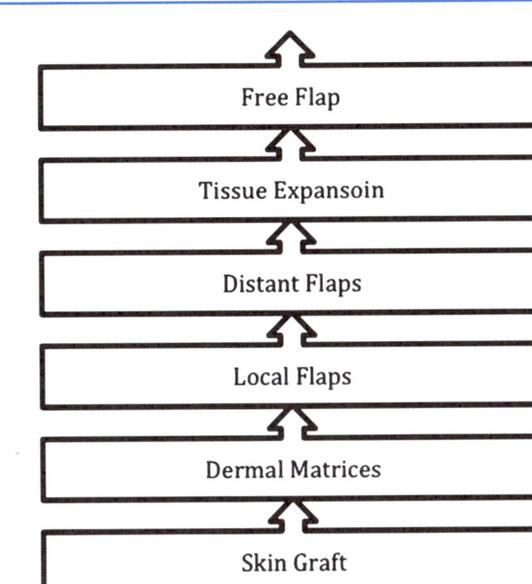

Fig. 10.3 Reconstructive ladder

surgical closure was associated with a reduced average healing time and no increase in postoperative complications [34]. However, in patients with DFOs that have extensive infection or late presentations, the preservation of soft tissue during surgical debridement and primary closure may not be possible. Significant tissue loss poses a challenge for reconstruction of the subsequent skeletal and soft tissue defects. These patients may be candidates for alternative soft tissue coverage using sking grafts, local/free muscle flaps or skeletal restoration and stabilization with bone grafts.

Primary closure or closure by secondary intention may not be an option and therefore a new addition to the reconstructive ladder was first described by Morykwat et al. in 1997 [35]. The success of NPWT in aiding wound healing is due to several different factors. Morykwat et al.'s original research on animal models noted an increased formation of granulation tissue in wounds treated with NPWT [35]. Zoch et al. then looked at the effect of NPWT on tissue perfusion in diabetic foot infections. They found a 31 % increase in perfusion to the wound and a 14 % increase in perfusion of surrounding tissue during NPWT therapy [36]. Additionally, Kamolz et al. concluded that NPWT had a reduction in periphcral cdcma, as a result of fluid removal [37]. These factors play a role in the therapeutic benefit of NPWT for wound closure. Some of the other alternative treatments for wound therapy include advanced moist wound therapy (AMWT), bioengineered tissue or skin substitutes, growth factors, and electric stimulation. In 2008 Blume et al. looked at the safety and efficacy of NPWT compared to AMWT specifically [38]. Their study was a multicenter randomized control trial, which enrolled 342 diabetic patients with foot ulcers who were followed up to 9 months. Findings showed a greater proportion of foot ulcers achieved complete closure with NPWT than with AMWT (43.2 % vs 28.9 %, $p=0.007$). The NPWT group also had significantly fewer secondary amputations ($p=0.035$). They concluded that NPWT is safe and more efficacious than AMWT. This study looked at diabetic ulcer healing and not specifically at patients with osteomyelitis. A Cochran Review published in 2013 evaluating the effects of NPWT compared with standard care echoed the results of Blume's study. They concluded that there is evidence to suggest that NPWT is more effective in healing postoperative foot wounds and ulcers of the foot in people with DM compared with moist dressings [39]. NPWT has not been directly compared to closure by secondary intention. There are many expanded therapeutic benefits in wounds beyond the scope of standard NPWT which can aid in healing of poorly vascularized tissue such as bone or tendon. These tissues are at increased risk to break down after closure by secondary intention and skin grafting leading to suboptimal results with thin, unstable coverage. Lee et al. published a small case series looking at 16 ankle wounds that had exposed bone and tendon. They were able to successfully granulate and graft 15 wounds with NPWT [40]. Bollero et al. similarly, described a series of 37 complex, high-risk, lower extremity wounds which were successfully reconstructed using NPWT [41]. Wound size, unfortunately still plays a limiting factor on the utilization of NPWT, with larger defects often requiring flap coverage for complete healing.

With large, complex wounds that are not amenable to primary closure or aided closure with NPWT, local flaps, and perforator flaps are the next sequential step up the reconstructive ladder. Local muscle flaps appeared in the late 1960s and were used exclusively for foot and ankle reconstructions until the late 1970s when microsurgical free flaps gained popularity [42]. Patients with large soft tissue defects that require aggressive bone resection in order to create an adequate soft-tissue envelope for primary closure can result in a mechanically unstable foot and ankle, which can be prone to future breakdown and tissue loss. The goal of limb preservation does require adequate coverage especially at anatomic sites at risk of failure such as weight bearing areas and mobile joints. Fasciocutaneous flaps are often inadequate due to limited size, mobility, and durability, while intrinsic muscle flaps are well-vascularized alternatives that are versatile and have shown to hold up better over time [43]. There are many muscle flaps that provide coverage for foot and ankle reconstruction. These include the abductor hallucis brevis for medial midfoot, heel and ankle defects; the abductor digiti minimi for lateral ankle and calcaneal defects; the flexor digiti minimi for midfoot defects; the flexor digitorum brevis for plantar heal defects; and the extensor digitorum brevis for anterior ankle defects [33, 44, 45]. There are many advantages for the use of intrinsic or local muscle flaps. They can be harvested with a simple ankle block, minimizing the anesthetic risk, and the donor site can almost always be closed primarily. A study by Ducic et al. looked at the effectiveness of pedicled muscle flaps in patients with diabetes for complex foot and ankle reconstruction. In this analysis, 32 patients received 34 pedicled muscle flaps with results showing a 91 % (31/34) success rate, and a 94 % limb salvage rate. Overall, only 15 complications were reported at the completion of all 45 reconstructive procedures. Compared to historical controls of nondiabetic patients, they did not find any difference in wound healing rates, flap success, limb salvage,

or ambulatory status. There was a slight difference in the number of operations and healing times, with diabetic patients requiring twice as many operations and twice as long to heal as nondiabetic patients. Diabetic patients also had slightly decreased long-term survival; however, it was still far superior to the long-term survival rates of amputees. Additional advantages of local muscle flaps include increased blood supply, improved oxygen transport, and direct delivery of host defense mechanisms or antibiotics. Also, vascularized tissue from these flaps are able to conform to a variety of spaces, eliminating dead space and decreasing local bacterial counts [44, 46]. Local or pedicled flaps, however, are handicapped by the pedicle which carries the blood supply and assures viability thus restricting their area of reach and arc of rotation. In conclusion, local tissue flaps have a significant utility in reconstruction of defects in patients with DFO (Fig. 10.4).

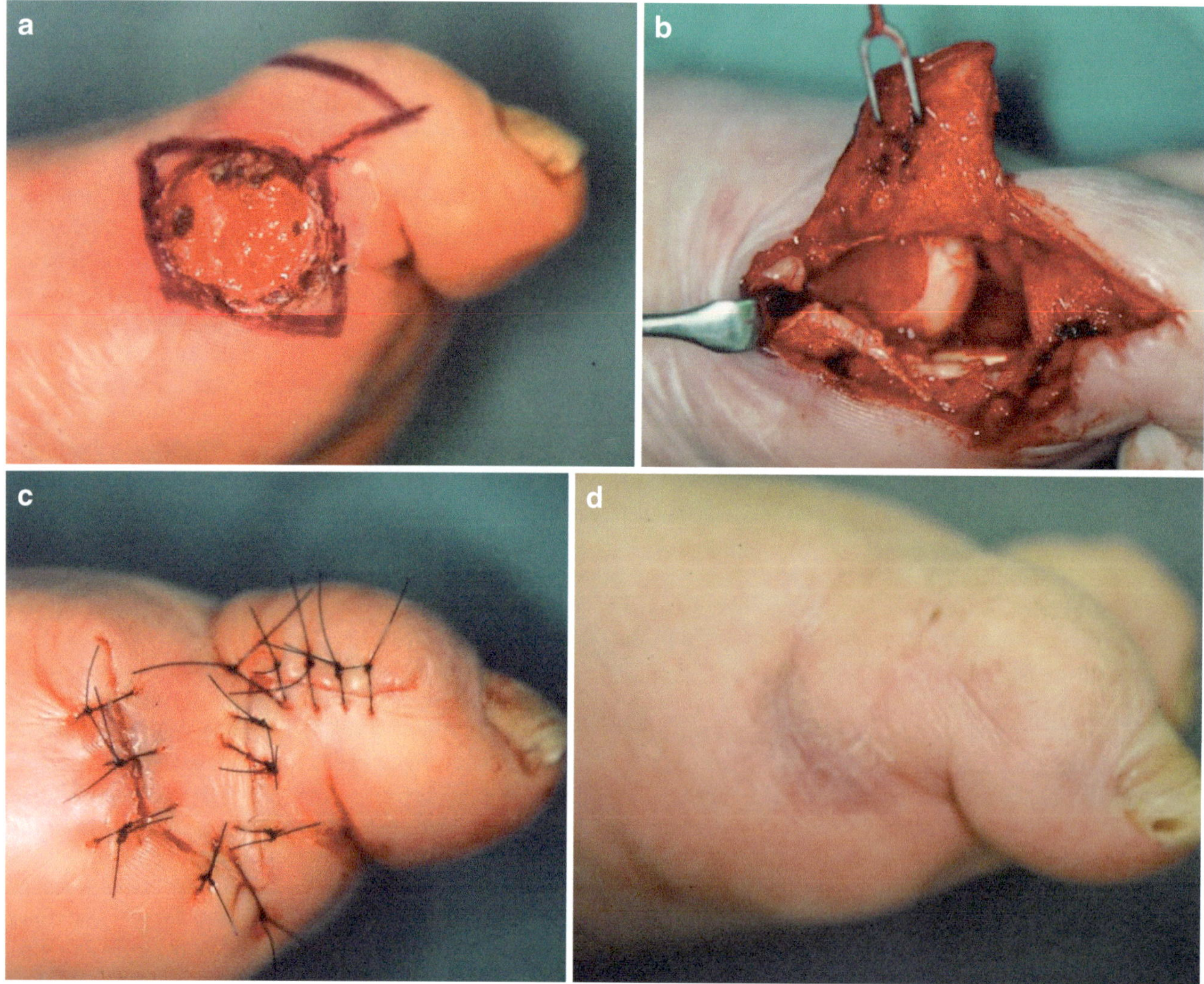

Fig. 10.4 (**a**) Osteomyelitis of first metatarsal phalangeal joint. (**b–d**) Single-stage resection approach including local flap reconstruction with biomechanical preservation

Although there are many advantages of using local flaps, each anatomic region of the foot and ankle has special reconstructive requirements that may preclude their use. The dorsum of the foot and ankle require thin, pliable, soft tissue for coverage of exposed tendons. Conversely, the skin over the plantar aspect must be flexible allowing for freedom of motion and enough durability in order to withstand constant pressure and force [47]. Free muscle flaps have provided an alternative method of tissue coverage to address these multiple considerations and sit at the top of the reconstructive ladder. Over four decades ago the first successful free composite tissue transfer was performed by McLean and Buncke in 1972 [48]. This was followed a year later by both Daniel and Taylor as well as O'Brien with the first transfer of island flaps from the groin to reconstruct traumatized lower extremities [49, 50]. The development and successful utilization of free-tissue transfer is especially important when planning intervention for patients with DFO, who require coverage after more radical excision of infected soft tissue and bone. Free flaps are highly vascularized via their own blood supply, enhancing the revascularization of a critically ischemic angiosome through the development of vascular connections between the flap and native tissue. Several different donor free flaps have been described in the literature. These include the lattismus dorsi perforator flap, antecubital flap, forearm flap, scapular flap, anterior lateral thigh flap, medial thigh flap, gracilis flap, and the deep inferior epigastric artery perforator flap (DIEP) [51–54]. Ohta et al. in 2006 reported on a small case series of 4 patients with DFO treated with free DIEP flaps. Their results showed that out of the four flaps, 3 took completely without any complications and one flap took with partial necrosis that healed with ointment treatment. Postoperatively, all patients were able to walk without difficulty [55]. In another small series by Omer et al., 13 patients with complications of DFO were treated with various free flaps. All reconstructed flaps survived well postoperatively, however they did have two major amputations reported due to persistent osteomyelitis. The overall limb salvage rate was 83 % [56]. In 2011, a meta-analysis and systematic review of free-tissue transfer in 528 diabetic patients with nonhealing wounds (55 % patients with specific mention of the presence of osteomyelitis) was reported by O'Conner et al. [57]. From the 18 studies evaluated, they found the overall flap survival rate was 92 % (primary patency rate was 86 %), and overall limb salvage rate was 83.4 % over a 28-month follow-up period. Only 16 studies reported on ambulation rate with a mean rate of 76 % (69.8–83.9, CI 95 %). In this review, the major cause of flap failure was infection, reinforcing the necessity for eradication of osteomyelitis as the priority in this population prior to reconstruction. Even though this review demonstrated successful wound healing and good functional outcomes after free-tissue transfer, it did not address the long-term impact on survival in patients with

DFO. In 2012 Suk Oh et al. looked specifically at 5-year survival rates and preoperative risk factors affecting outcomes after free-flap reconstruction in patients with diabetes [58]. Out of 121 cases, 111 Free-tissue transfers were successful (flap survival rate of 91 %). Limb preservation was 84.9 % and the 5-year survival was 86.8 %. Risk factors associated with higher rate of flap failure included history of one or more angioplasty procedures (OR 17.59, $p<0.001$), history of peripheral arterial disease (10.21, $p=0.032$), and patients using immunosuppressive agents after renal transplant (4.86, $p<0.041$). Patients who were treated for preoperative osteomyelitis did not show a statistically significant increased risk for flap failure in this series (OR 1.056, $p=0.935$). Free flaps do allow for closure of complex wounds but often complicate function of the limb due to size and type of tissue transformed. The paradigm shift in reconstructive strategies for these patients has really changed to focus on eradication of bone infection with local tissue reconstruction, with free flaps as a last resort (Fig. 10.5).

The strong evidence that supports tissue reconstruction in patients with DFO is based on the aforementioned concepts of debridement with eradication of infection. It is paramount that these patients have a suitable vascular supply to provide adequate blood flow to the tissue. The approach to revascularization in patients with foot wounds or ischemic ulcerations was traditionally based on the "best vessel" approach, with surgical techniques focusing on getting blood flow from a proximal blood vessel to the best available distal vessel regardless of location. Several studies however have reported high rates of unhealed wounds despite patent bypasses or restored in-line flow via endovascular methods [59, 60]. This evidence has supported investigation in a new model of revascularization based on angiosomes. Angiosomes are three-dimensional blocks of tissue fed by source arteries with functional vascular connections between muscles, fascia, and skin. The foot and ankle are composed of six distinct angiosomes with the main arteries having numerous direct arterial–arterial connections to provide alternative routes of blood flow if the direct route is disrupted [61]. An angiosome based revascularization strategy attempts to reestablish flow to the source artery of a lesion, rather than focusing on the most suitable artery as the target for revascularization. A systematic literature review was published by Sumpio et al. in 2013 to evaluate this strategy [62]. They found 11 papers to include in their outcomes analysis, most of which were retrospective case series or reviews of prospectively kept databases. Ten of these studies compared direct revascularization (angiosome model) to indirect revascularization (best vessel model). Of these, five reported significant increase in limb salvage rates with direct revascularization. In addition 5 out of 8 studies that reported wound-healing rates found a significant increase in healing when following the principles of the angiosome revascularization strategy. Even though there

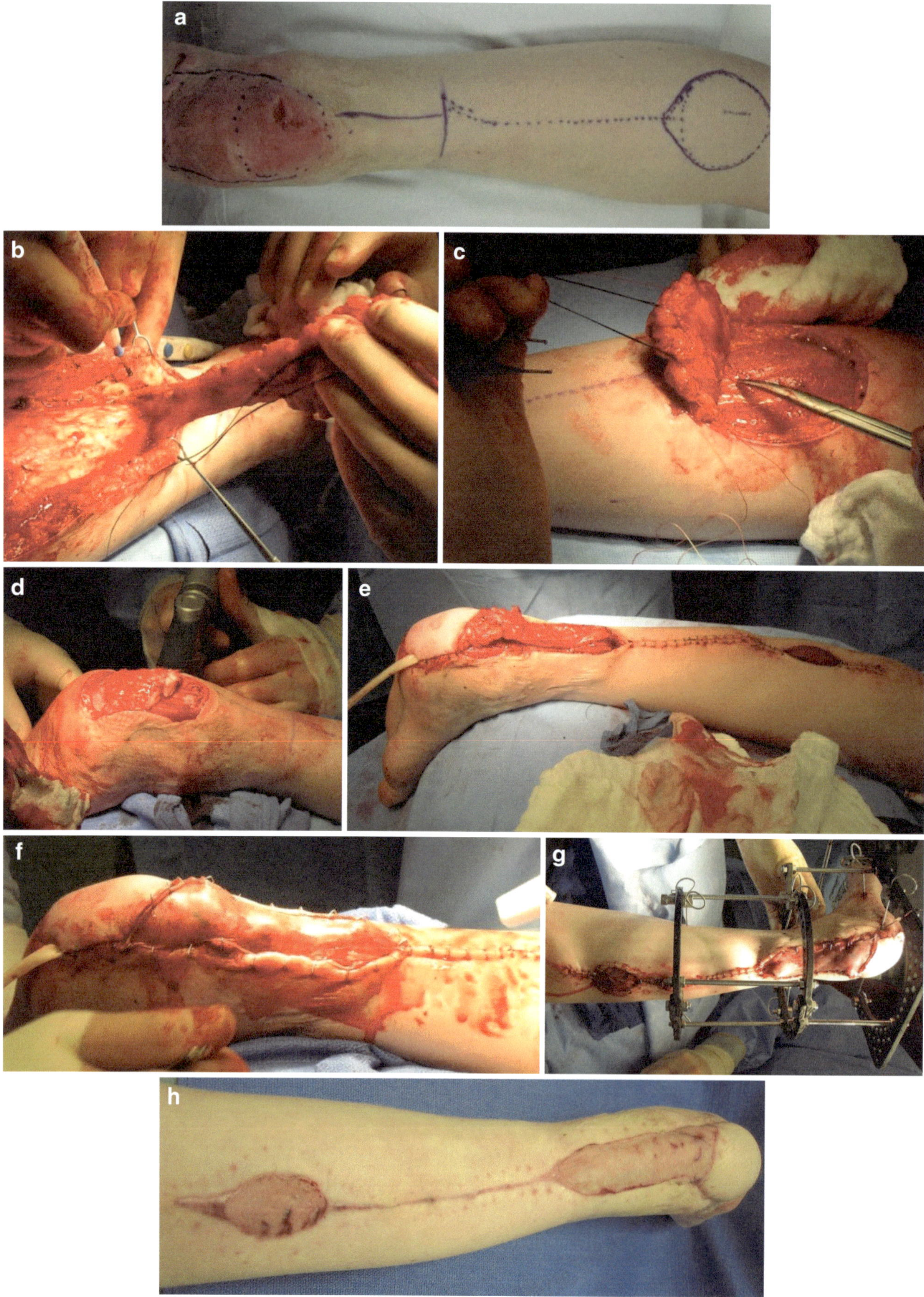

Fig. 10.5 (**a–h**): (**a**) Calcaneal osteomyelitis. (**b–f**) Resection and debridement of calcaneal osteomyelitis with Achilles tendon resection and reverse sural flap reconstruction. (**g**) External fixation placed for offloading. (**h**) Healed flap with mechanical preservation

is a limited amount of data available, these results support the ideal of attempting direct revascularization to the affected angiosome. Perhaps this is even more important in patients with diabetic foot wounds where they often have patchy atherosclerotic lesions, and destruction of collaterals, which will inhibit wound healing by indirect revascularization methods [63]. Another revascularization strategy for patients with significant peripheral arterial disease and inadequate inflow, is the use of combined vascular reconstruction and free-flap transfer for limb salvage. Vermassen et al. reported on 45 diabetic patients who underwent a combination of arterial revascularization and free-flap transfer [64]. The indications for all procedures were the presence of extensive gangrenous defects of the foot or lower leg with the exposure of bones or tendons. Patients were excluded in which treatment with a simple wound closure or split-thickness skin graft (STSG) wound have been possible or in whom postoperative ambulation wound not have been expected. In 45 patients, a total of 53 arterial reconstructions were performed, 37 of which the distal anastomosis was on a pedal or tibial vessel with either greater saphenous vein or cryopreserved homologous saphenous vein. Operative technique in these patients included a side-to-side anastomosis with the native vessel leaving a free end of the arterialized saphenous vein for an end-to end anastomosis with the flap artery. Venous anastomosis were performed on the concomitant deep veins in 38 patients with 3 patients having a superficial vein used as a second outflow, and 9 patients having superficial vein or mobilized lesser saphenous vein as primary outflow vessel. The remaining patients underwent a combination of two different levels either with bypass or percutaneous transluminal angioplasty plus bypass. At the conclusion of the study, reintervention was performed on 14 patients resulting in 5 flap losses (2 of which treated with new free flap, 3 were amputated), and 3 early postoperative deaths. Thirty-nine out of 45 patents (87 %) were discharged amputation free and 32/39 patients achieved independent ambulation. At 1-year followup, combined survival and limb-salvage rate was 84 % after 1 year. Subsequently in 2009 Random et al. published a similar study evaluating results and complication of combined simultaneous arterial revascularization and free-flap transfer in patients with critical limb ischemia and large soft-tissue defects. Only 70.5 % of their population was diabetic with 38 % presenting with osteomyelitis. They reported superior limb salvage at one year of 93 % decreasing to 71 % at 5-year follow-up. Combined 1-year limb salvage and survival was similar to Vermassen et al.'s results at 85 %. Some of the benefits of this combined approach is that free-flap transfer offers additional outflow to the bypass; as poor outflow and increased vascular resistance is a major cause for overall distal bypass failure. Lorenzetti et al. specifically investigated this concept and found that the low-resistance outflow bed of transferred muscle could increase graft flow by up to 50 % [65].

Based on these results, combined revascularization and tissue transfer in complicated diabetic patients with large defects not amenable to other reconstructive options, is a preferable option over primary major amputation with acceptable long-term survival and limb salvage rates. Whether a direct revascularization strategy based on an angiosome model or revascularization with combined tissue transfer is used, the importance of adequate blood flow available for wound healing cannot be stressed enough.

Adjuvant Agents

Total eradication of infection and reconstruction in patients with DFO was traditionally accomplished solely with surgical intervention as previously described. In many of these patients, however, there has been increasing evidence to support the addition of a few select adjuvant therapies in order to eradicate bone infection. Several adjunct treatments will be discussed including, super-oxidized solution, granulocyte colony-stimulating factor and antibiotic composites.

In addition to antibiotics and surgical debridement, the use of an antiseptic agent such as a stable super-oxidized solution (SOS) has been proposed to aid in treatment of osteomyelitis in diabetic foot infections. The use of antiseptics in tissue infections has historically been controversial due to sparse evidence available to support effective antibacterial activity, and reports of a few formulations which actually caused native tissue damage [66]. However, in 1996 Yahagi et al. looked at SOS, a new formulation of antiseptic, which was effective against bacteria but not on eukaryotic cells [67]. One limitation of Yahagi's research was that most of the solutions available were short acting making broad clinical application difficult [68]. Dermacyn wound care (DWC; Oculus Innovative Sciences, Petaluma, CA) subsequently appeared on the market as the first reported SOS that is stable at room temperature for up to 1 year [69]. Aragon-Sanchez et al. evaluated 14 patients who underwent conservative surgery for DFO, in whom clean bone margins could not be assured and had histopathologic confirmed osteomyelitis [70]. Intraoperatively, each patient received copious irrigation with DWC as well as daily irrigation with DWC either through a catheter inserted in the surgical cavity, between sutures, or via placing gauzes soaked with DWC over the open wound. All patients also received culture-directed antibiotic therapy. There were no reported side effects of the treatment and 100 % limb salvage was achieved in treated patient over an average healing period of 6.8 weeks. Later in 2010, Piaggesi et al. published a randomized controlled trial evaluating the safety and efficacy of DWC [71]. Forty patients with postsurgical lesions which were left open to heal by secondary intention were randomized into two groups: A, locally treated with DWC and B, povidone iodine as local medication.

Both groups received systemic antibiotic therapy and surgical debridement if needed. Patients were then followed weekly for 6 months. At the conclusion of their study, healing rates were significantly shorter in group A (90 %) than in group B (55 %; $p<0.01$). Time taken for cultures to become negative and duration of antibiotic therapy were also significantly shorter in group A than in group B. The number of interventions were also significantly higher in group B ($p<.05$) as well as reinfections ($p<0.01$). Based on current evidence, SOS antiseptics appear to be a safe and effective adjuvant to surgical debridement and antibiotic therapy creating an unfavorable environment for bacteria and assisting with accelerated wound healing. Nevertheless, additional research for their specific use in DFO is needed to completely understand their full therapeutic benefit and role in treatment.

The incidence and severity of infections in the diabetic population is partly enhanced by the dysfunction of the host antibacterial defense systems. In particular, defects in neutrophil function have been identified, including deficiencies in adherence, chemotaxis, phagocytosis, superoxide production, and intracellular killing [72–74]. To overcome these functional deficiencies, granulocyte colony-stimulating factor (G-CSF) has been used either alone or in combination with antibiotics to enhance the inflammatory response of patients with DFO. In 1997 Gough et al. enrolled 40 diabetic patients with foot infections in a double-blind placebo-controlled study where patients were randomly assigned to either G-CSF therapy or placebo therapy for 7 days along with antibiotic and insulin therapy [75]. They found that G-CSF therapy was associated with earlier eradication of pathogens ($p=0.02$), shorter duration of intravenous antibiotic treatment ($p=0.02$), quicker resolution of cellulitis ($p=0.03$), and shorter hospital stays ($p=0.02$). After 7 days of treatment, neutrophil superoxide production was measured in each group. Patients in the G-CSF group had a significantly higher level than those in the placebo group ($p<0.0001$). Their findings supported the use of G-CSF as an adjuvant to traditional treatment strategies for patients with DFO. Subsequently in 2001, de Lalla et al. also looked at the safety and efficacy of G-CSF as an adjunctive agent for the standard treatment of limb-threatening foot osteomyelitis in diabetic patients [76]. Forty-eight patients were enrolled in a prospective, randomized, controlled study to receive either conventional treatment alone (local treatment, consisting of debridement and wound care, plus systemic antibiotic therapy) or conventional treatment plus G-CSF. They found that at 9-week follow-up, patients who received G-CSF had a lower rate of amputation compared to standard treatment ($p=0.038$). The authors of this study speculated that these results may be due to a more effective response in the G-CSF group to infection and thus increased freedom from amputation. Although there has been promising data supporting the use of G-CSF in DFO, a preliminary meta-analysis of five randomized trials using G-CSF has not shown clinically significant evidence that G-CSF will accelerate resolution of infection [77]. It did show, however, that it may reduce the number of additional operative procedures.

Adjunct therapies to wound healing in DFO also include antibiotic-loaded cement and composites, which can be used as a temporary spacer or primary therapy for an elution of antibiotics. Calcium sulfate and calcium phosphate pellets with combinations of antibiotics are becoming increasingly more important in the eradication of bone infections. Large defects of bone and soft tissue often result from aggressive resection of osteomyelitis which can produce a dead space which can be a precursor to hematoma formation which is an ideal culture medium for bacteria. Antibiotic-containing polymethyl-methacrylate cement (PMMA) can be form-fitted for unique anatomic spaces but if left in place prevents bone growth over time. Additionally, once the antibiotic had fully eluted from the cement a risk of secondary infection could occur due to a reaction to the foreign body. These complications of antibiotic-loaded cement were the driving force in the development of a biodegradable antibiotic carrier. Stimulan (Biocomposites Ltd., Keele, UK) which is a synthetic crystallic semihydrate form of calcium sulfate which is biocompatible, completely reabsorbed and replaced by new bone as well as 100 % pure with no traces of potentially toxic impurities. It can be mixed with a variety of antibiotics such as Moxifloxacin, Tobramycin, and Vancomycin. This allows for use in patients with infections caused by a number of highly resistant organisms. This biocomposite can be formed into pellets of variable size that then are placed in the defect that remains after the debridement of vests amount of bone. It provides high local levels of antibiotic and then gradually dissolves, permitting infilling of the osseous defect with new bone. Over time the calcium sulfate is absorbed while concurrently stimulating new bone growth along with the continued elution of local antibiotics. Ferguson et al. reported their experience with the use of similar biodegradable calcium sulfate antibiotic spacers called Osteoset T (Wright Medical, Arlinton, Tennessee) in the surgical management of 195 cases of chronic osteomyelitis [78]. Osteoset T, is a hemihydrate calcium sulfate containing 4 % tobramycin made into 4.8 mm diameter pellets. Their results showed recurrent infection occurring in only 18 cases (9.2 %), with an overall resolution of infection in 97.9 % of their patients at the end of follow-up. Radiographic assessment showed no filling defect in 36.6 % of patients, partial defect in 59 %, and complete filling defects in only 4.4 % of patients. In another study by Chang et al., they evaluated 65 patients with chronic osteomyelitis and compared debridement to debridement with Osteoset T [79]. They found healing rates at 75-month follow-up to be 60 % and 80 % respectively. These results emphasize the impact and importance of incorporating bone cement and antibiotic products for local delivery in the surgical management of patients with complex DFO (Fig. 10.6).

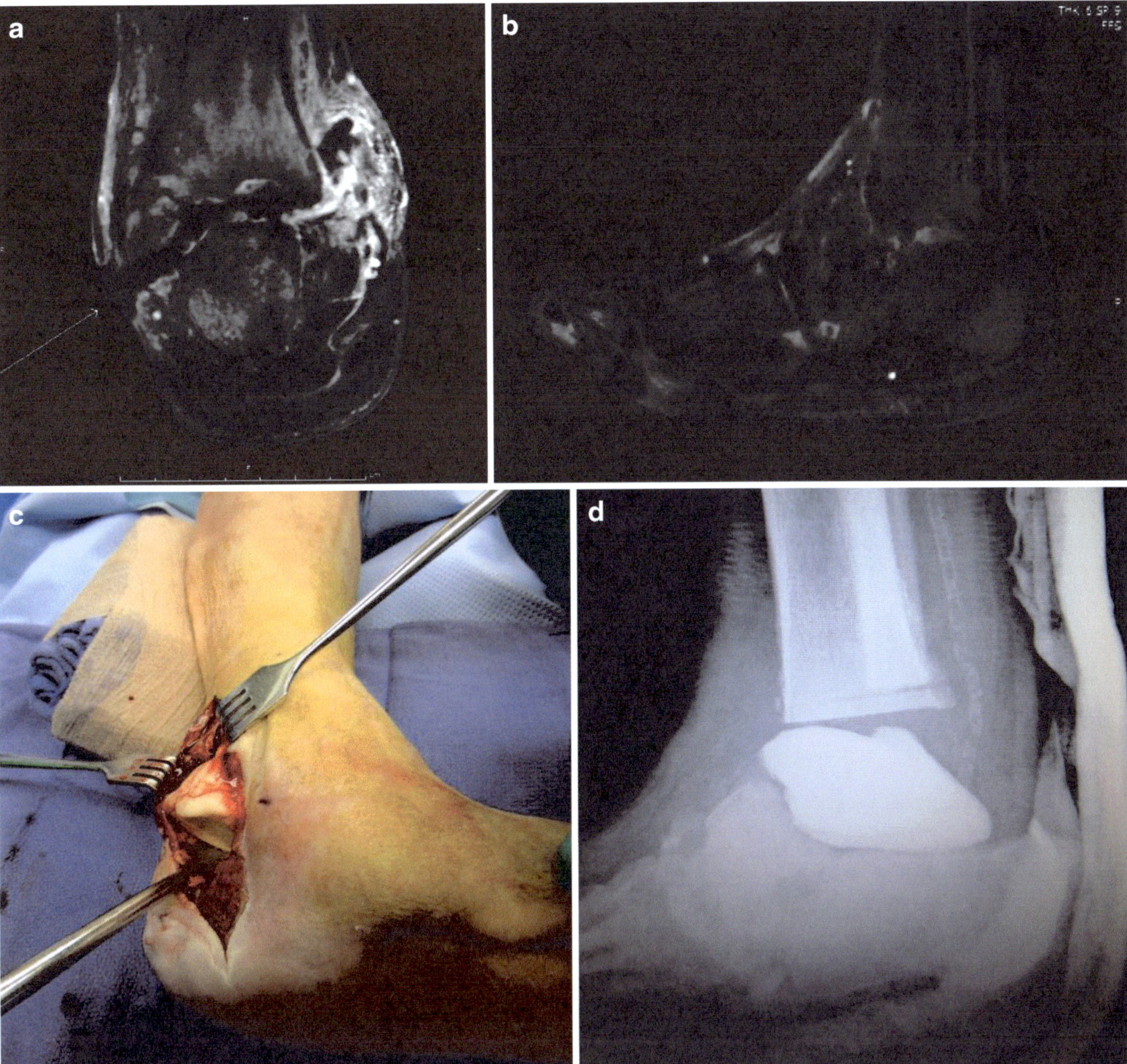

Fig. 10.6 A 50-year-old male presented with charcot arthropathy of the midfoot with osseous destruction and disorganization involving the distal tibia, fibula, talus, and majority of the calcaneus. Also seen on MRI imaging (**a**, **b**) peripherally rim-enhancing collection involving the ankle joint draining to a cutaneous ulceration distal to the lateral malleolus. (**c**) Taken to OR, resection of resection of osteomyelitic ankle with application of methy/methacrylate cement with 1.4 g of Tobramycin. (**b**) X-ray imaging of antibiotic spacer in place, spacer left in 6 weeks

Summary

In summary, eradication of bone infection is vital for soft tissue reconstruction in diabetic wounds. The surgical treatment principles for diabetic foot wounds that are complicated by osteomyelitis involve many disciplines and adjunct therapies. The ability to reconstruct a diabetic foot wound is dependent upon numerous principles. Surgical planning will typically involve surgical elimination of the wound with some form of bone and soft tissue debridement/resection. One must always plan for closure and reconstructive options using the reconstructive ladder as a framework. It is important to remember that po stoperative function of the limb is key to the success in this patient population. The use of free flaps allows for closure but often complicate function of these limbs. Bone resection with biomechanical stabilization and soft tissue closure in the simplest strategy and can often provide patients with a long-lasting and stable platform in order to ambulate. The biology of bone infection and the soft tissue component are also important considerations. Perfusion of the local tissues, which is required for healing, makes the angiosome concept and revascularization another paramount component for successful limb preservation. The ultimate goals of limb salvage in the at-risk population with diabetic foot and ankle osteomyelitis is the reestablishment of a functional limb that is free of wounds and infection thus preventing limb loss which reduces the rate of morbidity and mortality.

References

1. International Diabetes Federation. "Diabetes Atlas". http://da3.diabetesatlas.org/indexc419.html. Accessed 2 Jun 14.
2. Center for Disease Control. "National Diabetes Statistics Report". Last Updated 2 Jun 14. http://www.cdc.gov/diabetes/pubs/estimates14.htm. Accessed 15 Jun 2014.
3. Singh N, Armstrong DG, Lipsky BA. Preventing foot ulcers in patients with diabetes. JAMA. 2005;293(2):217–28.
4. Reiber GE. Epidemiology of foot ulcers and amputations in the diabetic foot. In: Bowker JH, Pfeifer MA, editors. The diabetic foot. St. Louis, MO: Mosby; 2001. p. 13–32.
5. American Cancer Society. Cancer facts and figures. http://www.cancer.org/research/cancerfactsstatistics/cancerfactsfigures2014/index. (2014). Accessed 4 Jun 2014.
6. Newman LG, Waller J, Palestro CJ, et al. Unsuspected osteomyelitis in diabetic foot ulcers. Diagnosis and monitoring by leukocyte scanning with indium in 111 oxyquinoline. JAMA. 1991;266: 1246–51.
7. Grayson ML, Gibbons GW, Habershaw GM, et al. Use of ampicillin/sulbactam versus imipenem/cilastatin in the treatment of limb-threatening foot infections in diabetic patients. Clin Infect Dis. 1997;25:1318–26.
8. Prompers L, Huijberts M, Apelqvist J, et al. High prevalence of ischaemia, infection and serious comorbidity in patients with diabetic foot disease in Europe. Baseline results from the Eurodiale study. Diabetologia. 2007;50:18–25.
9. Apelqvist J, Bakker K, van Houtum WH, et al. Practical guidelines on the management and prevention of the diabetic foot: based upon the International Consensus on the Diabetic Foot (2007) Prepared by the International Working Group on the Diabetic Foot. Diabetes Metab Res Rev. 2008;24 suppl 1:S181–7.
10. Berendt AR, Peters EG, Bakker K, et al. Diabetic foot osteomyelitis: a progress report on diagnosis and systematic review of treatment. Diabetes Metab Res Rev. 2008;24 Suppl 1:S1 45–S161.
11. Donegan R, Sumpio B, Blume P. Charcot foot and ankle with osteomyelitis. Diabet Foot Ankle. 2013;4:10. doi:10.3402/dfa.v4i0.21361.
12. Coneterno L, da Silva Filho. Antibiotics for treating chronic osteomyelitis in adults. Cochrane Database Syst Rev 2009, 3: CD004439.
13. Embil JM, Rose G, Trepman E, et al. Oral antimicrobial therapy for the diabetic foot osteomyelitis. Foot Ankle Int. 2006;27(10):771–9.
14. Senneville E, Legout L, Lombart A, et al. Outcome of diabetic foot osteomyelitis treated nonsurgically. Diabetes Care. 2008;31:637–42.
15. Yadlapalli N, Vaishnar A, Sheehan P. Conservative management of diabetic foot ulcers complicated by osteomyelitis. Wounds. 2002;14:31–5.
16. Senneville E, Yazdanpanah Y, Cazaubiel M, et al. Rifampin-ofloxacin oral regimen for the treatment of mild to moderate diabetic foot osteomyelitis. J Antimicrob Chemother. 2001;39:235–40.
17. Game F, Jeffcoate WJ. Primarily non-surgical management of osteomyelitis of the foot in diabetes. Diabetologia. 2008;51: 962–7.
18. Luis-Martinex J, Aragon-Sanchez J, Garcia-Morales E, et al. Antibiotics versus conservative surgery for treating diabetic foot osteomyelitis: a randomized comparative trial. Diabetes Care. 2014;37(3):789–95.
19. Ciampolini J, Harding KG. Pathophysiology of chronic bacterial osteomyelitis. Why do antibiotics fail so often? Postgrad Med J. 2000;76:479–83.
20. Lew DP, Waldvogel FA. Osteomyelitis. N Engl J Med. 1997;336:999–1007.
21. Faglia E, Clerici G, Caminiti M, et al. Influence of osteomyelitis location in the foot of diabetic patients with transtibial amputation. Foot Ankle Int. 2013;34:222–7.
22. Pinzur MS, Gil J, Belmares J. Treatment of osteomyelitis in charcot foot with single-stage resection of infection, correction of deformity and maintenance with ring fixation. Foot Ankle Int. 2012;33: 1069–74.
23. Dalla Paola L, Brocco E, Ceccacci T, et al. Limb salvage in charcot foot and ankle osteomyelitis: combined use single stage/double stage of arthrodesis and external fixation. Foot Ankle Int. 2009;30(11):1065–70.
24. Saltzman CL. Salvage of diffuse ankle osteomyelitis by single-stage resection and circumferential from compression arthrodesis. Iowa Orthop J. 2005;25:47–52.
25. Aragon-Sanchez F, Cabrerea-Galvan J, Quintana-Marrero Y, et al. Outcomes of surgical treatment of diabetic foot osteomyelitis: a series of 185 patients with histopathological confirmation of bone involvement. Diabetologia. 2008;51:1962–70.
26. Dalla Paola L, Ceccacci T, Ninkovic S, et al. Limb salvage in charcot foot and ankle osteomyelitis: combined use single stage/double stage of arthrodesis and external fixation. Foot Ankle Int. 2009;30:1065–70.
27. Thordarson DB, Patzakis MJ, Holtom P, et al. Salvage of the septic ankle with concomitant tibial osteomyelitis. Foot Ankle Int. 1997;18:151–6.
28. Richter D, Hahn MP, Laun RA, et al. Arthrodesis of the infected ankle and subtalar joint: technique, indications and results of 45 consecutive cases. J Trauma. 1999;47:1072–8.
29. Lipsky B, Peters E, Senneville E, et al. Expert opinion on the management of infections in the diabetic foot. Diabetes Metab Res Rev. 2012;28 Suppl 1:163–78.
30. Atway S, Nerone V, Springer K, et al. Rate of residual osteomyelitis after partial foot amputation in diabetic patiens: a standardized method of evaluating bone margins with intraoperative culture. J Foot Ankle Surg. 2012;51:749–52.
31. Janis JE, Kwon RK, Attinger CE. The new reconstructive ladder: modification to the traditional model. Plast Reconstr Surg. 2011;127(suppl):205S–12.
32. Blume P, Donegan R, Schmidt B. The role of plastic surgery for soft tissue coverage of the diabetic foot and ankle. Clin Podiatr Med Surg. 2014;31(1):127–50.
33. Hartrampf Jr CR, Scheflan M, Bostwick J. The flexor digitorum brevis muscle island pedicle flap: a new dimension in heel reconstruction. Plast Reconstr Surg. 1980;66:264–70.
34. Garcia-Morales E, Lazao-Martinex J, Aragon-Sanchez J, et al. Surgical complications associated with primary closure in patients with diabetic foot osteomyelitis. Diabetic Foot and Ankle. 2012;3. 10.3402/dfa.v3i0.19000.
35. Morykwas M, Argenta L, et al. Vacuum assisted closure: a new method for wound control and treatment: animal studies and basic foundation. Ann Plast Surg. 1997;38:553–62.
36. Zoch G. VAC-therapy and laser-induced fluorescence of indocyannine-green (IC-view), an assessment of wound perfusion in diabetic foot syndrome. Zentralbl Chir. 2004;129 Suppl 1:S80–1.
37. Kamolz L, Andel H, et al. Use of subatmospheric pressure therapy to prevent burn wound progression in human: first experiences. Burns. 2004;30:253–8.
38. Blume P, Walters J, Payne W, et al. Comparison of negative pressure wound therapy using vacuum-assisted closure with advanced moist wound therapy in the treatment of diabetic foot ulcers. Diabetes Care. 2008;31:631–6.

39. Dumville J, Hinchliffe R, Cullum N, et al. Negative pressure wound therapy for treating foot wound in people with diabetes mellitus. Cochrane Database Syst Rev. 2013;10:1–53.

40. Lee HJ, Kim JW, Oh CW, et al. Negative pressure wound therapy for soft tissue injuries around the foot and ankle. J Orthop Surg Res. 2009;4:14.

41. Bollero D, Carnino R, Risso D, et al. Acute complex traumas of the lower limbs: a modern reconstructive approach with negative pressure therapy. Wound Repair Regen. 2007;15:589–94.

42. Attinger C, Ducic I, Cooper P, et al. The role of intrinsic muscle flaps of the foot for bone coverage in foot and ankle defects in diabetic and non diabetic patients. Plast Reconstr Surg. 2002;110: 1047–54.

43. Attinger C, Ducic I, Zelen C. The use of local muscle flaps in foot and ankle reconstruction. Clin Podiatr Med Surg. 2000;17:681–711.

44. Ger R. The management of chronic ulcers of the dorsum of the foot by muscle transposition and free skin grafting. Br J Plast Surg. 1996;29:199–204.

45. Papp C, Hasenohrl C. Small toe muscles for defect coverage. Plast Reconstr Surg. 1990;86:941–5.

46. Schwabegger A, Shafighi M, Gurunluoglu R, et al. Versatility of the abductor halluces muscle as a conjoined or distally-based flap. J Trauma. 2005;59:1007–11.

47. Clark N, Sherman R. Soft-tissue reconstruction of the foot and ankle. Orthop Clin North Am. 1993;24:489–503.

48. McLean O, Buncke H. Autotransplant of omentum to a large scalp defect with microsurgical revascularization. Plast Reconstr Surg. 1972;41:268–73.

49. Daniel R, Taylor G. Distant transfer of an island flap by microvascular anastomoses: a clinical technique. Plast Reconstr Surg. 1973;52:11–6.

50. O'Brien B, MacLeod A, Hayhurst J, et al. Successful transfer of a large island flap from the groin to the foot by microvascular anastomosis. Plast Reconstr Surg. 1973;52:271–8.

51. Lai C, Lim S, et al. Limb salvage of infected diabetic foot ulcers with microsurgical free muscle transfer. Ann Plast Surg. 1991;26:212–20.

52. Rautio J, Asko-Seljavaara S, et al. Suitability of the scapular flap for reconstructions of the foot. Plast Reconstr Surg. 1990;85: 922–8.

53. Lamberty B, Cormack G. The antecubital fascio-cutaneous flap. Br J Plast Surg. 1993;36:428–33.

54. Koshima I, Saisho H, et al. Flow-through thin latissimus dorsi perforator flap for repair of soft-tissue defects in the legs. Plast Reconstr Surg. 1999;103:483–1490.

55. Ohta M, Ikeda M, et al. Limb Salvage of infected diabetic foot ulcers with free deep inferior epigastric perforator flaps. Microsurgery. 2006;26:87–92.

56. Ozkan O, Coskunfirat O, et al. Reliability of free-flap coverage in diabetic foot ulcers. Microsurgery. 2005;25:107–12.

57. Fitzgerald O'Connor E, Vessely M, et al. A systematic review of free tissue transfer in the management of non-traumatic lower extremity wounds in patients with diabetes. Eur J Vasc Endovasc Surg. 2011;4:391–9.

58. Suk Oh T, Seung Lee H, et al. Diabetic foot reconstruction using free flaps increases 5 year survival rate. Plast Reconstr Aesthetic Surg. 2013;66:243–50.

59. Berceli S, Chan A, Pomposelli F, et al. Efficacy of dorsal pedal artery bypass in limb salvage for ischemic heel ulcers. J Vasc Surg. 1999;30:499–508.

60. Dorros G, Jaff MR, Dorros AM, et al. Tibioperoneal (outflow lesion) angioplasty can be used as primary treatment in 235 patients with critical limb ischemia: five-year follow-up. Circulation. 2001;104:2057–62.

61. Attinger CE, Evans KK, Bulan E, Blume P, et al. Angiosomes of the foot and ankle and clinical implications for limb salvage: reconstruction, incisions, and revascularization. Plast Reconstr Surg. 2006;117(7 suppl):261–93.

62. Sumpio BE, Forsythe RO, Ziegler KR, et al. Clinical implications of the angiosome model in peripheral vascular disease. J Vasc Surg. 2013;58:814–26.

63. O'Neal LW. Surgical pathology of the foot and clinicopathological correlations. In: Bowker JH, Pfeifer MA, editors. Levin and O'Neal's the diabetic foot. 7th ed. Philadelphia, PA: Mosby Elsevier; 2008. p. 367–401.

64. Vermassen G, Van Landuyt K. Combined vascular reconstruction and free flap transfer in diabetic arterial disease. Diabetes Metab Res Rev. 2000;16:S33–6.

65. Lorenzetti F, Tukiainen E, et al. Blood flow in a pedal bypass combined with a free muscle flap. Eur J Vasc Endovasc Surg. 2001;22:161–4.

66. Lipsky B. Evidence-based antibiotic therapy of diabetic foot infections. FEMS Immunol Med Microbiol. 1999;26:267–76.

67. Yahagi N, Kono M, et al. Effect of electrolyzed water on wound healing. Artif Organs. 2001;24:984–7.

68. Sampson M, Muir A. Not all the super-oxidized waters are the same. J Hosp Infect. 2002;52:228–9.

69. Landa-Solis M, Gonzalez Espinosa D, et al. Microcyn, a novel super-oxidized water with neutral pH and disinfectant activity. J Hosp Infect. 2005;61(4):291–9.

70. Aragon-Sanchez J, Lazaro Martinex J, et al. Super-oxidized solution (dermacyn wound care) as an adjuvant treatment in the postoperative management of complicated diabetic foot osteomyelitis: preliminary experience in a specialized department. Int J Low Extrem Wounds. 2013;12:130–7.

71. Piaggesi A, Goretti C, et al. A randomized controlled trial to examine the efficacy and safety of a new super oxidized solution for the management of wide postsurgical lesions of the diabetic foot. Int J Low Extrem Wounds. 2010;9:10–5.

72. Marphoffer W, Stein M, et al. Impairment of polymorphonuclear leukocyte function and metabolic control of diabetes. Diabetes Care. 1992;15:256–60.

73. Marphhoffer W, Stein M, et al. Evidence of ex vivo and in vivo impaired neutrophil oxidative burst and phagocytic capacity in type 1 diabetes mellitus. Diabetes Res Clin Pract. 1993;19:183–8.

74. Tan JS, Anderson J, et al. Neutrophil dysfunction in diabetes mellitus. J Lab Clin Med. 1975;85:26–33.

75. Gough A, Clapperton M, Rolando N, et al. Randomised placebo-controlled trial or granulocyte-colony stimulating factor in diabetic foot infection. Lancet. 1997;350:855–9.

76. De Lalla F, Pellizzer GI, et al. Randomized prospective controlled trial of recombinant granulocyte colony-stimulating factor as adjunctive therapy for limb-threatening diabetic foot infection. Antimicrob Agents Chemother. 2001;45(4):1094–8.

77. Lipsky B, Berendt A, Embil A, et al. Diagnosing and treating diabetic foot infections. Diabetes Metab Res Rev. 2004;20 Suppl 1:S56–64.

78. Ferguson JY, Dudareva M, Riley ND, et al. The use of biodegradable antibiotic-loaded calcium sulphate carrier containing tobramycin for the treatment of chronic osteomyelitis: a series of 195 cases. Bone Joint J. 2014;96-B:829–36.

79. Chang W, Colangeli M, Colangeli S, et al. Adult osteomyelitis; debridement versus debridement plus osteoset T pellets. Acta Orthop Belg. 2007;73:238–44.

Use of Antibiotic Beads and Antibiotic Spacers in Limb Salvage

Noah G. Oliver, Corey M. Fidler, and John S. Steinberg

Introduction

The purpose of this chapter is to familiarize the reader with the use of antibiotic-impregnated bone cement in orthopedic foot and ankle surgery, particularly the scenario of diabetic limb salvage. Bacterial infections can be a devastating complication following primary orthopedic procedures, open traumatic fractures and injuries, and also in the field of diabetic limb salvage. Often, the effort to treat these infections through debridement of necrotic soft tissue and bone will leave a substantial deficit or "dead space." This defect can increase the risk of a hematoma, seroma, abscess, and other wound complications during the postoperative period. There are many options available to mitigate this "dead space" and reduce the rate of complications in these high-risk wounds. Some examples would include autogenous soft tissue graft, autogenous bone graft, as well as commercially available filler materials such as polymethylmethacrylate (PMMA) [1].

Acrylic bone cement offers mechanical and functional properties such as maintenance of length as well as providing local release of antibiotic in effective concentrations [2]. The benefits of local drug delivery are multifaceted. With increased regional distribution of antibiotics, the need for systemic antibiotics can be replaced or at least reduced. This local treatment can potentially decrease the risk of systemic drug reaction

complications and other concerns in this often complex patient population. Another advantage is that high levels of antibiotics acting locally can help facilitate the direct drug delivery to avascular segments of the wound by diffusion [3]. Additional vehicles for the delivery of local antibiotics include their addition to cancellous bone graft or other biodegradable products which will be discussed in length in the upcoming chapter.

History

Polymethylmethacrylate (PMMA) is a synthetic resin manufactured by the polymerization of methyl methacrylate [4] and has had an extensive history in the ophthalmological and dental fields before being bridged to orthopedics. The notion of using acrylic bone cement in orthopedic surgery was popularized by Charnley and his use of PMMA for the modern prosthetic hip implant in 1960 [5]. PMMA is created by the polymerization, exothermic reaction by mixing the monomer of methylmethacrylate powder to the catalyst benzoyl peroxide. This process is highly exothermic and can produce temperatures reaching 70–164 °C [6–8]. It is well known that care must be taken during this process in order to avoid osteonecrosis secondary to protein denaturation. Saline irrigation can be used to help reduce the damage to the local surrounding tissues, and the curing process can be completed outside of the wound during the PMMA preparation.

The notion of augmenting bone cement with antimicrobial agents as a proactive measure to reduce the incidence of prosthetic hip implant infection is credited to Buchholz and Engelbrecht in 1970 [9]. Klemm introduced the concept of adding PMMA beads to large soft tissue defects that were created after surgical excision of chronic osteomyelitis [10, 11]. Previous reports demonstrate a ratio of 3.6 g of antibiotic per 40 g of acrylic cement as the desired ratio that will provide sustained therapeutic levels of antibiotics while maintaining effective elution kinetics [12]. Other researchers have suggested upwards of 6–8 g of antibiotic per 40 g of cement in the presence of active infection [13].

N.G. Oliver, D.P.M., A.A.C.F.A.S. (✉)
Ochsner Medical Center, 1514 Jefferson Hwy., New Orleans, LA 70121, USA
e-mail: noaholiver@gmail.com

C.M. Fidler, D.P.M.
MedStar Washington Hospital Center, 110 Irving Street NW, Washington, DC 20010, USA
e-mail: coreyfids@gmail.com

J.S. Steinberg, D.P.M., F.A.C.F.A.S.
Georgetown University School of Medicine, 3800 Reservoir Road NW, Washington, DC 20007, USA
e-mail: jss5@gunet.georgetown.edu

© Springer International Publishing Switzerland 2015
T.J. Boffeli (ed.), *Osteomyelitis of the Foot and Ankle*, DOI 10.1007/978-3-319-18926-0_11

Antibiotic Selection

When selecting an antibiotic for incorporation into PMMA, its characteristics should include the following: small volume of powder for delivery, excellent solubility, heat stabile, possess low allergenic properties, and have a broad spectrum of antimicrobial coverage [14]. The aminoglycosides, particularly gentamycin and tobramycin, have traditionally been the antibiotic class of choice given their ability to encompass the majority of these characteristics, and accordingly gentamycin has been the most widely studied and utilized [4]. Aminoglycosides provide concentration-dependent bactericidal activity against aerobic gram-negative bacilli as well as some staphylococci and mycobacteria [15]. Administered parenterally, aminoglycosides are excreted by glomerular filtration in patients with normal renal function. The most common side effects include nephrotoxicity, due to accumulation in the renal cortex resulting in tubular cell degeneration (usually reversible) and ototoxicity, which is usually irreversible [16]. Vancomycin shares similar properties with aminoglycosides with the added benefit of providing methicillin-resistant *Staphylococcus aureus* (MRSA) coverage. However, there have been limitations regarding the difficulty of cement to polymerize if used in high doses and at low-release period [17]. This has been addressed and can be avoided by first mixing the PMMA monomer and powder together to form the liquid cement before adding the antibiotic powder [14]. In the presence of fungal infections, one can add up to 100–150 mg of amphoteracin B to the 40 g of bone cement [18].

Side Effects

Little research has been performed regarding the potential side effects of nephrotoxicity and ototoxicity in locally applied gentamycin graft materials. One study measured gentamycin levels in 38 patients following implantation of gentamycin-containing cement (0.5 g gentamycin per 40 g cement powder) and beads (4.5 mg gentamycin per bead.) Serum gentamycin levels remained less than 4 μg/mL immediately following surgery. Postoperative day one, local gentamycin levels were on average 37 μg/mL when beads were used and 15 μg/mL when cement was used. None of these patients exhibited any signs of nephrotoxicity or ototoxicity despite having local levels much higher than what can be achieved via parental administration [19].

Other potential side effects include the possibility of biofilm developing on the surface of the PMMA cement or beads themselves once the effective antibiotic elution is complete. This would indicate that not only has the bacteria developed resistance to the antibiotic but the PMMA is now serving to maintain the infection rather than combating it [20]. This

report by Neut et al. serves as a reminder to match an antibiotic according to the bacterial culture and susceptibility testing whenever possible.

There have also been reports during vertebral augmentation with PMMA of cardiopulmonary complications secondary to toxic effects of the monomer or anaphylaxis resulting in arterial hypotension, pulmonary infarction, oxygen desaturation, arrhythmia, and death [21].

In cases where absorbable beads are used in combination with primary closure, the natural degradation process of these materials can produce unwanted drainage from the wound which could lead to delayed coaptation. In addition, after 4–6 weeks the beads become enveloped by dense scar tissue and the ability to remove the beads if necessary can become quite challenging [4].

Antibiotic Elusion Properties

Elution of the antibiotic occurs in a biphasic manner, rapidly at first during the hours to days following implantation and then a slower yet sustained release with inhibitory concentrations maintained for 4–6 weeks [22, 23]. Wahlig and Dingeldein reported that gentamycin in certain cement delivery devices can provide sustained release for up to 5 years [24]. Diffusion of antibiotic is achieved either alone or by a combination of direct diffusion from the surface, the matrix, or through the cracks and voids within the cement [25]. Antibiotic elution is extremely reliant on the bone cement porosity as well as the type of antibiotic chosen. For instance, the decay rate of tobramycin elution is much faster than that of vancomycin, even though it elutes in much higher concentrations [26].

Delivery Vehicle Selection

When considering the use of an antibiotic-impregnated material traditionally there are nonabsorbable options such as PMMA and there are absorbable materials of various calcium-based compositions. The PMMA nonabsorbable material will provide stability and maintain length of the soft tissue envelope. The biodegradable alternatives can help to eradicate the infection, provide osteoconductive properties (in the case of calcium sulfate) and theoretically do not to require a second surgery for removal before bone grafting. There are a variety of bone cement alternatives that have been developed for the local delivery of antibiotics, and there are currently more in development. In addition to PMMA cement spacers and beads there are numerous biodegradable materials, with perhaps the most common being bone graft [27]. This has conventionally been used during a second procedure, after removal of antibiotic beads or cement in an effort to reduce soft tissue void or bone defect caused by resection of osteomyelitis. The autogenous or allograft bone is soaked in the antibiotic-loaded solution and then implanted into the defect which allows the antibiotic to be absorbed directly into the bone surfaces while eventually allowing incorporation of the bone graft [28]. Whether or not antibiotics affect the process of bone healing and regeneration is a topic of debate, and may be dependent on the class of antibiotic being used. Reports in animal and in vitro studies have shown that quinolones, when administered parentally, have a considerable adverse effect on fracture healing [29], while there was no apparent effect on fracture healing with the use of cefazolin, gentamycin, or vancomycin parentally. There is very little data referring to the actual concentration levels local antibiotics deliver and therefore the clinical effect this has on bone incorporation is still uncertain.

One of the more common bone graft substitutes is calcium sulfate, which has been used in the clinical setting of osteomyelitis [30]. The most suitable preparation noted by Hanssen, includes 1 g of vancomycin and 1.2 g of gentamycin per 25 g of calcium sulfate [4]. There are also reports of mixing bone cement with 6 % sodium fluoride, which has a direct stimulatory effect of osteoblast proliferation, and differentiation that can increase the volume of trabecular bone [31]. Another category of biomaterials includes the use of synthetic polymers such as polylactides-co-glycolides (PLGA) and others [32, 33] which provide the ability to carefully deliver antibiotics as well as other substances such as growth factors to augment bone regeneration. There are also combinations of the above materials in an effort to provide the best of either material: PMMA mixed with calcium carbonate and tricalcium phosphate particulate [34] and calcium sulfate beads coated with antibiotic-containing poly lactide-co-glycolide. The latter theoretically provides an initial burst of antibiotics followed by a sustained release of the coated antibiotic [35]. Regardless of the delivery vehicle chosen, there is still considerable research and development required to develop the most ideal biomaterial that provides reproducible antibiotic delivery while successfully contributing to the bone regeneration process. Many of the absorbable materials have frustrated surgeons over the years due to wound site drainage that can be generated as part of their degradation, but newer biomaterials promise to resolve that concern.

Foot and Ankle Applications

Foot and ankle osteomyelitis (OM) is most often treated with antibiotics and operative excisional debridement. Antibiotic-loaded bone cement (ABLC) is the gold standard for local antibiotic delivery and dead space management resulting from aggressive operative debridement [1].

ABLC provides a sustained release of local, highly concentrated antibiotics at the site of infection, independent of the host's vascular supply, which is often compromised by peripheral arterial disease (PAD), diabetes, or trauma [25, 36]. This quality is important because even patients with seemingly robust lower extremity perfusion may suffer from undiagnosed microvascular disease or zones of avascularity as a result of local infection [37]. These potential local vascular compromise zones can further compromise systemic antibiotic delivery due to poor bone penetration [36]. In addition, the amount of effective systemic antibiotics reaching the foot may be limited because of the uniquely avascular nature of the foot's osseous anatomy, which has a high ratio of cortical to cancellous bone [38].

Implanted ABLC can play an important mechanical role in soft tissue and osseous reconstruction. The implanted ABLC may maintain the length and tension of surrounding soft tissues, joint and skeletal alignment, and weight bearing ability. These qualities allow aggressive debridement of infected soft tissue and bone while minimizing the secondary functional compromise [39].

Masquelet et al. [40] described a technique using an ABLC spacer to induce a vascular membrane at the site of bone loss. Pelissier et al. [41] reported that these induced membranes secrete growth factors including vascular and osteoinductive factors and could stimulate bone regeneration. The biologically active membrane develops and matures 3–5 weeks after ABLC placement, improving the local environment for bone graft incorporation and corticalization [42]. Antibiotic-loaded cement has several applications for treatment of OM in the foot and ankle.

Diabetic Foot

Diabetic foot osteomyelitis (DFO) often requires a combination of medical and surgical treatment. While complete resection of the affected bone is the surest way to eliminate the infection and prevent recurrence, aggressive resection may cause structural instability and altered mechanics increasing the risk for future transfer lesions, re-ulceration, and infection. As discussed above, ABLC plays a vital role in dead space management after aggressive debridement and can be considered when treating DFO (Fig. 11.1).

Several case series have reported success using ABLC as an adjunct to partial foot amputation or as part of a staged limb salvage protocol [43–45]. Krause et al. [43] used absorbable ABLC beads in 46 diabetic patients undergoing a single-staged transmetatarsal amputation and reported a significantly lower complication rate in comparison to 16 transmetatarsal amputation patients that were not treated with ABLC beads.

Schade and Roukis [38] analyzed 29 patients with diabetic foot infections that were treated with parenteral antibiotics, aggressive surgical debridement, and PMMA beads impregnated with 500 mg of gentamicin and 2.4 g of tobramycin.

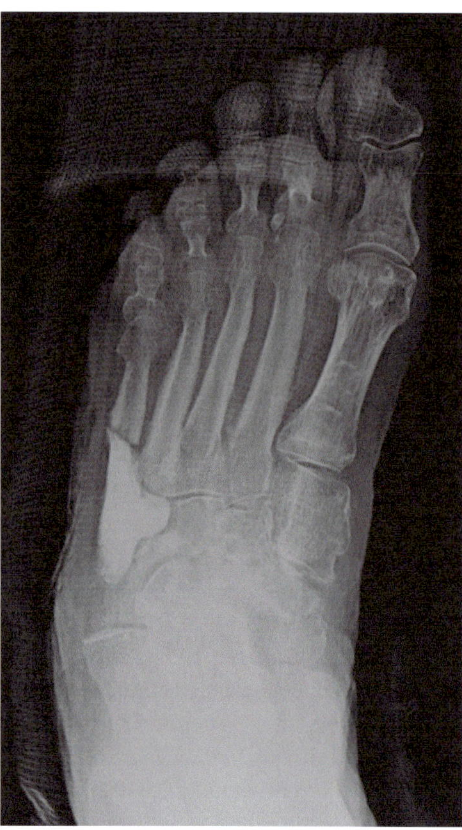

Fig. 11.1 ABLC spacer inserted into deadspace after debridement of diabetic foot osteomyelitis

Patients underwent repeat debridement and bead exchange approximately 3 days post implantation as needed before definitive closure. Cultures taken at the time of bead removal revealed positive bacterial growth in only five patients. They theorized that the reason for this persistent infection was inadequate debridement at the index surgery and suggested that the role of ABLC appeared to be maintenance of an aseptic environment instead of complete infection eradication.

Some patients have local and/or systemic factors that make them poor candidates for additional revision surgery [46]. A permanent ABLC spacer (Fig. 11.2) may provide adequate stability for these patients in lieu of amputation or long-term systemic antibiotics. Melamed and Peled [47] reported a 91 % success rate in treating 23 cases of forefoot DFO with debridement and placement of an ABLC spacer as an alternative to toe or partial ray amputation. They hypothesized that the ABLC would resolve the deep infection and temporarily or permanently fill the void, maintaining structural stability at the area created by extensive debridement. The spacer was retained permanently in ten patients and removed with conversion to successful resection arthroplasty/pseudoarthrosis in six patients and fusion in five patients, respectively. The authors concluded that when left

as a permanent spacer at the metatarsal head location, the spacer appears to participate in weightbearing and stability and may provide a viable alternative to amputation or additional reconstruction.

Trauma

Given the foot and ankle's thin soft tissue envelope and limited vascular perfusion, lower extremity trauma often results in open wounds. In addition, open fractures may result in segmental bone defects with or without OM. These cases require sequential debridement to eradicate infection before wound closure, fracture repair, or reconstruction. Adjunctively, ABLC has been used for decades to control infection and manage dead space resulting from traumatic injury.

As first described by Masquelet et al. [40], defects requiring delayed bone grafting can be temporarily filled with an ABLC spacer for 4–5 weeks to decrease the risk of infection, allow healing of soft tissues and induce the formation of a vascularized membrane around the ABLC. This induced-membrane optimizes the local environment for delayed bone grafting and prevents fibrous ingrowth and graft reabsorption [48]. While this technique is commonly used for segmental bone loss from high-energy trauma [42], few cases specific to the foot and ankle have been published.

Huffman et al. [49] used the Masquelet technique to treat a patient with complex open fractures and bone loss at the medial column secondary to a gunshot. Two weeks following initial debridement and ORIF, the patient underwent repeat debridement, insertion of an ABLC spacer into the medical column defect and wound closure with a microsurgical free flap. They performed the second stage of the Masquelet technique several months later. This involved removing the ABLC, filling the encapsulated defect (5 cm×3 cm) with autograft and fixating the fusion site with a locking plate. At the 1-year follow-up, graft incorporation and fusion were noted and the patient was able to ambulate with a custom-molded shoe.

Malizos et al. [50] retrospectively reviewed the outcomes of 84 consecutive patients that were treated for posttraumatic or postoperative OM at the foot or ankle. All patients were treated with a limited course of parenteral antibiotics and a surgical protocol of aggressive debridement and an ABLC spacer or bead pouch (4 g of vancomycin per 40 g of PMMA cement power and 3 g of fucidic acid), which was placed into the open wound and wrapped and sealed with an impermeable adhesive membrane. External fixation was used in cases involving segmental defects at the distal tibia. A "second-look" debridement and ABLC exchange was performed 48–72 h after the initial debridement and repeated until the

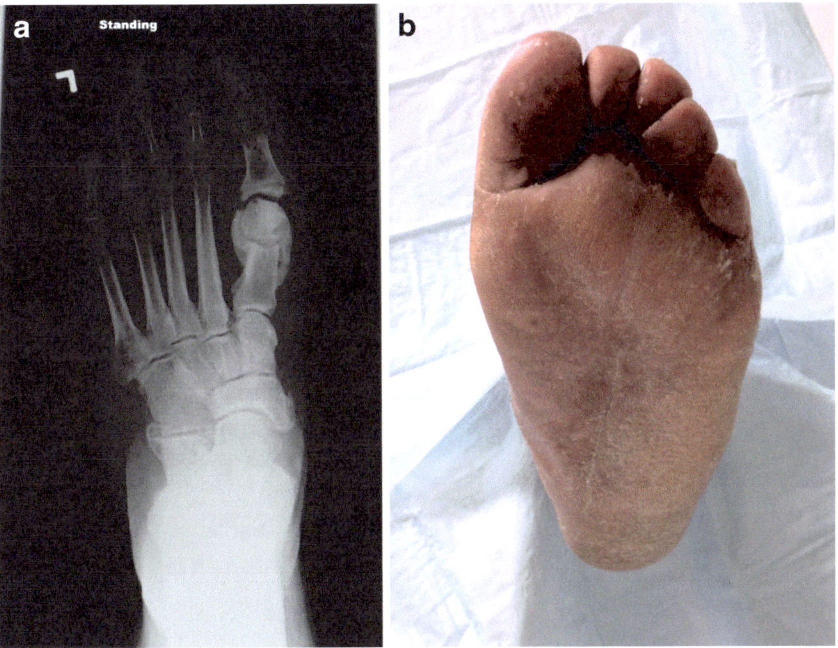

Fig. 11.2 (**a**) Regenerate bone growth surrounding and stabilizing the ABLC spacer, (**b**) Preservation of the hallux and no re-ulceration in patient with a permanently retained ABLC spacer at the first MTP joint

wound was clean. Once the wound was deemed clean, they performed bony reconstruction using autograft (Ten patients), distraction osteogenesis (Eight patients), or joint fusion (11 patients) and soft tissue closure following the reconstructive ladder.

They achieved limb salvage and infection control without an amputation in 69/84 (82 %) cases. They performed a primary below-knee amputation (five patients) or ray amputation (six patients) for Cierny-Mader type B and C hosts with a non-salvageable infection. A mean of three operative procedures per patient were performed. Host-type B and C patients required significantly more operative procedures than host-type A patients ($P = 0.02$). Additionally, the risk of complications was significantly greater for type-B and -C hosts versus type-A ($p < 0.001$). They concluded that a staged surgical management protocol combining radical debridement, local antibiotic delivery, and short-term systemic antibiotics efficiently controlled infection and achieved functional limb salvage in the majority of patients.

Postoperative Infection/Septic Joint

Postoperative bone or joint infection is a challenging and potentially limb-threatening complication of reconstructive surgery. Treatment goals include eradication of the infection and restoration of a painless functional limb through revision of initial surgery or salvage procedure [51].

Treatment options for surgical revision and limb salvage include: debridement with retention of hardware and long-term antibiotic suppression, debridement with removal of all hardware, insertion of a temporary ABLC spacer with a one- or two- stage implant exchange or arthrodesis procedure, or amputation [46, 50–52] (Fig. 11.3).

While the literature and outcomes data specific to the foot and ankle are limited [53], multiple joint replacement centers have reported good clinical and functional results using a two-stage procedure for the treatment of hip and knee infections [54–57]. The preferred, two-stage revision starts with removal of the infected implant, joint debridement, irrigation, and placement of an ABLC in the implant site. The second stage typically follows a few (2–4) months later and consists of ABLC removal and replanting of a revision prosthetic or an arthrodesis-type procedure [2].

Not all patients are good candidates for additional surgical revision.

Ferrao et al. [51] used an ABLC spacer as definitive management for postoperative ankle infections following total ankle replacement ($n = 6$). They used ankle arthrodesis ($n = 3$) for patients who, following insertion of the cement spacer, either did not desire further surgery or were medically unfit for further surgery. Two patients eventually underwent BKA for wound complication and pain as a result of the ABLC loosening. All patients with a retained spacer were able to ambulate and perform basic activities with minimal discomfort.

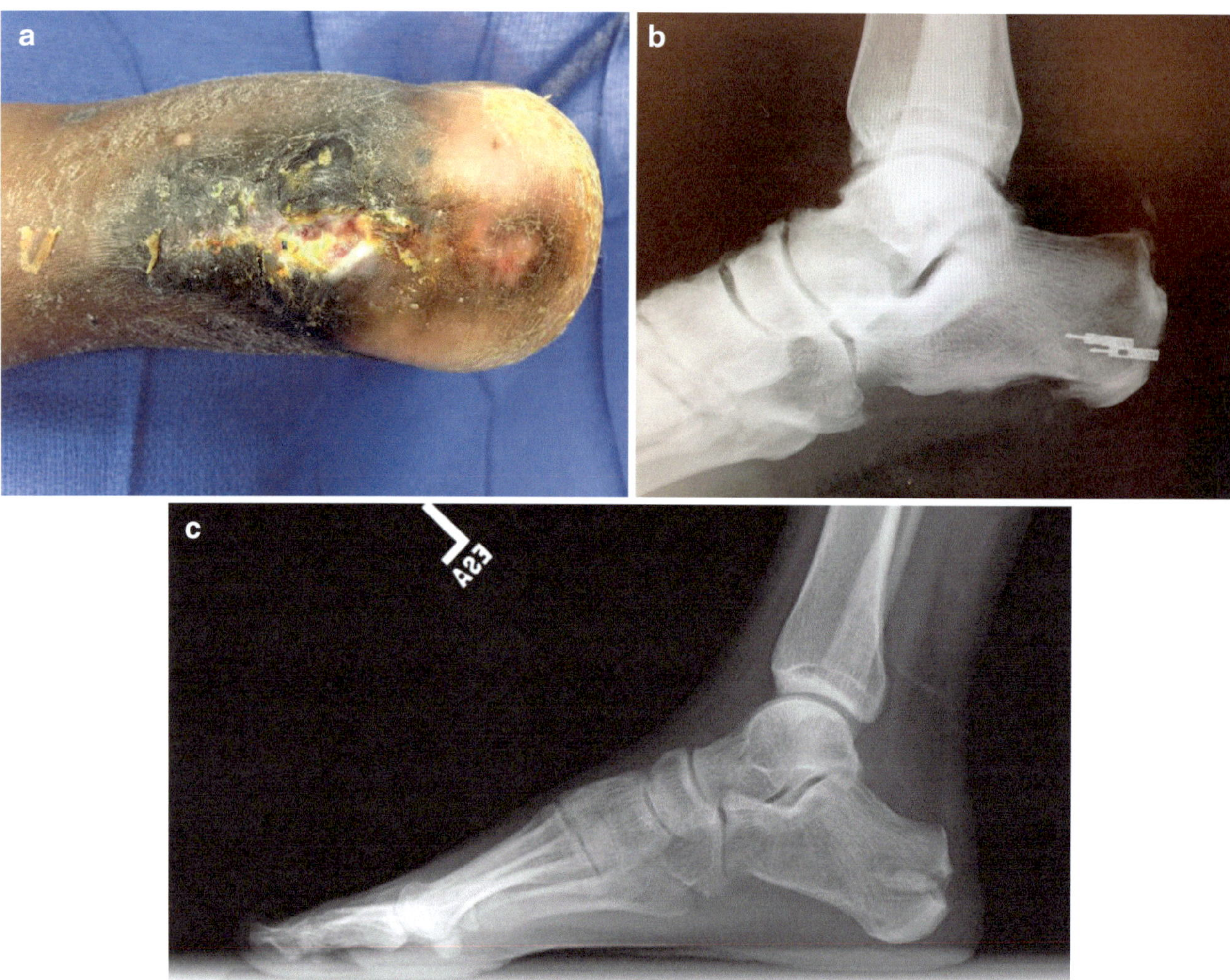

Fig. 11.3 (**a**) Postoperative dehiscence and infection of Achilles tendon and calcaneous, (**b**) Retained suture anchors in posterior calcaneous with osteomyelitis, (**c**) ABLC spacer used to treat osteomyelitis and fill void after removal of anchors and debridement of infected bone

Management Protocol/Surgical Algorithm (Chart 1)

Foot and ankle osteomyelitis is an often complex and limb-threatening condition that requires a team of specialists (infectious disease, vascular surgery, etc.) to optimize healing potential and maximize the patient's chance of limb salvage. A systematic management protocol is imperative to maximize systemic and local host factors, eradicate infection, manage dead space, and optimize lower extremity mechanics and function.

Debridement

The first and most critical step in our management protocol is aggressive and wide resection of all infected, necrotic, and nonviable bone and soft tissue until only normal, well-perfused tissue remains. Necrotic or dead bone has a discolored, avascular appearance and soft consistency. Bone should be debrided back to a hard consistency with punctate bleeding on the cortex (Haversian) and normal-looking marrow in cancellous (sinusoidal) bone (paprika sign). A sagittal saw is useful for serially sawing off bone slices until exposed surfaces bleed in uniform and the transition from necrotic infected bone to viable bone is observed [46]. *Atraumatic* surgical technique should be used throughout debridement to avoid damaging adjacent healthy tissues [58].

We prefer to perform debridement without an inflated tourniquet so that the quality of bleeding at the debrided wound edges and bone margins can be continually assessed. When a tourniquet is utilized for hemostasis during debridement, it is important to deflate the tourniquet before performing a final wound assessment [58]. Inadequate debridement can result from concerns about how to close and reconstruct the resultant defect, highlighting the importance of access to a multidisciplinary team of surgeons. The removal of all

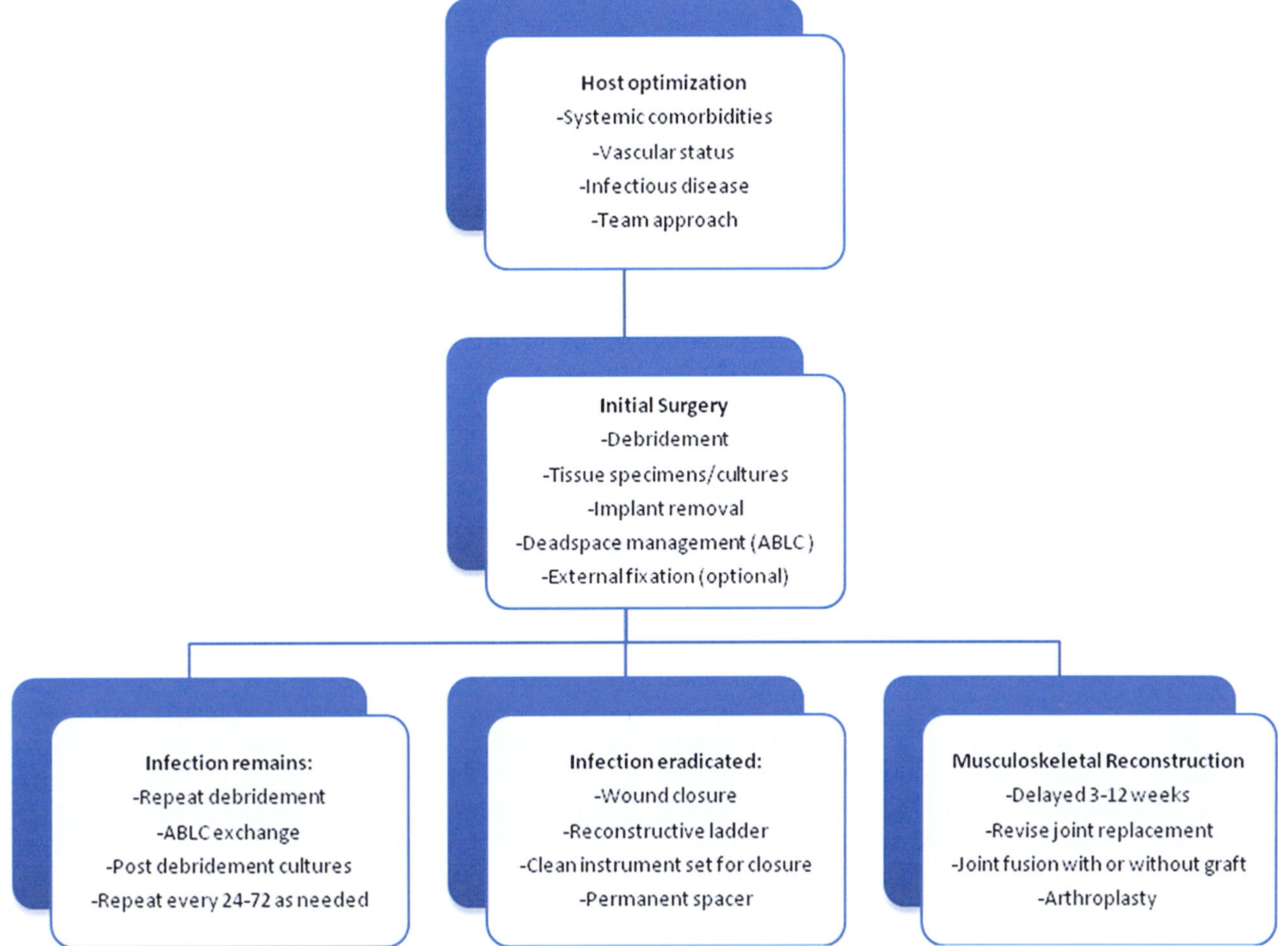

Chart 1 Staged surgical treatment of foot and ankle osteomyelitis with antibiotic-loaded cement

osteomyelitic bone takes precedence over the preservation of normal, bony architecture [46].

Multiple studies demonstrate that the quality of debridement plays a vital role to eradicate and prevent the recurrence of infection [38, 59]. Simpson et al. [59] found a significantly lower infection recurrence rate in patients with osteomyelitis who underwent wide resection—5 mm beyond the normal margin of infected bone—compared to those that underwent a less aggressive, marginal debridement. After debridement, the wound is irrigated with a pulsed lavage system, using 3–6 L of normal saline, taking care to avoid unwanted irritation to the healthy tissues.

Hardware Removal

Hardware and implants are carefully evaluated during the initial debridement and removed when any suspicion for looscning or dcep infection exist. Internal hardware is a nidus for infection and early biofilm formation. The surest way to eliminate biofilms in orthopaedic infection is to remove the affected device that harbors the biofilm completely [60].

Cultures and Biopsy

Multiple, deep soft tissue and bone specimens should be sent for microbiologic culture (aerobic, anaerobic, fungal, acid-fast) to obtain antibiotic sensitivities and confirm findings consistent with osteomyelitis through histologic analysis. These samples should be taken from representative tissue at the zone of infection before and after debridement and irrigation. Additionally, it is important to obtain cultures of both the debrided osteomyelitic bone and the normal bone proximal to the area of debridement. Analysis of this normal bone or "clean margin" and the post-debridement wound cultures are used to guide antibiotic therapy, confirm the irradiation of infection, and determine whether further debridement or wound closure is appropriate [46, 58]. When possible, the initiation of empiric, broad-spectrum antibiotics should be delayed until these deep cultures are obtained [46].

Antibiotic-Loaded Cement Implantation

High-dose ABLC (>1 g antibiotic per batch of cement) is effective and indicated for treating infection, but the only commercially available ABLC products are low dose (≤1 g of antibiotic per batch of cement) and are indicated for prophylactic with revision joint replacements. Because the FDA has not approved a reformulated high-dose ABLC (2–8 g antibiotic per 40 g of bone cement), the formation and use of high-dose ABLC requires hand mixing by surgeons, resulting in a wide variation of dosages and types of antibiotics used to treat infection [13, 61]. Although antibiotics dosage is not yet standardized for high-dose ALBC, at least 3.6 g of tobramycin and 1 g of vancomycin per 40 g package of bone cement has been recommended for effective elution levels [13].

Technique

The ABLC is created using sterile technique on the back table according to the manufacturer's instructions. Methylmethacrylate can be dry mixed with the appropriate antibiotic powder—we prefer approximately 2 g aminoglycoside and/or 2 g vancomycin per 40 g of cement prepared, depending on the patient's infection history and risk factors. The liquid monomer is then added and the combination is mixed until the cement is semirigid. Alternatively, Hanssen [13] recommends first mixing the PMMA monomer and powder together to form the liquid cement before adding the antibiotic power, in order to make mixing easier when using high volumes of antibiotic.

Beads vs. Spacer

Once the ABLC is semirigid, it is molded into beads or a spacer. Beads are often used to treat osteomyelitis in small areas or when structural stability is not as important (partial foot amputation). Spacers are custom-molded to fit the size and shape of the defect (block, sphere, intramedullary rod) providing improved stability, maintenance of musculoskeletal alignment, and soft tissue tension, which is important when planning a revision [62] (Fig. 11.4).

Spacers are inserted into the defect when still slightly moldable. Care is taken to ensure that the defect is not overstuffed and no prominences are felt to prevent excess pressure to the skin and wound-healing problems (Fig. 11.5). Although the majority of the hardening process should take place on the back table, saline irrigation can be used while the cement hardens to prevent exothermic damage at the adjacent skin [38].

Beads measuring 5–8 mm in diameter can be formed and strung on a strong monofilament suture or wire when the ABLC is moderately viscous. They should be allowed to cure completely (15–20 min) before insertion into the defect. The bead pouch technique [63] or negative pressure wound therapy can be used to cover the wound when the overlying soft tissue defect is too large for closure.

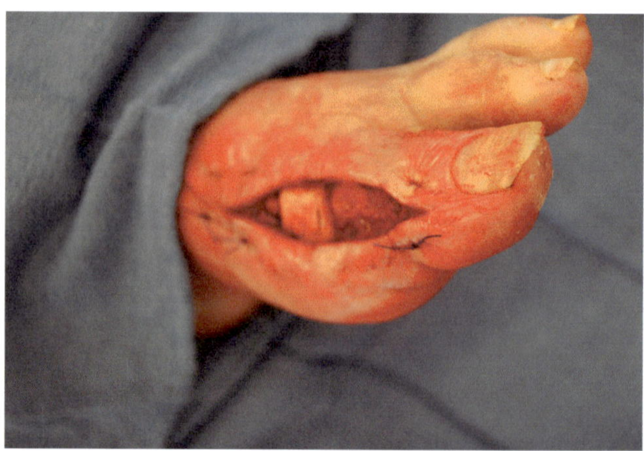

Fig. 11.4 Antibiotic-loaded cement spacer inserted into the defect resulting from debridement of osteomyelitis. Note that first MTP joint alignment is maintained

External Fixation

Temporary external fixation may be applied when additional stability is needed in cases of large segmental defects to maintain anatomic alignment. Monorails (Fig. 11.6) are typically used to span the forefoot and midfoot while static ring fixation is used to stabilize the ankle and hind foot.

Soft Tissue Closure

Wound closure is performed when infection eradication is noted with clinical findings, laboratory data as well as postdebridement culture and biopsy results. When confirmed clean at take-back evaluation and debridement, wound closure is performed following irrigation using a double instrument setup to avoid recontamination [58]. When possible, the soft tissues are closed primarily over the spacer or beads using an interrupted technique with monofilament.

The reconstructive ladder is used to guide wound closure when large- or difficult-to-close defects are present. Although several modifications of the concept have been described, most descriptions start with direct closure, followed by skin graft, local flap, and finally free flap. In addition, negative pressure wound therapy (Fig. 11.7) can be used as an adjunct to any method of reconstruction [64]. Before wound closure, drain insertion should be considered to prevent dehiscence [61].

Spacer Removal or Exchange

Patients typically return to surgery 24–72 h after the initial debridement for a repeat debridement and ABLC exchange, or ABLC removal and wound closure based on the clinical response to therapy and surgical goals. Serial debridement and spacer exchange every few days may be repeated until all infection is eradicated [61] (Fig. 11.8).

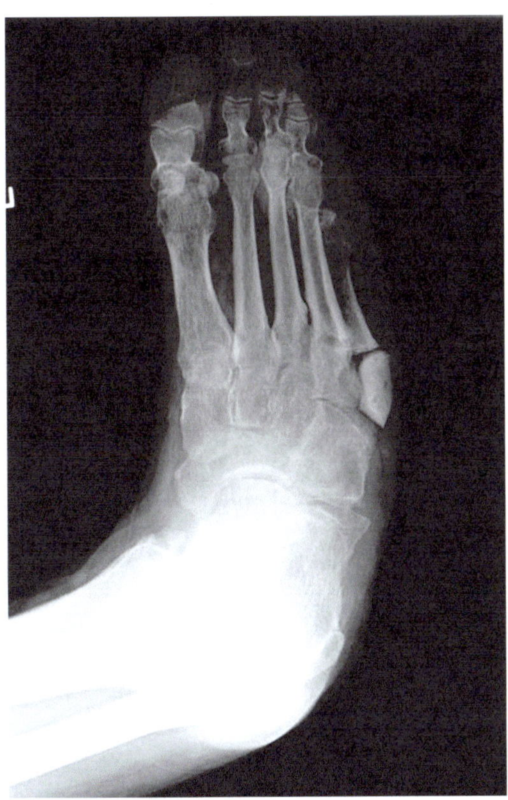

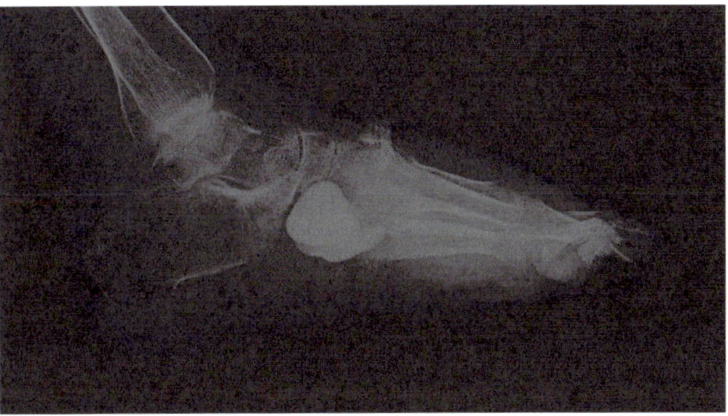

Fig. 11.7 Negative pressure wound therapy used for wound management in a patient with an ABLC spacer implanted to fill the void left after removal of the infected cuboid

When planning a musculoskeletal reconstruction, the ABLC removal and final procedure should be performed after 3–12 weeks to allow adequate time for soft tissue healing. ABLC implanted within the medullary canal must be removed earlier as tissue overgrowth makes removal difficult in as soon as 2 weeks [19].

Skeletal Reconstruction

The second stage, skeletal reconstruction including revision of joint prosthesis, bone grafting, arthroplasty and arthrodesis is performed 3–12 weeks following the initial debridement upon confirmation that infection has resolved and soft tissues have healed. Once the ABLC is removed, the defect should be inspected and optimized by preserving healthy, granular tissue and removing devitalized tissues. The type of skeletal reconstruction is chosen based on the location of defect and host factors [46, 50].

Examples

Case 1: ABLC Spacer Revised to Fusion A healthy, 68-year-old male presented with surgical site dehiscence, osteomyelitis, and nonunion at first metatarsal head 1-month status post-bunionectomy. During the initial debridement, hardware was removed, nonviable bone was resected, PMMA ABLC spacer was inserted into the defect, and partial wound closure with adjunctive negative pressure wound therapy was applied. The patient was taken back to surgery for debridement and closure 3 days later. The second stage reconstruction, first metatarsophalangeal (MTP) joint fusion, was performed 5 months later utilizing tibial autograft to replace the ABLC spacer (Fig. 11.9).

Case 2: ABLC Spacer Revised to Arthroplasty A 62-year-old male with diabetes mellitus presented with an

Fig. 11.5 Antibiotic-loaded cement spacer at the fifth TMT joint. A larger, more prominent spacer could cause wound-healing problems to the adjacent skin

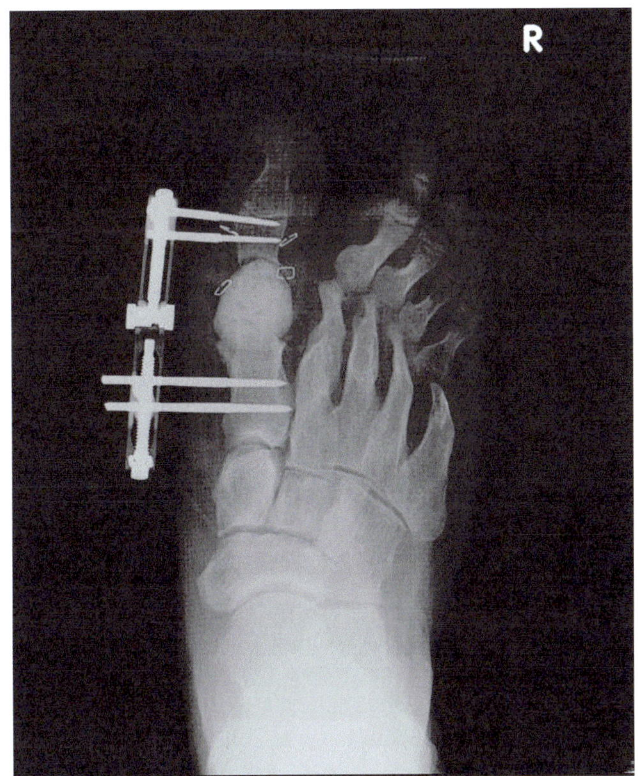

Fig. 11.6 Monorail external fixation used to stabilize and maintain position of the first MTP joint and ABLC spacer

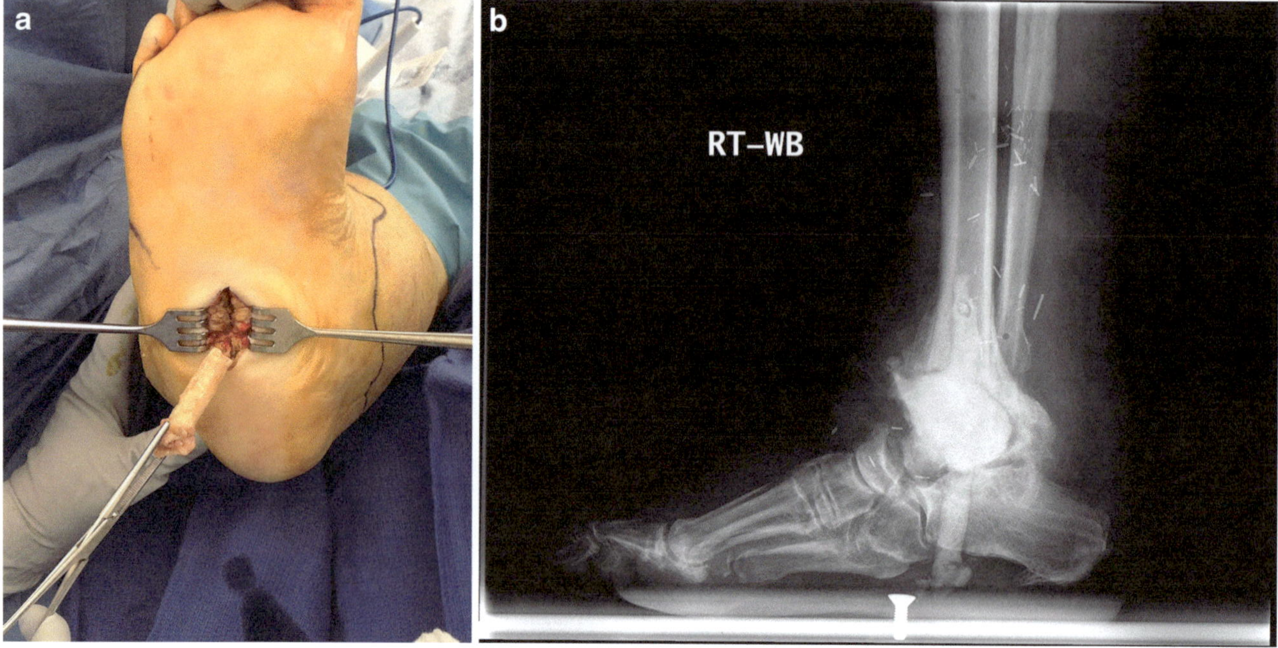

Fig. 11.8 (a) Removal of an antibiotic rod, (b) ABLC spacer implanted in the ankle and within the medullary canal for management of a septic ankle post-Charcot reconstruction

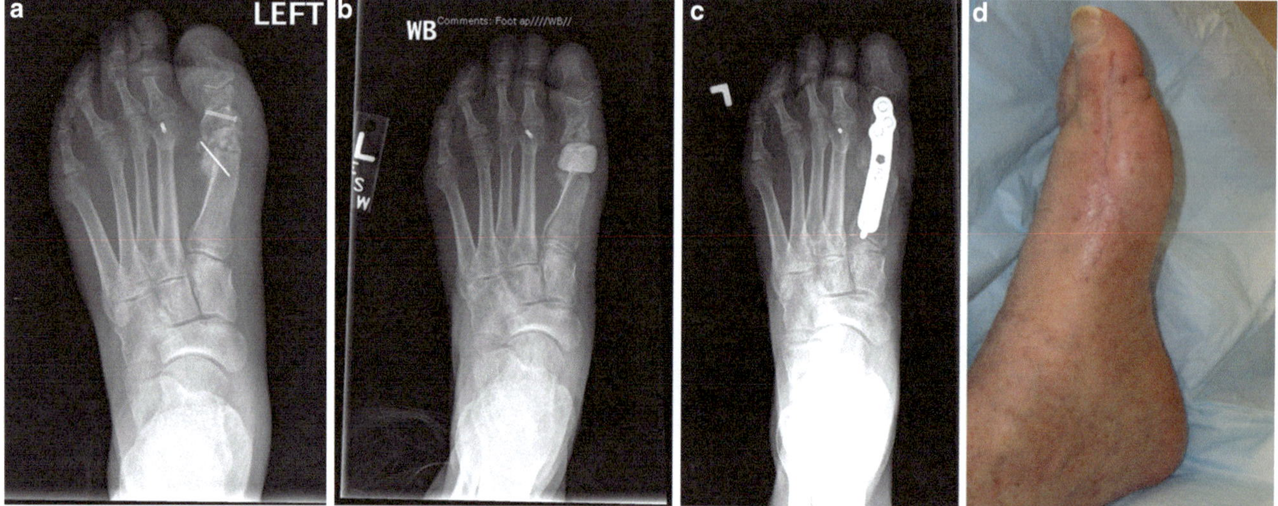

Fig. 11.9 (a) Osteomyelitis and nonunion at first metatarsal head 1-month status post bunionectomy, (b) following hardware removal and resection of nonviable bone, PMMA ABLC spacer was inserted into the defect, (c) five months later, the ABLC was removed and the first MTPJ was fused using autograft, (d) salvage of forefoot following MTP joint arthrodesis

infected plantar forefoot ulcer with contiguous osteomyelitis at the first MTP joint. Surgical debridement and ABLC spacer insertion was performed and repeated twice before the infection resolved. Once the infection was eradicated and the defect managed with an ABLC spacer, a minirail external fixator was applied to stabilize the joint, the wound was closed, and an Achilles tendon lengthening was performed.

The spacer was removed approximately 6 months later, after the soft tissues were healed with no signs of infection. The patient currently ambulates using a custom-molded orthotic and remains ulcer-free (Fig. 11.10).

Case 3: Permanent ABLC Spacer This 54-year-old female with diabetes mellitus and history of contralateral Charcot reconstruction presented with cellulitis and first MTP joint osteomyelitis. The initial surgical debridement consisted of ulcer excision and MTP joint resection. Three days later, debridement was repeated, an ABLC spacer was inserted, minirail external fixator applied, and delayed primary closure performed. The external fixator was removed in the office approximately 3 weeks later. The ABLC was retained as a permanent spacer. Now 4 years later, the joint is stable and the patient is ambulatory with no ulceration or reinfection (Fig. 11.11).

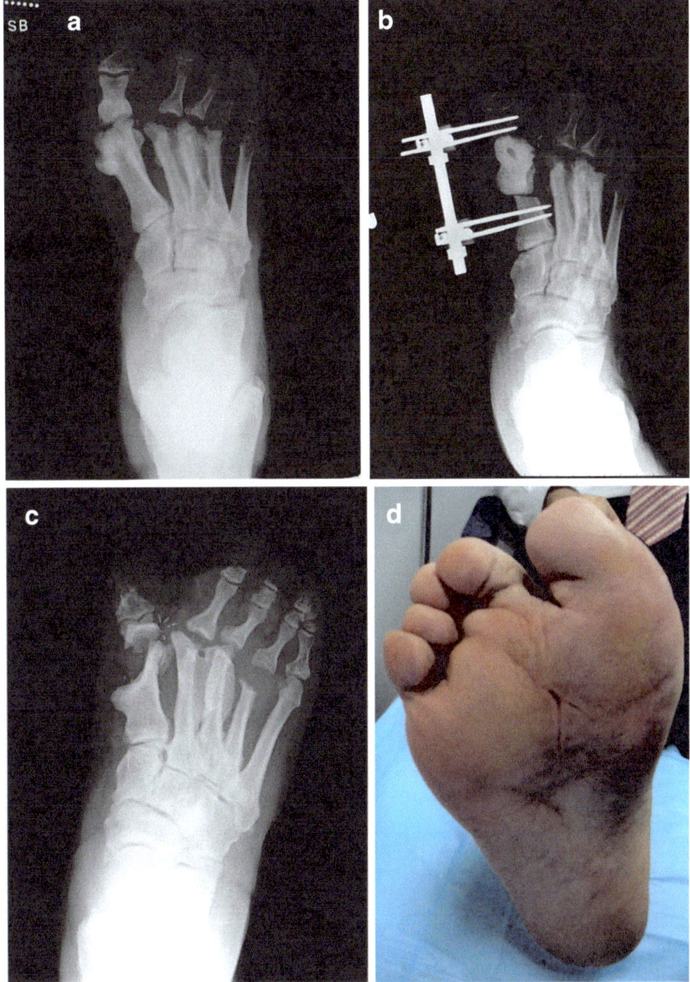

Fig. 11.10 (**a**) Osteomyelitis at the first MTP joint contiguous to a plantar diabetic foot ulcer, (**b**) following aggressive debridement, an ABLC spacer was inserted into the bony defect and the MTPJ was stabilized with monorail external fixator, (**c**) note the regenerated bone at the arthroplasty site approximately 4 years following the original surgery, (**d**) ulcer-free foot 4 years later

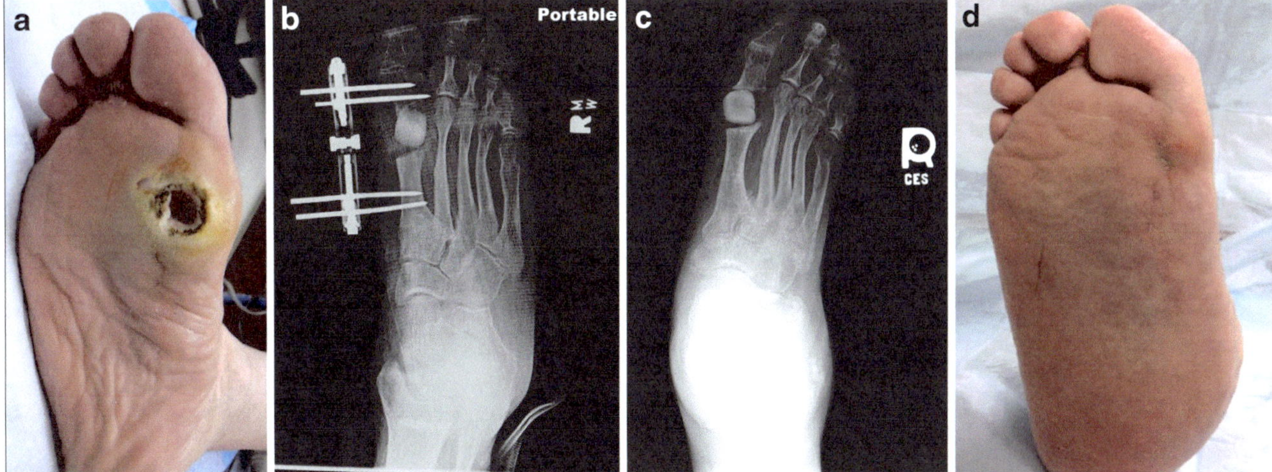

Fig. 11.11 (**a**) Diabetic foot ulcer with contiguous first MTP joint osteomyelitis, (**b**) following first MTP joint resection, an ABLC spacer was inserted and minirail external fixator applied, (**c**) 3-year follow-up with retained ABLC spacer and rectus first MTP joint alignment, (**d**) stable forefoot with no re-ulceration at 4-year follow-up

References

1. Nelson CL. The current status of material used for depot delivery of drugs. Clin Orthop Relat Res. 2004;427:72–8.
2. Magnan B, Bondi M, et al. Acrylic bone cement: current concept review. Musculoskelet Surg. 2013;97:93–100.
3. Hanssen AD. Local antibiotic delivery vehicles in the treatment of musculoskeletal infection. Clin Orthop Relat Res. 2005;437:91–6.
4. Polymethyl methacrylate (PMMA). Encyclopedia Britannica. Encyclopedia Britannica Online. Encyclopedia Britannica Inc., 2014. Web. 31 Aug. 2014.
5. Charnley J. Surgery of the hip-joint: present and future developments. Br Med J. 1960;19:821–6.
6. Webb JC, Spencer RF. The role of polymethylmethacrylate bone cement in modern orthopaedic surgery. J Bone Joint Surg Br. 2007;89:851–7.
7. Haas SS, Brauer GM, et al. A characterization of polymethylmethacrylate bone cement. J Bone Joint Surg Am. 1975;57:380–91.
8. Bibbo C. Treatment of the infected extended ankle arthrodesis after tibiotalocalcaneal retrograde nailing. Tech Foot Ankle Surg. 2002;1:74–86.
9. Buchholz HW, Engelbrecht H. Depot effects of various antibiotics mixed with Palacos resins. Chirurg. 1970;41:511–5.
10. Klemm K. Gentamicin-PMMA-beads in treating bone and soft tissue infections. Zentralbl Chir. 1979;104:934–42.
11. Klemm K. The treatment of infected osteosynthesis using gentamicin-PMMA-bead chains. Hefte Unfallheilkd. 1979;138: 197–200.
12. Penner MJ, Masri BA, Duncan CP. Elution characteristics of vancomycin and tobramycin combined in acrylic bone-cement. J Arthroplasty. 1996;11:939–44.
13. Hanssen AD, Spangehl MJ. Practical applications of antibiotic-loaded bone cement for treatment of infected joint replacements. Clin Orthop Relat Res. 2004;427:79–85.
14. Wininger DA, Fass RJ. Antibiotic-impregnated cement beads for orthopedic infections. Antimicrob Agents Chemother. 1996;40: 2675–9.
15. Gonzalez US, Spencer JP. Aminoglycosides: a practical review. Am Fam Physician. 1998;58:1811–20.
16. Tran Ba Huy P, Deffrennes D. Aminoglycoside ototoxicity: influence of dosage regimen on drug uptake and correlation between membrane binding and some clinical features. Acta Otolaryngol. 1988;105:511–5.
17. Chohfi M, Langlais F, Fourastier J, et al. Pharmacokinetics, uses, and limitations of vancomycin-loaded bone cement. Int Orthop. 1998;22:171–7.
18. Phelan DM, Osmon DR, Keating MR, Hanssen AD. Delayed reimplantation arthroplasty for candidal prosthetic joint infection: a report of 4 cases and review of the literature. Clin Infect Dis. 2002;34:930–8.
19. Salvati EA, Callaghan JJ, Brause BD, Klein RF, Small RD. Reimplantation in infection: elution of gentamycin from cement and beads. Clin Orthop Relat Res. 1986;207:83–93.
20. Neut D, van de Belt H, Stokroos I, van Horn JR, van der Mei HC, Busscher HJ. Biomaterial-associated infection of gentamicin-loaded PMMA beads in orthopedic revision surgery. J Antimicrob Chemother. 2001;47:885–91.
21. Nussbaum DA, Gailloud P, Murphy K. A review of complications associated with vertebroplasty and kyphoplasty as reported to the Food and Drug Administration medical device related web site. J Vasc Interv Radiol. 2004;15:1185–92.
22. Klemm K. The use of antibiotic-containing bead chains in the treatment of chronic bone infections. Clin Microbiol Infect. 2001;7:28–31.
23. Masri BA, Duncan CP, Beauchamp CP. Long-term elution of antibiotics from bone-cement: an in vivo study using the prosthesis of antibiotic-loaded acrylic cement (PROSTALAC) system. J Arthroplasty. 1998;13:331–8.
24. Wahlig H, Dingeldein E. Antibiotics and bone cements. Experimental and clinical long-term observation. Acta Orthop Scand. 1980;51:49–56.
25. Calhoun JG, Mader JT. Antibiotic beads in the management of surgical infections. Am J Surg. 1989;157:443–9.
26. Duncan CP, Masri BA. The role of antibiotic-loaded cement in the treatment of an infection after a hip replacement. Instr Course Lect. 1995;44:305–13.
27. McLaren AC. Alternative materials to acrylic bone cement for delivery of depot antibiotics in orthopedic infections. Clin Orthop. 2004;427:101–6.
28. Cierny G, Mader JT. Approach to adult osteomyelitis. Orthop Rev. 1987;16:259–70.
29. Huddleston PM, Steckelberg JM, Hanssen AD, et al. Ciprofloxacin inhibition of experimental fracture healing. J Bone Joint Surg Am. 2000;82:161–73.
30. Gitelis S, Brebach GT. The treatment of chronic osteomyelitis with a biodegradable antibiotic-impregnated implant. J Orthop Surg (Hong Kong). 2002;10:53–60.
31. Magnan B, Gabbi C, Regis D. Sodium fluoride sustained release bone cement: an experimental study in vitro and in vivo. Acta Orthop Belg. 1994;60:72–80.
32. Ramchandani MA, Robinson D. In vitro and in vivo release of ciprofloxacin from PLGA 50:50 implants. J Control Release. 1998;54:167–75.
33. Shi M, Kretlow JD, Nguyen A, et al. Antibiotic-releasing porus polymethylmethacrylate constructs for osseous space maintenance and infection control. Biomaterials. 2010;31:4146–56.
34. Frazier DD, Lathi VK, Gerhart TN, Hayes WC. Ex vivo degradation of a polypropylene glycol-fumarate biodegradable particulate composite bone cement. J Biomed Mater Res. 1997;35:383–9.
35. Benoit MA, Mousset B, Delloye C, Bouillet R, Gillard J. Antibiotic loaded plaster of Paris implants coated with poly lactide-co-glycolide as a controlled release delivery system for the treatment of bone infections. Int Orthop. 1997;21:403–8.
36. Decoster TA, Bozorgnia S. Antibiotic beads. J Am Acad Orthop Surg. 2008;16(11):674–8.
37. Cierny III G. Infected tibial nonunions (1981–1995). The evolution of change. Clin Orthop Relat Res. 1999;360:97–105.
38. Schade VL, Roukis TS. The role of polymethylmethacrylate antibiotic-loaded cement in addition to debridement for the treatment of soft tissue and osseous infections of the foot and ankle. J Foot Ankle Surg. 2010;49(1):55–62.
39. Sagray BA, Malhotra S, Steinberg JS. Current therapies for diabetic foot infections and osteomyelitis. Clin Podiatr Med Surg. 2014;31(1):57–70.
40. Masquelet AC, Fitoussi F, Begue T, Muller GP. Reconstruction of the long bones by the induced membrane and spongy autograft. Ann Chir Plast Esthet. 2000;45(3):346–53.
41. Pelissier P, Masquelet AC, Bareille R, Pelissier SM, Amedee J. Induced membranes secrete growth factors including vascular and osteoinductive factors and could stimulate bone regeneration. J Orthop Res. 2004;22(1):73–9.
42. Masquelet AC, Begue T. The concept of induced membrane for reconstruction of long bone defects. Orthop Clin North Am. 2010;41(1):27–37.
43. Krause FG, deVries G, Meakin C, Kalla TP, Younger AS. Outcome of transmetatarsal amputations in diabetics using antibiotic beads. Foot Ankle Int. 2009;30:486–93.
44. Roeder B, Van Gils CC, Maling S. Antibiotic beads in the treatment of diabetic pedal osteomyelitis. J Foot Ankle Surg. 2000;39:124–30.
45. Roukis TS, Landsman AS. Salvage of the first ray in a diabetic patient with osteomyelitis. J Am Podiatr Med Assoc. 2004;94:492–8.

46. Cierny 3rd G. Surgical treatment of osteomyelitis. Plast Reconstr Surg. 2011;127 Suppl 1:190S–204.
47. Melamed EA, Peled E. Antibiotic impregnated cement spacer for salvage of diabetic osteomyelitis. Foot Ankle Int. 2012;33(3):213–9.
48. McCall TA, Brokaw DS, Jelen BA, Scheid DK, Scharfenberger AV, Maar DC, Green JM, Shipps MR, Stone MB, Musapatika D, Weber TG. Treatment of large segmental bone defects with reamer-irrigator-aspirator bone graft: technique and case series. Orthop Clin North Am. 2010;41(1):63–73.
49. Huffman LK, Harris JG, Suk M. Using the bi-masquelet technique and reamer-irrigator-aspirator for post-traumatic foot reconstruction. Foot Ankle Int. 2009;30(9):895–9.
50. Malizos KN, Gougoulias NE, Dailiana ZH, Varitimidis S, Bargiotas KA, Paridis D. Ankle and foot osteomyelitis: treatment protocol and clinical results. Injury. 2010;41(3):285–93.
51. Ferrao P, Myerson MS, Schuberth JM, McCourt MJ. Cement spacer as definitive management for postoperative ankle infection. Foot Ankle Int. 2012;33(3):173–8.
52. Cierny 3rd G, Cook WG, Mader JT. Ankle arthrodesis in the presence of continuous sepsis. Indications, methods, and results. Clin Podiatr Med Surg. 1990;7(3):545–63.
53. Shapiro SE, Spurling DC, Cavaliere R. Infections following implant arthroplasties of the forefoot. Clin Podiatr Med Surg. 1996;13:767–91.
54. Romanò CL, Romanò D, Albisetti A, Meani E. Preformed antibiotic-loaded cement spacers for two-stage revision of infected total hip arthroplasty. Long-term results. Hip Int. 2012;22 Suppl 8:S46–53.
55. Degen RM, Davey JR, Davey JR, Howard JL, McCalden RW, Naudie DD. Does a prefabricated gentamicin-impregnated, load-bearing spacer control periprosthetic hip infection? Clin Orthop Relat Res. 2012;470(10):2724–9.
56. Pitto RP, Castelli CC, Ferrari R, Munro J. Pre-formed articulating knee spacer in two-stage revision for the infected total knee arthroplasty. Int Orthop. 2005;29(5):305–8.
57. Wan Z, Karim A, Momaya A, Incavo SJ, Mathis KB. Preformed articulating knee spacers in 2-stage total knee revision arthroplasty: minimum 2-year follow-up. J Arthroplasty. 2012;27(8):1469–73.
58. Attinger CE, Janis JE, Steinberg J, Schwartz J, Al-Attar A, Couch K. Clinical approach to wounds: débridement and wound bed preparation including the use of dressings and wound-healing adjuvants. Plast Reconstr Surg. 2006;117(7 Suppl):72S–109. Review.
59. Simpson AH, Deakin M, Latham JM. Chronic osteomyelitis. The effect of the extent of surgical resection on infection-free survival. J Bone Joint Surg Br. 2001;83(3):403–7.
60. Gristina AG, Shibata Y, Giridhar G, Kreger A, Myrvik QN. The glycocalyx, biofilm, microbes, and resistant infection. Semin Arthroplasty. 1994;5:160–70.
61. Adams K, Couch L, Cierny G, Calhoun J, Mader JT. In vitro and in vivo evaluation of antibiotic diffusion from antibiotic-impregnated polymethylmethacrylate beads. Clin Orthop Relat Res. 1992;278:244–52.
62. Hsieh PH, Shih CH, Chang YH, Lee MS, Shih HN, Yang WE. Two-stage revision hip arthroplasty for infection: comparison between the interim use of antibiotic-loaded cement beads and a spacer prosthesis. J Bone Joint Surg Am. 2004;86-A(9):1989–97.
63. Henry SL, Ostermann PA, Seligson D. The antibiotic bead pouch technique. The management of severe compound fractures. Clin Orthop Relat Res. 1993;295:54–62.
64. Janis JE, Kwon RK, Attinger CE. The new reconstructive ladder: modifications to the traditional model. Plast Reconstr Surg. 2011;127 Suppl 1:205S–12.

Troy J. Boffeli and Jonathan C. Thompson

Introduction

Neuropathic ulcerations of the plantar foot are a common nidus for the development of osteomyelitis. These ulcers typically form due to an underlying structural deformity or prominence that causes increased peak plantar pressure in a concentrated region that leads to tissue breakdown during weight bearing. One relatively common cause of such prominence is heterotopic bone growth that frequently forms at the surgical resection site following partial foot amputation. Heterotopic ossification (HO) is the formation of mature, lamellar bone in the soft tissues adjacent to bone that is exacerbated by trauma or surgery [1]. Moderate- to high-grade HO formation can create an iatrogenic prominence on the foot, placing the neuropathic patient who has already undergone partial foot amputation at risk for recurrent ulceration. While HO can occur in a number of locations, we have most frequently appreciated clinically relevant formation at the resection site of partial metatarsal amputations, which may lead to subsequent plantar forefoot ulcerations (Figs. 12.1 and 12.2). Clinically relevant HO refers to HO that causes ulceration or pre-ulcerative lesions as a result of its prominence. Such HO-related ulcerations are many times full-thickness due to an often well-defined underlying osseous prominence. This concentration of peak plantar pressure increases the likelihood of full-thickness tissue breakdown and can lead to exposed heterotopic bone that is at high risk

for developing osteomyelitis. Such a complication may be devastating in diabetic neuropathic patients already considered at high risk for proximal limb loss, which is the typical profile of patients requiring initial partial foot amputation.

Heterotopic ossification is a phenomenon that has been well described in the hip, knee, and upper extremities [2–12]. It can be classified into the following categories based on etiology: posttraumatic, nontraumatic or neurogenic, and myositis ossificans progressiva or fibrodysplasia ossificans progressive [13–29]. Posttraumatic HO includes surgically induced etiologies and is the focus of this chapter. It has been documented as the most common complication following total hip arthroplasty with a mean incidence of 53 % [22]. Prophylactic measures are often employed in such settings. While being well recognized throughout the body, HO following local amputation in the foot has historically received little attention from a clinical or research standpoint. However, in a retrospective cohort of 72 patients who underwent amputation consisting of partial metatarsal or transmetatarsal amputation, Boffeli and colleagues found a 75 % incidence of postoperative HO formation by 10 weeks postoperatively. Nearly three-quarters of patients who formed HO exhibited mid- to high-grade bone growth with 18.5 % of patients exhibiting an HO-associated ulcer requiring repeat surgical resection [30]. Similarly, the incidence of heterotopic bone growth after metatarsal head resection in the setting of rheumatoid arthritis has been reported as high as 72 %, most commonly on the second and third metatarsals [31].

Several medical and surgical prophylactic measures are available to decrease the potential for HO. Medical prophylaxis mainly consists of nonsteroidal anti-inflammatory medications or single-dose radiation treatment, which are often advocated in patients deemed at high risk for developing HO. Radiation is performed perioperatively in conjunction with surgical intervention. Additionally, certain surgical techniques and practices can minimize the potential for complicating HO. Given the high incidence and potential for complication, such prophylactic measures are important in limiting local amputation-associated morbidity.

T.J. Boffeli, D.P.M., F.A.C.F.A.S. (✉)
Regions Hospital/HealthPartners Institute for Education and Research, 640 Jackson Street, Saint Paul, MN 55101, USA
e-mail: troy.j.boffeli@healthpartners.com

J.C. Thompson, D.P.M., M.H.A., A.A.C.F.A.S.
Mayo Clinic Health System, Orthopedic Center,
1400 Bellinger Street, Eau Claire, WI 54702, USA
e-mail: thompson.jonathan@mayo.edu

© Springer International Publishing Switzerland 2015
T.J. Boffeli (ed.), *Osteomyelitis of the Foot and Ankle*, DOI 10.1007/978-3-319-18926-0_12

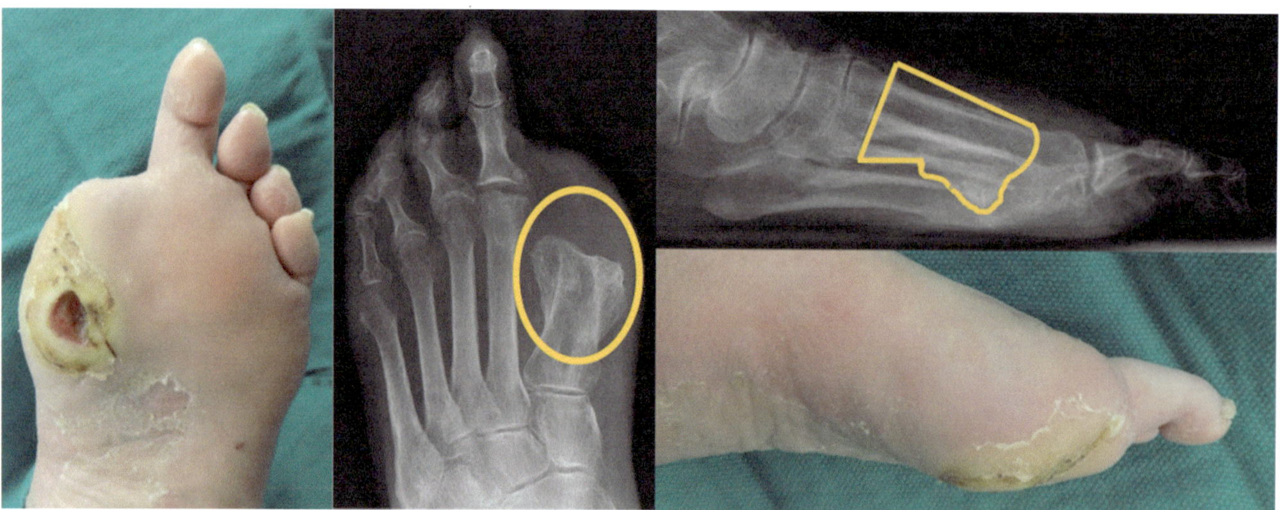

Fig. 12.1 Heterotopic ossification is most frequently appreciated at partial metatarsal amputation sites. It becomes clinically relevant when mid- to high-grade ossification forms on the plantar weight bearing aspect of the foot. *Re-published with permission of the Journal of Foot and Ankle Surgery* [30]

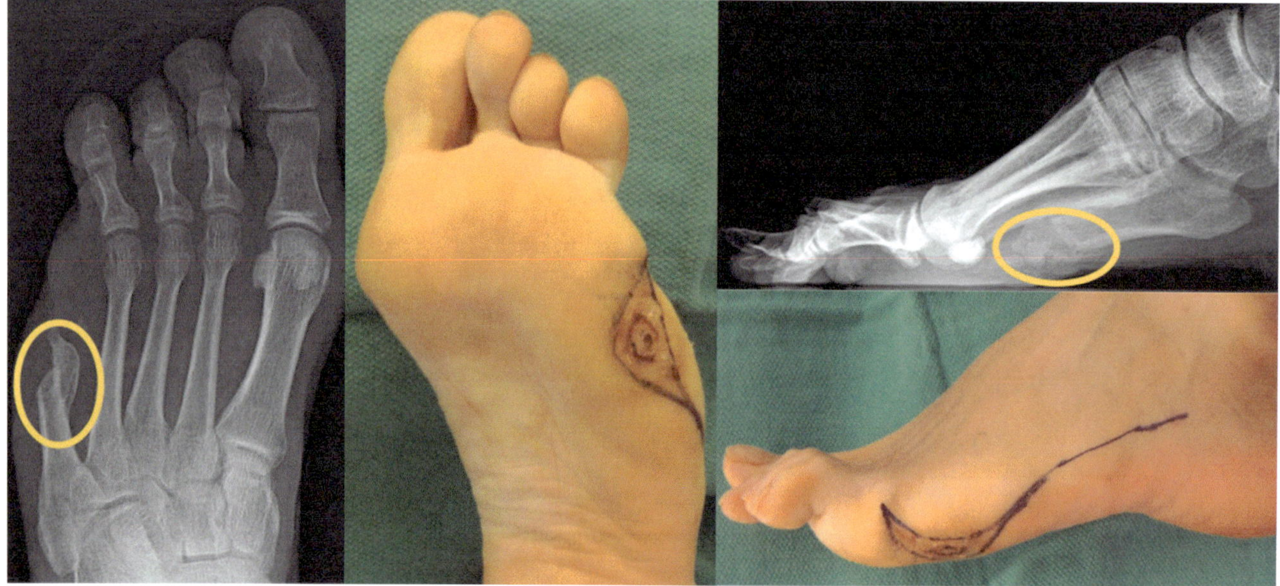

Fig. 12.2 Clinically relevant heterotopic ossification is appreciated at a previous partial fifth metatarsal amputation site. Complete fifth ray resection with staged surgery requiring peroneal tendon transfer into the cuboid was performed due to the development of osteomyelitis at the initial resection site

Etiology of Heterotopic Ossification

The specific cause of heterotopic ossification remains elusive. It is felt that mesenchymal stem cells are introduced into the soft tissues secondary to violation of bone and exposure of bone marrow from trauma or surgery, although these pluripotent cells can also be derived from adjacent muscle. These stem cells then differentiate into osteoblasts in the soft tissues and undergo osteogenesis [32]. While the impetus for stem cell differentiation remains unclear, the likely responsible factor is bone morphogenetic protein derived from traumatized tissue [33]. This differentiation appears to begin at approximately 16 h and peaks at 32 h postoperatively [34].

The typical scenario for clinically relevant HO involves a patient undergoing partial foot amputations secondary to

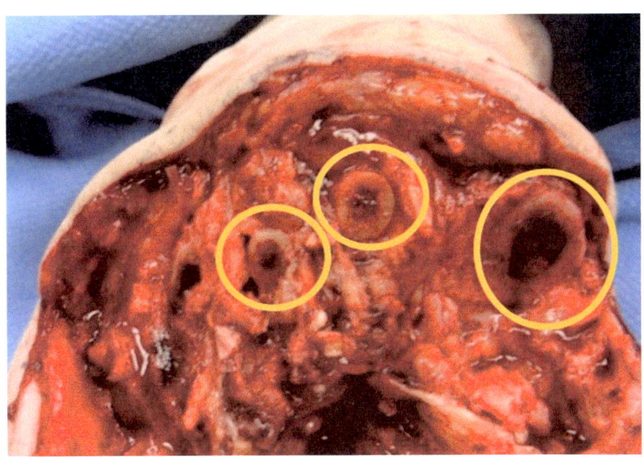

Fig. 12.3 Exposed medullary bone at the amputation site creates a portal for osteoprogenitor cells from the endosteum to extravasate into the soft tissues and differentiate into bone-forming osteoblasts

Table 12.1 Metatarsal resection HO staging

Grade 0—No heterotopic ossification	
Grade I—Isolated bone island adjacent to resection site	*a*—No adjacent ulceration
Grade II—Adhered bone spur formation <1cm	*b*—Adjacent ulceration
Grade III—Adhered bone spur formation >1cm	

These staging criteria help to establish the extent of radiographic HO formation and associated clinical relevance [30]

osteomyelitis, soft tissue infection, gangrene, or trauma with exposed medullary bone at the amputation site (Fig. 12.3). The periosteum and endosteum of bone contain the main supply of osteoprogenitor cells [35]. When performing a bone cut, the periosteum is often stripped before the cut is advanced through the medullary canal. Thus the periosteum and endosteum are both violated by the local trauma associated with the amputation, exposing a maximal amount of osteoprogenitor cells to the adjacent soft tissue. Hematoma derived from the medullary canal likely provides a vehicle for transfer of the osteoprogenitor cells into the soft tissues immediately adjacent to the amputation site, placing patients with robust vascular status at higher risk of HO formation [35].

Clinical Presentation

In order to appreciate the clinical presentation of HO, it is important to have an understanding of the risk factors that predispose the patient to heterotopic bone growth. The top predictor for whether HO can be anticipated is a prior history of formation [36]. Sufficient vascular status to the extremity may place the patient at higher risk as well, as those with peripheral vascular disease have exhibited a 30 % lower risk [37]. Furthermore, while diabetes and peripheral neuropathy are not independent risk factors [37], these are relative risk factors as diabetic neuropathic patients are at higher risk for amputation [38]. Less common risk factors are alkaline phosphatase and bone-forming disorders, such as ankylosing spondylitis or Paget's disease. Race and age have not been shown to be strong predisposing factors [39].

Signs and symptoms of actively forming HO can present from 3 to 12 weeks postoperatively [40]. There is often more swelling and erythema at the surgical site that persists longer and to a greater extent than would be anticipated with normal healing. Such findings may appear similar to postoperative infection, which should be ruled out. Serial postoperative radiographs are instrumental in monitoring for HO. We have appreciated radiographic changes as early as 4 weeks and as late as 10 weeks postoperatively [37]. For the purpose of determining the extent of HO involvement, Boffeli and colleagues developed a staging system similar to those created for the hip [30, 41, 42] (Table 12.1). The first radiographic sign of HO may be a soft tissue mass near the amputation site. Ossification typically begins in the soft tissues adjacent to the bone resection site, so early radiographic appearance of bone is often circumferential radiodensity with a lucent center [39]. There may be several foci of ossification within the osteoid. At this stage, bone frequently resembles an isolated bone island and is characterized as grade I (Fig. 12.4a). As the callus continues to ossify, it often adjoins to the original bone and the radiodense portion continues to enlarge (Grades II and III) (Fig. 12.4b, c) [30]. The bone continues to remodel until approximately 30 months postoperatively, when the pattern of heterotopic bone closely resembles that of normal bone [23].

Patients who have previously undergone partial foot amputation and develop subsequent neuropathic ulcers or pre-ulcerative lesions should be assessed for the presence of HO as a possible etiology. In particular, bone formation on the plantar weight bearing portion of the foot would pose the most substantial threat. HO-related ulcers are often full thickness in depth due to the concentrated peak plantar foot pressure created during weight bearing by relatively discrete HO prominences. Thus concomitant osteomyelitis may be present as well. The practitioner should not assume that radiographic appearance consistent with HO precludes the diagnosis of osteomyelitis, as both can be present in conjunction with one another. Laboratory analysis and advanced imaging may be warranted in this situation. While bone scans, ultrasonography, and computed-tomography imaging has been used for diagnosis of HO in the hip, this has not been assessed in the foot. We do not routinely use such modalities but will consider magnetic resonance imaging (MRI) to determine the presence of soft tissue abscess or osteomyelitis. The typical appearance of heterotopic ossification on MRI is a low-signal-intensity rim with a heterogeneous, high-signal-intensity tissue structure [43].

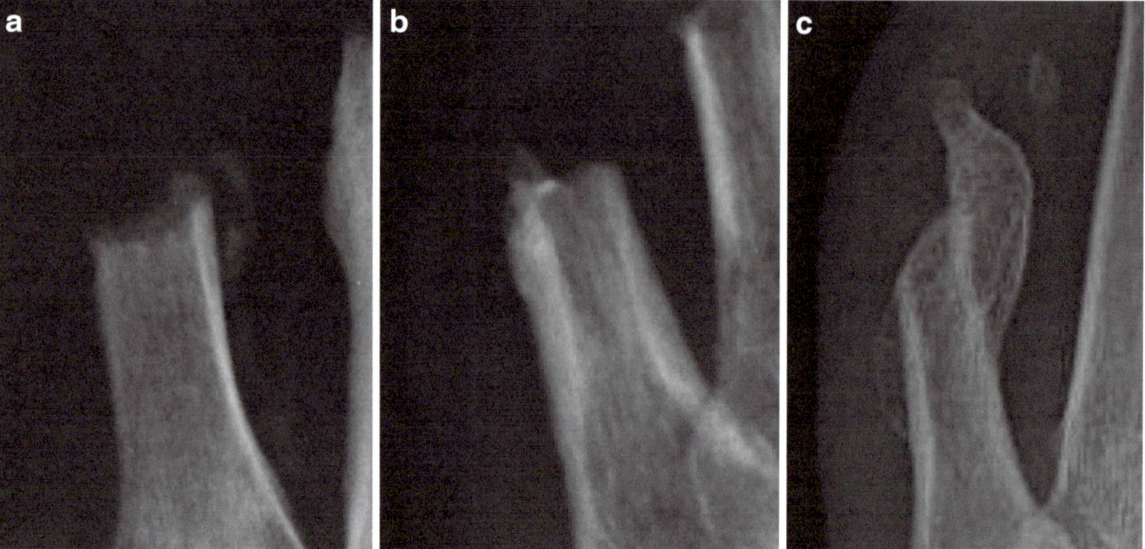

Fig. 12.4 (**a**) Grade I heterotopic ossification exhibits a rim of radiodense bone formation with a center of lucency. (**b**) As heterotopic ossification progresses, it may attach to the original bone, indicated as Grade II formation. (**c**) Advanced Grade III heterotopic ossification is classified as bone growth greater than 1 cm on radiograph

Treatment and Prophylactic Measures

Clinically relevant heterotopic ossification often requires surgical intervention either for non-healing wounds that have failed appropriate offloading measures or in patients who have developed secondary osteomyelitis. In our experience, while offloading measures may allow the wound to improve or heal, the re-ulceration rate is high in patients with HO-induced neuropathic ulceration. In the patient with acute soft tissue infection or osteomyelitis, surgical resection is the mainstay of treatment. Goals of surgery are to correct structural deformity, resect potentially infected bone for biopsy purposes, avoid recurrent HO, and allow for primary closure of soft tissues. Intraoperatively, it is often difficult to dissect heterotopic bone growth from adjacent soft tissues as the two are intimately affixed. Care is taken to ensure that all bone growth is excised not only when attached to the adjacent bone but also when isolated islands are present in the soft tissues as these could be a source of pressure if not removed. Oftentimes during direct intraoperative inspection, the degree of involvement appreciated at the HO site appears much more extensive than preoperative radiographs would indicate as abnormal tissue that fails to fully ossify may not be evident on radiograph (Fig. 12.5). When excising heterotopic bone, it is often necessary to resect proximal to the previous resection site in order to obtain a clean margin in the event of osteomyelitis and for sufficient soft tissue coverage if necessary (Figs. 12.6 and 12.7).

The resected bone is sent for pathologic analysis to confirm heterotopic ossification and possible concomitant osteomyelitis.

Histologically, well-developed HO appears as cancellous and mature lamellar bone with associated blood vessels and bone marrow as well as low-grade hematopoiesis. Edema, hypersensitivity, muscle necrosis, and osteoporosis may surround HO and be a consequence of it rather than a cause (Fig. 12.8) [44]. The medical and surgical preventative measures discussed below should routinely be applied at this time to avoid repeat heterotopic bone growth. Two main preventative measures have traditionally been advocated for patients deemed at particular risk for HO formation: nonsteroidal anti-inflammatory drugs (NSAIDs) and radiation therapy. Furthermore, certain routine surgical techniques and approaches can minimize the potential for developing HO.

Surgical Prophylaxis

Appropriate surgical technique during the initial amputation procedure can help minimize the development of complicating HO and should be the standard for all amputation procedures. While there is higher potential for heterotopic bone growth in any region where the medullary canal is exposed to adjacent soft tissues, there should be a higher level of concern when amputating through the metatarsals. This level of amputation seems particularly prone to clinically relevant HO likely due to the void left adjacent to an open medullary canal, which predisposes the patient to hematoma formation. Extravasation of hematoma from the medullary canal likely carries osteoprogenitor cells that will ultimately differentiate into bone-forming osteoblasts, so any efforts to minimize local hematoma formation at the resection site will be beneficial.

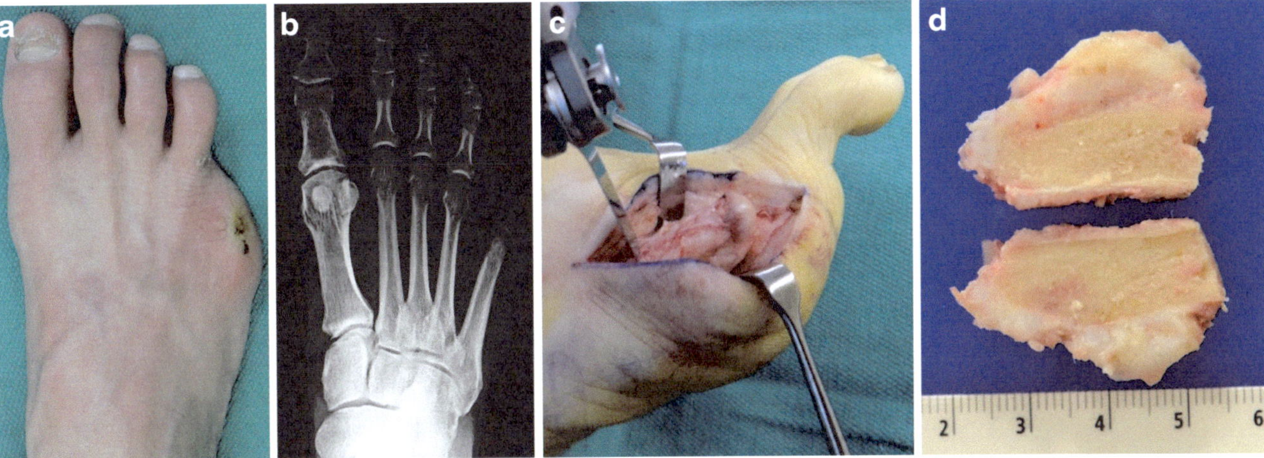

Fig. 12.5 (**a**) Clinical appearance of a patient who had undergone previous partial fifth ray resection whose surgical wound never fully epithelialized and became a source of pain postoperatively. (**b**) Radiographs would suggest minimal HO involvement, but (**c**) intraoperative findings revealed abnormal tissue with extensive involvement at the previous resection site. (**d**) Sectioning of the metatarsal resection site reveals a large prominence on the plantar aspect of the bone not fully appreciated on preoperative radiographs. Pathologic analysis revealed no signs of osteomyelitis at the resection site

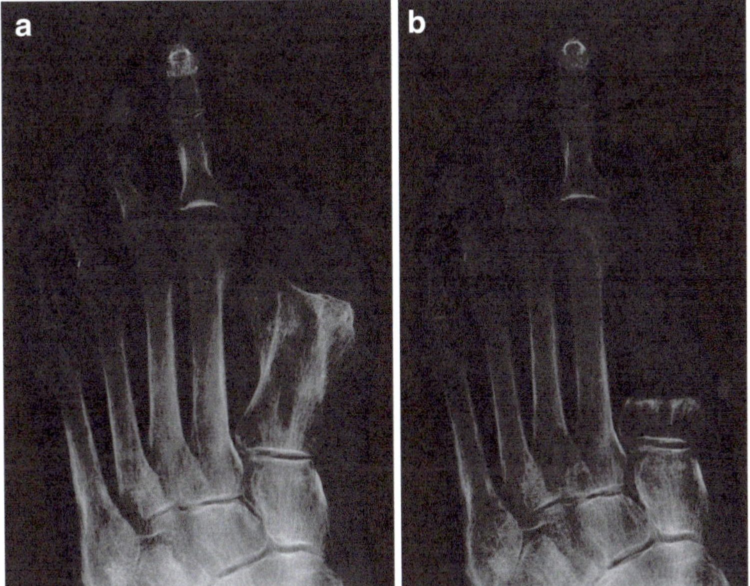

Fig. 12.6 (**a**) Preoperative radiographs of extensive heterotopic bone growth with associated full-thickness neuropathic ulcer and osteomyelitis. (**b**) Postoperative radiographs reveal the level of resection required in this situation to allow sufficient soft tissue closure and obtain noninfected margins as confirmed by pathology. While disarticulation at the first tarsometatarsal joint can decrease the likelihood of forming HO, retaining the metatarsal base serves to maintain stability by preserving the insertion of the tibialis anterior and peroneus longus tendons. Subsequent postoperative radiographs revealed no signs of HO recurrence when treated with single-dose radiation therapy. *Republished with permission of the Journal of Foot and Ankle Surgery* [30]

We often utilize a staged surgical approach, with the majority of bone being resected in the initial surgery for purposes of infection source control. This often allows cellulitis to resolve prior to subsequent repeat irrigation and hematoma evacuation followed by delayed primary closure within a few days. In patients deemed at high risk for hematoma formation, such as in the setting of anticoagulation therapy or robust vascular status, staged surgery with dead space management using antibiotic beads can be employed. This approach can also be utilized when residual osteomyelitis persists after resection when parenteral antibiotics in isolation may not be sufficient. After initial incision and drainage

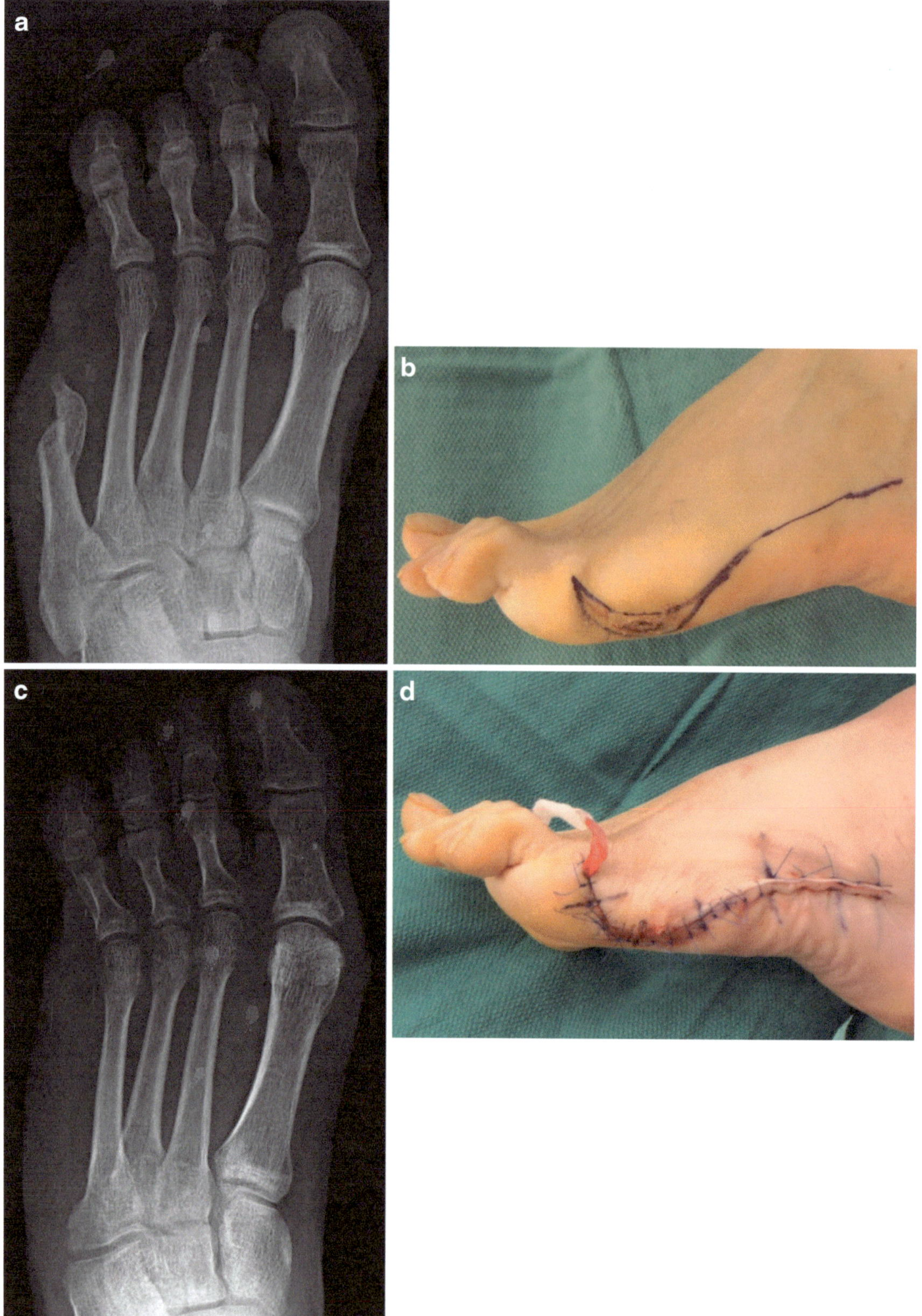

Fig. 12.7 (**a**, **b**) Preoperative clinical and radiographic appearance of clinically relevant heterotopic ossification. (**c**, **d**) Postoperative clinical and radiographic appearance following complete fifth ray resection with staged surgery requiring peroneal tendon transfer into the cuboid. Disarticulation decreases the likelihood for recurrent heterotopic ossification as opposed to repeat resection through the metatarsal.

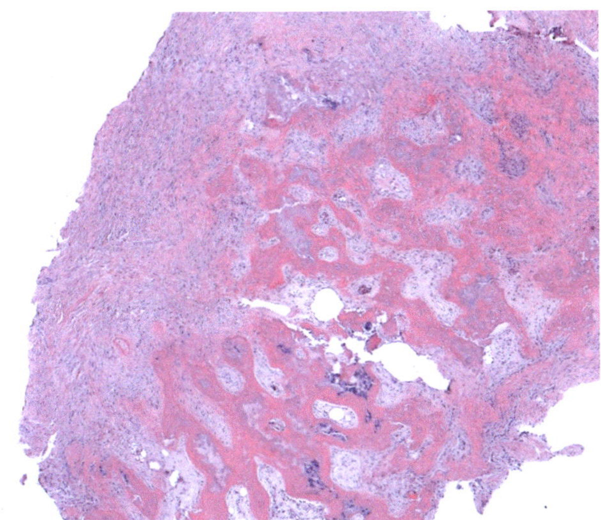

Fig. 12.8 Histologic features of heterotopic ossification. Culture and pathology specimens should be collected intraoperatively to confirm the diagnosis of heterotopic ossification and possible concomitant osteomyelitis

and antibiotic bead application, stage 2 typically occurs 2 weeks later and consists of antibiotic bead removal with irrigation and evacuation of hematoma (Fig. 12.9).

Developing osteoid that may be forming is debrided at that time as well. The portion of the incision site that is most likely to heal uneventfully is reopened, and the chain of antibiotic beads that were initially left prominent near the incision are removed prior to debridement. The adjacent medullary canal is often curetted in order to obtain a proximal margin specimen while not further shortening the cortical rim. A variety of other standard surgical techniques can be employed to minimize the potential for HO. Because osteoprogenitor cells are contained within the periosteum, excessive stripping of the periosteum should be avoided when performing dissection or bone cuts (Fig. 12.10a). Similarly, osteoprogenitor-rich bone fragments generated from saw cuts should be thoroughly irrigated and removed intraoperatively as well (Fig. 12.10b). Generally, care should be taken to achieve satisfactory hemostasis to diminish the potential for hematoma. While we do not regularly apply electrocautery to the exposed medullary canal to avoid further devitalizing bone in the setting of infection, this may help prevent medullary canal-derived hematoma in certain settings. To avoid violating the medullary canal altogether, disarticulation can be performed when feasible in patients at risk of developing HO (Fig. 12.10c). When a cut through the bone is necessary, it should be performed with a saw rather than a blunt bone-crushing instrument to avoid further trauma at the amputation site. Postoperative activity restrictions including non-weight bearing and strict elevation help decrease the potential for hematoma formation.

Radiation Therapy Prophylaxis

Radiation therapy has long been recognized as a method for inhibiting HO formation, first being reported by Craven and Urist in 1971 [33]. Radiation acts by bombarding radiosensitive osteoprogenitor cells with radiation prior to differentiation, after which these cells become relatively radioresistant [1]. The targeting of these pluripotent cells prevents them from differentiating into bone-forming osteoblasts. Administration consists of a single dose of radiation given from 24 h preoperatively to 72 h postoperatively. In the event of staged surgery, radiation should target the surgery requiring the most amount of dissection and invasive bone work. Administration can be performed in the inpatient or outpatient setting by a radiation therapy department. The foot is placed on a tissue-equivalent surface while a single-fraction dose of 700 cGy radiation is administered to the affected region, typically the forefoot (Fig. 12.11) [30]. This is a brief procedure that does not require weight bearing or removal of the dressing. Preoperative administration of radiation is ideal for several reasons if feasible. It avoids unnecessary transport during the first few days postoperatively that could place the patient at higher risk for HO-forming hematoma. Furthermore, if insurance issues or other factors preclude the patient from receiving radiation, appropriate changes can be made intraoperatively if necessary, such as disarticulation or intentional staging of the procedure. Preoperative administration is not always feasible, however, as emergent surgery secondary to acute infection is relatively common in this patient population.

While formal indications for radiation after partial foot amputation have yet to be established, we routinely advocate for treatment in patients deemed at higher than typical risk. This would consist of patients with a previous history of HO and those felt to be at high risk for primary heterotopic bone growth due to concomitant bone disorders. The risks associated with single-fraction, relatively low-dose radiation are low [45, 46]. While the negative effects of multiple-fraction radiation therapy on wound healing are well documented [47], uneventful wound healing has been appreciated in partial foot amputation patients receiving single-fraction administration [30]. Given the low risk of prophylactic treatment and the potential for HO-related re-ulceration and reamputation, our threshold for performing radiation treatment is relatively low.

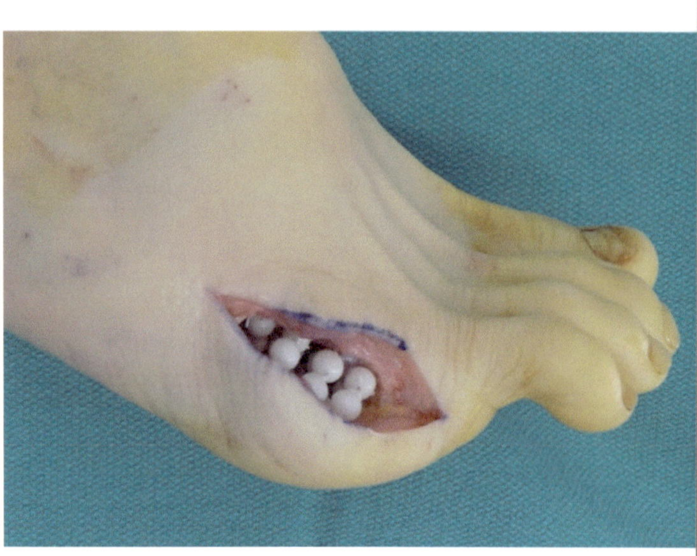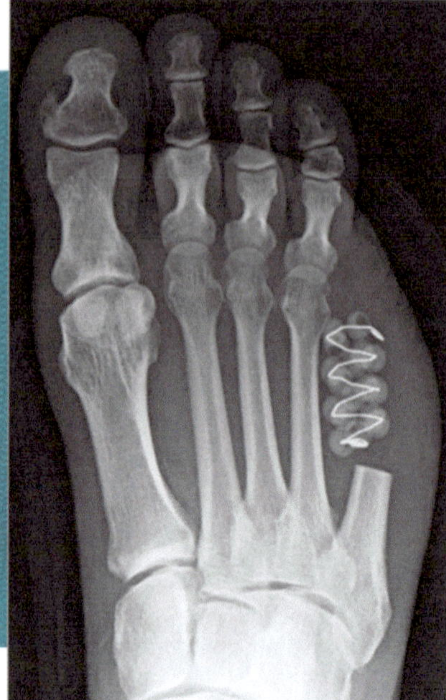

Fig. 12.9 A staged surgical approach is a valuable adjunct to avoiding heterotopic ossification. Antibiotic-impregnated beads are applied in the dead space created at the resection site during the initial surgery. The secondary staged surgery typically occurs 2 weeks later and involves bead removal, evacuation of organized hematoma that could promote HO formation, proximal margin biopsy, minimal soft tissue debridement as needed, and delayed primary closure. Oftentimes the proximal margin biopsy is obtained from curettage of the medullary canal as opposed to resection of a segment cortical bone in order to preserve metatarsal length

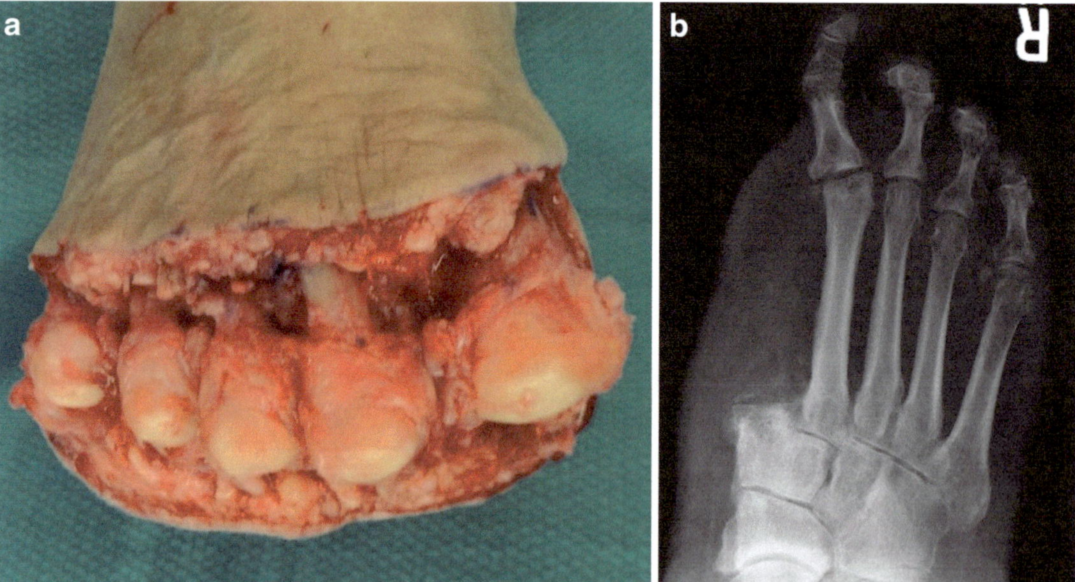

Fig. 12.10 Surgical techniques for avoiding heterotopic ossification. (**a**) As the periosteum is a source of osteoprogenitor cells, excessive periosteal elevation should be avoided during amputation. Care should be taken to remove osseous debris created during bone cuts that may contain pluripotent cells. (**b**) In the patient with previous history of HO, disarticulation may be a preferable option to avoid the potential for repeat bone formation at the resection site, although this may not always be practical from a biomechanical standpoint

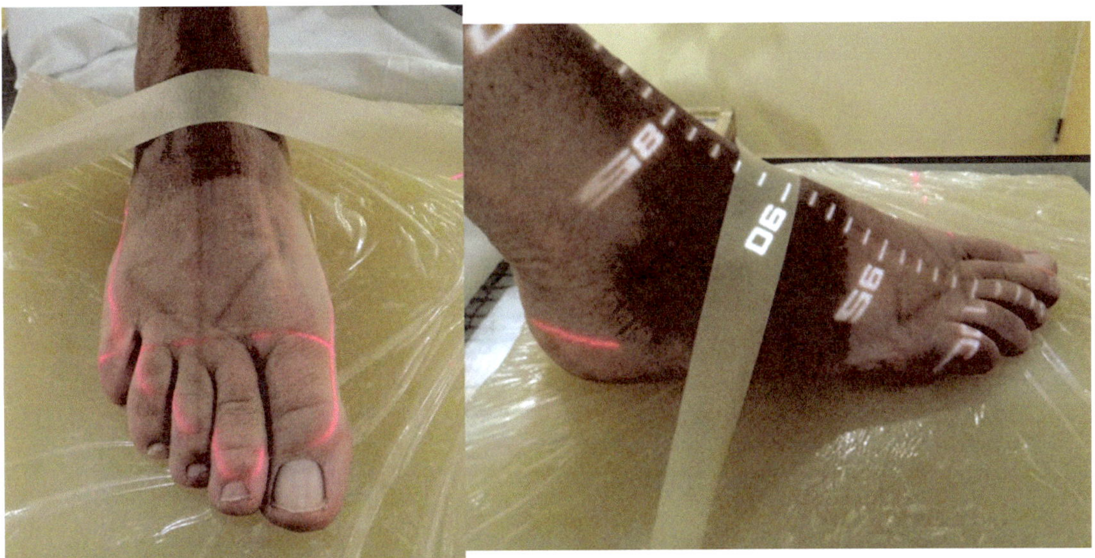

Fig. 12.11 Perioperative radiation therapy. A single fraction of relatively low-dose radiation is directed to the operative region within 24 h preoperatively to 72 h postoperatively to prevent heterotopic bone formation. In the event of staged surgery, radiation should be coordinated with the surgery requiring the most extensive dissection. We prefer preoperative administration to avoid additional transportation and manipulation of the foot postoperatively. Our practice utilizes radiation therapy in the high-risk patient with previous history of HO in the ipsilateral limb, contralateral limb, or elsewhere in the body. *Re-published with permission of the Journal of Foot and Ankle Surgery* [30]

Pharmacological Prophylaxis

The mainstay pharmacological option for heterotopic bone prevention is NSAID therapy. This is a well-described prophylactic measure in the hip and other regions, but it is not well documented in the foot and ankle. NSAIDs serve to inhibit the formation of HO via two pathways. It provides an inhibitory effect on the differentiation of pluripotent mesenchymal cells to osteoblasts. Secondly, NSAIDs suppress the prostaglandin-mediated inflammatory response, which is normally an important aspect of osteogenesis [39]. Indomethacin has been described as the gold standard for heterotopic ossification prophylaxis in the setting of total hip arthroplasty. However, naproxen and diclofenac have been shown to be equally as effective [39]. Cyclooxygenase-2 inhibitors are a similarly effective option with fewer gastrointestinal side effects, but concern has been raised regarding cardiovascular risks [48]. While there have been several recommendations regarding duration of therapy, it is typically believed that prophylaxis should be initiated within 3 days postoperatively. Duration following total hip arthroplasty has ranged from 7 days to 6 weeks [9, 39]. While many medications, dosages, and durations have been determined to be effective, common protocols consist of indomethacin 25 mg three times a day or diclofenac 50 mg three times a day. While a duration as short as seven days has proven effective, it is typically extended to 3–6 weeks [9, 11]. Side effects that have been associated with NSAIDs are gastromucosal irritation, prolonged bleeding time, and increased nonunion rates [49].

Bisphosphonates are a less common prophylactic measure that has been applied in the setting of total hip arthroplasty but has not been evaluated in the foot. The most studied medication in this category is etidronate disodium, which acts by inhibiting the precipitation of calcium phosphate and preventing its conversion into hydroxyapatite (Macfarlane). One concern with bisphosphonates are that once the drug is discontinued, mineralization of the bone matrix can resume [26]. We do not utilize bisphosphonates as part of our treatment protocol.

The efficacy of prophylactic single-dose radiation compared to NSAID pharmacotherapy has been well studied. Vavken and colleagues performed a systematic review and meta-analysis of nine studies regarding prophylaxis in the hip and found no evidence for a statistically significant or clinically relevant difference between NSAIDs and radiation therapy [50]. However, Blokhuis performed a systematic review of five prospective studies comparing prophylactic radiation versus indomethacin after acetabular fractures and found a significantly lower incidence of HO when radiation was used, leading them to advocate for radiation until further information is available [51]. When providing prophylaxis following partial foot amputation, we prefer to utilize radiation therapy in high-risk patients as opposed to NSAIDs for several reasons. Radiation therapy is not dependent on patient compliance, as pharmacotherapy is contingent on the patient taking the prescribed medication. Furthermore, radiation avoids renal toxicity in the often renally impaired patient population requiring partial foot amputation. Finally, gastrointestinal disturbances are avoided with radiation, and it is not dependent on vascular perfusion for permeation to the distal aspect of the lower extremity. While the cost of radiation administration is certainly higher, this is justifiable when considering the direct and indirect costs associated with revisional surgery and potential for limb loss.

Conclusions

Heterotopic ossification is a common and sometimes detrimental complication in the setting of partial foot amputations. It has the potential for re-ulceration, which can lead to recurrent infection and repeat amputation. Local reamputation options are often much more limited than the initial procedure, increasing patient morbidity and potential for eventual limb loss. This is not ideal in the already-impaired patient population that often requires partial foot amputation. Patients with a history of previous HO formation or those with profound neuropathy and robust vascular status should be considered at higher risk for development. Given the high incidence of heterotopic ossification and the potential for damaging side effects after partial foot amputation, surgical prophylactic measures should routinely be employed, and pharmacological or radiation prophylaxis should be utilized in the high-risk patient in an effort to minimize patient morbidity.

References

1. Balboni TA, Gobezie R, Mamon HJ. Heterotopic ossification: pathophysiology, clinical features, and the role of radiotherapy for prophylaxis. Int J Radiat Oncol Biol Phys. 2006;65:1289–99.
2. Martini F, Sell S, Reize P, Jani R, et al. Perioperative side effects of preventative measures against heterotopic ossification: diclofenac versus irradiation. Aktuelle Rheumatol. 1995;20:61–5.
3. Bremen-Kühne R, Stock D, Franke C. Indomethacin: short-term therapy versus single low dosage radiation for prevention of periarticular ossifications after total hip endoprosthesis [in German]. Z Orthop Ihre Grenzgeb. 1997;135:422–9.
4. Kölbl O, Knelles D, Barthel T, et al. Preoperative irradiation versus the use of nonsteroidal anti-inflammatory drugs for prevention of heterotopic ossification following total hip replacement: the results of a randomized trial. Int J Radiat Oncol Biol Phys. 1998;42:397–401.
5. Kienapfel H, Koller M, Wust A, et al. Prevention of heterotopic bone formation after total hip arthroplasty: a prospective randomised study comparing postoperative radiation therapy with indomethacin medication. Arch Orthop Trauma Surg. 1999;119:296–302.
6. Chao ST, Joyce MJ, Suh JH. Treatment of heterotopic ossification. Orthopedics. 2007;30(6):457–64.
7. Burd TA, Lowry KJ, Anglen JO. Indomethacin compared with localized irradiation for the prevention of heterotopic ossification following surgical treatment of acetabular fractures. J Bone Joint Surg Am. 2001;83-A:1783–8.
8. Schafer SJ, Schafer LO, Anglen JO, et al. Heterotopic ossification in rehabilitation patients who have had internal fixation of an acetabular fracture. J Rehabil Res Dev. 2000;37:389–93.
9. Moore KD, Goss K, Anglen JO. Indomethacin versus radiation therapy for prophylaxis against heterotopic ossification in acetabular fractures: a randomised, prospective study. J Bone Joint Surg Br. 1998;80:259–63.
10. Kölbl O, Knelles D, Barthel T, et al. Randomized trial comparing early postoperative irradiation vs. the use of nonsteroidal antiinflammatory drugs for prevention of heterotopic ossification following prosthetic total hip replacement. Int J Radiat Oncol Biol Phys. 1997;39(5):961–6.
11. Sell S, Willms R, Jany R, et al. The suppression of heterotopic ossifications: radiation versus NSAID therapy—a prospective study. J Arthroplasty. 1998;13:854–9.
12. Knelles D, Barthel T, Karrer A, Kraus U, et al. Prevention of heterotopic ossification after total hip replacement. A prospective, randomised study using acetyl-salicylic acid, indomethacin and fractional or single-dose irradiation. J Bone Joint Surg Br. 1997;79:596–602.
13. Nuovo MA, Norman A, Chumas J, et al. Myositis ossificans with atypical clinical, radiographic, or pathologic findings: a review of 23 cases. Skeletal Radiol. 1992;21(2):87–101.
14. Garland DE. A clinical perspective on common forms of acquired heterotopic ossification. Clin Orthop Relat Res. 1991;263:13–29.
15. Singer BR. Heterotopic ossification. Br J Hosp Med. 1993;49(4):247–55.
16. Thomas BJ. Heterotopic bone formation after total hip arthroplasty. Orthop Clin North Am. 1992;23(2):347–58.
17. Allard MM, Thomas RL, Nicholas Jr RW. Myositis ossificans: an unusual presentation in the foot. Foot Ankle Int. 1997;18(1):39–42.
18. Jacobs JE, Birnbaum BA, Siegelman ES. Heterotopic ossification of midline abdominal incisions: CT and MR imaging findings. AJR Am J Roentgenol. 1996;166(3):579–84.
19. Reardon MJ, Tillou A, Mody DR, Reardon PR. Heterotopic calcification in abdominal wounds. Am J Surg. 1997;173(2):145–7.
20. Haque S, Eisen RN, West AB. Heterotopic formation in the gastrointestinal tract. Arch Pathol Lab Med. 1996;120(7):666–70.
21. Naraghl FF, DeCoster TA, Moneim MS, et al. Heterotopic ossification. Orthopedics. 1996;19(2):145–51.
22. Thomas BJ, Amstutz HC. Prevention of heterotopic bone formation: clinical experience with diphosphonates. Hip. 1987: 59–69.
23. Rossier AB, Bussat P, Infante F, et al. Current facts of para-osteoarthropathy (POA). Paraplegia. 1973;11(1):38–78.
24. Subbarao JV, Garrison SJ. Heterotopic ossification: diagnosis and management, current concepts and controversies. J Spinal Cord Med. 1999;22(4):273–83.
25. Gibson CJ, Poduri KR. Heterotopic ossification as a complication of toxic epidermal necrolysis. Arch Phys Med Rehabil. 1997;78(7):774–6.
26. Stover SL, Niemann KM, Tulloss JR. Experience with surgical resection of heterotopic bone in spinal cord injury patients. Clin Orthop Relat Res. 1991;263:71–7.
27. Inan M, Chan G, Dabney K, Miller F. Heterotopic ossification following hip osteotomies in cerebral palsy: incidence and risk factors. J Pediatr Orthop. 2006;26(4):551–6.
28. Benetos IS, Mavrogenis AF, Themistocleous GC, et al. Optimal treatment of fibrodysplasia ossificans progressiva with surgical excision of heterotopic bone, indomethacin, and irradiation. J Surg Orthop Adv. 2006;15(2):99–104.
29. Kaplan FS, Xu M, Glaser DL, et al. Early diagnosis of fibrodysplasia ossificans progressive. Pediatrics. 2008;121(5):1295–300.
30. Boffeli TJ, Pfannenstein RR, Thompson JC. Radiation therapy for recurrent heterotopic ossification following partial metatarsal ray resection. J Foot Ankle Surg. 2015;54:345–9.
31. Vahvanen V, Piirainen H, Kettunen P. Resection arthroplasty of the metatarsophalangeal joints in rheumatoid arthritis: a follow-up study of 100 patients. Scand J Rheumatol. 1980;9:257–65.
32. Buring K. On the origin of cells in heterotopic bone formation. Clin Orthop Relat Res. 1975;110:293–302.

33. Craven PL, Urist MR. Osteogenesis by radioisotope labelled cell populations in implants of bone matrix under the influence of ionizing radiation. Clin Orthop Relat Res. 1971;76:231–3.

34. Tonna EA, Cronkite EP. Autoradiographic studies of cell proliferation in the periosteum of intact and fractured femora of mice utilizing DNA labeling with H3-thymidine. Proc Soc Exp Biol Med. 1961;107:719–21.

35. Ross MH, Pawlina W. Chapter 8, Cells of bone tissue. In: Histology: a text and atlas, with correlated cell and molecular biology. 6th ed. Baltimore: Wolters Kluwer; 2009.

36. Eggli S, Woo A. Risk factors for heterotopic ossification in total hip arthroplasty. Arch Orthop Trauma Surg. 2001;121:531–5.

37. Boffeli TB, Pfannenstein RR, Thompson JC, Mahoney KM, Waverly BJ. Incidence and clinical significance of heterotopic ossification following partial metatarsal ray resection. Poster presentation at the American College of Foot and Ankle Surgeons' Annual Scientific Conference in Kissimmee, Florida, February 2014.

38. Morbach S, Quante C, Ochs HR, et al. Increased risk of lower-extremity amputation among Caucasian diabetic patients on dialysis. Diabetes Care. 2001;24(9):1689–90.

39. Mavrogenis A, Soucacos P, Papagelopoulos P. Heterotopic ossification revisited. Orthopedics. 2011;34(3):177.

40. Downing MR, Knox D, Gibson P, Reid DM, Polter A, Ashcroft GP. Impact of trochanteric heterotopic ossification on measurement of femoral bone density following cemented total hip replacement. J Orthop Res. 2008;26(10):1334–9.

41. Brooker AF, Bowerman JW, Robinson RA, et al. Ectopic ossification following total hip replacement: incidence and a method of classification. J Bone Joint Surg Am. 1973;55(8):1629–32.

42. Schmidt J, Hackenbroch MH. A new classification for heterotopic ossification in total hip arthroplasty considering the surgical approach. Arch Orthop Trauma Surg. 1996;115(6):339–43.

43. De Smet AA, Norris MA, Risher DR. Magnetic resonance imaging of myositis ossificans: analysis of seven cases. Skeletal Radiol. 1992;21(8):503–7.

44. Vanden Bossche L, Vanderstraeten G. Heterotopic ossification: a review. J Rehabil Med. 2005;37:129–36.

45. Lo TC, Pfeifer BA, Smiley PM, Gumley GJ. Case report: radiation prevention of heterotopic ossification after bone and joint surgery in sites other than hips. Br J Radiol. 1996;69:673–7.

46. Healy WL, LO TC, DeSimone AA. Single-dose irradiation for the prevention of heterotopic ossification after total hip arthroplasty. A comparison of doses of five hundred and fifty and seven hundred centigray. J Bone Joint Surg Am. 1995;77:590–5.

47. Haubner F, Ohmann E, Pohl F, Strutz J, et al. Wound healing after radiation therapy: review of the literature. Radiat Oncol. 2012;7: 162–71.

48. Macfarlane RJ, Ng BH, Gamie Z, et al. Parmacological treatment of heterotopic ossification following hip and acetabular surgery. Expert Opin Pharmacother. 2008;9(5):767–86.

49. Burd TA, Hughes MS, Anglen JO. Heterotopic ossification prophylaxis with indomethacin increases the risk of long-bone nonunion. J Bone Joint Surg Br. 2003;85:700–5.

50. Vavken P, Castellani L, Sculco TP. Prophylaxis of heterotopic ossification of the hip. Clin Orthop Relat Res. 2009;467:3283–9.

51. Blokhuis TJ, Frolke PM. Is radiation superior to indomethacin to prevent heterotopic ossification in acetabular fractures?: a systematic review. Clin Orthop Relat Res. 2009;467:526–30.

Prevention of Osteomyelitis in Traumatic Injuries

Rachel C. Collier and Jessica A. Tabatt

Introduction

Traumatic injuries of the foot and ankle can be challenging to manage due to the relative subcutaneous nature of bone and joint structures and the environmental factors associated with lower extremity trauma that predispose to posttraumatic infection. This chapter will focus on infection prevention when treating traumatic injuries of the foot and ankle. Early and prompt management is imperative for prevention of infection with initial focus on limiting soft tissue damage and stabilization of the limb. A delay in treatment or inadequate initial treatment may substantially increase the risk for development of osteomyelitis [1].

The skin has a critical role in infection prevention by providing a protective barrier. The effectiveness of the skin at preventing infection is severely compromised with open injuries, which allows inoculation with a potentially high concentration of organisms. The lower extremity has been shown to be immunocompromised compared to other regions of the body, and trauma itself can alter the effectiveness of the immune system in regard to neutrophil function and ability to react to stimuli [2, 3]. The foot is often placed in a variety of environmental conditions leading to various potential pathogens. Wounds contaminated by dirt, soil, or feces are more prone to infection [4–6]. Furthermore, devitalized tissue which is commonly found in open fractures and other traumatic injuries will act as a nidus for infection if not appropriately removed from the injured region.

Infection prevention is important for both immediate and long-term outcomes. Posttraumatic osteomyelitis has the potential to turn an otherwise treatable injury into a debilitating and possibly limb-threatening disorder requiring multiple operations and long-term antibiotic therapy. Prevention of osteomyelitis in children is especially important as it can cause growth plate arrest leading to altered growth [7]. The risk of osteomyelitis associated with plantar puncture wounds has been described as 0.1–2 %, with a greater prevalence in forefoot injuries through athletic shoes [8]. Clinical infection rates in open fractures types I, II, and III based on the Gustilo and Anderson classification (Table 13.1) [9, 10] have been described as 1.4 %, 3.6 %, and 10–50 %, respectively [11]. The focus of this chapter is to discuss infection prevention protocols for traumatic injuries involving the foot and ankle. Case examples demonstrate our preferred treatment protocols for the management of puncture wounds, open fractures, crush injuries, degloving injuries, and traumatic amputation associated with industrial, recreational, and lawn mower injuries.

Initial Workup

Initial evaluation and management of a trauma patient is similar regardless of the mechanism of injury. A detailed history is necessary with special considerations given to various factors such as time elapsed since the injury, mechanism of injury, environment where the injury occurred, and any initial treatments that have been performed. These variables have an impact on treatment decisions and can play a role in the potential for osteomyelitis. Specifically, the type of injury and environmental factors are useful for determining appropriate initial antibiotic coverage (Table 13.2). Tetanus status should be established with puncture wounds and open fractures. Recommended tetanus prophylaxis is dependent upon previous immunization history as described in Table 13.3 [12–14]. A detailed lower extremity physical examination is performed to evaluate soft tissue viability, neurovascular

R.C. Collier, FACFAOM (✉)
Regions Hospital/HealthPartners Institute for Education
and Research, 640 Jackson Street, St. Paul, MN 55101, USA
e-mail: Rachel.C.Collier@healthpartners.com

J.A. Tabatt, DPM
Essentia Health, St. Joseph's Brainerd Clinic,
2024 South 6th Street, Brainerd, MN 56401, USA
e-mail: jatabatt@gmail.com

© Springer International Publishing Switzerland 2015
T.J. Boffeli (ed.), *Osteomyelitis of the Foot and Ankle*, DOI 10.1007/978-3-319-18926-0_13

Table 13.1 Gustilo–Anderson classification for open fractures [9, 10]

Type I	Open fracture, wound <1 cm in length and clean
Type II	Open fracture, wound >1 cm in length without extensive soft tissue damage, flaps, avulsions
Type III	Open segmental fracture; open fracture with extensive soft tissue damage; traumatic amputation (including gunshot injuries, open fractures caused by farm injuries, fractures requiring vascular repair)
A	Adequate periosteal coverage of the fractured bone despite the extensive soft tissue laceration or damage; high-energy trauma regardless of wound size
B	Extensive soft tissue loss with periosteal stripping and bone exposure, usually associated with massive contamination
C	Arterial injury requiring repair, irrespective of degree of soft tissue injury

Table 13.2 Injury presentations and primary bacterial concerns

Injury type	Bacteria concern	Antibiotic options
Lawn mower/chain saw injuries (farm/soil environment)	*Pseudomonas* spp.	Ciprofloxacin Levofloxacin Aminoglycosides
	Anaerobic (*Clostridium* spp.)	Penicillins Amoxicillin/clavulanic acid Piperacillin/tazobactam
Boating injuries (water environment)	*Vibrio* spp., *Aeromonas hydrophila*, *Mycobacterium marinum*	Tetracyclines

Acute presentation puncture wound *Consider broad spectrum choices for heavily contaminated wounds and diabetics*	Gram positive: *Staphylococcus aureus*, Alpha hemolytic *Streptococcus*, *Staphylococcus epidermidis*
	Gram negative: *E. coli*, *Klebsiella* spp., *Proteus* spp.
		PO
		  Cephalexin
		  Amoxicillin/clavulanic acid
		  Trimethoprim/sulfamethoxazole
		  Clindamycin/ciprofloxacin
		IV
		  Cefazolin
		  Ampicillin/sulbactam
		  Piperacillin/tazobactam
		  Clindamycin
		  Ciprofloxacin

Chronic presentation puncture wound *Consider osteomyelitis, especially when through rubber-soled shoe*	*Pseudomonas* spp.	Ciprofloxacin Levofloxacin Aminoglycosides Piperacillin/tazobactam
Gustilo–Anderson Type I	Gram positive	Cephalosporins Piperacillin/tazobactam Aminoglycosides Clindamycin (PCN alternative)
Gustilo–Anderson Type II	Gram positive > gram negative	Cefazolin Piperacillin/tazobactam
Gustilo–Anderson Type III	Gram negative > gram positive	Cefazolin or piperacillin/tazobactam, + Gentamicin/tobramycin, + Penicillin with severe contamination

Table 13.3 Tetanus prophylaxis [12–14]

	Clean and minor wounds		All other wounds[a]	
Vaccination history	Tdap	TIG	Tdap	TIG
Incomplete series[b]/unknown	Yes	No	Yes	Yes
Complete series <5 years	No	No	No	No
Completes series 5–10 years	No	No	Yes	No
Completes series ≥10 years	Yes	No	Yes	No

[a]Puncture wounds, avulsions, burns, frostbite, wounds from missiles (i.e., gunshot wounds); wounds contaminated with dirt, soil, feces, and saliva
[b]A complete series is three doses of a tetanus toxoid
DTaP Diphtheria, Tetanus, Pertussis, for children <7 years; *Tdap* Tetanus, Diphtheria, Pertussis, for children and adults ≥11 years; *TIG* Human Tetanus Immune Globulin

status, tendon function, and extent of open wounds. Radiographs are necessary to evaluate for retained foreign bodies and to identify any fractures. MRI, ultrasound, or CT scans are adjunctive modalities that may be needed to assist in further assessing damage and identifying any foreign objects. Initial laboratory testing for infection is optional depending on the time lapsed since injury which includes complete blood count (CBC) with differential, erythrocyte sedimentation rate (ESR), and C-reactive protein (CRP). Inflammatory marker labs are useful to follow the progress of therapy if there is concern for infection.

Initial Irrigation and Debridement for Open Trauma

Prompt and thorough irrigation and debridement of open traumatic injuries is a simple and effective approach for infection prevention. Local, regional, or general anesthesia may be necessary, and early determination should be made in the acute care setting regarding the need for surgical treatment in the operating room (OR). Open fractures are considered a surgical emergency, and the care teams should be mindful to reduce the time elapsed between injury and OR management. Historically, debridement of an open fracture was recommended within 6 h of the injury. Recent literature describes timely management is important; however, a larger emphasis is placed on taking into account the grade of the open fracture [15–19]. A recent study by Hull evaluated a series of 364 patients with open fractures and confirmed that higher grade Gustilo–Anderson fractures (Table 13.1) are more likely to develop a deep infection than lower grade fractures. Furthermore, a delay in treatment has a greater effect on these higher grade fractures and those that are grossly contaminated [18]. Thus, heightened awareness of the time to the OR is necessary in the higher grade and grossly contaminated injuries.

Prompt irrigation and debridement allows initial removal of debris or foreign objects and aids in reduction of the total bacterial load [5]. Secondary and staged irrigation and debridement is often indicated to further remove devitalized soft tissue and residual debris. Devitalized soft tissue reduces the effectiveness of the host immune system, thus attempts are made to remove any necrotic or devitalized tissue from the traumatized wound [4, 20]. The viability of skin and soft tissue is determined by color and bleeding, whereas muscle should be inspected for contractility in addition to color and bleeding. Irrigation solution is frequently based on surgeon preference, but adding povidone-iodine solution or antibiotics to normal saline or lactated ringers solution may not add value and perhaps has undesirable side effects [21, 22]. Detergent solutions have been shown to be effective at removing bacteria and dirt from bone [21, 22]. It is our preference to utilize saline alone, with the principle of copious irrigation for removal of bacteria and organic contaminants. Each traumatic wound or open fracture may require a varying amount of irrigation depending on the extent of injury and degree of contamination. Data is lacking to validate the exact volume of fluid that should be utilized for irrigation. Historically, 3 L is recommended for type I fractures, 6 L for type II, and 9 L for type III fractures [23]. Primary wound closure may be performed under conditions of prompt and appropriate antibiotic treatment, thorough debridement with healthy appearance of local tissues post debridement, and a good host immune system [20, 24–28]. Primary closure may prevent secondary contamination; however, the surgeon should not rush to close a wound if it does not appear ready. Inadequate debridement, inadequate antibiotics, and premature primary closure can increase the risk of complications. Early closure in patients with continued wound contamination with dirt, feces, and nonviable tissue can increase the risk of infection with *Clostridium*. The second stage procedure is planned 2–3 days later allowing secondary irrigation and debridement with hopeful partial or complete closure. The surgeon should not hesitate to perform staged procedures. Ideally, soft tissue coverage is performed within 3 days as a delay in closure beyond 7–10 days increases the risk of infection [29, 30]. Fracture management may be performed acutely or delayed depending on the fracture pattern and condition of the soft tissues. External fixation is useful for temporary stabilization in an unstable fracture when there is concern regarding the soft tissue envelope. If primary closure cannot be achieved, alternative coverage options such as negative pressure wound therapy (NPWT) may be valuable in patients with extensive loss of soft tissue followed by staged skin grafting at a later date. Case examples with treatment protocols are presented below regarding management of puncture wounds, open fractures, and crush injuries associated with industrial, recreational, and lawn mower injuries with the intent to avoid poor outcomes associated with posttraumatic osteomyelitis.

Puncture Wounds

Puncture wounds represent unique traumatic injuries as the wound is small, but there is potential for heavy contamination, internal injury, and retained foreign bodies. Secondary osteomyelitis can develop acutely due to direct inoculation of bacteria into bone or in a delayed manner due to contiguous spread of infection from local abscess formation. Pedal puncture wounds are common injuries that account for 7 % of lower extremity trauma emergency department visits [31]. The majority of puncture wounds heal without complications, but a delay in medical treatment may lead to problems including cellulitis, abscess formation, septic arthritis, and osteomyelitis. The location of the injury, type of footwear worn at the time of injury, and time elapsed before initial treatment will influence the incidence of infection development and osteomyelitis. The Patzaki classification system for puncture wounds divides the foot into three zones: zone 1 extends from the metatarsal neck to the toes, zone 2 is from the metatarsal neck to the distal calcaneus, and zone 3 includes the calcaneus [1]. The risk of osteomyelitis associated with plantar puncture wounds has been described as 0.1–2 %, with a greater prevalence in forefoot injuries (zone 1) through athletic shoes [8]. The distance between the soft tissue and bone is narrow in this weight bearing portion of the foot, and it is common for puncture wounds in this location to cause direct inoculation to a bone or joint depending on the length, rigidity, and sharpness of the penetrating object. Pedal puncture wounds are particularly concerning in the diabetic population since neuropathic patients frequently have a delay in treatment which commonly results in increased morbidity associated with puncture wounds [32]. Diabetic patients are five times more likely to have multiple operations and 46 times more likely to have lower extremity amputations after puncture wounds [33].

Imaging for Puncture Wounds

Imaging is valuable for foreign body evaluation in the presence of a puncture wound. Standard radiographs are useful for metal objects, large wooden objects that cast a shadow, and glass (Fig. 13.1). Foreign bodies with low radiopacity that are located in muscle tissue, or between bone and muscle tissue, can be difficult to visualize with standard radiographs or CT and are better seen on ultrasound imaging [34]. Thus, ultrasound can be useful to identify radiolucent objects such as plastic or wood and can identify the size and depth of the foreign object as well [35, 36] (Fig. 13.2a). An ultrasound technician can place a skin marker at the approximate location of the object for ease of foreign body removal which is particularly useful in lake presentation injuries when the wound is no longer visible. The amount of information obtained from an ultrasound however remains highly dependent on the skill of the user. An MRI is an alternative imaging option if there is a suspicion for foreign body despite negative radiographs or with late presentation puncture wound injuries with concern for abscess formation or osteomyelitis. It is not uncommon for a chronic and infected plantar puncture wound to develop an abscess that can track dorsally or plantarly along the tendon sheaths, in which case, an MRI is helpful for preoperative planning (Fig. 13.2b).

Antibiotic Considerations for Puncture Wounds

Acute presentation of minor or superficial puncture wounds without clinical signs of contamination may not require antibiotics. However, puncture wounds with a delayed presentation, contamination, necrotic tissue, or known infection require antibiotic therapy. This is initiated after thorough irrigation, debridement, and culture. *Staphylococcus aureus* is the most common organism involved in soft tissue infections

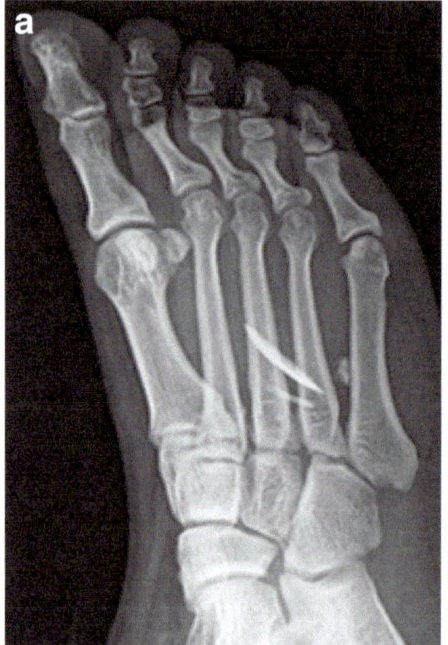
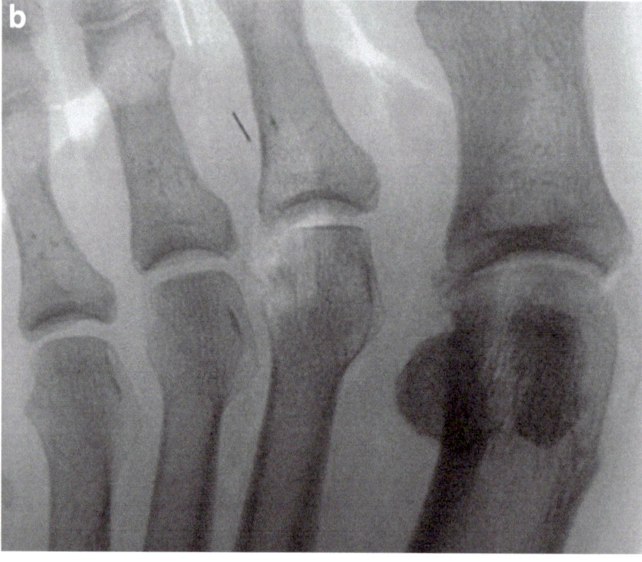

Fig. 13.1 X-ray evaluation for retained foreign body. Standard X-rays are the go-to imaging modality for puncture wounds. (**a**) Modern digital imaging is effective at identifying most fragments of glass regardless of lead content. (**b**) Identification of a foreign body on X-ray is the most useful tool for intraoperative guidance since the surgeon is able to directly view the X-ray during attempted removal. X-rays also provide baseline assessment of bone integrity for future comparison should infection develop

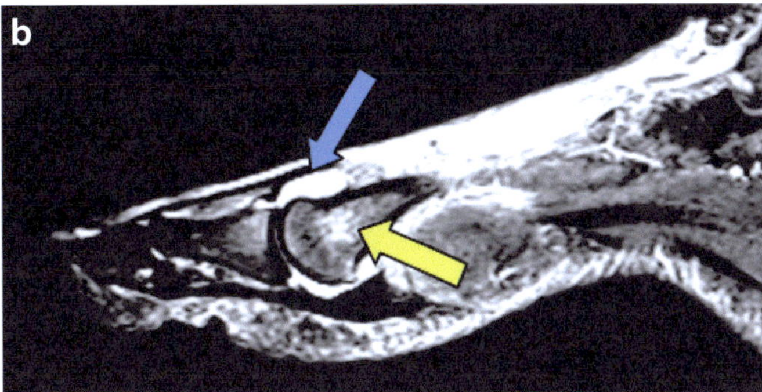

Fig. 13.2 Advanced imaging for puncture wounds and foreign bodies. Diagnostic ultrasound is useful to identify radiolucent foreign bodies or local abscess, although small shards of glass or wood may not be visible. (**a**) Ultrasound images may not be as useful to the surgeon although skin marking over the identified foreign body is quite benefi- cial for incision planning. (**b**) MRI imaging is used in cases of small foreign bodies, potential abscess formation, or joint sepsis associated with puncture wound injuries. Joint effusion is indicated by the *blue arrow*, and bone marrow edema is identified by the *yellow arrow*

following acute puncture wounds. Empiric treatment with a first-generation cephalosporin is the drug of choice in acute puncture wounds without concern for other environmental factors. *Pseudomonas* is frequently found in soil, water, skin flora, and rubber-soled shoes. Thus, penetrating injuries that occur through rubber-soled tennis shoes require coverage for *Pseudomonas* [35]. In wounds that occur in brackish water, consideration for coverage of *Aeromonas hydrophila* and *Mycobacterium marinum* should be considered [37, 38] (Table 13.2). In delayed presentation puncture wounds or when there is a concern for development of underlying osteo- myelitis, *Pseudomonas* coverage is important. *Pseudomonas* is the most common organism associated with puncture wound related osteomyelitis [35, 39]. If osteomyelitis occurs following a puncture wound, management follows basic prin- ciples including a combined medical and surgical approach with 4–6 weeks of antibiotics after bone biopsy and adequate debridement.

Initial Debridement of Puncture Wounds and Foreign Body Removal at Acute Presentation

Many acute presentation puncture wounds can be treated in an office setting or emergency department with a minor inci- sion and drainage procedure. An attempt is made to remove any retained foreign body if present since this will act as a nidus for infection and frequently results in pain while walking. Inspection of the wound is needed to determine the depth as a deeper wound is more likely to involve tendon, bone, and joint structures. In younger children that cannot tolerate a local injection, procedural sedation is an option if available otherwise a traditional OR procedure should be considered.

The approach to removal of the foreign body depends on the depth within the soft tissue. A visible splinter or shard of glass can be easily removed in the office with or without a local block. The author's preferred technique is to use the sharp tip of a 1.5 in. long 18 gauge needle to peel away the skin surrounding the foreign body. The needle acts as a tiny scalpel which minimizes unwanted injury. Loupe magnifica- tion is helpful for improved visualization.

Deeper foreign bodies typically require an incision below the dermis which also serves to drain any infection. A small (less than 1 cm) transverse plantar foot incision will typically heal within 7–14 days even without sutures; therefore, sutures are generally not needed. A local infiltrative block is utilized for anesthesia, and standard skin prep is performed. A technique that we have found beneficial is to first utilize a 1–3 mm dermal curette to inspect the deep wound in a methodical manor. The curette acts as a blunt probe and allows for initial inspection with both tactile and audible sen- sation. One should have a clear understanding of the location of the foreign body as demonstrated by radiographs or ultra- sound prior to probing. Care is taken to avoid pushing the object deeper or into a new location. If the foreign body is located with the curette, a small hemostat is placed into the

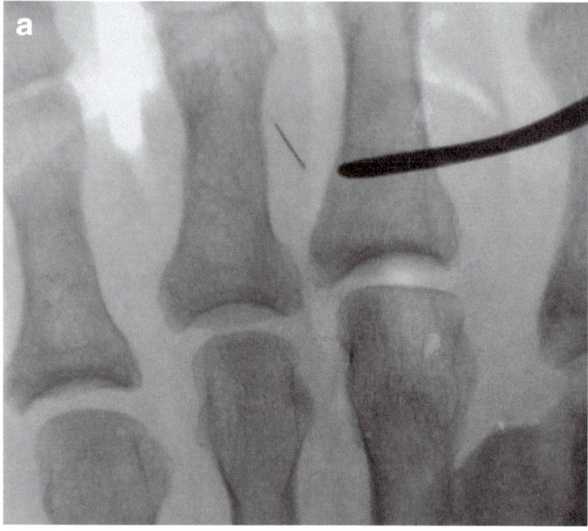
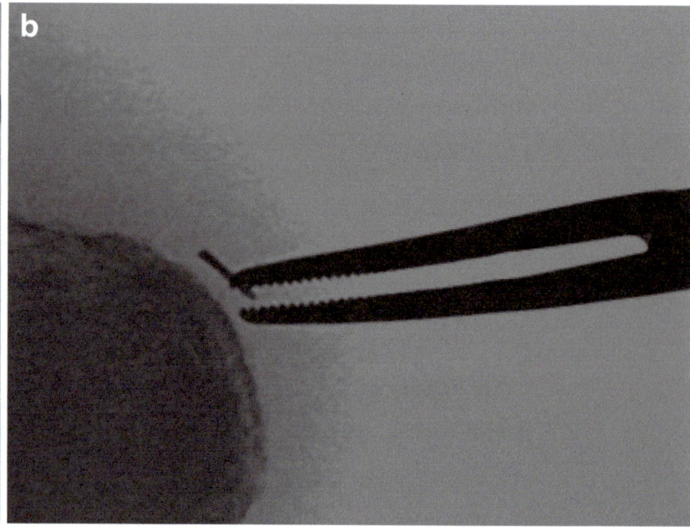

Fig. 13.3 Fluoroscopy-assisted foreign body removal. (**a**) A curette or freer can be utilized as a blunt probe for foreign body location using fluoroscopy. Care is taken to avoid pushing the object deeper or into a new location. (**b**) A small hemostat can be placed into the wound for extraction under fluoroscopic guidance

wound for retrieval. If needed and available, a fluoroscan can be useful to assist with location of the foreign object (Fig. 13.3). After removal of the foreign object, the wound is irrigated and culture swabs are obtained from the deep wound if appropriate. Depending on the size, depth, and observed cleanliness of the wound, a decision is made regarding primary closure, packing the wound, or to simply bandage and allow healing by secondary intention. Acute presentation with timely debridement and removal of the foreign body typically allows primary closure without subsequent development of infection.

Surgical Treatment of Complex Puncture Wounds

Puncture wounds that require surgical treatment include failed retrieval with initial minor procedure, deep foreign bodies or deep penetrating wounds, foreign bodies near vital structures, delayed presentation puncture wounds, significant contamination, and concern for abscess or infection. Diabetes-related foot infections associated with puncture wounds and foreign bodies can be limb threatening and often present as surgical emergencies. Intraoperative fluoroscopy is typically beneficial to locate the object. Incision considerations involve the desire for adequate exposure and avoidance of incisions on the weight bearing surface, although achieving both goals is frequently not possible. Partial foot amputation may be necessary, and consideration should be given to flap closure options when planning incisions.

Two cases are presented to highlight surgical management protocols for complex puncture wounds. Case 1 is a patient with a retained foreign body and joint sepsis following a dorsal puncture wound from a nail gun (Figs. 13.4 and 13.5). Case 2 involves a delayed presentation puncture wound with abscess formation and significant soft tissue loss (Figs. 13.6, 13.7, 13.8, and 13.9). Removal of the foreign object is performed first if possible although exploration may be required for deep objects. Inspection for abscess, necrotic tissue, and bone exposure assists in determining the extent of surgery, need for staged surgery, closure options, and postoperative antibiotics. If an abscess is tracking in a direction away from the initial incision, one may consider a counter incision to aid in drainage. Intraoperative cultures are obtained after irrigation. The decision to close the wound primarily is based on the intraoperative appearance of the wound. If the nidus of infection is removed, no purulence was encountered, and remaining tissues are healthy in appearance, primary closure can be performed [26]. If an abscess or cellulitis is present, a staged approach to surgery is often best. The surgeon should not hesitate to perform repeat incision and drainage procedures approximately every 3 days until the infection is under control at which point the wound can be closed. If significant tissue debridement was necessary, the surgeon may decide for wound closure by secondary intention. NPWT with delayed skin graft closure is an option under these conditions. Antibiotic management is based on intraoperative appearance of the wound, likelihood of bone involvement, inflammatory marker labs, and culture results.

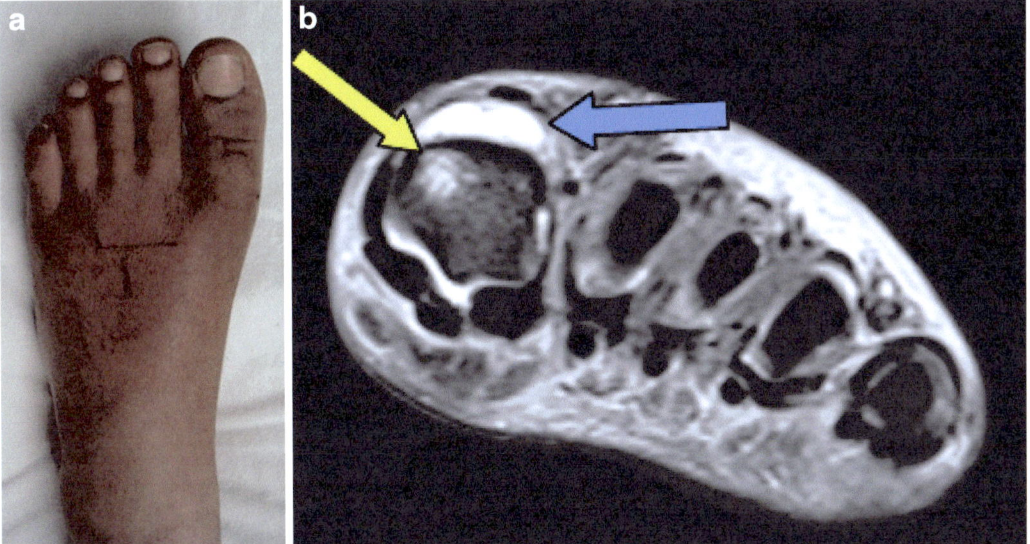

Fig. 13.4 Case 1: Penetrating injury with resultant first metatarsophalangeal joint (MPJ) sepsis. A roofing nail gun injury to the first MPJ was initially treated in the emergency department. X-rays were negative for residual foreign body. The injury occurred through a rubber shoe, and thus antibiotic coverage was provided for pseudomonas. (**a**) Outpatient follow-up 4 days later identified fever and chills, localized edema, erythema centered over the first MPJ, and a healed wound without drainage. (**b**) MRI showed first metatarsophalangeal joint effusion (*blue arrow*) and increased signal within the first metatarsal head (*yellow arrow*)

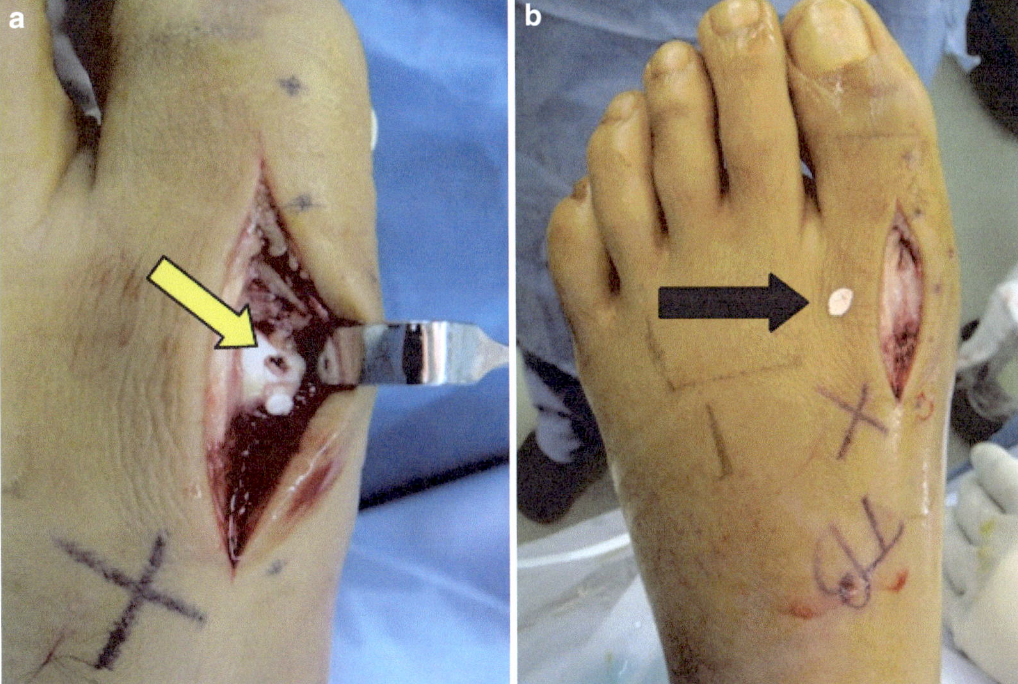

Fig. 13.5 Case 1: Single-stage emergency incision and drainage (I&D) of joint infection. Dorsal first MPJ incision allowed open I&D of infection, curettage of traumatic bone injury, and bone biopsy. (**a**) The nail punctured directly through the head of the first metatarsal without purulence or necrosis (*yellow arrow*). (**b**) A small piece of rubber was found within the joint (*black arrow*). Immediate closure allowed prompt healing and return to range of motion to minimize chance of mobility restriction. Pathology was negative for osteomyelitis, and no long-term sequelae was encountered

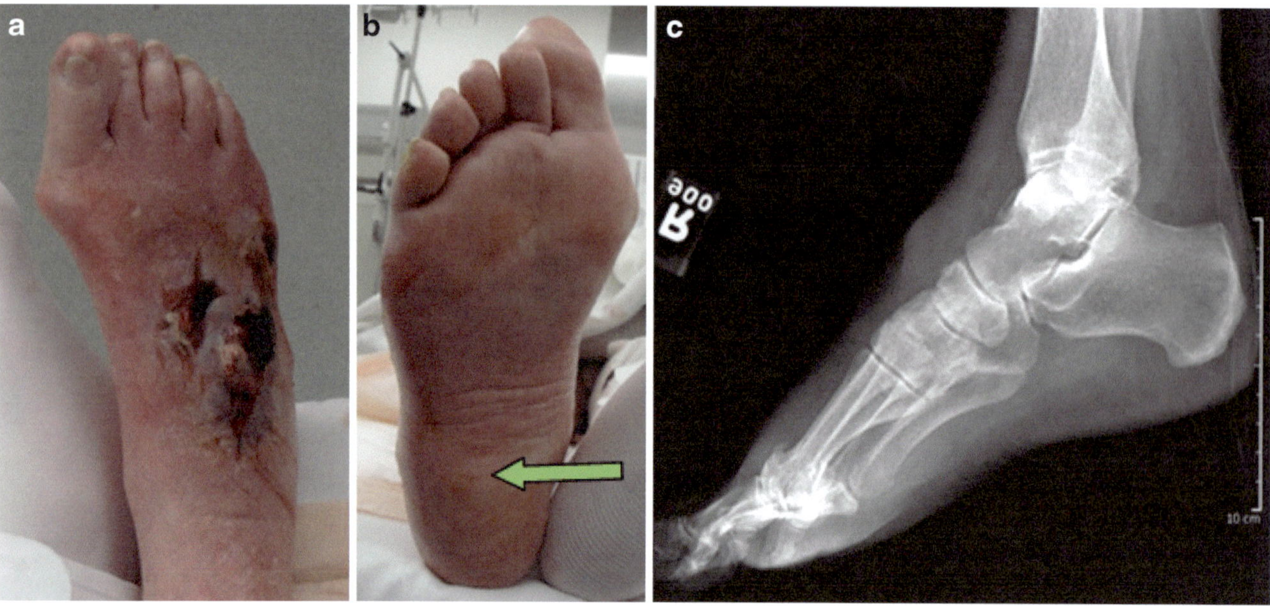

Fig. 13.6 Case 2: Delayed presentation puncture wound with limb-threatening infection. (**a**) Elderly nondiabetic female with a limb-threatening infection after stepping on a toothpick. (**b**) The initial injury involved puncture wound to the plantar heel (*arrow*). Initial treatment 4 days prior involved irrigation of the wound in urgent care and 4 days of oral antibiotics. (**c**) X-rays demonstrated no retained foreign body or soft tissue gas

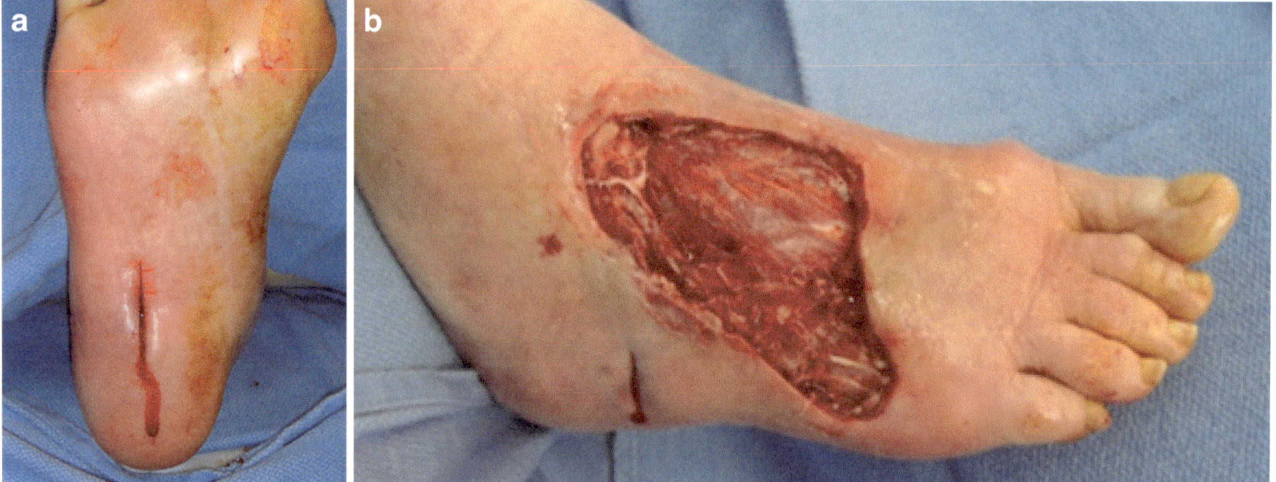

Fig. 13.7 Case 2: Stage 1 incision and drainage with wide resection of necrotic tissue. (**a**) Surgery was performed emergently for incision and drainage of the plantar wound and wide resection of the dorsal necrotic tissue. Extensor tendons were widely exposed after debridement of the necrotic extensor retinaculum. The exposed tendons were completely excised to expose viable underlying periosteum. (**b**) Note that very thin tissue is now covering a broad area of the tarsal and metatarsal bones. An attempt to preserve the tendons under these conditions is often fruitless and leads to poor wound healing with predisposition for proximal spread of infection

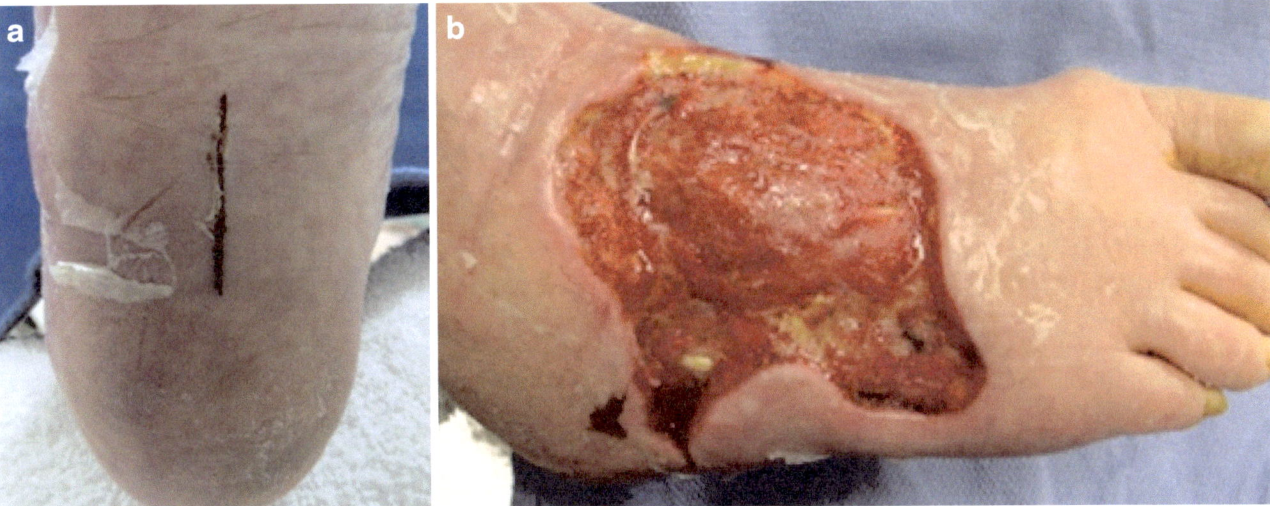

Fig. 13.8 Case 2: Stage 2 debridement was performed 3 days later. (**a**) The plantar wound healed secondarily within 11 days, and no sutures were needed. (**b**) The dorsal wound promptly developed granulation tissue with the aid of negative pressure wound therapy. Broad coverage with granulation tissue is the best hope to avoid slough of the periosteum and ultimately osteomyelitis of the midfoot. This also prepares the wound for skin grafting

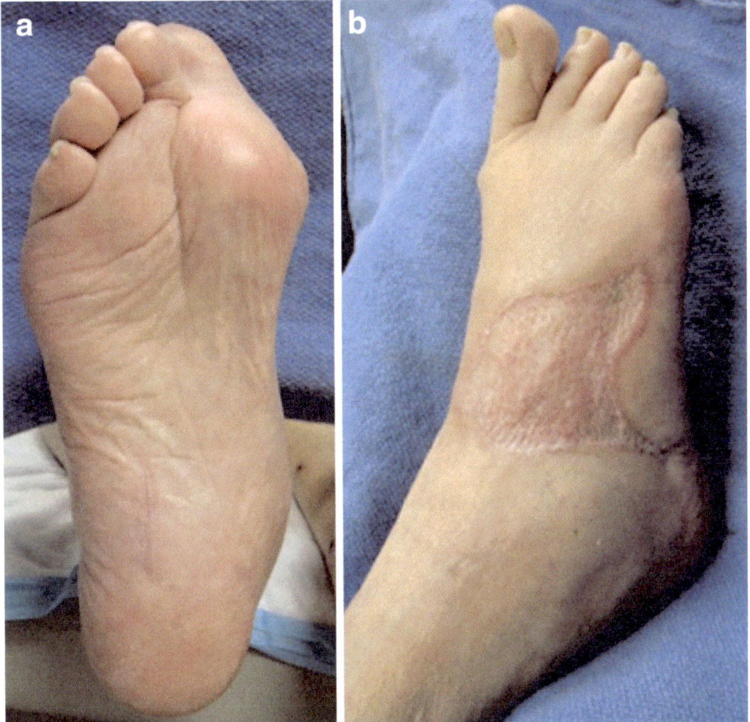

Fig. 13.9 Case 2: (**a**, **b**) Three month postoperative clinical photos demonstrating complete healing of the dorsal and plantar wounds. Spilt thickness skin grafting allowed prompt healing without additional complications. (**b**) Note that the lesser toes are slightly plantar positioned and flexor tendon release could be performed if this were to become problematic. Extensive dorsal scar tissue typically prevents progressive digital deformity

Open Fractures

The primary goals in the surgical management of open fractures are to stabilize the limb, restore function, and prevent infection. Open fractures involve contaminated wounds, and the immediate goal is to convert to clean wounds [40, 41]. Open fractures associated with high-energy industrial, recreational, and lawn mower injuries often involve significant soft tissue damage. Crush injuries, degloving injuries, and traumatic amputations present unique treatment challenges, and initial treatment is focused on avoidance of infection, preservation of limb function, or prevention of loss of limb. Preoperative planning regarding soft tissue viability for coverage or flap creation is necessary for these traumatic open fractures with significant soft tissue involvement. Internal fixation may not be possible depending on the condition of the local soft tissues, and alternative fixation methods may be necessary. In some cases with a significant degree of comminution and soft tissue destruction, the surgeon must decide between reconstruction and amputation. This situation is frequently encountered when an incomplete amputation is present and the distal part of the limb has extensive injury, contamination, and soft tissue damage. Three major types of open fractures have been described by Gustilo and Anderson and are based on soft tissue involvement (Table 13.1). Infection risk has been described as 10–50 % in type III injuries, 2–10 % in type II, and 0–2 % in type I [9, 10].

Antibiotic Considerations for Open Fractures

Infection prevention is of paramount importance in the treatment of open fractures. Antibiotic administration should begin in a timely fashion as a delay of more than 3 h increases the risk of infection [11]. Antibiotic coverage for open fractures is guided by the work performed by Gustilo and Anderson (Table 13.2). A high incidence of *S. aureus* is present in open fractures. As the severity of the injury increases, the risk of *Pseudomonas* and other gram-negative infections increases, and additional coverage is added in type II and III injuries [9, 10, 42]. Open fractures involving lawn mower injuries are frequently contaminated with soil and are at increased risk for anaerobic bacteria and *Clostridium* [4] (Table 13.2). Antibiotic therapy should be limited to 24–72 h based on the severity of the injury or until closure is achieved, as prolonged therapy raises concern for development of resistance [20, 41]. Additional courses of up to 72 h of antibiotics should be initiated with subsequent surgical procedures. Wound cultures before and after debridement for open fractures have been shown to have a low predictive value of postoperative infections [43, 44]. Appropriate prophylactic antibiotics are of more importance for infection prevention. Coverage for both gram-positive and gram-negative bacteria should be considered, especially in type III injuries [42].

Surgical Considerations for Infection Prevention

The quality and extent of the debridement is one of the most important factors for infection prevention. As discussed, removal of devitalized tissue and debris is necessary as any foreign debris or devitalized tissue remaining in the open wound can promote the growth of organisms and increase the risk of deeper infection. When treating open fractures associated with industrial, recreational, and lawn mower injuries, soft tissue assessment is a large component of the initial evaluation and management for proper preoperative planning of soft tissue coverage options. Planning for timely tissue closure is important as prolonged exposure with an open wound can increase the risk of infection. Thus, soft tissue coverage is ideally performed within 3 days [29, 30]. Fractures are frequently comminuted, and small bone fragments without soft tissue attachment are not preserved, except if they involve the joint surface and reconstruction is a possibility. When digits are involved, the degree of fracture, comminution, and soft tissue destruction may necessitate amputation as the most viable option. Stabilization with external fixation or external pinning is advantageous in circumstances where internal fixation is not possible due to lack of soft tissue coverage or heavy contamination. External fixation avoids the need to leave fixation long term, can easily be removed if complications develop, limits the amount of dissection needed, provides desired stability, and can be replaced with interval fixation at a later date if necessary. Cases 3–7 are presented to demonstrate management and surgical pearls for infection prevention with open fractures.

Case 3: Road Rash Injury Road rash injuries present with unique challenges associated with widespread compromise of soft tissue with exposed tendon, bone, and joint structures with high propensity for post-injury infection. The term road rash is typically used to describe a deep abrasion from falling on asphalt/cement off of motorcycles, bicycles, skateboards, or other recreational vehicles. Debris from the environment and asphalt is often deeply imbedded within the injured soft tissues (Fig. 13.10a). Thorough irrigation is necessary for removal of this nidus of infection, and often a staged approach is necessary which allows progressive debridement as the injured tissue demarcates (Fig. 13.10b–e). Widespread injury to the soft tissue creates challenges for closure and coverage options. When this involves the digits, toe amputation may be necessary which allows closure over exposed bones and joints. In other locations of the foot, NPWT with future skin grafting is often a viable and useful option to provide coverage where primary healing is not possible. The surgeon should be creative with preserving or creating tissue flaps in traumatic injuries involving degloving and traumatic amputation. Survival of seemingly thin tissue is common in young, healthy trauma patients (Fig. 13.10f).

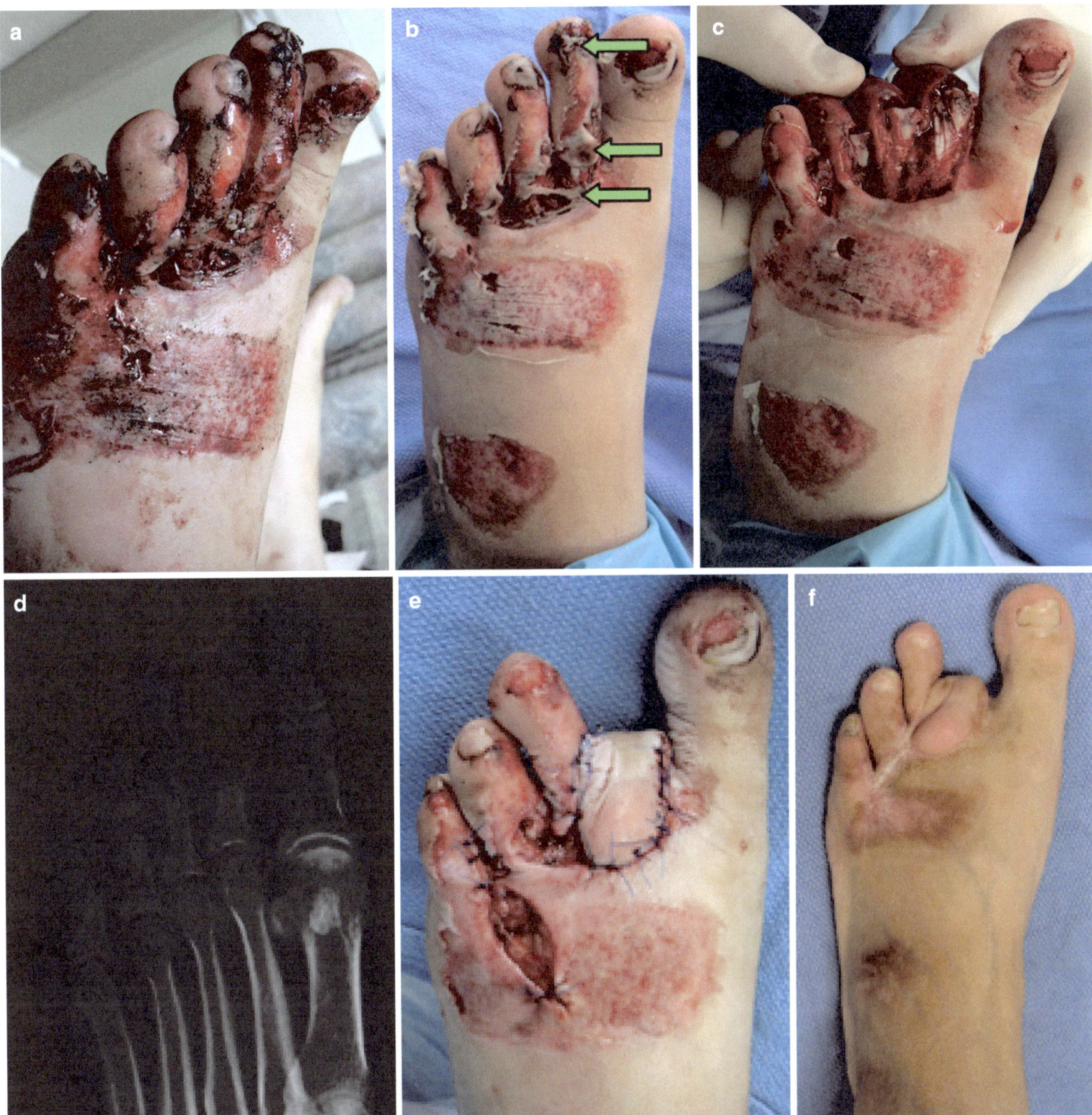

Fig. 13.10 Case 3: Road rash injury. Degloving injury associated with motor vehicle vs. pedestrian accident. (**a**) Road rash injuries as shown are uniquely prone to debris embedded within the compromised soft tissue. There is often exposed tendon, bone, and joint structures given the significant soft tissue loss. The amount of tissue injury and contamination with foreign debris increases infection risk in these injuries. (**b**) Initial management involved irrigation and debridement followed by removal of devitalized tissue and foreign material. Green arrows indicate nonviable tissue that will not survive. (**c**) Initial debridement unroofed damaged tendons with exposure of the proximal phalanges and interphalangeal joints of the involved toes. (**d, e**) Broad exposure of bone was treated with delayed second toe amputation incorporating a plantar digital fillet flap to cover the main dorsal wound deficit. Early arthroplasty of the third, fourth, and fifth proximal interphalangeal joints also minimized ongoing bone exposure allowing prompt healing of the digital wounds. (**f**) Clinical photograph 1 year after injury with complete healing of the wounds and preservation of four functional toes

Case 4: Chainsaw Injury Chainsaw injuries create large and irregular areas of soft tissue damage with underlying bone deficits and fragmentation. Patients frequently present with near amputation of the involved region (Fig. 13.11a, b). Heightened concern for contamination with soil dwelling organisms directs antibiotic selection (Table 13.2) and necessitates appropriate and thorough irrigation. It has been described that soil has infection-potentiating fractions including organic components and clay, and the ability of these fractions to cause infection is related to the damage to host defenses [4, 5]. A staged approach may be necessary if there is any uncertainty regarding the extent of soil or fecal matter removal. Stabilization of fractures

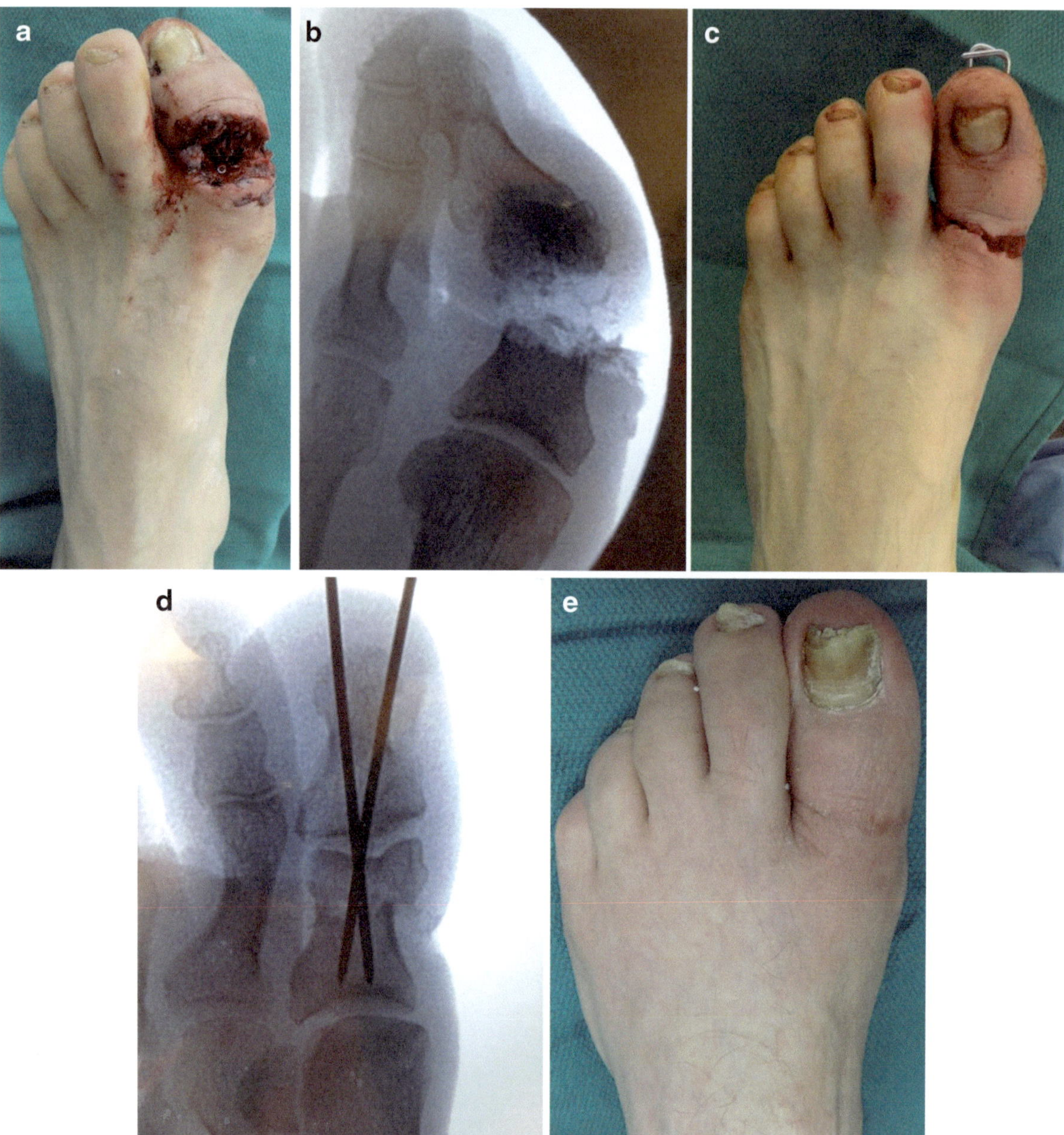

Fig. 13.11 Case 4: Chainsaw injury with open fracture of the first toe. (**a**) Near complete hallux amputation from a chainsaw injury with open fracture creates challenges with surgical management. (**b**) Loss of bone substance and wide fragmentation are common with chainsaw injuries. (**c**, **d**) Emergent washout, debridement, and external pin fixation allowed stabilization of the soft tissues with hopeful distal perfusion through the plantar vasculature. The shortened bone structure allowed primary closure of the wound margin. Primary amputation with plantar advancement flap would have been a reasonable alternative under these circumstances. (**e**) Clinical photograph at 4 months postoperatively demonstrates a well-healed injury without infection complications

with external pin fixation is beneficial and allows stabilization of not only the bony segment but also reduces tension on the injured soft tissues to allow closure (Fig. 13.11c, d). Primary amputation in these injuries may be necessary if autoamputation is near completed from the chainsaw and the distal portion has significant tissue destruction or vascular compromise.

Case 5: Lawn Mower Injury Lawn mower injuries have similar concerns as chainsaw injuries in regard to significant soft tissue loss, bone fragmentation, contamination with soil, and antibiotic considerations (Table 13.2). However, the mechanism of injury from this type of machinery involves repeated impact of the limb with a rotary blade which leads to an increased capacity to create traumatic amputations (Fig. 13.12a, b) [45, 46]. According to the National Hospital Discharge Summary Data from 1996 to 2004, fractures to the phalanges were noted to be the most common lawn mower injury at 34.4 %, followed by traumatic amputation of the toe at 32.4 % [47]. Given the dirty environment of the injury, timely surgical intervention is beneficial to reduce the risk of

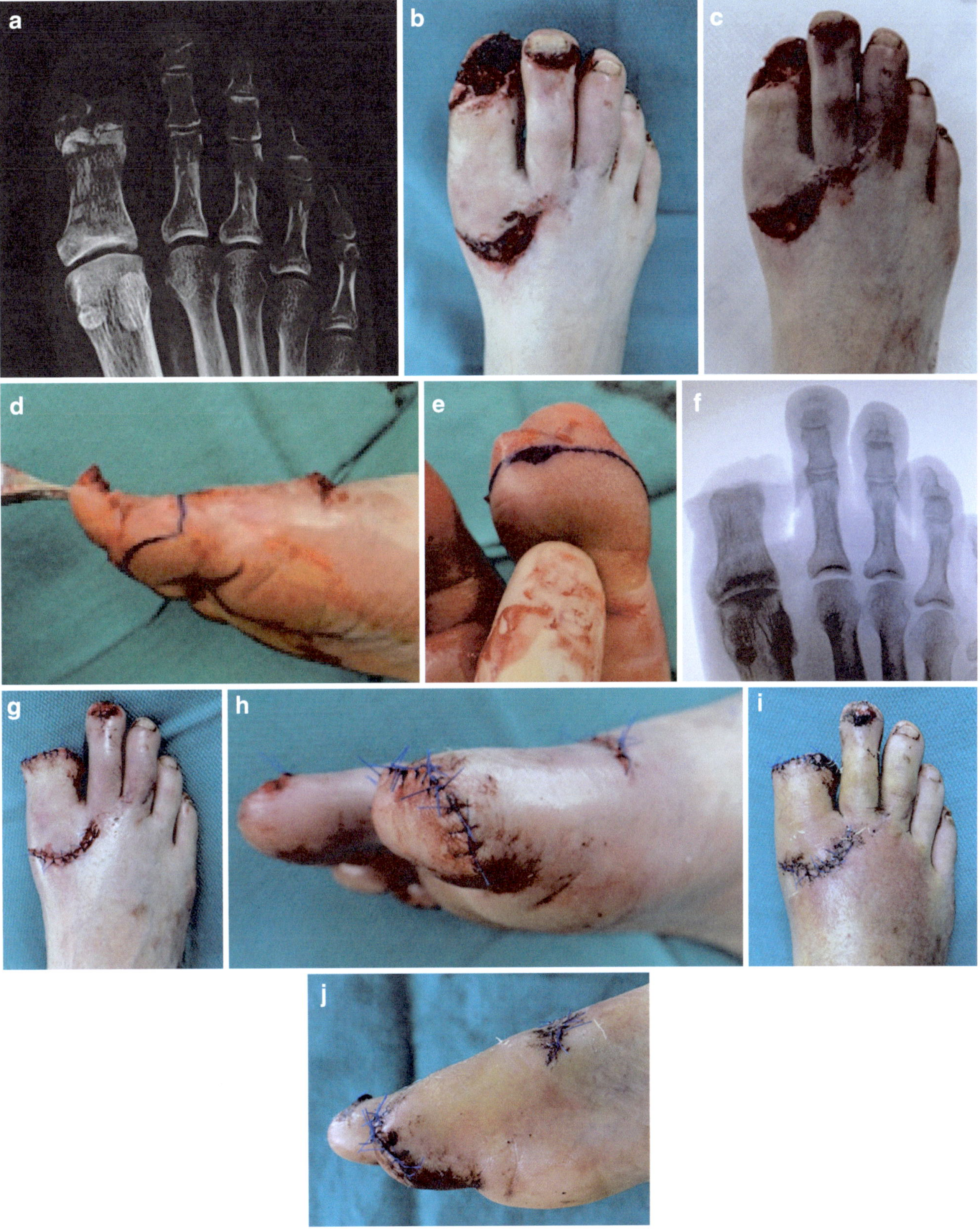

Fig. 13.12 Case 5: Lawn mower injury with traumatic amputation. (**a, b**) Lawn mower injury with open fractures of the tips of the first and second toes and open fracture with exposed first metatarsophalangeal joint. Most of the first distal phalanx bone fragments are missing. (**c**) Immediate presentation to the emergency department allowed emergent washout with debridement of devitalized bone fragments and removal of foreign material. (**d–f**) Single-stage conversion to distal Symes hallux amputation allowed preservation of the intact plantar flap to cover the remodeled tip of the proximal phalanx. Note how the proximal pha-

lanx has an appearance similar to distal phalanx with regard to a rounded distal weight bearing surface. Open fractures at the base of the first proximal phalanx and tip of the second toe were washed out and closed primarily. (**g, h**) Single-staged closure of all wounds allowed a short course of antibiotics directed at pseudomonas and potential anaerobic infection considering the environmental exposure. (**i, j**) A short course of IV antibiotics during overnight hospitalization followed by 2 weeks of oral antibiotics avoided infection despite heavily contaminated open fractures with compromised soft tissue infection. Recent literature supports primary closure when appropriate antibiotic treatment has been initiated, thorough debridement is performed in a timely fashion, healthy appearance of local tissues is present post debridement, and the patient has a good host immune system [26]. When local amputation is needed for definitive closure purposes, much of the contaminated tissue is discarded, decreasing the chance of leaving remaining soil or debris behind (Fig. 13.12d–f).

Case 6: Motor Vehicle Collision and Open Fracture Motor vehicle collisions (MVC) often cause high-energy trauma without significant wound contamination. However, the location of wound lacerations may compromise traditional approaches for fracture visualization. Alternative treatment methods for repair may be needed to limit soft tissue compromise (Fig. 13.13a–d). In a recent study, drivers and passengers that sustained foot and ankle injuries had a higher

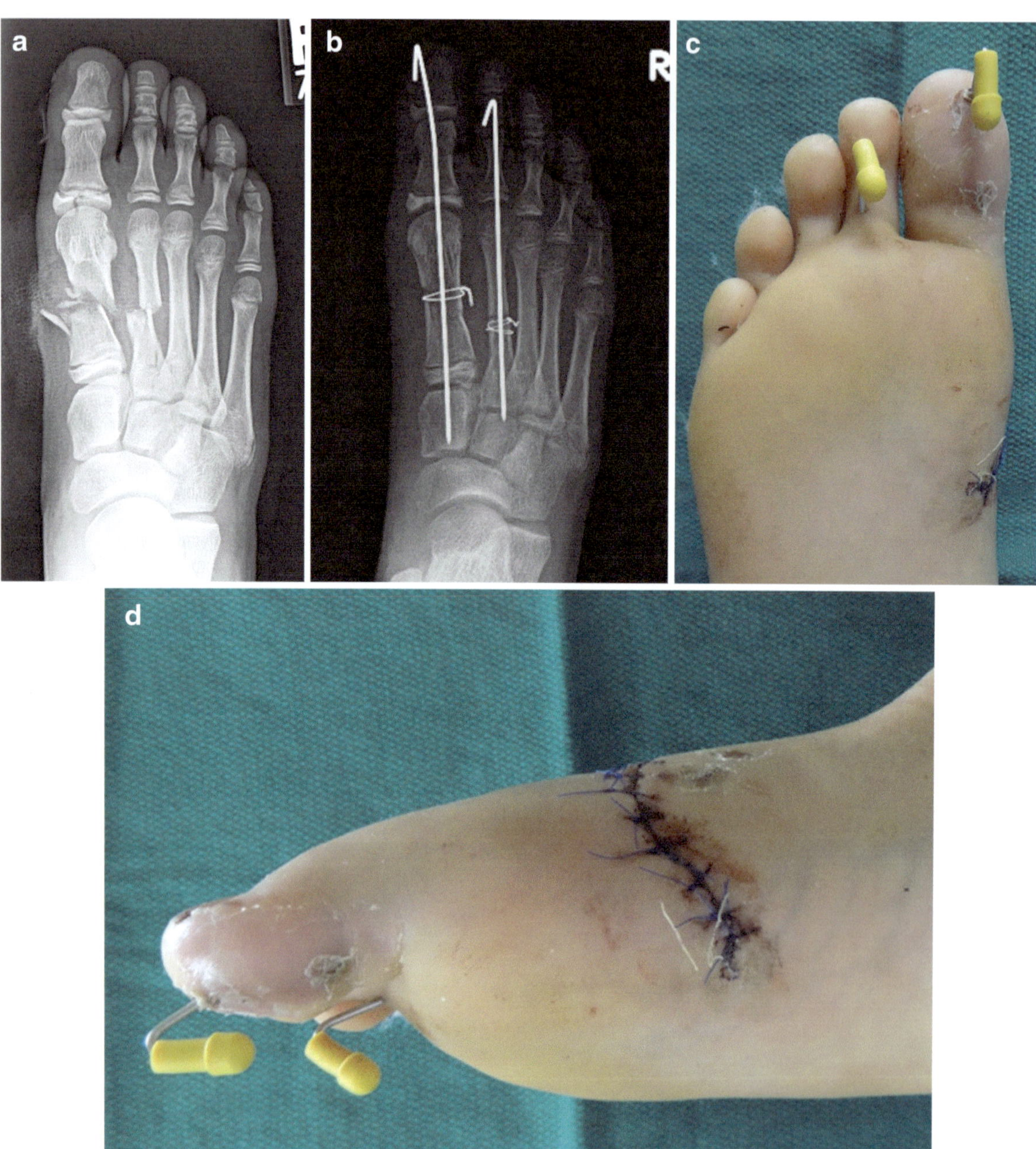

Fig. 13.13 Case 6: Motor vehicle collision with open fracture. (**a**) A pediatric patient sustained a large laceration across her dorsal medial foot as well as comminuted metatarsal fractures after a motor vehicle collision. Transverse laceration at the level of the metatarsal shaft fractures created challenges with open surgical repair and internal fixation. Plate fixation to restore metatarsal length would have been ideal; however, the transverse laceration was not easily amenable to this approach. (**b–d**) Intramedullary pin fixation is useful under these circumstances. Monofilament wire was used internally to circumferentially reduce small fracture fragments to support against telescopic shortening of the metatarsals. External fixation would have been an alternative treatment measure to hold the metatarsals out to length. Early washout, prompt healing of the laceration, and stabilization of the fractures with minimally invasive fixation helped to avoid complications like infection

amount of associated serious injuries when compared to drivers and passengers without foot and ankle injuries [48]. This is an important consideration when planning surgery on polytrauma patients after a MVC. The other more serious injuries take precedence over the foot and ankle, and appropriate preoperative planning to limit any unnecessary time under anesthesia is important. Given the often lack of wound contamination in these types of injuries after quality debridement and irrigation, our preference is for primary closure for infection prevention (Fig. 13.13d).

Case 7: Industrial Crush and Degloving Injury Industrial injuries commonly involve heavy machinery which can create complex trauma involving crush injuries, large lacerations, open fractures, and degloving injuries (Fig. 13.14a–e). Crush injuries are typically caused by high impact forces and are at increased risk for infection. It has been described that the impact of the injury reduces the ability of the tissue to resist infection, and therefore infection may develop at a lower rate of bacterial count than injuries from a simple laceration [49]. Furthermore, degloving injuries occur from a high-energy force, most often a run-over accident involving detachment of the skin and subcutaneous tissues from the underlying fascia [50, 51]. Early management is focused on infection prevention, limiting skin and flap necrosis, stabilizing fractures, and controlling edema. Immediate reduction and stabilization of fractures with external fixation (Fig. 13.15a–c) is beneficial for edema control which has an impact on soft tissue viability which influences infection prevention. Staged surgery allows definitive fracture repair and wound closure once soft tissues are amenable to open treatment and internal fixation (Fig. 13.16a–d). This staged approach combines both internal and external fixation to maximize infection prevention while preserving foot function with definitive surgery (Fig. 13.17a–c).

Conclusion

The unique anatomy of the foot and ankle, environmental factors associated with lower extremity trauma, and various injury patterns predispose this region to challenges with regard to infection prevention. Prompt and thorough evaluation and management are important for osteomyelitis prevention in traumatic open injuries. Specifically in open fractures, early administration of antibiotics and the quality of the debridement are important factors for infection prevention. In addition, early closure of traumatic wounds when appropriate may be of benefit for infection prevention. Posttraumatic infection and osteomyelitis can have significant sequela including the need for long-term IV antibiotic therapy, multiple staged surgeries, chronic pain, and potential amputation. Early and thorough management in open injuries is imperative for prevention of infection, as a delay in treatment or inadequate initial treatment may substantially increase the risk for the development of osteomyelitis.

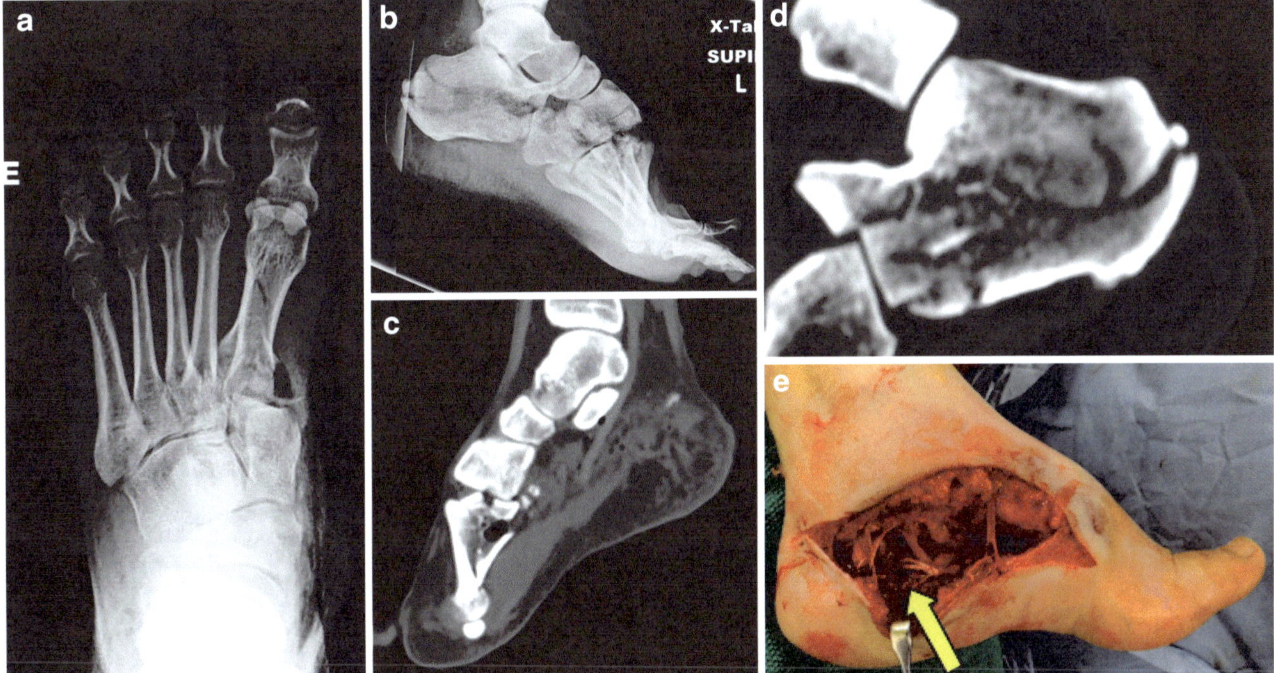

Fig. 13.14 Case 7: Industrial crush injury with open midfoot and rearfoot fractures with wide plantar foot degloving injury. (**a–d**) Forklift-related crush injury resulting in open Lisfranc fracture dislocation, midfoot tarsal dislocation, and displaced calcaneus fracture. (**e**) The open wound is not an incision but rather a degloving traumatic laceration with wide exposure of the plantar neurovascular structures (*yellow arrow*)

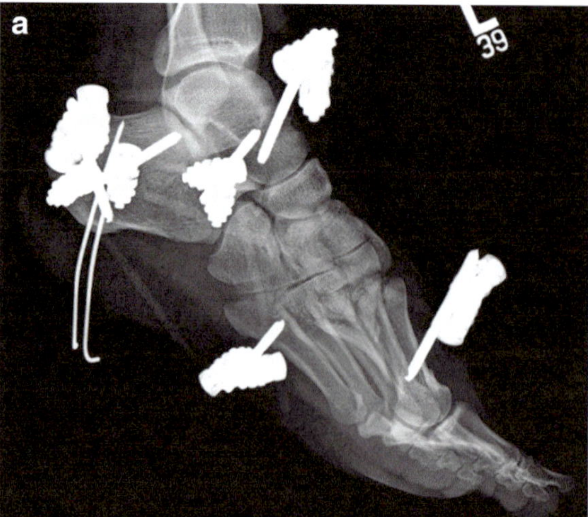

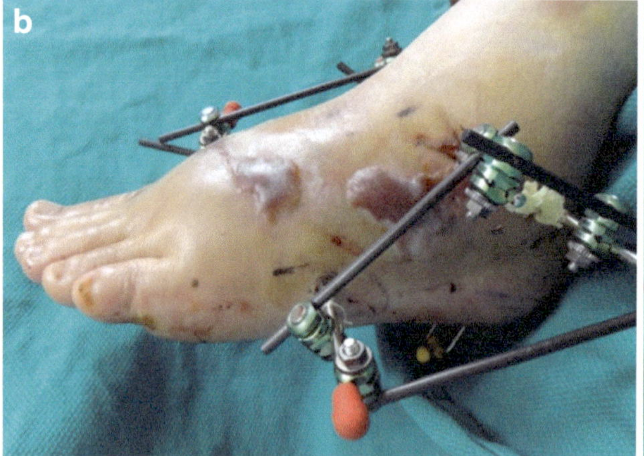

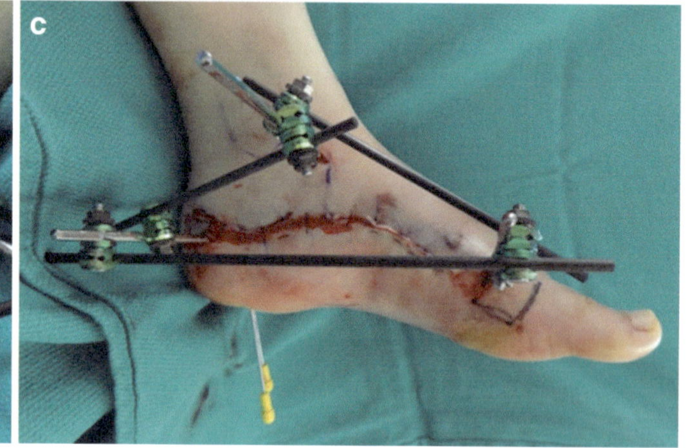

Fig. 13.15 Case 7: Initial surgical management. (**a**, **b**) Treatment for this Stage IIIA open fracture involved immediate irrigation and debridement in the operating room followed by primary closure of the wound and external fixation of the fractures. Medial and lateral delta frame external fixation was applied to reduce and stabilize the complex open fractures. Fixation was applied in a manner that could become a definitive fracture treatment in the event of progressive soft tissue compromise. Immediate reduction and stabilization of the fractures allows prompt control of edema which has broad implications with regard to postoperative pain, survival of the soft tissues, and ultimately avoidance of soft tissue compromise which would predispose to infection. (**c**) Note the development of fracture blisters on the dorsal and lateral foot

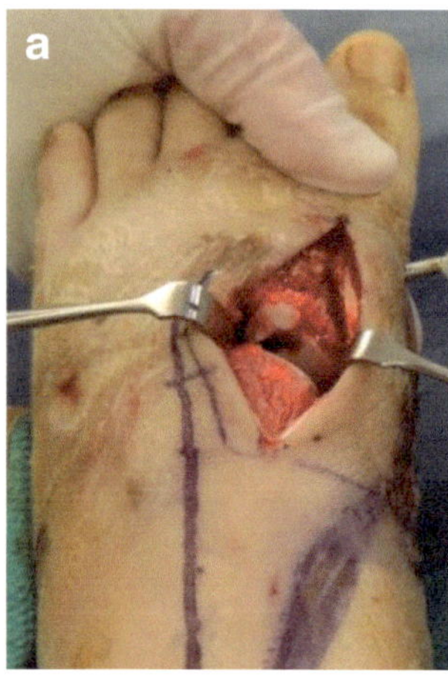

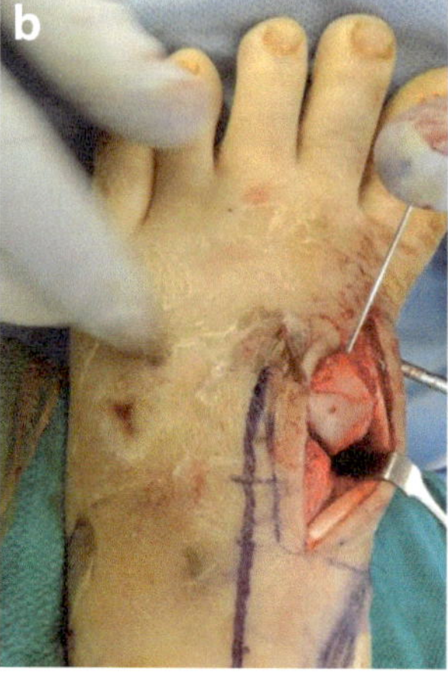

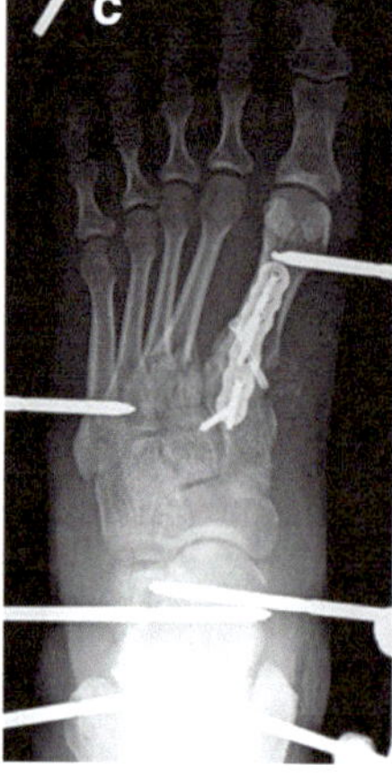

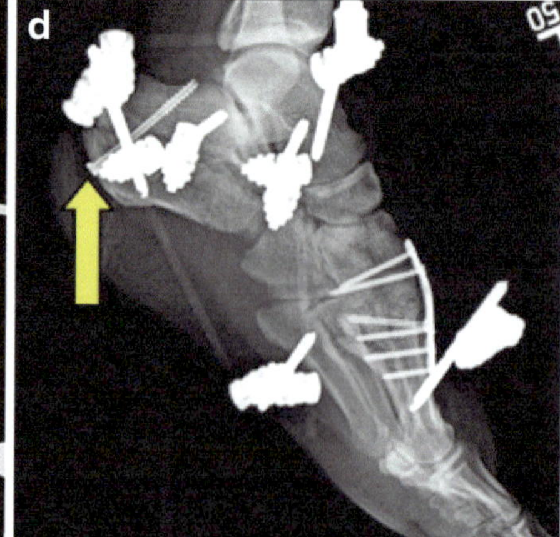

Fig. 13.16 Case 7: (**a–d**) Stage II surgery 3 weeks later with conversion to partial open reduction and internal fixation. Delayed ORIF allowed healing of extensive fracture blisters. The lateral delta frame was left in place during surgery, while the medial frame was disconnected but half pins were left for later reapplication of the frame. A minimally invasive approach to stabilization of the Lisfranc injury involved first metatarsal cuneiform primary fusion. The plantar calcaneal external pins were converted to screw fixation through minimal incision techniques (*yellow arrow*). The frames were removed 6 weeks later

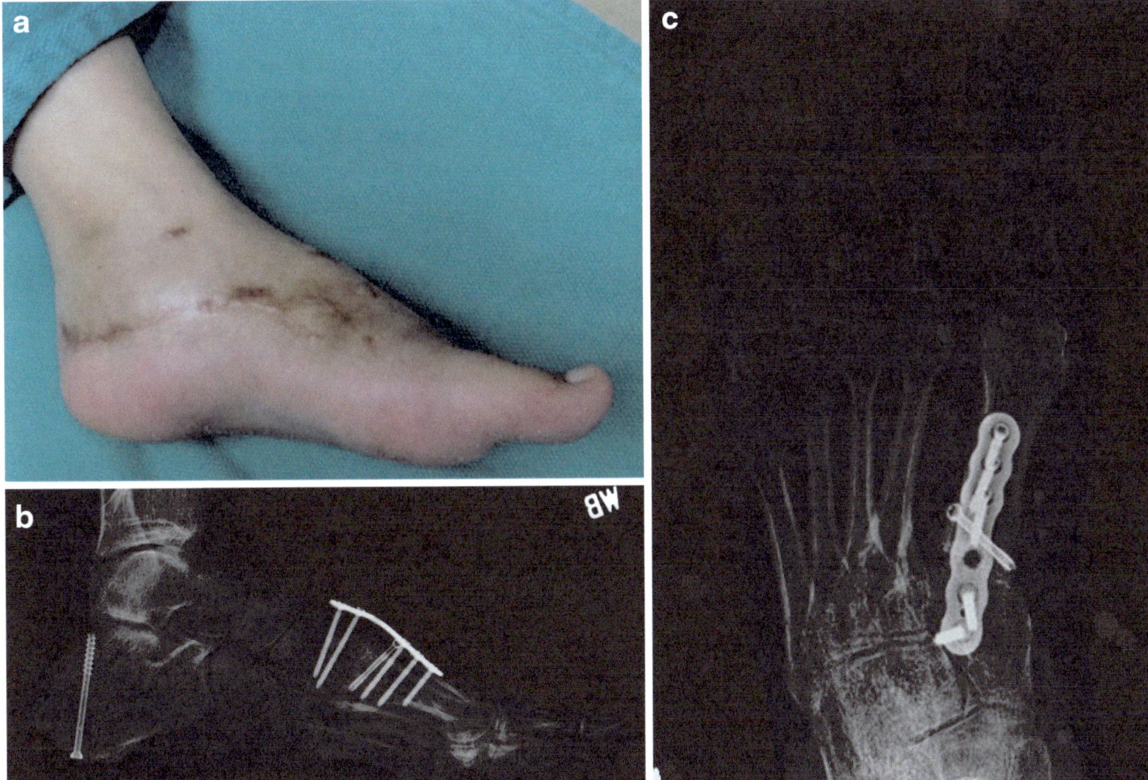

Fig. 13.17 Case 7: (**a–c**) Six month postoperative clinical photo and radiographs. This staged approach to open fracture repair with compromising soft tissue injury allowed complete healing without infection or tissue necrosis. The combined internal and external fixation approach preserved foot function without predisposing to infection. Primary fusion was achieved at the midfoot which helped to preserve foot architecture

References

1. Patzakis MJ, Wilkins J, Brien WW, et al. Wound site as a predictor of complications following deep nail punctures o the foot. West J Med. 1989;150(5):545–7.
2. Howard RJ. Effect of burn injury, mechanical trauma and operation on immune defenses. Surg Clin North Am. 1979;59:199.
3. Lineaweaver W, Seeger J, Andel A, Rumley T, Howard R. Neutrophil delivery to wounds of the upper and lower extremities. Arch Surg. 1985;120:430–1.
4. Edlich RF, Rodeheaver GT, Morgan RF, et al. Principles of emergency wound management. Ann Emerg Med. 1988;17:1248–302.
5. Haury B, Rodeheaver G, Vensko J, et al. Debridement an essential component of traumatic wound care. Am J Surg. 1978;135:238.
6. Roberts AH, Rye DG, Edgerton MT. Activity of antibiotics in contaminated wounds containing clay soil. Am J Surg. 1979;137:381.
7. Dabov GD. Osteomyelitis. In: Canale TS, Beaty JH, editors. Campbell's operative orthopaedics. Philadelphia: Mosby; 2013. p. 725–47. Chapter 21.
8. Schwab RA, Powers RD. Conservative therapy of plantar puncture wounds. J Emerg Med. 1995;13(3):291–5.
9. Gustilo RB, Anderson JT. Prevention of infection in the treatment of one thousand and twenty-five open fractures of long bones: retrospective and prospective analyses. J Bone Joint Surg Am. 1976;58:453–8.
10. Gustilo RB, Mendoza RM, Williams DN. Problems in management of type III (severe) open fractures: a new classification of type III open fractures. J Trauma. 1984;24:742–6.
11. Patzakis MJ, Wilkins J. Factors influencing infection rate in open fracture wounds. Clin Orthop Relat Res. 1989;243:36–40.
12. Centers for Disease Control and Prevention (CDC). Updated recommendations for use of tetanus toxoid, reduced diphtheria toxoid and acellular pertussis (Tdap) vaccine from the Advisory Committee on Immunization Practices, 2010. MMWR Morb Mortal Wkly Rep. 2011;60(1):13–5.
13. Centers for Disease Control and Prevention. Updated recommendations for use of tetanus toxoid, reduced diphtheria toxoid, and acellular pertussis (Tdap) vaccine in adults aged 65 years and older—Advisory Committee on Immunization Practices (ACIP), 2012. MMWR Morb Mortal Wkly Rep. 2012;61(25):468–70.
14. Centers for Disease Control and Prevention (CDC). Updated recommendations for use of tetanus toxoid, reduced diphtheria toxoid, and acellular pertussis vaccine (Tdap) in pregnant women—Advisory Committee on Immunization Practices (ACIP), 2012. MMWR Morb Mortal Wkly Rep. 2013;62(7):131–5.
15. Ak M, Goldberg S, Graham J, et al. Open extremity fractures: impact of delay in operative debridement and irrigation. J Trauma Acute Care Surg. 2014;76:1201–7.
16. Crowley DJ, Kanakaris NK, Giannoudis PV. Debridement and wound closure of open fractures: the impact of the time factor on infection rates. Injury. 2007;38:879–89.
17. Harley BJ, Beaupre LA, Jones CA, et al. The effect of time to definitive treatment on the rate of nonunion and infection in open fractures. J Orthop Trauma. 2002;16(7):484–90.
18. Hull PD, Johnson SC, Stephen DJG, et al. Delayed debridement of sever open fractures is associated with a higher rate of deep infection. Bone Joint J. 2014;96-B(3):379–84.

19. Al-Arabi YB, Nader M, Hamidian-Jahromi AR, Woods DA. The effect of the timing of antibiotics and surgical treatment on infection rates in open long-bone fractures: a 9-year prospective study from a district general hospital. Injury. 2007;38:900–5.

20. Zalavras CG, Patzakis MJ, Holtom PD, Sherman R. Management of open fractures. Infect Dis Clin North Am. 2005;19(4):915–29.

21. Anglen JO. Comparison of soap and antibiotic solutions for irrigation of lower-limb open fracture wounds: a prospective, randomized study. J Bone Joint Surg Am. 2005;87(7):1415–22.

22. Bhandari M, Adili A, Schemitsch E. The efficacy of low-pressure lavage with different irrigating solutions to remove adherent bacteria from bone. J Bone Joint Surg Am. 2001;83(3):412–9.

23. Anglen J. Wound irrigation in musculoskeletal injury. J Am Acad Orthop Surg. 2001;9:219–26.

24. Davis AG, Erie MD. Primary closure of compound fracture wounds. J Bone Joint Surg Am. 1948;30:405–15.

25. De Long Jr WG, Born CT, Wei SY, et al. Aggressive treatment of 119 open fracture wounds. J Trauma. 1999;46(6):1049–54.

26. Goldsmith JR, Massa ER. Primary closure of lawn mower injuries to the foot: a case series. J Foot Ankle Surg. 2007;46(5):366–71.

27. Jenkinson RJ, Kiss A, Johnson S, et al. Delayed wound closure increases deep-infection rate associated with lower-grade open fracture: a propensity-matched cohort study. J Bone Joint Surg Am. 2014;96:380–6.

28. Patzakis MJ, Dorr LD, Ivler D, et al. The early management of open joint injuries. A prospective study of one hundred and forty patients. J Bone Joint Surg Am. 1975;57(8):1065–70.

29. Liu DSH, Sofiadellis F, Ashton M, et al. Early soft tissue coverage and negative pressure wound therapy optimizes patient outcomes in lower limb trauma. Injury. 2012;43:772–8.

30. Small JO, Mollan RA. Management of open tibial fractures. Acta Orthop Belg. 1996;62:188–92.

31. Reinherz RP, Hong DT, Tisa LM, et al. Management of puncture wounds in the foot. J Foot Surg. 1985;24:288.

32. Lavery LA, Harkless LB, Ashry HR, et al. Infected puncture wounds in adults with diabetes: risk factors for osteomyelitis. J Foot Ankle Surg. 1994;33(6):561–6.

33. Armstrong DG, Lavery LA, Quebedeaux TL, et al. Surgical morbidity and the risk of amputation due to infected puncture wounds in diabetic versus nondiabetic adults. J Am Podiatr Med Assoc. 1997;87(7):321–6.

34. Aras MH, Miloglu O, Barutcugil C, Kantarci M, Ozcan E, Harorli A. Comparison of the sensitivity for detecting foreign bodies among conventional plain radiography, computed tomography and ultrasonography. Dentomaxillofac Radiol. 2010;39(2):72–8.

35. Haverstock BD. Puncture wounds of the foot. Clin Podiatr Med Surg. 2012;29:311–22.

36. Lyon M, Brannam L, Johnson D, Blaivas M, Duggal S. Detection of soft tissue foreign bodies in the presence of soft tissue gas. J Ultrasound Med. 2004;23:677–81.

37. Joseph WS. Infections following lower extremity trauma. In: Scurran B, editor. Foot and ankle trauma. New York: Churchill Livingstone; 1989. p. 639–54.

38. Weber CA, Wertheimer SJ, Ognjan A. Aeromonas hydrophila-its implications in freshwater injuries. J Foot Ankle Surg. 1995;34(5):442–6.

39. Laughlin TJ, Armstrong DG, Caporusso J, et al. Soft tissue and bone infections from puncture wounds in children. West J Med. 1997;166(2):126–8.

40. Karlin JM. Management of open fractures. In: Scurran B, editor. Foot and ankle trauma. New York: Churchill Livingstone; 1989. p. 39–58.

41. Healy KM, Danis KM. Treatment of open fractures. Clin Podiatr Med Surg. 1995;12(4):791–800.

42. Price C, Mauffrey C, Hak D, et al. Acute management of open fracture: proposal of a new multidisciplinary algorithm. Orthopedics. 2012;35(10):877–81.

43. Lee J. Efficacy of cultures in the management of open fractures. Clin Orthop Relat Res. 1997;339:71–5.

44. Valenziano CP, Chattar-Cora D, O'Neill A, et al. Efficacy of primary wound cultures in long bone open extremity fractures: are they of any value? Arch Orthop Trauma Surg. 2002;122(5):259–61.

45. Robertson Jr WW. Power lawnmower injuries. Clin Orthop Relat Res. 2003;409:37–42.

46. Anger DM, Ledbetter BR, Stasikelis PJ, Calhoun JH. Injuries of the foot related to the use of lawn mowers. J Bone Joint Surg Am. 1995;77(5):719–25.

47. Costilla V, Bishai DM. Lawnmower injuries in the United States: 1996 to 2004. Ann Emerg Med. 2006;47(6):567–73.

48. Wilson Jr LS, Mizel MS, Michelson JD. Foot and ankle injuries in motor vehicle accidents. Foot Ankle Int. 2001;22(8):649–52.

49. Cardany C, Rodeheaver G, Thacker J, et al. The crush injury: a high risk wound. JACEP. 1976;5:965–70.

50. Yan H, Gao W, Li Z, Wang C, et al. The management of degloving injury of lower extremities: technical refinement and classification. J Trauma Acute Care Surg. 2013;74(2):604–10.

51. Latifi R, El-Hennaway H, El-Menyar A, Peralat R, et al. The therapeutic challenges of degloving soft-tissue injuries. J Emerg Trauma Shock. 2014;7(3):228–32.

Osteomyelitis Associated with Charcot Arthropathy

Laurence G. Rubin and Allen M. Jacobs

Introduction

Osteomyelitis associated with Charcot arthropathy is almost always associated with an ulcer or tissue breakdown secondary to pressure from a boney prominence, especially in a neuropathic patient. Charcot arthropathy, particularly during its early presentation, is typically characterized by unilateral erythema, warmth, and edema (Fig. 14.1). The presence of a local ulceration raises the concern that the clinical manifestations may be the result of a septic process. Four distinct clinical circumstances may exist in a patient with acute or chronic Charcot joint deformity:

1. Isolated Charcot arthropathy
2. Charcot arthropathy with noninfected ulceration
3. Charcot arthropathy with soft tissue infection
4. Charcot arthropathy with osteomyelitis

The differential diagnosis in the presence of unilateral edema, erythema, and increased temperature includes cellulitis or other soft tissue infection, thrombophlebitis, or acute arthropathy such as gouty arthritis. Additionally, stress fractures or insufficiency fractures may also present with the same clinical symptoms. This is usually secondary to diabetes-associated bone disease with continued ambulation on the fracture due to the inability of the patient to perceive the fracture especially in the presence of sensory neuropathy. It has been suggested that the unperceived bony injury may represent an initial inciting factor for the development of Charcot arthropathy [1].

Charcot arthropathy often leads to boney prominence associated with destruction and collapse along the medial or lateral borders of the foot or through the ankle. This prominence can lead to local ulceration which compromises the skin envelope and creates an environment for soft tissue infection (Fig. 14.2). The adjacent bone eventually becomes exposed to organisms and osteomyelitis is a common sequella. The Charcot deformity and resultant boney prominence that created the ulceration will have to be dealt with along with the infection. This can be done as a staged procedure or as a single-stage reconstruction. Osteomyelitis through a hematogenous route can also occur in patients with both the acute and chronic Charcot arthropathy [2]. Osteomyelitis can also be the cause of the Charcot arthropathy due to weakening of the bone structure [2, 3].

Clinical Evaluation

As with most clinical disorders, evaluation of a patient with Charcot arthropathy and potential infection involves a careful history, clinical examination, the judicial utilization of laboratory studies, and bone and joint imaging studies.

In a patient with Eichenholtz stage 0 or stage I Charcot joint deformity, the patient may recall unilateral swelling preceding the development of an open wound. Under such circumstances, the edema may be complicated by other causes of swelling, such as venous insufficiency, lymphedema, or neuropathic edema commonly encountered in the patient with diabetic autonomic neuropathy. Lower extremity edema may result in pressure against shoes or the supporting surface, following which the ulceration noted was subsequent to the edema.

The patient with chronic Charcot arthropathy manifesting as Eichenholtz stage II or stage III deformity may recall initial swelling and deformity of the foot, following which an ulceration of the skin envelope occurred. Charcot arthropathy is not associated with a history of fever, chills, or systemic inflammatory response to sepsis. In those circumstances in which the patient recalls the ulceration preceding swelling, redness, and warmth, a consideration that the manifestations

L.G. Rubin, D.P.M., F.A.C.F.A.S. (✉)
3808 Hackamore Lane, Richmond, VA 23233, USA
e-mail: lgrubin@comcast.net

A.M. Jacobs, D.P.M., F.A.C.F.A.S.
6400 Clayton Rd #402, St. Louis, MO, USA

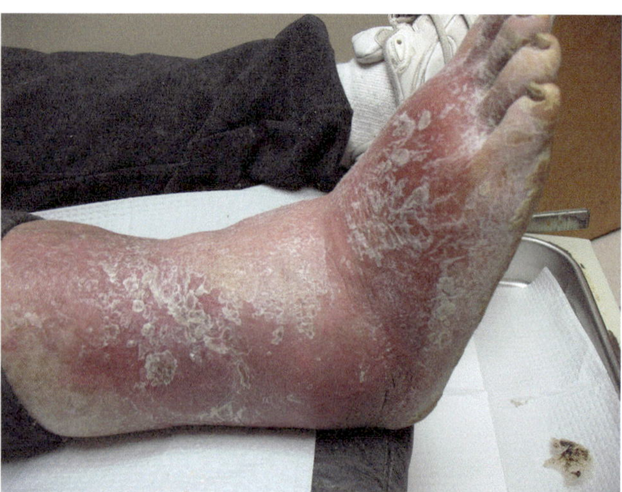

Fig. 14.1 Acute Charcot arthropathy. Note severe swelling and erythema which is difficult to differentiate from acute infection

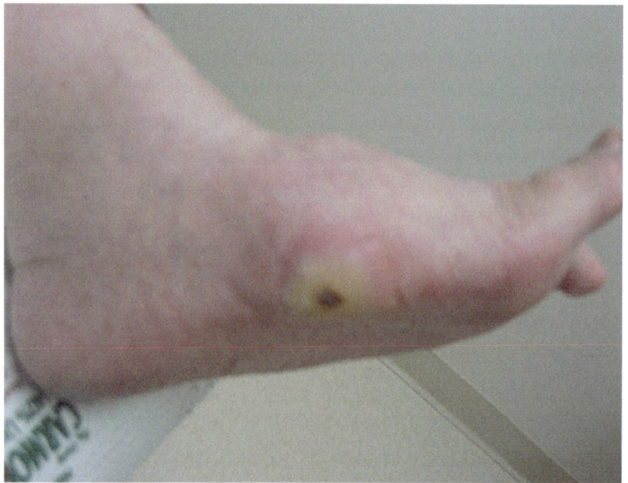

Fig. 14.2 Ulceration of medial aspect of the foot secondary to deformity associated with midfoot Charcot arthropathy

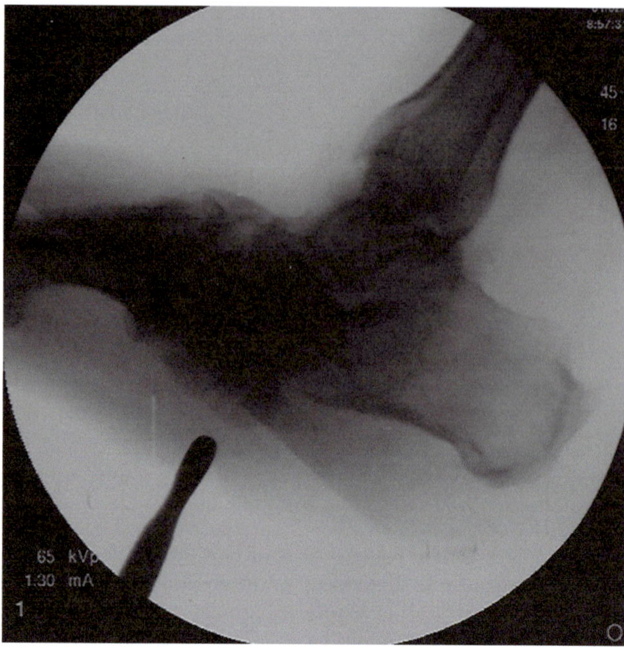

Fig. 14.3 Probe to bone test. Note that the wound is located directly over the prominent midfoot bone associated with Charcot arthropathy

noted represent an infectious process is raised. It should be noted that local infection including osteomyelitis in a patient with diabetes can occur absent systemic signs or symptoms of sepsis. Although pain may be present in a patient with Charcot arthropathy, the deformity is typically painless. Significant pain is usually present with local sepsis.

There is an association of ulceration and infection including osteomyelitis in the Charcot foot, but the relationship is not well defined in the literature. Ulceration in the Charcot foot typically occurs adjacent to prominent and palpable osseous structures such as the cuboid, fifth metatarsal base, or below the first metatarsal-cuneiform joint. There is no specific data available evaluating the incidence of osteomyelitis in a patient with diabetic ulceration associated with Charcot arthropathy. Generally, references are sited which examine the incidence of osteomyelitis association with diabetic ulceration. Studies have demonstrated that greater than 50 %

of chronic diabetic ulcerations are infected, and of those ulcerations, 20–60 % of infected ulcerations can be demonstrated as having an underlying osteitis or osteomyelitis. Ulcerations of longer duration are more likely to be associated with underlying osteitis or osteomyelitis. It has also been generally reported that ulcerations greater than 2.0–4.5 cm^2, and deeper than 3 mm, are more likely to be associated with underlying osteitis or osteomyelitis [4–7].

The presence of exposed bone at the base of an ulceration in a patient with Charcot arthropathy increases the likelihood of associated osteitis or osteomyelitis. When not directly visible within the ulceration itself, probing of the ulcer with a metallic probe is frequently employed in order to determine the likelihood of osteomyelitis (Fig. 14.3). This maneuver is commonly referred to as the "probe to bone test." There are no specific studies on the utilization of the probe to bone test for the diagnosis of osteomyelitis in ulcers associated with Charcot arthropathy. Reported rates of sensitivity of the probe to bone test ranged from 38 to 94 % and specificity 85 %–98 % [8–13]. A positive probe to bone test is most valuable when placed in proper clinical context; in many patients contamination of the outer portion of the bone, osteitis rather than osteomyelitis is present. Given the presence of either a positive probe to bone test or radiographs suggestive of osteomyelitis, one study demonstrated that 72.4 % of patients demonstrated histologically proven osteomyelitis, of which 82.5 % demonstrated a positive bone culture [11]. In general, osteomyelitis may be diagnosed with confidence when the probe to bone test is positive in a patient whose clinical presentation is consistent with osteomyelitis or when the radiographs are consistent with osteomyelitis.

Laboratory Evaluation

Although characterized by clinical evidence of inflammatory changes such as redness, swelling, and warmth, laboratory studies with Charcot arthropathy are generally not reflective of a systemic response to infection or other inflammatory process. Markers for inflammation such as elevated procalcitonin, elevated erythrocyte sedimentation rate (ESR), elevated C. reactive protein (CRP), and presence of a leukocytosis are not present and, when present, should raise the concern for underlying infection. The utilization of procalcitonin to determine the presence of osteomyelitis in patients with infected diabetic foot ulcers has been examined. Elevation in procalcitonin levels was noted in patients both with osteomyelitis (66.7 pg/mg) and without osteomyelitis (58.6 pg/mL) [14]. In general, erythrocyte sedimentation rates and elevation in WBC are significantly higher in the presence of osteomyelitis. C. reactive protein has not been demonstrated to be of significant assistance in the differentiation of soft tissue versus bone infection in a patient with diabetic foot ulceration. However, posttreatment persistent elevation of CRP is associated with increased risk of amputation [15].

Bone Biopsy

Bone biopsy and histology have long been considered the "gold standard" for the diagnosis of osteomyelitis associated with diabetic ulceration. Bone histology along with bone culture is also used for the discrimination of Charcot arthropathy from osteomyelitis. The areas that should be biopsied are based on radiologic examination: MRI, CT scan, and X-ray, as well as intraoperative clinical findings. Multiple areas of the bone in question should be biopsied and labeled by their anatomic orientation. Possible contamination of the specimens obtained and difficulty in histologic discrimination of osteomyelitis from Charcot arthropathy with the associated bony changes require careful interpretation of bone histology and bone culture reports. In one study, pathologists blinded to the source of specimens obtained from diabetic patients and asked to diagnose either osteomyelitis or no osteomyelitis were in complete agreement in only 33.33 % of cases and were in disagreement as to the presence or absence of osteomyelitis in 41.03 % of cases [16]. Another study found that the results of specimens divided and sent for culture and histology demonstrated that a positive culture and a negative histology are just as likely to occur as are a positive histology and a negative culture. The study further concluded that microbiologic testing is equivalent to histologic testing for the diagnosis of osteomyelitis associated with diabetic ulceration [17]. The usefulness of obtaining both a bone culture and histology is reflected by a study demonstrating that culture demonstrates a 42 % sensitivity for the diagnosis of osteomyelitis, whereas the combination of culture and histology is associated with 84 % sensitivity with a diagnosis of osteomyelitis [18]. Biopsy of the bone directly under an ulceration by approaching the bone directly through the wound itself has been reported [19]. Although the potential for contamination exists with this approach, successful resolution of underlying osteomyelitis, present in 96 % of bone cultures obtained through the wound, was reported utilizing treatment based upon the wound culture. Cultures obtained directly from exposed bone for the treatment of osteomyelitis has been examined, although not specifically for ulceration in diabetic ulceration associated with Charcot arthropathy. Bone contact swabs were compared with bone biopsy in one study, demonstrating 82.35 % agreement with swabbing of the exposed bone and true bone biopsy. Swabbing of the exposed bone was 96 % sensitive for the causative pathogen, with a 79 % specificity and a positive predictive value of 92 % [20]. Evaluation of osteomyelitis by culturing through a sinus tract has also been examined. In one study, two different cultures were obtained from a sinus tract taken at different times. The concordance of the sinus tract cultures with true bone cultures was reported as 96 %, with a sensitivity of 91 % and a specificity of 86 %. Accuracy of sinus tract cultures was reported as 90 %, particularly when the infection was monomicrobial in etiology [21]. The techniques of needle biopsy versus transcutaneous biopsy for the diagnosis of osteomyelitis have also been examined. Needle biopsy has been demonstrated to be associated with a 16.1 % false-positive and 38.1 % false-negative rates. Overall, bone biopsies have been reported as associated with a 67.7 % recovery rate, bone needle biopsy 58 % recovery rate, and bone swabs 96.7 % recovery rate [22].

Circumstances have been proposed in which biopsy should be considered [23]. These circumstances include concern for the presence of a drug-resistant organism, the presence of continuing bone destruction or elevated markers of inflammation in the presence of ongoing antibiotic therapy, in circumstances where a definitive diagnosis is required, and finally in those circumstances wherein there is a plan for the utilization of internal or external fixation secured within a bone which is potentially infected.

Bone cultures and histological specimens are frequently obtained from patients who have received prior antibiotic therapy for presumed soft tissue or bone infection. Ideally, bone cultures are obtained when the patient is either antibiotic naïve or has not received antibiotics for at least 2 weeks. Discontinuation of antibiotics for 48 h has been associated with acceptable bone cultures [24].

All techniques of bone culture and histology are associated with both false-positive and false-negative results. The practitioner faced with the possibility of Charcot arthropathy with associated soft tissue or bone infection should consider the results of testing in a clinical scenario as "likely associated with osteomyelitis" versus "not likely to be associated with osteomyelitis."

In summary, bone cultures and histology are associated with a significant incidence of false-positive and false-negative results. Studies available for the evaluation of bone cultures and histology associated with diabetic ulceration are not studies specifically entered for the treatment of possible osteomyelitis in the patient with Charcot arthropathy. All such studies must be interpreted carefully in the patient with Charcot arthropathy. This is of particular concern given the fact that many diabetic ulcerations, unlike the patient with Charcot arthropathy, do not present with significant signs of inflammation such as erythema, warmth, and acute edema.

Bone and Joint Imaging

Charcot arthropathy, particularly during its acute phase, is characterized by variable presentation of osteopenia, joint effusion, the presence of bone debris, as well as erosive and destructive bone changes on X-ray. At times, the distribution of such changes particularly when limited to Lisfranc joint, or the midtarsal joint, strongly suggests the presence of Charcot arthropathy to the experienced clinician. However, the radiographic changes, which characterize Charcot arthropathy, may also be demonstrated in a patient with osteomyelitis. Given the presence of an open wound, particularly with exposed bone, in a warm and swollen foot in the patient with diabetes, the presence of disruptive or resorptive bone changes is concerning. The differential diagnosis of such changes includes Charcot arthropathy, osteomyelitis, inflammatory arthritis, or reactive bone changes secondary to adjacent soft tissue inflammation.

Focal destruction, involving an isolated bone rather than a more global joint destruction process, is more concerning for osteomyelitis. Diffuse osseous and articular changes involving an entire joint structure, such as Lisfranc joint, the ankle joint, the midtarsal joint, and the subtalar joint, are more consistent with, although not diagnostic of, Charcot arthropathy. The presence of isolated bone destruction contiguous to an existing ulceration or other soft tissue defect is concerning for osteomyelitis. The presence of air or gas density within soft tissues is similarly concerning for an ongoing infectious process. MRI studies are frequently utilized for the discrimination of Charcot arthropathy from osteomyelitis, reactive marrow edema, or osteomyelitis superimposed on a prior existing Charcot joint deformity. Osteomyelitis is characterized by increased T2 signal and decreased T1 signal in bone marrow, with changes localized or contiguous to a soft tissue ulcer or abscess [25]. Conversely, polyarticular distribution of bone changes, or distribution along periarticular structures in the absence of a continuous ulceration or soft tissue defect, is more likely associated with Charcot arthropathy. Diffuse bone marrow signal abnormalities, progressive subarticular enhancement, and the presence of an MRI "ghost sign" are highly suggestive of an acute infectious process superimposed on preexisting Charcot arthropathy [25].

Radionuclide imaging is helpful for initial screening and localization of the sites of bone pathology. However, radionuclide imaging with technetium is nonspecific although sensitive, as it may be reflective of fracture, neuropathic bone changes, Charcot arthropathy, avulsion fracture, inflammatory arthritis, stress fracture, or reactive osteitis. FDG-PET scanning has been examined in several studies for the discrimination of soft tissue infection from osteomyelitis. In general, FDG-PET scans are expensive and frequently not readily available. The results are inconsistent when compared to either MRI or WBC scintigraphy and clear superiority over MRI has not been consistently demonstrated [26–28].

Making the Diagnosis

A classification system has been proposed [7] for the diagnosis of osteomyelitis as being definite, probable, possible, or unlikely. Definite osteomyelitis is diagnosed as obtaining a positive culture and histology, or the presence of purulence observed within the bone at surgery, or the presence of an intraosseous abscess on MRI, or any two probable, or possible, or one probable and two possible findings. Probable osteomyelitis has been defined as the presence of viable cancellous bone within an ulcer, and an MRI demonstrating bone edema or other signs of osteomyelitis, a positive bone culture with negative bone histology, or a positive bone histology with negative bone culture or any two findings within the category of probable bone infection. Possible osteomyelitis is felt to exist when X-rays are consistent with osteomyelitis, or an MRI demonstrates bone edema or cloaca, or there is a positive probing to bone test, where there is visible cortical bone within an ulceration, or when an erythrocyte sedimentation rate is greater than 70 mm/h, where there is a nonhealing ulceration of greater than 6 weeks, where there is an ulceration of greater than 2 weeks duration with local signs and symptoms of infection. Osteomyelitis is considered unlikely when there are no signs or symptoms of inflammation, a normal X-ray, an ulceration of less than a 2-week duration, a superficial ulceration, a normal MRI, and a normal bone scan.

General Preoperative Evaluation

The preoperative medical evaluation consists of advanced imaging, vascular evaluation, and endocrine and laboratory workup. It is advisable to do a thorough patient workup if time permits for nonemergency surgical treatment. An MRI or CT scan should be obtained if one has not already been ordered as part of the diagnostic evaluation. This will help determine which bones will need to be addressed and provide the surgeon a 3-plane evaluation of the deformity to help determine the best treatment options for the Charcot deformity and the boney prominence.

Preoperative vascular evaluation is critical since vascular disease can contribute to the development of infection and have a direct effect on the ability to heal [2]. It is preferable to revascularize the patient prior to doing any foot or ankle surgery, but if the patient requires vascular surgery, the timing will usually depend on the presence of infection. There is a 25 % risk of major amputation and a 35 % chance of morbidity and mortality when there is severe infection in the diabetic population [29, 30]. A bone endocrine evaluation consisting of Vitamin D, PTH, and a 24 urine calcium should be ordered. These values will help determine the bone healing potential. This may help determine whether the patient is a good candidate for a single-stage procedure or a better candidate for delaying the fusion until the endocrine issues have been corrected. The renal status of the patient should also be evaluated. An elevated creatinine can have an effect on the choice of antibiotic and the dosing regimen. The creatinine level will also determine whether the patient can have contrast dye for an arteriogram or for an MRI with contrast.

Treatment

The treatment of osteomyelitis superimposed on Charcot arthropathy is dependent on multiple factors. The surgeon must treat the infection as well as the Charcot arthropathy. The osteomyelitis will need to be treated with antibiotic therapy and thorough debridement of the necrotic and infected tissue. The Charcot arthropathy will need to be stabilized or treated.

Culture- and sensitivity-based antibiotics are the major component for the treatment of osteomyelitis. Antibiotics are held if possible until intraoperative cultures are accomplished. Oral antibiotics may be utilized in place of parenteral antibiotics, provided the antibiotic utilized has appropriate pharmacologic and pharmacokinetic properties including bone penetration in concentrations that are adequate to treat osteomyelitis. In many circumstances, there does not appear to be any advantage offered by the use of parenteral antibiotics over oral antibiotics. Both are associated with a chronic osteomyelitis recurrence rate of approximately 20–30 % [31]. Local antibiotic delivery systems created from antibiotic-impregnated bone cement or bone graft substitutes have been successfully utilized in conjunction with systemic antibiotic coverage [32] (see Fig. 14.4). The antibiotic cement beads/spacers allow concentrated delivery of the antibiotics without adding to the systemic toxicity of the parenteral antibiotics. They can also provide stability to the surrounding structures and help maintain length and alignment of the bone structure.

Antibiotic treatment is typically combined with the surgical debridement of the infected or necrotic soft tissue and bone. The intraoperative cultures should be performed after debridement of the necrotic tissue. The necrotic bone can be from osteomyelitis or Charcot arthropathy; either way, the necrotic bone must be completely excised through surgical debridement (see Fig. 14.5).

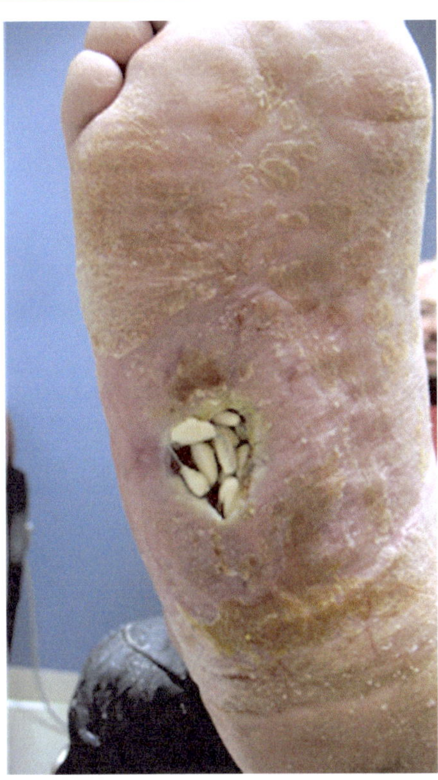

Fig. 14.4 Antibiotic beads in a plantar ulcer that was caused by deformity associated with Charcot arthropathy

If a bone prominence created the ulcer, this should also be debrided to help prevent recurrence of the ulcer. Bone biopsies should be obtained during the debridement from several different areas. Osteomyelitis and Charcot arthropathy can have similar findings on histopathological specimens, therefore it is advisable to discuss the biopsy with the pathologist and give them a "heads up" on the possible diagnosis of Charcot bone versus osteomyelitis.

Along with the treatment of the osteomyelitis, the Charcot arthropathy should be treated. The boney prominence that created the ulcer should be dealt with to prevent recurrence. Maintaining the foot in the deformed position, that created the original ulcer, will likely result in another ulceration once the patient is weight bearing. In the setting of acute Charcot arthropathy, the lower extremity must be stabilized. Splinting, total contact casting, or external fixation along with non-weight bearing can achieve stabilization. Splints are initially used until the edema has stabilized. Total contact casting is often used as the first line of treatment [33–35]. There is controversy as to whether the patient can bear weight in the total contact cast or must remain non-weight bearing. This should be based on the stage of the Charcot arthropathy the patient is in, as well as the inherent stability of the lower extremity. Weight bearing in a cast or boot in an unstable patient can create ulcerations and further bone destruction. This has been most prevalent at the malleoli. The length of time of non-weight bearing may depend on the anatomic location of the Charcot arthropathy with the

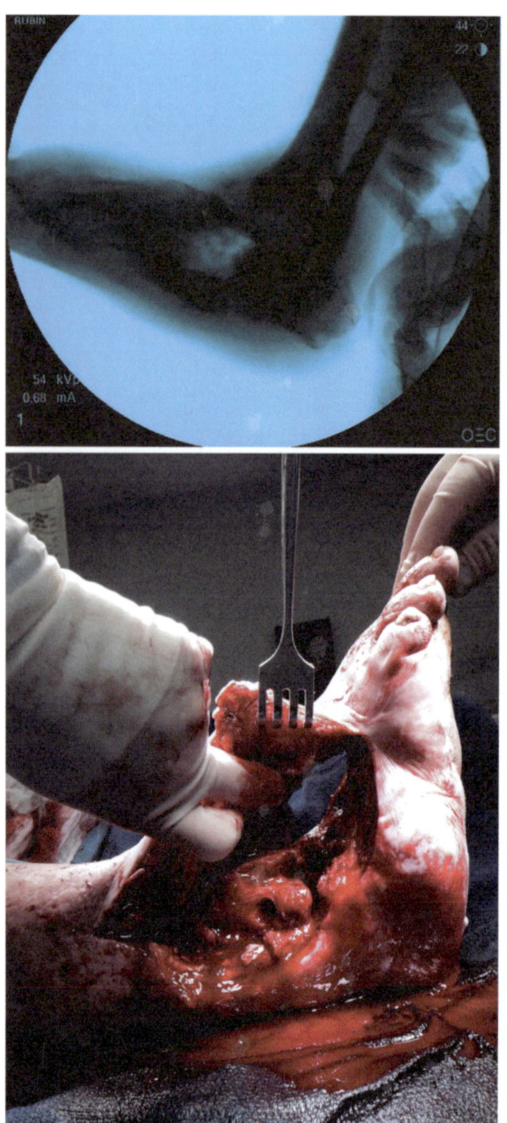

Fig. 14.5 Intraoperative imaging and operative photo after debridement of bone for Charcot arthropathy complicated by osteomyelitis

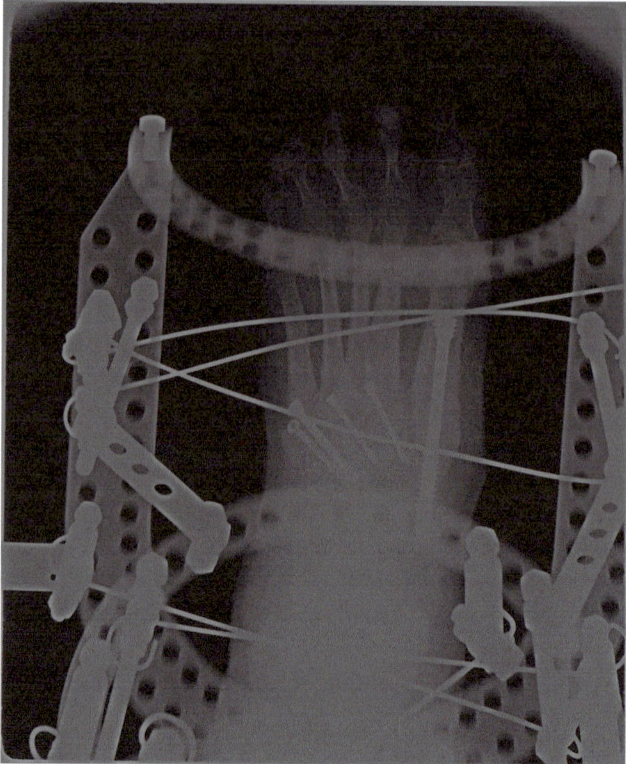

Fig. 14.6 Combined internal and external fixation in Charcot reconstruction

forefoot requiring the least amount of time [36]. The period of non-weight bearing can last up to 6 months [34]. Total contact casting has been shown to be a safe and effective technique to immobilize Charcot arthropathy [37, 38]. Guyton studied 70 patients with 389 total contact cast changes and concluded that there was a 6 % per cast complication rate [37]. In patients that cannot be accommodated with a splint or with total contact casting, external fixation has been used to stabilize the lower extremity. Although this will provide good stabilization and allows for accommodation of most deformities, it does increase the complication rate. Care should be taken during the application of the external fixator to prevent the wires or half pins from enter-

ing areas of active infection. Ideally the wires and pins should be placed remotely to the area of active infection and not contiguous or through the infected area. This will allow for stabilization of the Charcot arthropathy without contributing to the infection.

In a plantigrade foot without significant deformity, the prominent bone can be resected or protected with padding. In cases where the prominence cannot be treated with local excision, or protection with padding because the deformity is too great, or the foot/ankle is unstable or not plantigrade, the deformity will need to be corrected. This is accomplished by osteotomy and arthrodesis using internal fixation, external fixation, or the combination of both internal and external fixation. This is usually performed after the infection has been treated and eliminated with debridement of soft tissue and bone along with appropriate antibiotic coverage. When inflammatory signs and symptoms as well as laboratory markers for inflammation have stabilized, deformity reconstruction has been traditionally approached. Arthrodesis is the most commonly used reconstructive procedure for Charcot arthropathy with concomitant osteomyelitis after resolution of the infection [39, 40]. It is often necessary to use negative pressure therapy and grafts to heal the soft tissue defects prior to the reconstruction. Negative pressure therapy with antibiotic beads and external fixation has been described

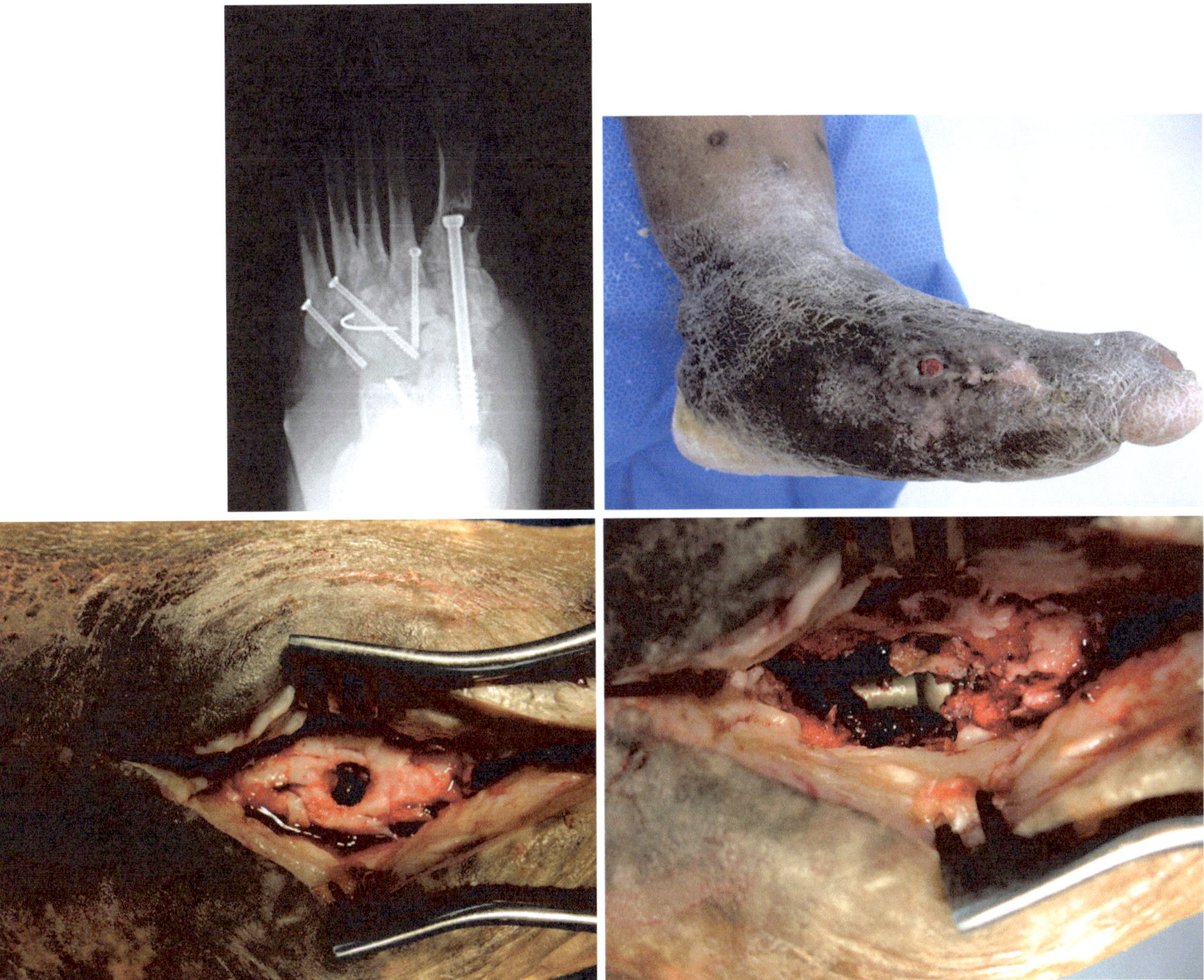

Fig. 14.7 Postoperative infection of the medial column beaming screw. Note bone resorption on X-ray at the screw head and draining sinus tract. There is a cloaca at the screw head present intraoperatively

in the literature for the treatment of complex wounds along with bone defects in patients with Charcot arthropathy and osteomyelitis [41]. The goal of the reconstructive procedure is to attain a stable plantigrade foot through osteotomies and arthrodesis. Stabilization of the arthrodesis is achieved by internal fixation, external fixation, or a combination of internal and external fixation (Fig. 14.6). Placing fixation into the area of previous infection before there has been complete resolution of the infection can create a flare-up of the previous infection (Fig. 14.7). Pinzur et al. [33] reported on 26 feet with Charcot arthropathy and open ulcers and/or chronic osteomyelitis. Twenty-two patients had 32 surgical procedures. Sixteen patients had debridement of bone and soft tissue, eight underwent an exostectomy, and seven had partial excision with attempted arthrodesis. At an average follow-up of 3.6 years, only one patient was nonambulatory. None of the patients required a below-knee amputation, but three had

a proximal Syme's amputation, one had a Chopart's amputation, and one had a midfoot amputation.

Several authors have described a single-stage procedure where the debridement and reconstruction/arthrodesis are done at the same setting (Fig. 14.8). Pinzur et al. [42] reported on 73 cases of concomitant osteomyelitis and Charcot arthropathy. The technique involved debridement of the infected bone, intraoperative correction of deformity and placement of percutaneous pins, placement of three level external fixator, and parenteral antibiotics based on intraoperative cultures. Patients were in the external fixator for 8–12 weeks followed by weight bearing in a total contact cast for 4–6 weeks. This protocol achieved a 95.7 % limb salvage with patients able to ambulate in commercially available therapeutic footwear. Dalla Paola et al. [43] reported on 45 patients with Charcot arthropathy and osteomyelitis treated with debridement and external fixation. Thirty-nine of the patients healed. Two

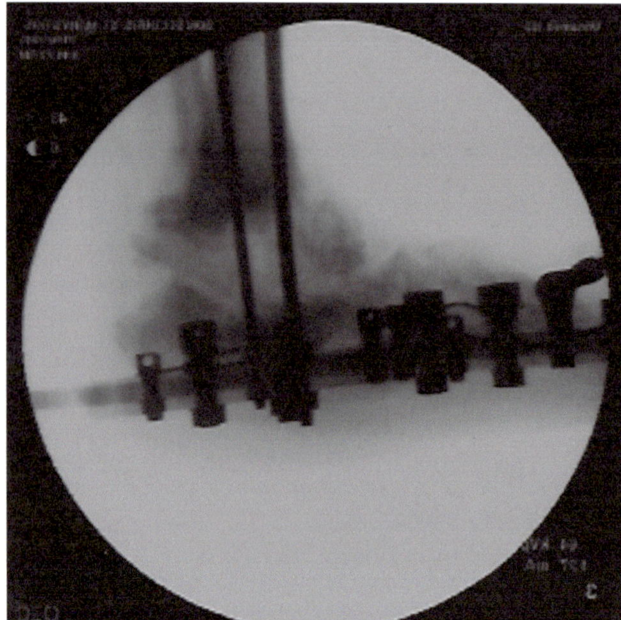

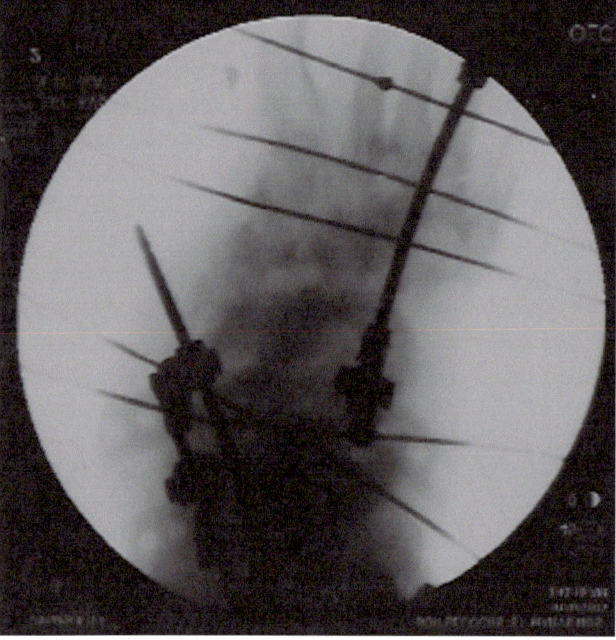

Fig. 14.8 Osteomyelitis of the talus in a Charcot patient treated with debridement and external fixation in a single-stage procedure

patients had a subsequent surgery requiring an intramedullary nail and four required a major amputation.

Pawar et al. [40] treated five patients with infected Charcot arthropathy of the ankle by debridement and insertion of an antibiotic-coated, locked intramedullary nail. Three of the patients had a previously failed treatment with an external fixator; the two remaining patients were treated primarily. All patients were infection free and achieved union with an average radiologic healing time of 4.1 months.

Summary

Charcot arthropathy with concomitant osteomyelitis can be a difficult diagnosis to treat and has a high rate of complications and major amputations. The first step is to make the diagnosis since Charcot arthropathy and osteomyelitis can have similar clinical presentations, laboratory and radiographic findings, and histopathological features. This can make diagnosing Charcot arthropathy versus Charcot arthropathy with osteomyelitis extremely challenging, especially when there is an open wound present. There are no generally accepted guidelines for the treatment of osteomyelitis in a patient with Charcot arthropathy. The treatment for osteomyelitis includes complete eradication of the infection through antibiotics and thorough debridement of the soft tissues and bone. Stabilization of the lower extremity should also be achieved while treating the infection. The reconstructive surgery can be done after the infection is cured as a staged procedure or as a single-stage procedure at the time of the debridement.

References

1. Chantelau E, Richter A, Ghassem-Zadeh H, Poll LW. "Silent" bone stress injuries in the feet of diabetic patients with polyneuropathy: a report on 12 cases. Arch Orthop Trauma Surg. 2007;127(3):171–7.
2. Ramanujam CL, Stapleton JJ, Zgonis T. Diabetic Charcot neuroarthropathy of the foot and ankle with osteomyelitis. Clin Podiatr Med Surg. 2014;31:487–92.
3. Zgonis T, Stapleton JJ, Shibuya N, et al. Surgically induced Charcot neuroarthropathy following partial forefoot amputation in diabetes. J Wound Care. 2007;16:57–9.
4. Lavery LA, Peters EJ, Armstrong DG, Wendel CS, Murdoch DP, Lipsky BA. Risk factors for developing osteomyelitis in patients with diabetic foot wounds. Diabetes Res Clin Pract. 2009;83:347–52.
5. Lipsky BA, Peters EJ, Senneville E, Berendt AR, Embril JM, Lavery LA, et al. Expert opinion on the management of infection in the diabetic foot. Diabetes Metab Res Rev. 2012;28 Suppl 1:163–78.
6. Newman LG, Waller J, Palestro CJ, Schwartz M, Klein MJ, Hermann G, et al. Unsuspected osteomyelitis in diabetic foot ulcers. Diagnosis and monitoring by leukocytes scanning with Indium 111 oxyyquinoline. JAMA. 1991;266:1246–51.
7. Ertugrel BM, Oncul O, Turlek N, Willke A, Sacar S, Tunxxan OG, et al. A prospective, multi center study: factors related to the management of diabetic foot ulcers. Eur J Clin Microbiol Infect Dis. 2012;31:2345–52.
8. Grayson ML, Gibbons GW, Balogh K, Levin E, Karchmer AW. Probing to bone in infected pedal ulcers. A clinical sign of underlying osteomyelitis in diabetic patients. JAMA. 1995;273:721–3.
9. Shone A, Burnside J, Chipchase S, Game F, Jeffcoate W. probing the validity of the probe–to–bone test in the diagnosis of osteomyelitis of the foot in diabetes. Diabetes Care. 2006;29:945.
10. Lavery LA, Armstrong DG, Peters EJ, Lipsky BA. Probe-to-bone test for diagnosing diabetic foot osteomyelitis: reliable or relic? Diabetes Care. 2007;30:270–4.
11. Aragon-Sanchez J, Lipsky BA, Lazaro-Martinez JL. Diagnosing diabetic foot osteomyelitis: is the combination of probe-to-bone test and plain radiography sufficient for high-risk inpatients. Diabet Med. 2011;28(2):191–4.

12. Mutuoglu M, Uzun G, Sildirulgu O, Turhan V, Mutlu H, Yildiz S. Performance of the probe-to-bone test in a population suspected of having osteomyelitis of the foot in diabetes. J Am Podiatr Med Assoc. 2012;102:369–72.

13. Morales Lozano R, Gonzalez Fernandez ML, Martinez Hernandez D, Beneit Montesinos JV, et al. Validating the probe-to-bone test and other tests for diagnosing chronic osteomyelitis in the diabetic foot. Diabetes Care. 2010;33:2140–5.

14. Mutluoglu M, Uzun G, Ipcioglu OM, et al. Can procalcitonin predict bone infection in people with diabetes with infected foot ulcers? A pilot study. Diabetes Res Clin Pract. 2011;94(1):53–6.

15. Akinci B, Yener S, Yesil S, et al. Acute phase reactants predict the risk of amputation in diabetic foot infection. J Am Podiatr Med Assoc. 2011;101(1):1–6.

16. Meyr AJ, Singh S, Zhang X, et al. Statistical reliability of bone biopsy for the diagnosis of diabetic foot osteomyelitis. J Foot Ankle Surg. 2011;50:663–7.

17. Weiner RD, Viselli SJ, Fulkert KA, Accetta P. Histology versus microbiology for accuracy in identification of osteomyelitis in the diabetic foot. J Foot Ankle Surg. 2011;50(2):197–200.

18. White LM, Schweitzer ME, Deely DM, Gannon F. Study of osteomyelitis: utility of combined histologic and microbiologic evaluation of percutaneous biopsy samples. Radiology. 1995;197(3):840–2.

19. Lesens O, Desbiez F, Vidal M, et al. Culture of per–wound bone specimens: A simplified approach for the medical management of diabetic foot osteomyelitis. Clin Microbiol Infect. 2011;17(2):285–91.

20. Bernard L, Assal M, Garzoni C, Uckay I. Predicting the pathogen of diabetic toe osteomyelitis by two consecutive ulcer cultures with bone contact. Eur J Clin Microbiol Infect Dis. 2011;30(2):279–81.

21. Bernard L, Uckay I, Vuagnat A, et al. Two consecutive deep sinus tract cultures predict the pathogen of osteomyelitis. Int J Infect Dis. 2010;14(5):e390–3.

22. Senneville E, Morant H, Descamps D, et al. Needle puncture and transcutaneous bone biopsy cultures are inconsistent in patients with diabetes and suspected osteomyelitis of the foot. Clin Infect Dis. 2009;48(7):888–93.

23. Erugrul BM, Lipsky BA, Savk O. Osteomyelitis or Charcot neuroosteoarthropathy? Differentiating these disorders in diabetic patients with a foot problem. Diabet Foot Ankle. 2013;4:32. doi:10.3402/dfa.v4i0.21855.

24. Wu JS, Gorbachova T, et al. Imaging-guided bone biopsy for osteomyelitis: are there factors associated with positive or negative cultures. AJR Am J Roentgenol. 2007;188:1529–34.

25. Toledano TR, Fatone EA, Weis A, Cotton A, Beltran J. MRI evaluation of bone marrow changes in the diabetic foot: a practical approach. Semin Musculoskelet Radiol. 2011;15(3):257–68.

26. Familiari D, et al. Can sequential 18F-FDG PET/CT replace WBC imaging in the diabetic foot? J Nucl Med. 2011;52(7):1012–9.

27. Schwegler B, Stumpe KD, Weishaupt D, Strobel K, et al. Unsuspected osteomyelitis is frequent in persistent diabetic foot ulcer and better diagnose by MRI then by18F-FDG PET or 99mTc-MOAB. J Intern Med. 2008;263(1):99–106.

28. Heiba SI, Kolker D, Mocheria B, Kapoor K, et al. The optimized evaluation of diabetic foot infection by dual isotope SPECT/CT imaging protocol. J Foot Ankle Surg. 2010;49(6):529–36.

29. Zgonis T, Stapleton JJ, Roukis TS. A stepwise approach to the surgical management of severe diabetic foot infections. Foot Ankle Spec. 2008;1:46–53.

30. Jeffcoate W, Lima J, Nobrega L. The Charcot Foot. Diabet Med. 2000;17:253–8.

31. Conterno LO, da Silva Filho CR. Antibiotics for treating chronic osteomyelitis in adults. Cochrane Database Syst Rev. 2009;3, CD004439. doi: 10.1002/14651858.CD004439.pub2.

32. Ramanujam CL, Zgonis T. Antibiotic-loaded cement beads for Charcot ankle osteomyelitis. Foot Ankle Spec. 2010;3(5):274–7.

33. Pinzur MS, Sage R, Stuck R, Kaminsky S, Zmuda A. A treatment algorithm for neuropathic (Charcot) midfoot deformity. Foot Ankle. 1993;14:189–97.

34. Frykberg RG, Zgonis T, Armstrong DG, Driver VR, Giurini JM, et al. Diabetic foot disorders. A clinical practice guideline (2006 revision). J Foot Ankle Surg. 2006;45:S1–66.

35. Myerson M, Papa J, Eaton K, Wilson K. The total-contact cast for management of neuropathic plantar ulceration of the foot. J Bone Joint Surg Am. 1992;74:261–9.

36. Sinacore DR. Acute Charcot arthropathy in patients with diabetes mellitus: healing times by foot location. J Diabetes Complications. 1998;12:287–93.

37. Guyton GP. An analysis of iatrogenic complications from the total contact cast. Foot Ankle Int. 2005;26:903–7.

38. Wukich DK, Motko J. Safety of total contact casting in high-risk patients with neuropathic foot ulcers. Foot Ankle Int. 2004;25:556–60.

39. Stapleton JJ, Zgonis T. Surgical reconstruction of the diabetic Charcot foot: internal, external or combined fixation? Clin Podiatr Med Surg. 2012;29:425–33.

40. Pawar A, Dikmen G, Fragomen A, Rozbruch SR. Antibiotic-coated nail for fusion of infected Charcot ankles. Foot Ankle Int. 2013;34:80–4.

41. Ramanujam CL, Facaros Z, Zgonis T. An overview of conservative treatment options for diabetic Charcot foot neuroarthropathy. Diabet Foot Ankle. 2011;2:56.

42. Pinzur MS, Gil J, Belmares J. Treatment of osteomyelitis and charcot foot with single-stage resection of infection, correction deformity, and maintenance with ring fixation. Foot Ankle Int. 2012;33:1069–74.

43. Dalla Paola L, Brocco E, Ceccacci T, et al. Limb salvage in Charcot foot and ankle osteomyelitis: combined use single stage/ double stage of arthrodesis and external fixation. Foot Ankle Int. 2009; 30:1065–70.

First Ray Osteomyelitis

Troy J. Boffeli, Shelby B. Hyllengren, and Matthew C. Peterson

Introduction

Osteomyelitis of the first ray may be localized or extensive involving the distal phalanx, the proximal phalanx, the first metatarsal, or the sesamoids. First ray osteomyelitis is generally associated with contiguous spread of infection from neuropathic ulcers located at the distal tip of the hallux, around the first interphalangeal joint (IPJ), or at the first metatarsal phalangeal joint (MPJ) (Fig. 15.1). Proximal infection at the base of the first metatarsal is not as common and is typically associated with recurrent or persistent osteomyelitis following partial first ray amputation. Midfoot ulceration caused by Charcot deformity may also lead to infection at the base of the first metatarsal. Contiguous spread from infected gangrene of the hallux is also common, while decubitus ulceration over a bunion is less common.

Osteomyelitis along the medial column is a frequently encountered problem in the diabetic foot which directly correlates with the high incidence of hallux ulceration [1, 2]. Although neuropathy is the leading risk factor for first ray ulceration, other factors play a role in the etiology of tissue breakdown including deformity and poor circulation. Abnormal mechanics and structural deformities cause pathologic stress on the local tissues and significantly influence ulcer location, propensity for poor healing, and ultimately the development of osteomyelitis [3, 4]. Foot and ankle deformities including hallux limitus, hallux valgus, hallux hammertoe, and ankle equinus are known risk factors for first ray ulceration [3]. Although not as common, nonstructural etiologies such as gout, gangrene, septic joint, toenail trauma, puncture wounds, and open fractures can also lead to the formation of osteomyelitis (Fig. 15.2).

A combined medical and surgical treatment protocol is generally preferred for first ray osteomyelitis in an effort to address not only bone infection but also the soft tissue wound defect and underlying mechanical or structural issues. The ideal surgical plan should also attempt to preserve the important weight bearing function of the first ray when possible. Incision and drainage of infection, excision of the ulcer, conservative bone resection or amputation, implantation of antibiotic beads, immediate or delayed wound closure, and antibiotic therapy are commonly incorporated to provide a global approach to this potentially limb-threatening condition. Staged surgery and integration of rotational flaps are common in the surgical treatment of first ray osteomyelitis since continued bone exposure at the site of a nonhealing wound often leads to persistent or recurrent osteomyelitis despite long-term postoperative antibiotic therapy. Failure to address the source of abnormal pressure predisposes to the dilemma of recurrent wound breakdown which is detrimental to the pursuit of a clinical cure of osteomyelitis. Conservative bone resection at the site of osteomyelitis allows removal of the nidus of infection, provides specimen for bone biopsy, and has the potential to address the source of bone prominence or abnormal mechanics [5]. A biomechanically sound procedure could actually improve the function of the first ray or at least decrease the likelihood of recurrent ulceration which goes against the commonly held belief that surgery should be a last resort option.

Some degree of first ray amputation is commonly performed for osteomyelitis and ranges from partial hallux amputation to complete first ray amputation. Compared with amputation of other toes, there are added undesirable consequences associated with first ray amputation including transfer ulcers at adjacent areas leading to repeat infection and further

T.J. Boffeli, D.P.M., F.A.C.F.A.S. (✉)
Regions Hospital/HealthPartners Institute for Education and Research, 640 Jackson Street, St. Paul, MN 55101, USA
e-mail: troy.j.boffeli@healthpartners.com

S.B. Hyllengren, D.P.M.
Allina Health Cambridge Clinic, 701 South Dellwood Street, Cambridge, MN 55008, USA
e-mail: shelby.b.hyllengren@gmail.com

M.C. Peterson, D.P.M., A.A.C.F.A.S.
Fairview Health Servces, 6545 France Ave, Ste. 150, Edina, MN 55435, USA
e-mail: mpeter11@fairview.org

© Springer International Publishing Switzerland 2015
T.J. Boffeli (ed.), *Osteomyelitis of the Foot and Ankle*, DOI 10.1007/978-3-319-18926-0_15

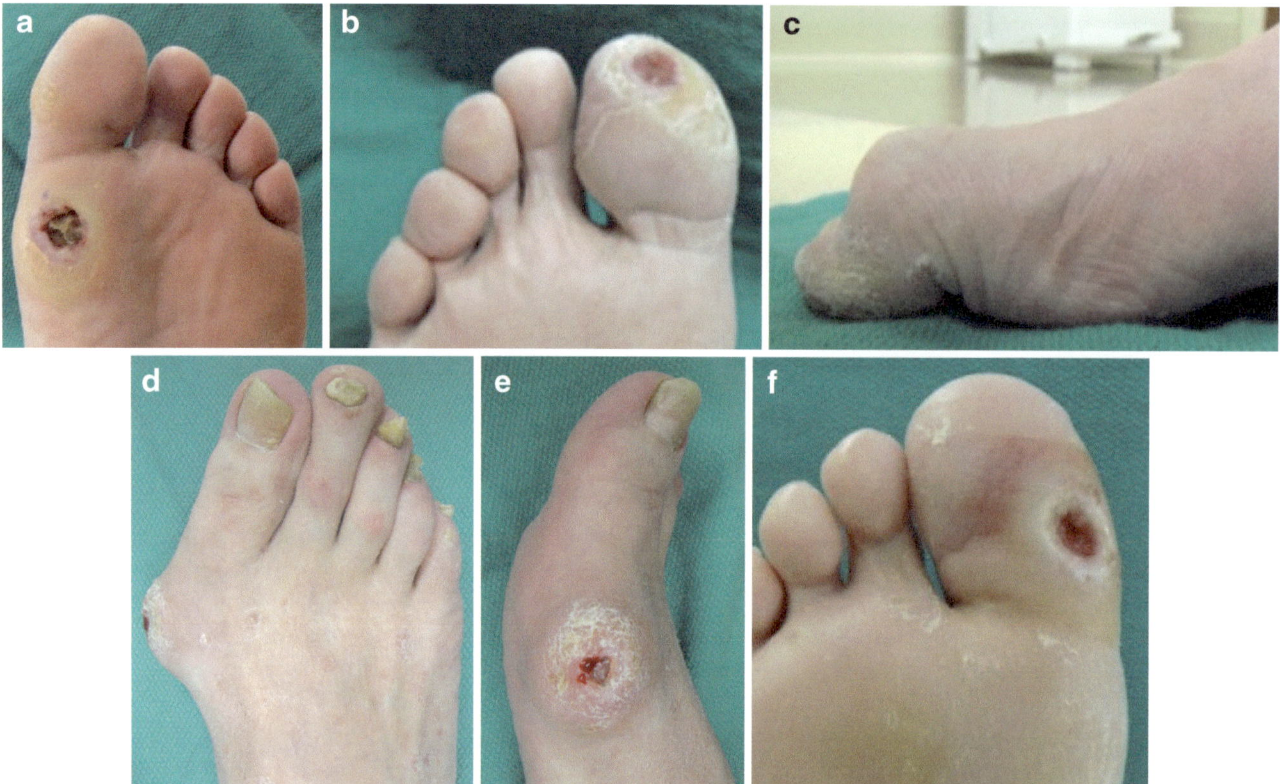

Fig. 15.1 First ray osteomyelitis is most commonly associated with contiguous spread of infection from adjacent neuropathic ulcers. Neuropathic ulcers are classically located over points of boney prominence or excessive pressure including (**a**) the plantar aspect of the first metatarsal head and sesamoids, (**b**, **c**) distally at the tip of the first toe or dorsally over the first interphalangeal joint associated with hallux hammertoe, (**d**, **e**) along the medial first metatarsal head associated with hallux valgus, and (**f**) plantar to the first interphalangeal joint associated with hallux rigidus, hallux valgus, or hallux interphalangeus

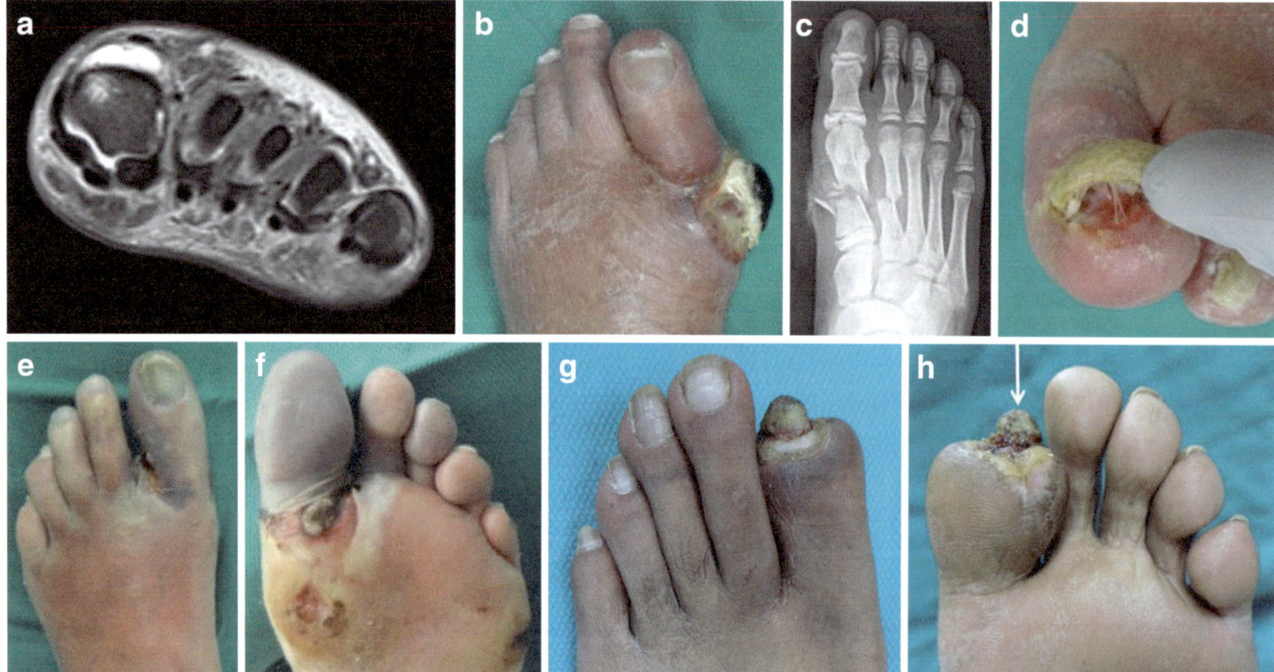

Fig. 15.2 Non-neuropathic ulcer related first ray osteomyelitis. (**a**) First ray osteomyelitis is rarely associated with hematogenous osteomyelitis although the first metatarsal phalangeal joint can develop hematogenous joint sepsis with secondary adjacent osteomyelitis seen here on MRI. (**b**) Ulcerated tophaceous gout commonly leads to contiguous spread of infection. (**c**) Direct inoculation may occur through puncture wound or open fractures. (**d**) Toenail-related infections and nail bed wounds can lead to osteomyelitis of the distal phalanx. (**e**, **f**) Infected gangrene commonly results in osteomyelitis. (**g**, **h**) Autoamputation of full thickness dry gangrene will commonly lead to bone exposure and secondary osteomyelitis (note exposed bone at tip of *arrow*)

amputation [6, 7]. Reconstructive podiatric procedures are oftentimes appropriate for nonhealing wounds with suspected osteomyelitis provided that surgery is performed early while the local soft tissues remain viable. Reconstructive approaches commonly involve limited bone resection which allows early bone biopsy and creates laxity in the tissue allowing use of a rotational flap to close the wound. Amputation is more likely in the setting of tissue necrosis, extensive bone infection, severe deformity, and failed prior procedures. This may be the consequence of waiting too long to address a seemingly stable first ray ulcer. Amputation may be prevented by an early decision to pursue elective surgical treatment after a reasonable period of conservative wound management has been unsuccessful due to underlying mechanical issues. The surgeon ultimately needs to decide what is best for an individual patient based on his or her unique set of circumstances.

The extent and location of both the wound and the osteomyelitis are important factors when selecting the ideal surgical treatment plan. The bone immediately adjacent to the ulcer is most prone to contiguous spread of infection. Neuropathic ulcers frequently develop over joints which predisposes to infection from contiguous spread to one or both of the adjacent bones. Common first ray wound locations include the tip of the hallux, the dorsal IPJ, the plantar IPJ, the medial MPJ, and the plantar MPJ. Figure 15.3 is a flowchart of common first ray surgical treatment pathways based on location of the wound and expectation of osteomyelitis based on clinical, laboratory, and radiographic workup. Elective procedure pathways are also provided for nonhealing wounds with low likelihood of bone infection or early and localized osteomyelitis. Early intervention with elective, reconstructive wound surgery provides bone biopsy and may allow resolution of the wound prior to the onset of osteomyelitis. Short first ray resection near the metatarsal base has a significant impact on foot stability, medial column function, and second ray overload. Resection near the base may also add risk for future conversion to transmetatarsal amputation (TMA) and is avoided when possible. Procedure and patient selection criteria including surgical technique and staging pearls are detailed below.

Reconstructive Procedures

Hallux Hammertoe Procedures

Hallux hammertoe deformity is frequently associated with tip-of-toe ulcers, dorsal IPJ ulcers, and plantar MPJ ulcers. It is reasonable to pursue elective hammertoe surgery in an attempt to address the underlying structural deformity before osteomyelitis develops, which puts the toe at risk for amputation. The open wound would ideally be healed prior to elective surgery, but this is not always practical as deformity

correction may be necessary to resolve the wound. Hallux hammertoe repair typically consists of flexor hallucis longus (FHL) tenotomy, IPJ fusion, or IPJ arthroplasty. Extensor hallucis longus (EHL) lengthening or transfer to the first metatarsal head is added if the EHL is a contributing deforming force. Ideal procedure selection depends on the flexibility of IPJ and MPJ deformity, location and depth of the ulcer, and suspicion for osteomyelitis. Elective surgery frequently allows procurement of bone for biopsy and primary or flap closure of the wound. The simplest approach is an office-based FHL tenotomy which is indicated for reducible IPJ contracture without bone or soft tissue infection, as shown in case 1 (Figs. 15.4, 15.5, 15.6, and 15.7). This ambulatory procedure is highly amenable to the office setting in patients with neuropathy, and there is no need to hold anticoagulation therapy as bleeding is minimal. Immediate weight bearing is preferred to promote stretch after tendon and joint release. Deep and complicated tip-of-toe ulceration is often best treated with hallux distal Symes amputation as described later.

Rigid deformity of the IPJ is generally treated with joint fusion or arthroplasty (Fig. 15.8). Interphalangeal joint fusion requires internal fixation or pin fixation which is less practical in patients with open wounds or suspected osteomyelitis. If uncomplicated wounds can be healed preoperatively and the risk of osteomyelitis is low, elective hallux fusion is preferred. This approach leads to a more stable and functional toe. A staged approach is also possible with initial FHL tenotomy followed by delayed fusion once the distal ulcer heals.

Hallux IPJ Arthroplasty with Unilobed Rotational Plantar Flap

A primary indication for hallux IPJ arthroplasty is a nonhealing IPJ plantar ulceration with suspected or imminent osteomyelitis within the head of the proximal phalanx, as demonstrated in case 2 (Figs. 15.9, 15.10, 15.11, 15.12, 15.13, 15.14, 15.15, 15.16, 15.17, 15.18, and 15.19). We commonly incorporate a unilobed flap with or without a secondary dorsal incision for bone resection [8]. A dorsal incision is helpful when patients present with cellulitis and inflammation on the dorsum of the hallux despite the wound being plantar as these clinical signs likely indicate violation of the joint capsule. Since infection most commonly spreads from an area of higher pressure (plantar foot) to an area of lower pressure (dorsal foot), the spread of infection to the dorsum of the foot is common once the joint capsule is compromised [9]. A course of conservative wound treatment is warranted but often ineffective for IPJ ulcer treatment due to abnormal biomechanical forces. Surgical intervention would ideally be implemented before cellulitis or osteomyelitis develops, but a staged approach is common with acute infection.

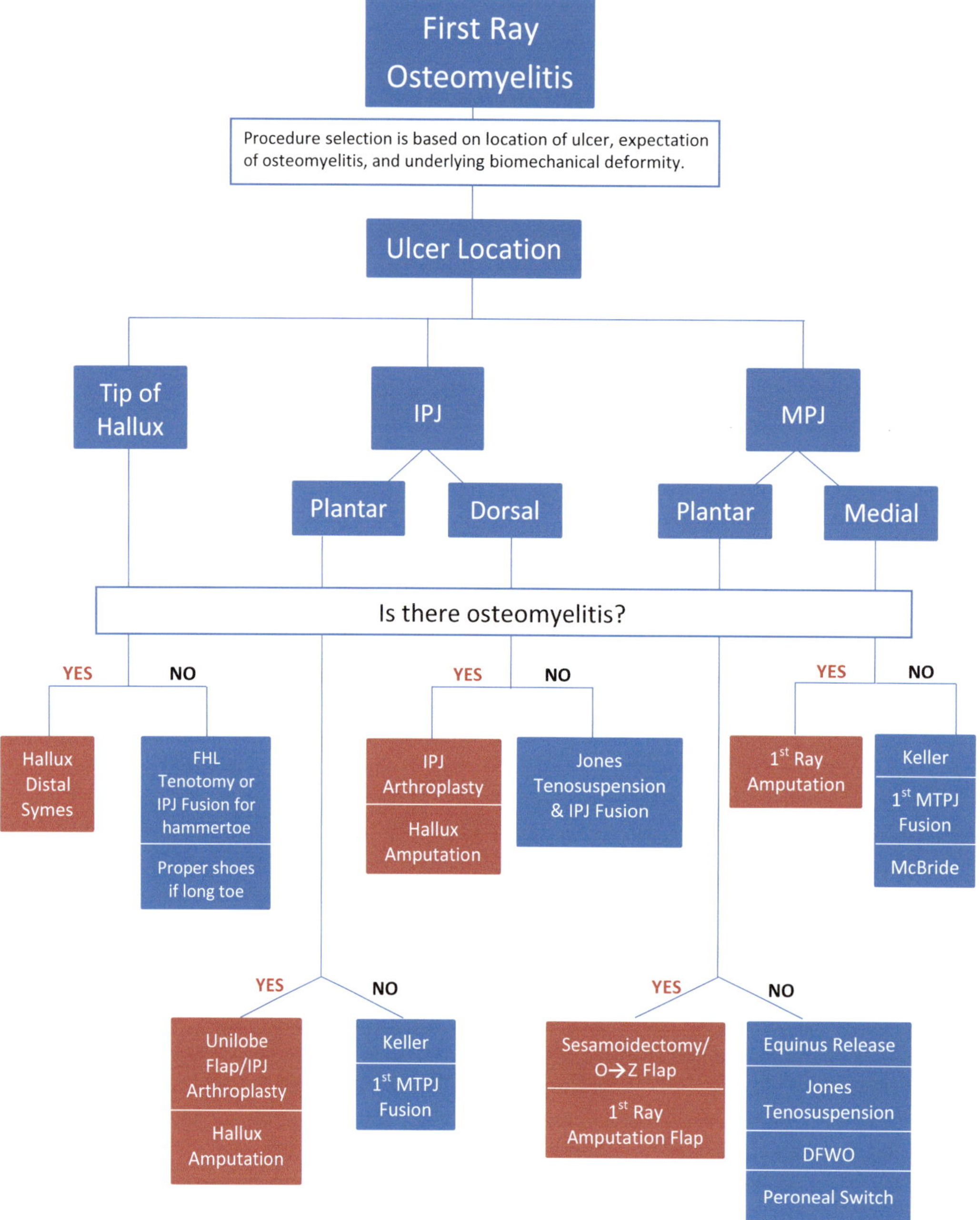

Fig. 15.3 Procedure selection flowchart for first ray osteomyelitis. This flowchart outlines common first ray surgical treatment pathways based on location of the wound, expectation of osteomyelitis, and underlying biomechanical deformity. Elective procedure pathways are also provided for nonhealing wounds with low likelihood of bone infection or early and localized osteomyelitis. The ideal procedure for a given patient should address abnormal mechanics and structural deformities yet minimize the potential for transfer ulcers

The benefits of this digital salvage procedure include complete ulcer excision, early bone resection and biopsy, flap coverage with viable soft tissue, and offloading of mechanical pressure at the plantar hallux IPJ. Care is taken to select patients with adequate MPJ dorsiflexion and healthy surrounding soft tissue which is more likely with early intervention before the onset of extensive soft tissue or bone infection. Clinical exam of patients with ulcers at the plantar IPJ location commonly identifies hyperextension of the IPJ associated with functional hallux limitus. Plantar IPJ bone prominence is also common along with ankle equinus deformity. A weight bearing stress dorsiflexion lateral hallux view is helpful to assess for functional MPJ range of motion [10]. Standard weight bearing X-rays are also useful to evaluate for osteomyelitis, a prominent plantar IPJ sesamoid, or other causes of excessive plantar pressure at the IPJ. MRI may also

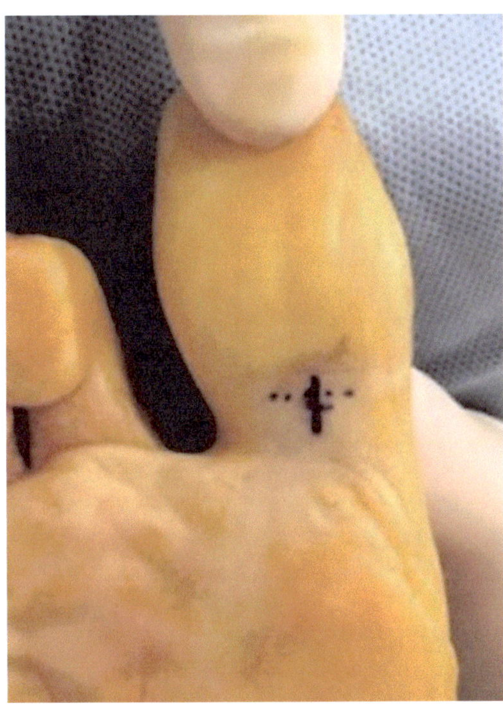

Fig. 15.4 Case 1: Tip-of-toe hallux ulceration associated with hammertoe contracture. (**a**, **b**) A contracted first toe placed substantial pressure at the tip of the toe where the distal phalanx is fairly superficial. Neuropathic ulcers related to hammertoe deformity tend to become chronic and eventually deepen which results in osteomyelitis and loss of the toe. Early intervention to address the deformity may allow prompt wound healing and preservation of the digit. Consideration was given to interphalangeal joint arthroplasty or fusion although FHL tendon release was performed since the contracture was flexible. Reconstructive procedures are best performed prior to the onset of osteomyelitis or soft tissue infection. A course of orthotic treatment and wound care is reasonable, but significant deformity may be best treated with surgery. Note that longer shoes do not solve ulcers caused by hammertoe contracture and tenotomy may make the toe longer

Fig. 15.5 Flexor hallucis longus tenotomy was performed through a percutaneous plantar incision in case 1. The plantar incision was placed approximately mid-proximal phalanx where the FHL tendon (*linear line*) is subcutaneous, narrow, and easily accessible. A more distal IPJ incision is possible, but the tendon widens at the insertion point on the base of the distal phalanx. The transverse incision (*dotted line*) was within the skin lines which healed within 1 week and no suture was required

thus does not preserve digital function or cosmetic appearance. A Schrudde Type 1 unilobed rotational flap design is used with the size of the flap being approximately 75 % of the total soft tissue defect after wound excision (Fig. 15.11c) [11]. This is typically a single-stage outpatient procedure that is performed supine without the use of a tourniquet. Staged surgery is possible with initial excision of the wound followed by debridement and biopsy of the proximal phalanx. Final bone resection and delayed flap closure of the wound is performed once cellulitis and abscess resolve. Persistent infection despite initial bone resection could always be converted to hallux amputation, especially if the soft tissues remain compromised by infection or poor circulation. Staged surgery also allows time for vascular intervention if indicated.

Sesamoidectomy with O-to-Z Flap or Bilobed Flap Closure of Plantar MPJ Ulceration

Plantar first MPJ ulcers are difficult to heal due to significant stress applied during gait. This stress is amplified in patients with diabetic peripheral neuropathy combined with certain biomechanical alterations that contribute to plantar MPJ ulcer formation. A recent study found that diabetics with peripheral neuropathy and foot ulcer formation demonstrated a significantly lower range of motion at the hips, knees, ankles, and first MPJ compared to diabetics without ulcer formation [12]. Previous studies have shown abnormally high pressure under the metatarsal heads in diabetic patients with peripheral neuropathy. Patry also reported that forefoot pressure was 2.3 times higher than rearfoot pressure in those patients [13]. These findings help explain why ulcers at this location are common and difficult to heal with propensity to progress to the point of osteomyelitis.

help determine the extent of osteomyelitis to assess whether the toe is amenable to IPJ arthroplasty. If osteomyelitis extends throughout the entire proximal phalanx or both the proximal and distal phalanges, hallux amputation may be a better option. Excessive bone debridement for necrosis or digital deformity causes instability of the tip of the toe and

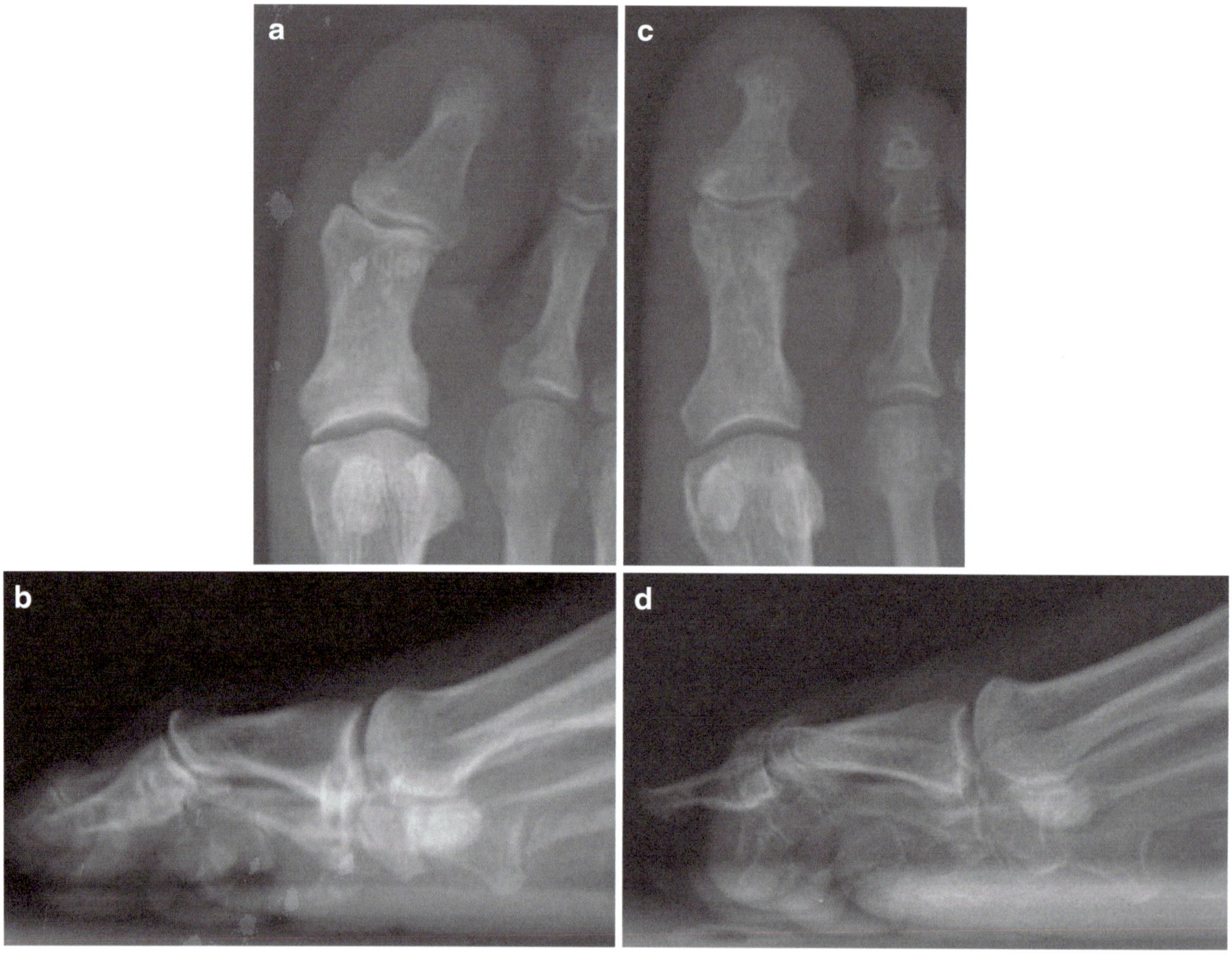

Fig. 15.6 Preoperative and post-FHL tenotomy radiographs involving tip of hallux ulceration in case 1. (**a, b**) Preoperative AP and lateral weight bearing radiographs show contracture deformity at the hallux interphalangeal joint (IPJ). No signs of osteomyelitis were seen at the tip of the distal phalanx. (**c, d**) Postoperative AP and lateral weight bearing radiographs show fairly normal positioning of the IPJ with pressure now applied to the plantar digital pulp which is well padded

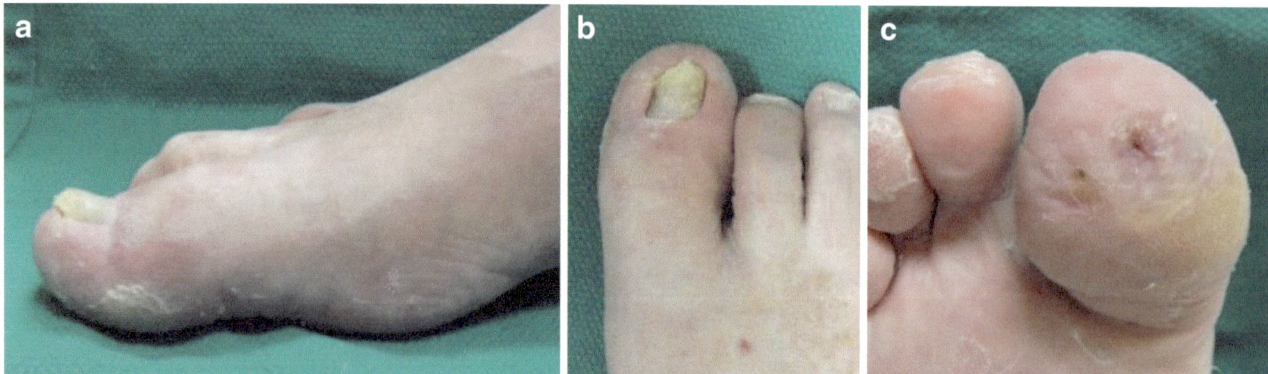

Fig. 15.7 Clinical appearance 4 weeks after flexor hallucis longus tenotomy in case 1. (**a, b**) Weight bearing clinical photos show a straight first toe that no longer placed pressure on the distal tip of the hallux. Note that the second toe had contracted slightly which is commonly seen and thought to be related to interconnection between the flexor hallucis longus and flexor digitorum longus at the master knot of Henry. Prophylactic lengthening of the second toe is common to avoid transfer lesions. (**c**) The tip of the toe hallux ulcer was nearly healed at 4 weeks postoperatively despite full weight bearing which helped to stretch the lengthened tendon

Fig. 15.8 Hallux IPJ fusion or arthroplasty for hallux hammertoe deformity. (**a**, **b**) Joint fusion requires internal fixation or percutaneous pins, which is not always practical in patients with complicated wounds or suspected osteomyelitis. Uncomplicated wounds can oftentimes be healed preoperatively allowing successful fusion. Infection can also be ruled out preoperatively with bone biopsy or advanced imaging including bone scan or MRI. (**c**) Hallux IPJ arthroplasty involves removal of the head of the proximal phalanx. This releases contracted soft tissues to reduce pressure dorsal, plantar, or medially at the IPJ and at the tip of the toe

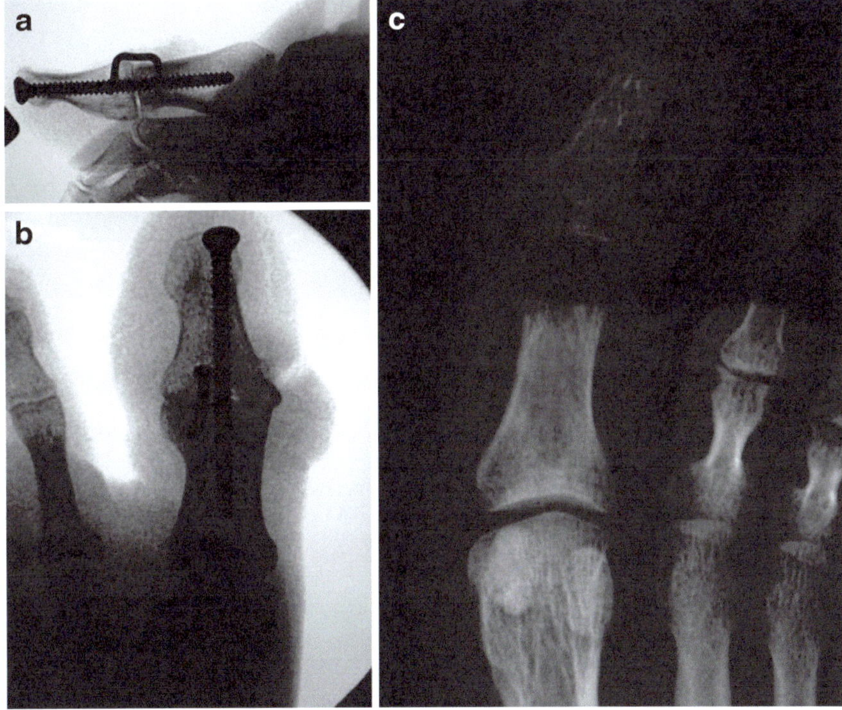

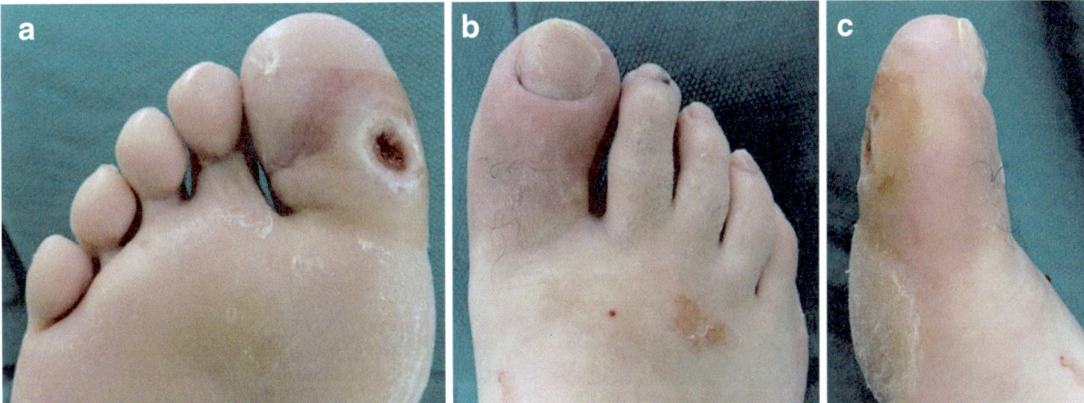

Fig. 15.9 Case 2: Hallux IPJ plantar ulcer. (**a**) A typical nonhealing plantar medial hallux IPJ neuropathic ulcer is shown. (**b**, **c**) Slight valgus deformity of the toe and functional hallux limitus contributed to excessive pressure and wound formation. Note low-grade, but persistent, erythema to the dorsal IPJ area despite the plantar wound location raising suspicion for joint infection and osteomyelitis

Chronic wounds under the first MPJ frequently develop osteomyelitis of the sesamoid bones prior to extension of infection into the MPJ and the adjacent metatarsal and proximal phalanx (Fig. 15.20). Early surgical intervention with sesamoidectomy for nonhealing or recurrent wounds can be effective to avoid partial first ray amputation which is often necessary once the joint becomes exposed. The procedure is most effective when performed early before the onset of soft tissue infection. Our typical approach is to employ standard wound healing measures until the point when the wound probes to bone, which is the primary indication for surgery. It is important to evaluate patients with chronic or recurrent plantar first MPJ ulcers for related deformities including ankle equinus, plantar displacement of the first metatarsal, or hallux hammertoe contracture. These deformities can be addressed surgically prior to onset of infection.

The O-to-Z flap, outlined in case 3 (Figs. 15.20, 15.21, 15.22, and 15.23), and the bilobed flap, shown in case 4 (Fig. 15.24), both allow complete excision of the ulcer, widespread access to the plantar joint structures for bone resection, and immediate soft tissue coverage with viable tissue. Flap closure of the wound is a key component of this semi-elective procedure because persistent postoperative exposure of the metatarsal head is undesirable.

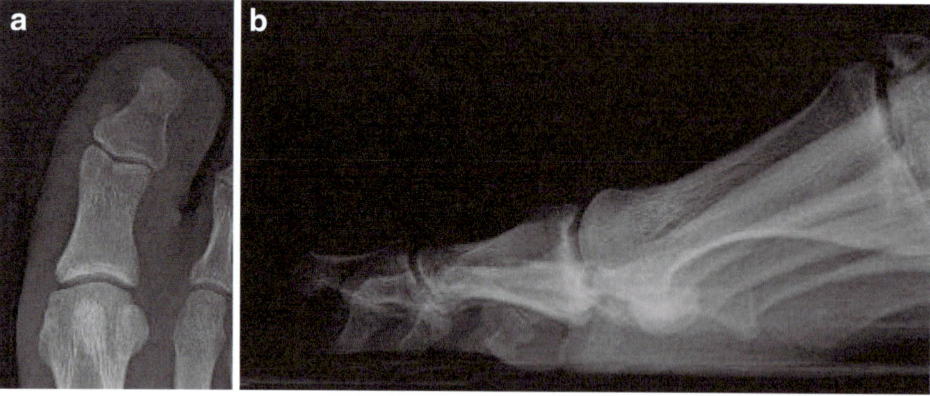

Fig. 15.10 Preoperative imaging in case 2. (**a, b**) X-rays were fairly unremarkable with the exception of lateral deformity at the IPJ. Radiographic changes consistent with osteomyelitis are a relatively delayed finding. Early diagnosis of osteomyelitis requires clinical suspicion based on the nonhealing nature of the wound, local soft tissue infection, positive probe to bone, laboratory workup including infection marker labs, and advanced imaging. X-rays are useful to evaluate for structural deformity such as hallux interphalangeus, interphalangeal joint sesamoid bone, hallux limitus, hallux valgus, bone spurs, malaligned fractures, and degenerative joint disease. Early radiographs also serve as a baseline for later comparison

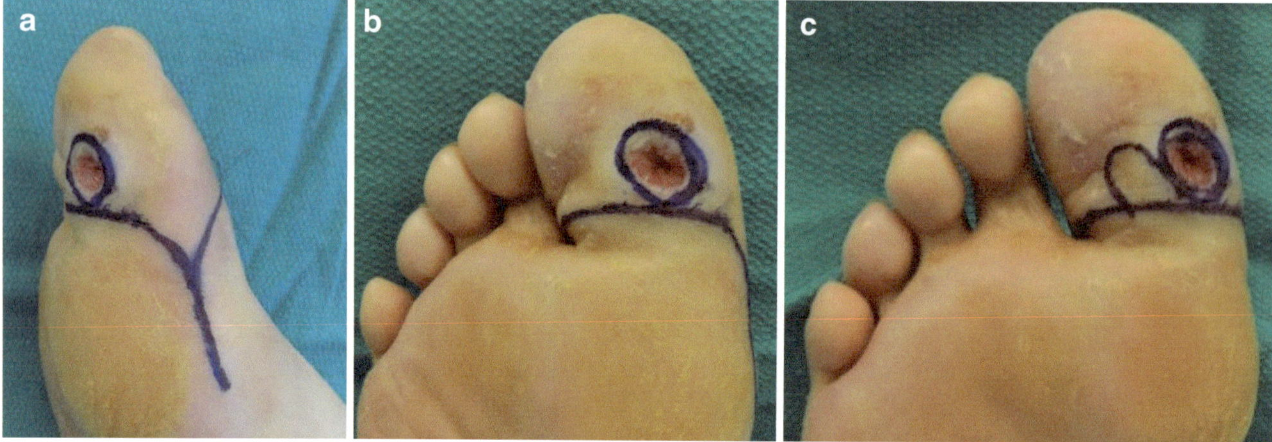

Fig. 15.11 Incision plan for hallux IPJ arthroplasty and unilobed rotational flap in case 2. (**a, b**) The incision for hallux amputation was drawn prior to making the flap incision. This ensures that the flap donor site does not compromise later conversion to hallux amputation as this is the fallback procedure depending on intraoperative findings or postoperative healing process. (**c**) The unilobed flap was then drawn lateral to the plantar medial IPJ ulcer. The length and width of the flap should roughly match the size of the wound defect left after excision of the ulcer but can be approximately 25 % smaller in both dimensions due to secondary movement of the surrounding tissues upon flap rotation and closure of the donor site

Hallux Amputation Procedures

Hallux amputation traditionally involves disarticulation at the first MPJ which remains the primary technique, especially for extensive osteomyelitis of the proximal phalanx or localized soft tissue gangrene or infection. Timely removal of the hallux under these conditions eliminates the source of infection which allows prompt recovery of an acutely ill patient and stabilization of the more proximal tissues. The immediate goal of complete hallux amputation is to preserve the weight bearing function of the first metatarsal head although open amputation is commonly performed as stage 1 surgery with the intent to convert to first ray amputation once the soft tissue infection is under control.

Localized phalangeal osteomyelitis associated with viable digital soft tissues creates an opportunity to preserve partial function of the proximal phalanx with partial hallux amputation. The hallux distal Symes amputation procedure preserves a reasonably normal toe appearance and post-op function which is primarily indicated for wound complications associated with hammertoe deformity or an elongated first toe. These structural abnormalities typically lead to ulceration at the tip of the toe which commonly results in osteomyelitis of the distal phalanx. The hallux distal Symes amputation procedure allows resection and biopsy of the infected distal phalanx, margin biopsy of the proximal phalanx, and correction of underlying toe deformity. Partial hallux amputation through the middle of the proximal phalanx is appropriate for ulcers at or distal to the IPJ. Partial hallux amputation avoids exposure of the first metatarsal head in an effort to limit the risk of cross contamination. This procedure also maintains the intrinsic flexor and extensor attachments important for normal first ray function and prevents proximal migration of the sesamoid apparatus in an effort to minimize the risk of transfer ulcers at the second MPJ. The downside of preserving a portion of the proximal phalanx is re-ulceration at the digital stump which is most likely to occur in situations where preexisting hallux equinus and plantarflexed positioning of the first MPJ creates ongoing plantar pressure points.

Hallux Distal Symes Amputation

Tip-of-toe distal hallux ulcers often become complicated with osteomyelitis that is localized to the distal phalanx (Fig. 15.25). This is seen in patients with hallux malleus or hallux hammertoe deformity. When osteomyelitis is contained within the distal phalanx, the hallux distal Symes amputation procedure is a viable surgical option that allows removal of infected bone, correction of digital deformity, excision of the ulcer, and removal of the often deformed toenail. This procedure also maintains digital length for improved cosmesis and preservation of first ray function.

Case 5 demonstrates how the hallux distal Symes technique was utilized to treat osteomyelitis associated with an infected ischemic ulcer on the medial tip of the hallux (Figs. 15.26, 15.27, 15.28, 15.29, 15.30, 15.31, 15.32, and 15.33). Stage 1 of the procedure was an in-office incision and drainage procedure which included bone biopsy confirming osteomyelitis of the distal phalanx bone. The patient returned 1 week later after outpatient vascular intervention with complete wound bed necrosis indicating the need for partial toe amputation. Staged surgery allowed resolution of cellulitis prior to definitive surgery. Stage 2 was then completed with resection of the distal phalanx, remodeling of the proximal phalanx, and wound closure.

Partial Hallux Amputation

Partial hallux amputation through the middle of the proximal phalanx is an alternative for tip-of-toe gangrene or ulcers at or distal to the IPJ, as shown in case 6 (Fig. 15.34). The extent of osteomyelitis within the proximal phalanx, the size and location of the wound, and the condition of the surrounding soft tissues largely determine the level of amputation.

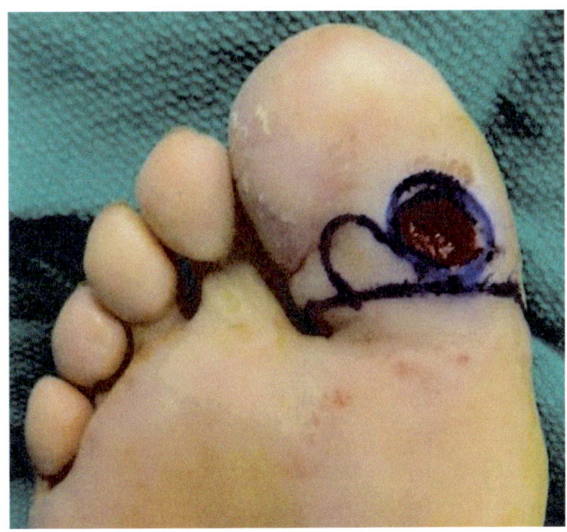

Fig. 15.12 Wound excision technique in case 2. The wound was excised full depth with a no-touch technique. The flexor hallucis longus tendon is preserved if it appears healthy and functional. Gloves were changed at this point and the wound was re-prepped prior to raising the flap

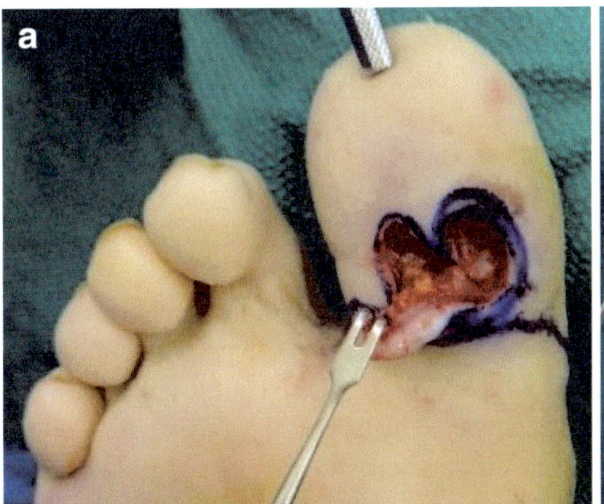
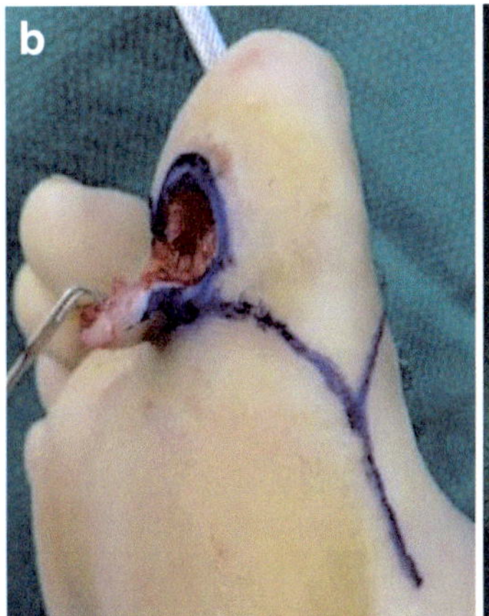
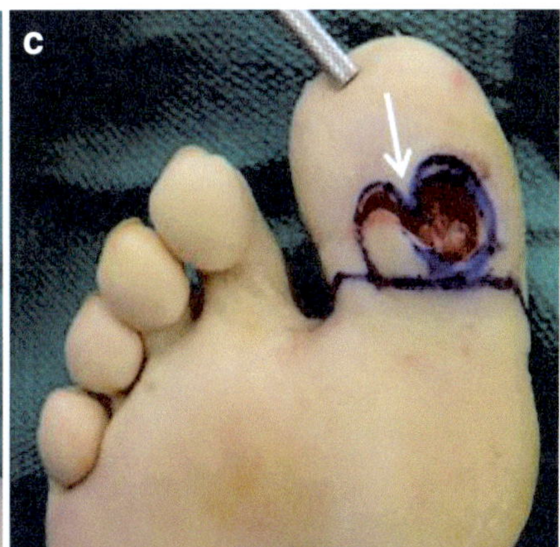

Fig. 15.13 Raising the unilobe flap in case 2. (**a**, **b**) The flap is incised and raised full thickness using a skin hook for a no-touch technique. (**c**) It is important to preserve the central frenulum (*arrow*) as this will help with closure of the flap donor site. Bone resection can be performed through the plantar wound, but a secondary dorsal approach is common with smaller flaps

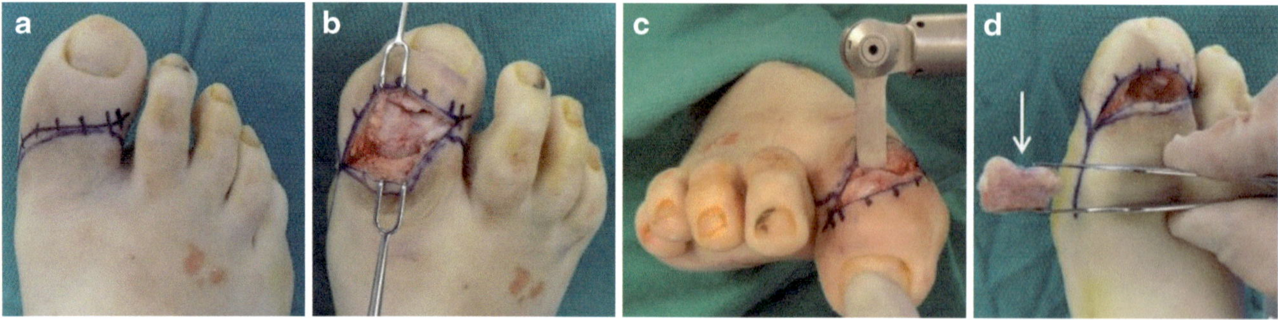

Fig. 15.14 IPJ arthroplasty through a secondary dorsal incision in case 2. (**a**) A lazy S-type transverse dorsal incision was made over the IPJ. Note how the incision did not compromise the dorsal flap should conversion to toe amputation becomes necessary. (**b**) The EHL tendon was cut transversely and repaired after bone resection. (**c**) A sagittal saw was utilized for bone resection, and (**d**) the head of the proximal phalanx (*arrow*) was removed

Fig. 15.15 Intraoperative imaging to confirm adequate bone resection in case 2. (**a**, **b**) Intraoperative imaging is helpful to ensure adequate resection proximal to the metaphyseal flare on the proximal phalanx. Inadequate bone resection increases the risk of re-ulceration, especially if the plantar flare remains. Excessive bone resection leads to instability and loss of function of the distal toe

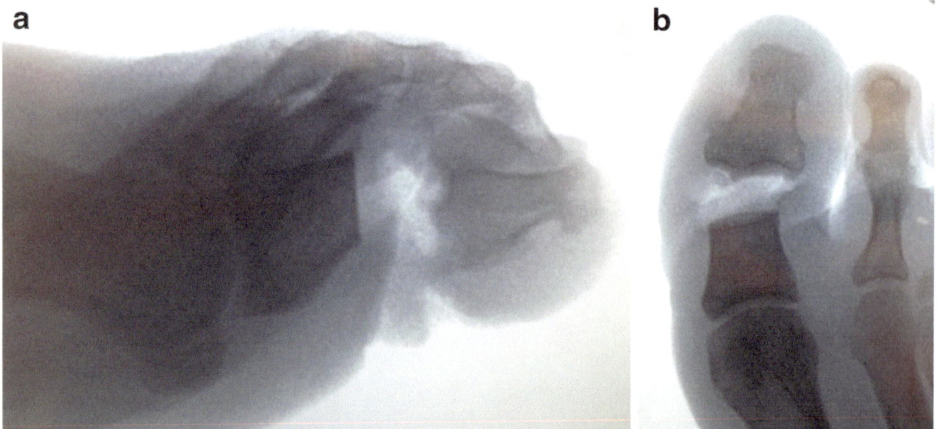

These factors also dictate whether or not reconstructive toe sparing techniques including IPJ arthroplasty are possible. The goals of preserving the base of the proximal phalanx are to avoid exposure of the metatarsal head and maintain function of the sesamoids. Figure 15.35 highlights the advantage of using a bone saw versus other instrumentation when performing amputation. A jagged edge at the amputation stump increases the likelihood of persistent pressure points and recurrent ulceration.

Complete Hallux Amputation with First MPJ Disarticulation

Complete amputation of the hallux is common as the typical clinical presentation of infected hallux wounds frequently requires wide resection of the toe. This decision is often due to the poor condition of the soft tissues including extensive ulceration or necrosis from abscess or gangrene. Deformity at the MPJ is also a major factor leading to the decision for MPJ disarticulation including hallux limitus, hallux valgus, and hallux hammertoe. There is no benefit to preserving a portion of the proximal phalanx if MPJ deformity is contributing to hallux ulceration.

Complete hallux amputation is largely an alternative to partial first ray amputation with the intent to preserve the metatarsal head. There is debate among surgeons regarding the ideal level of amputation to avoid transfer ulcers. It is important to consider that no level of foot amputation is definitive and ulcer recurrence is possible whether the metatarsal head is left intact or not. Borkosky et al. systematically reviewed the literature regarding the re-ulceration incidence following partial first ray amputation in diabetic patients [6]. The initial amputation level along the first ray varied from the base of the proximal phalanx to the base of the first metatarsal. They found an overall reamputation rate of 19.8 % (86/435). They concluded that 1 out of 5 patients undergoing a partial first ray amputation will require a more proximal amputation. We prefer to preserve the first metatarsal head when not infected as demonstrated in Fig. 15.36. This approach requires that the surrounding tissues allow primary closure over the metatarsal head. First MPJ disarticulation

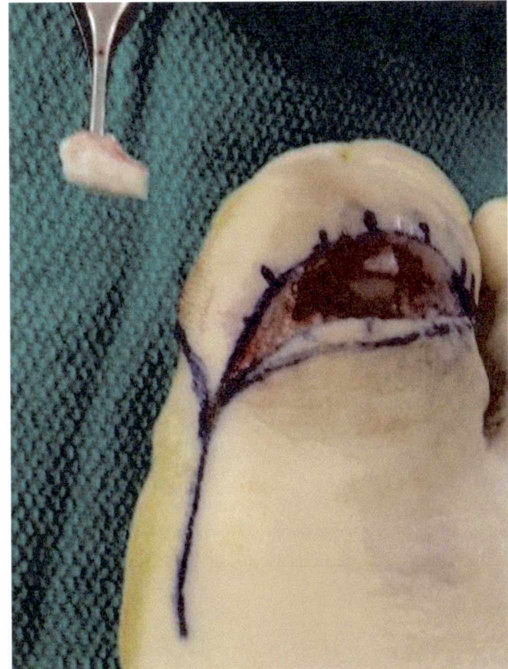

Fig. 15.16 Removal of the IPJ sesamoid bone in case 2. An IPJ sesamoid bone is almost always located beneath the head of the proximal phalanx at the IPJ which likely contributes to plantar prominence. This may or may not be visible on X-ray depending on imaging technique and degree of ossification. The IPJ sesamoid was resected, taking care not to disrupt the long flexor tendon

also retains function of the sesamoids, preserves functional length of the medial column, and improves cosmetic appearance of the foot. Our preference is to leave the metatarsal cartilage intact when performing complete hallux amputation in an effort to minimize the chance of cross contamination of infection to the metatarsal head.

First Ray Amputation Procedures

First ray amputation is ideally contained at the distal neck of the metatarsal in an effort to preserve function and stability of the medial column. Osteomyelitis of the first metatarsal often necessitates partial amputation of the first ray which involves hallux amputation, first metatarsal head resection, and removal of the sesamoids. When addressing osteomyelitis of the first metatarsal, the hallux is typically sacrificed to aid in soft tissue closure, but more often the digit is removed due to lack of function once the first metatarsal head is resected. Osteomyelitis and gangrene of the hallux are also commonly treated with first ray amputation since metatarsal head resection allows primary closure in the event that the digital soft tissues are compromised.

Beyond the location and extent of osteomyelitis, ulcer size and location are paramount when deciding on the ideal incisional approach. The traditional first ray amputation

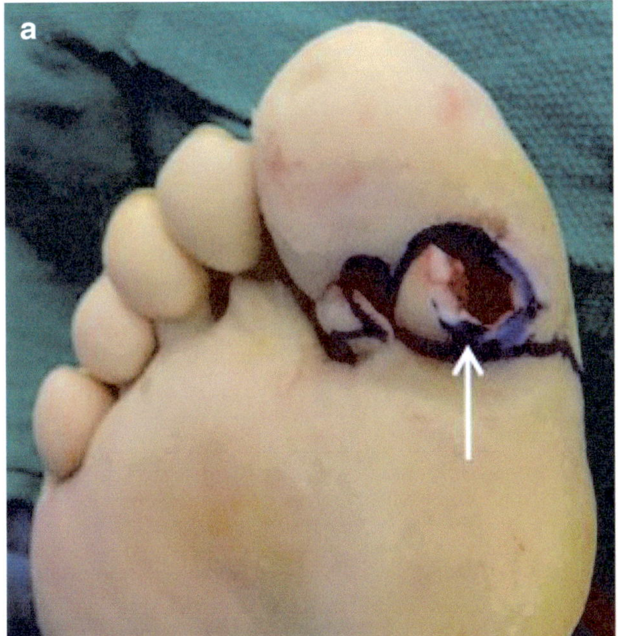
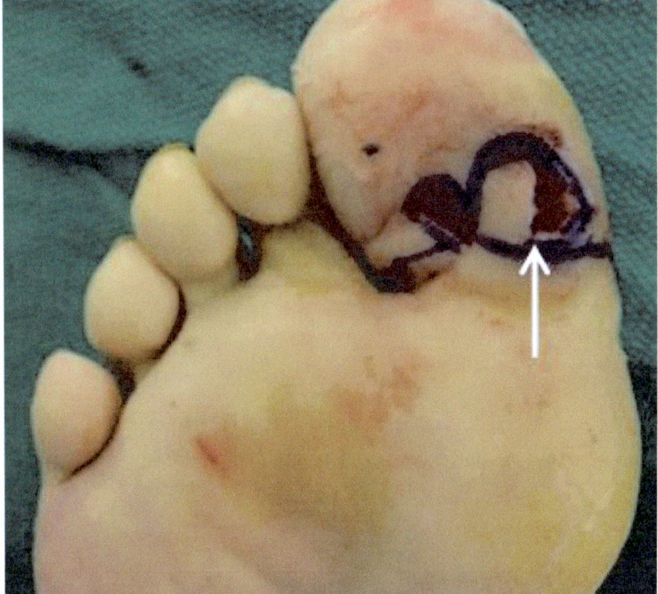

Fig. 15.17 Rotation of the unilobed flap into wound defect in case 2. (**a**) Using a minimal touch technique, the unilobe flap was rotated medially into the wound defect. Note that a curved point of rotation creates a dog ear (*arrow*). (**b**) The flap rotated without creating a dog ear after the point of rotation (*arrow*) was converted to a 90° angle

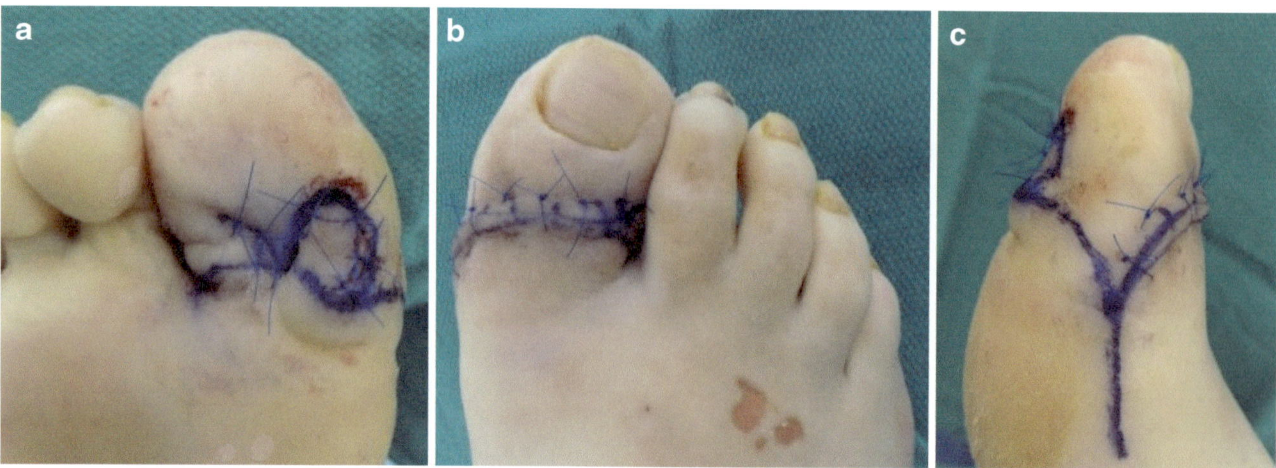

Fig. 15.18 Unilobed rotational flap closure in case 2. (**a–c**) The plantar flap, donor site, and dorsal incisions were closed with simple interrupted sutures. Dorsal sutures are removed at 2 weeks, but plantar sutures are typically removed at 4–6 weeks depending on healing

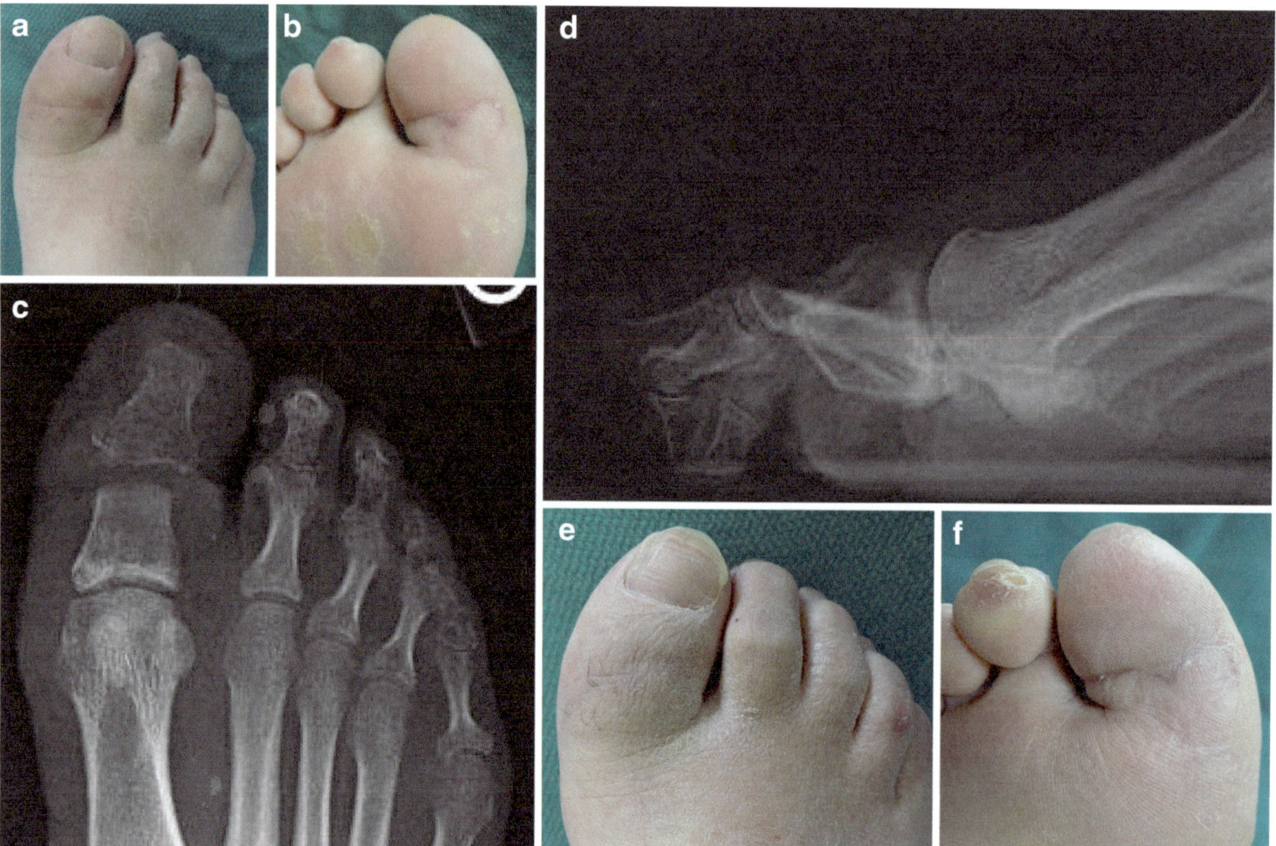

Fig. 15.19 Postoperative results after IPJ arthroplasty and unilobed rotational flap in case 2. (**a, b**) Ten week postoperative clinical presentation and (**c, d**) X-rays with apparent resolution of osteomyelitis and chronic ulceration based on clinical, laboratory, and radiographic evaluation. Osteomyelitis was confirmed on microbiologic and pathologic biopsy, but no clean margin was taken. Inflammatory marker labs had returned to normal. Concomitant gastrocnemius recession was performed to reduce the risk of recurrent ulceration. (**e, f**) Six-month postoperative clinical presentation

technique using dorsal and plantar flaps is appropriate when the ulcer is located near the IPJ or medially at the level of the first MPJ. Medial ulceration is often found with concomitant hallux valgus deformity. The standard incision approach can also be considered when dealing with partial thickness ulcers plantar to the MPJ, which may heal secondarily upon removal of any underlying bony prominence through a medial approach. We commonly incorporate advanced incision techniques including rotational flaps for full thickness wounds at the plantar aspect of the first MPJ.

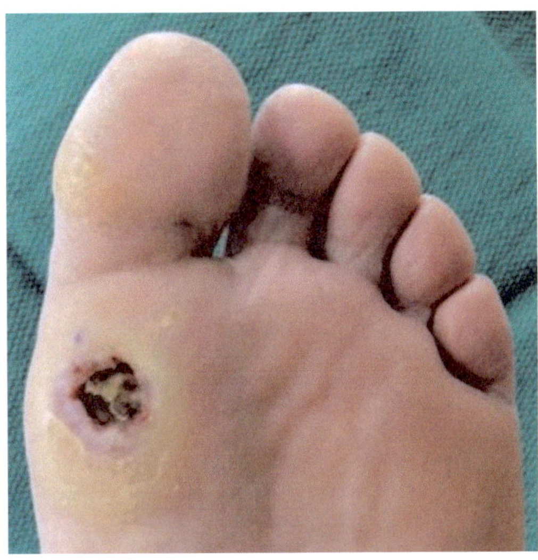

Fig. 15.20 Case 3: Chronic full thickness plantar neuropathic ulceration at the first metatarsophalangeal joint. Nonhealing neuropathic ulcers of the first metatarsophalangeal joint (MPJ) with persistent sesamoid bone exposure commonly results in osteomyelitis of the sesamoids, first metatarsal, or proximal phalanx. First MPJ joint sepsis is also a common sequela. Removal of the sesamoids is possible; however, this size and location of wound defect is not very amenable to primary wound closure. Leaving the plantar metatarsal head exposed after sesamoid excision will almost certainly result in bone or joint infection. Note poor quality tissue at the base of the wound. Probe to bone test was positive

Traditional Partial First Ray Amputation Technique

The traditional first ray amputation technique is outlined in case 7 (Figs. 15.37, 15.38, 15.39, 15.40, 15.41, 15.42, 15.43, and 15.44). A medially placed tennis racquet-type incision is used to create dorsal and plantar flaps. The proximal arm of the incision extents to the mid portion of the first metatarsal and is placed midway from dorsal to plantar along the medial side of the foot. The lateral convergence of the incision is deep in the interdigital space at the base of the hallux. This technique allows complete removal of a medial wound centered over the first metatarsal head. A no-touch technique is utilized to minimize contamination. The blade should be oriented at 90° to the skin surface to avoid beveling the incision. The flaps are raised off of the underlying proximal phalanx in a full thickness manner to include periosteum. The hallux is disarticulated at the MPJ and set on the back table for later biopsy. If staged surgery is necessary due to acute infection, retention sutures can hold the dorsal and plantar flaps loosely approximated which provides temporary metatarsal head coverage and maintains flap length. Stage 2 is performed several days later depending on readiness of the soft tissues.

The first metatarsal is cut with a sagittal saw oriented distal dorsal to proximal plantar to minimize any plantar

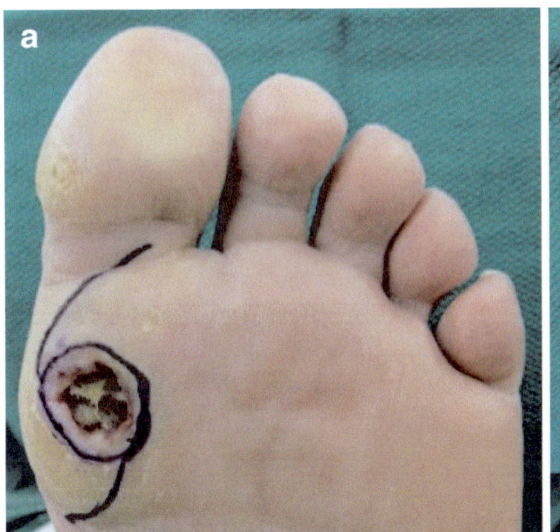
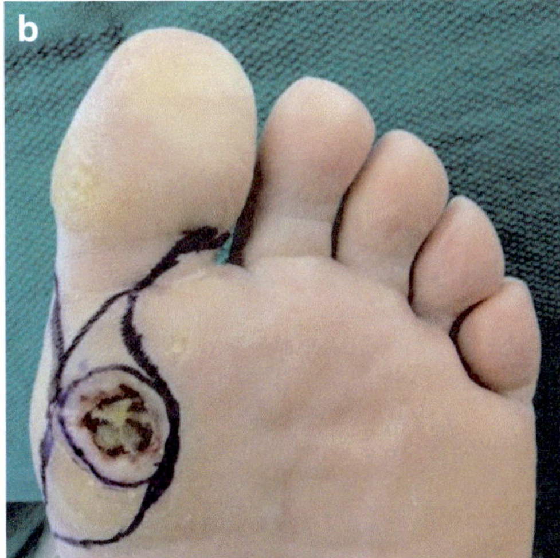
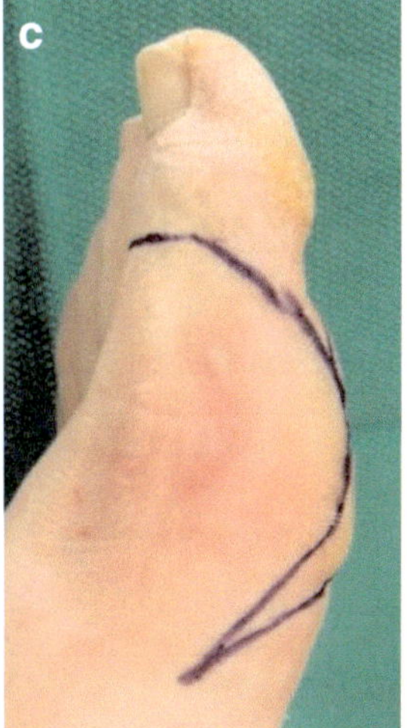

Fig. 15.21 O-to-Z flap for plantar first metatarsal head ulceration in case 3. (**a**) The O-to-Z flap technique (or O to S as shown) allowed complete excision of the ulcer, wide access to the plantar joint structures for removal of the sesamoids, and immediate soft tissue coverage with viable soft tissue. (**b**, **c**) This incision design also allows conversion to first ray amputation with rotational flap closure which is discussed later in case 8. Note that the O-to-Z flaps fall within the tissue excised at the time of amputation

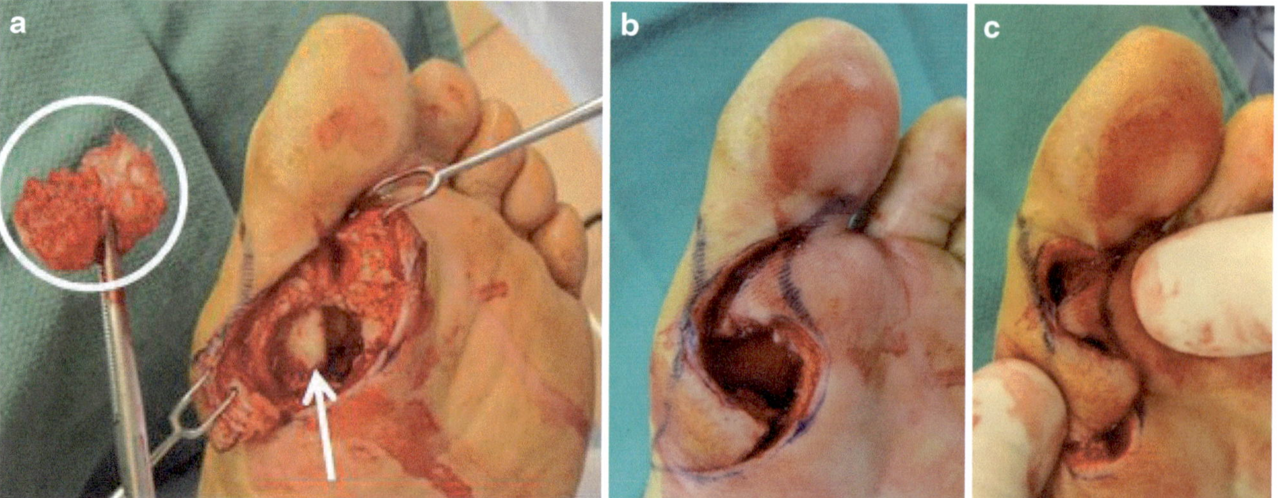

Fig. 15.22 O-to-Z flap with sesamoidectomy surgical technique in case 3. (**a**) The flaps were raised full thickness with careful attention to preserve the long flexor tendon. Raising the flaps provided access to the sesamoids which were removed as one unit (*circle*). Note how the plantar aspect of the metatarsal head was quite prominent after sesamoid removal (*arrow*). (**b**) A bone saw and rongeur were used to remodel the plantar aspect of the metatarsal head in an effort to remove the cartilage, recontour the bone structure, and procure margin biopsy. Bone resection exposed cancellous bone which contributes to the formation of granulation tissue and flap adherence. (**c**) Bone resection also allowed improved mobility of the flaps which are shown here rotated into position

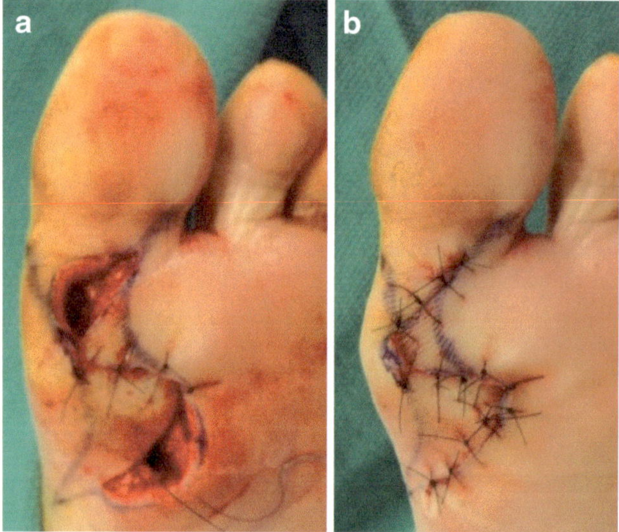

Fig. 15.23 Closure of the O-to-Z flap was performed without tension on the wound in case 3. (**a**) The central arm of the flap was sutured, allowing coverage of the original wound defect. (**b**) The proximal and distal arms of the flap were then closed with simple sutures

There is no functional benefit to partial metatarsal head resection, and this approach seems to predispose to recurrent wound breakdown. The wound is copiously irrigated during and after bone resection in an effort to remove bone debris as heterotopic ossification is common with this procedure [14]. The metatarsal head serves as the primary biopsy specimen if metatarsal osteomyelitis is suspected. The proximal medullary canal is inspected for viability with the hope to find healthy cancellous bone. It is common to see medullary bone that appears liquefied, which may be from infection, but is also common after sawing through osteoporotic bone. The canal can be reamed using a bone curette if there is suspicion for infection and clean margin biopsy can be taken from deep within the canal. We commonly fill the canal with antibiotic beads if performing staged surgery. The medullary canal can also be filled with antibiotic-loaded cement prior to hardening if there is concern that the canal will serve as a harbinger of infection.

The procedure is frequently performed without a tourniquet, but one is being utilized it should be released prior to closure and hemostasis obtained with selective electrocautery. The wound is then closed with or without a drain using simple sutures. Deep sutures are not routinely used.

prominence. The cut is also beveled from medial to lateral in an effort to minimize medial prominence. The resected head of the metatarsal is dissected free with caution to avoid cutting the plantar intermetatarsal artery which runs along the plantar lateral aspect of the metatarsal neck. Imaging confirms the desired level and angle of metatarsal resection. It is the author's preference to perform the osteotomy at the metatarsal neck just proximal to the metaphyseal flare in order to preserve metatarsal length yet avoid bone prominence.

Partial First Ray Amputation with Rotational Flap Closure of a Plantar MPJ Wound

Osteomyelitis of the sesamoids and first metatarsal head associated with plantar first MPJ ulceration may not be amenable to the traditional partial ray amputation incision

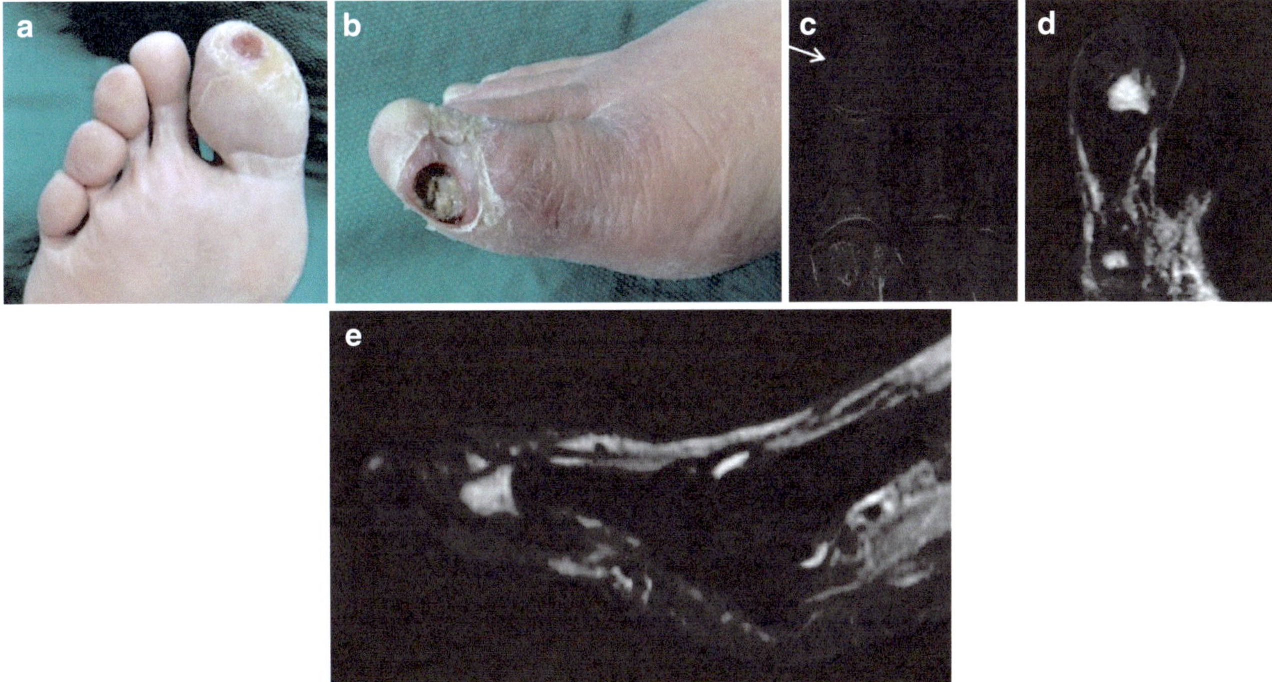

Fig. 15.24 Case 4: First metatarsophalangeal joint (MPJ) sesamoidectomy with bilobed rotational flap. (**a**, **b**) An alternative plantar first MPJ ulcer technique involves a bilobed rotational flap. The bilobed flap is a random flap that can be harvested from any location around the periphery of the wound defect. Axial flow into the flap is not necessary for "random" flaps. Harvesting the flap from the distal soft tissues has several advantages including a relatively non-weight bearing donor site and avoidance of compromising the proximal or lateral tissues that would be necessary for conversion to ray amputation or transmetatarsal amputation. (**c**) The bilobed flap also provided wide access for sesamoidectomy and remodeling of the first metatarsal head plantar surface. (**d**) Initial wound coverage and (**e**) intermediate-term result 1 year postoperatively are shown. Note the lack of a recurrent wound which is attributed to the removal of prominent sesamoids which were positive for osteomyelitis on biopsy

Fig. 15.25 Patient selection for distal Symes hallux amputation. (**a**) Neuropathic and (**b**) ischemic ulcers located at the tip of the hallux and medial to the toenail commonly result in osteomyelitis of the distal phalanx. (**c**) Early diagnosis of osteomyelitis within the distal phalanx on standard X-ray is difficult since the cortex at the distal tuft is naturally irregular (*arrow*). (**d**, **e**) MRI is most useful to confirm clinical suspicion or determine extent of bone involvement which may be helpful for procedure selection. Distal Symes amputation allows interphalangeal joint disarticulation and partial preservation of digital length and function

design described above unless the plantar wound is left to heal secondarily. Our first ray amputation flap technique allows for removal of the plantar ulcer with immediate or delayed flap closure [15]. This flap design takes advantage of dorsal and medial tissue that would otherwise be discarded with traditional ray amputation, as shown in case 8 (Figs. 15.45, 15.46, 15.47, and 15.48). The first ray amputation is easily converted to TMA if needed in the near or distant future since the proximal extension of the incision curves toward the medial midline of the foot, as opposed to extension along the plantar arch. Incision planning is vital and the flap margins should be drawn prior to any early stage incision and drainage procedures in an effort to preserve the flap donor site.

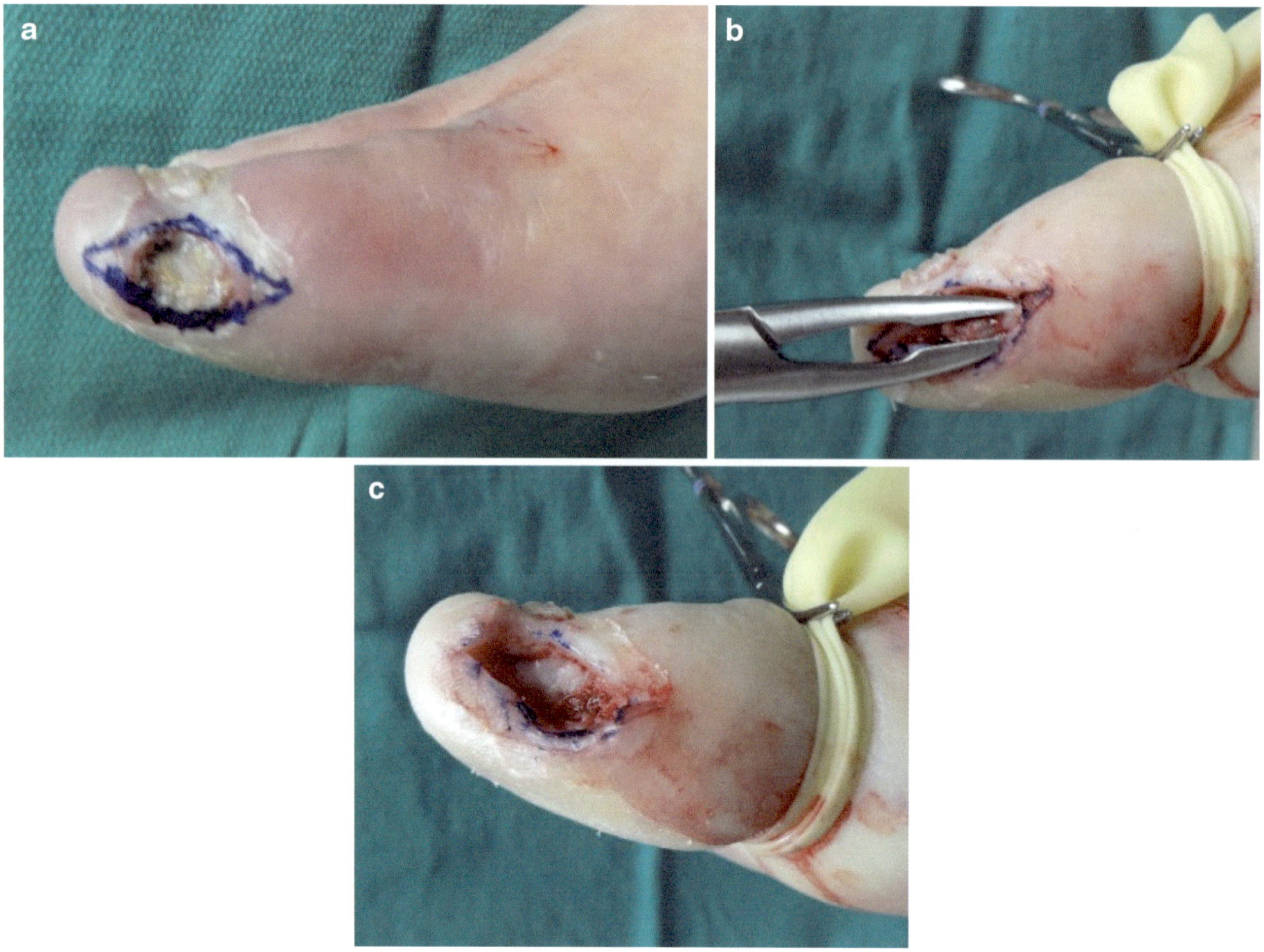

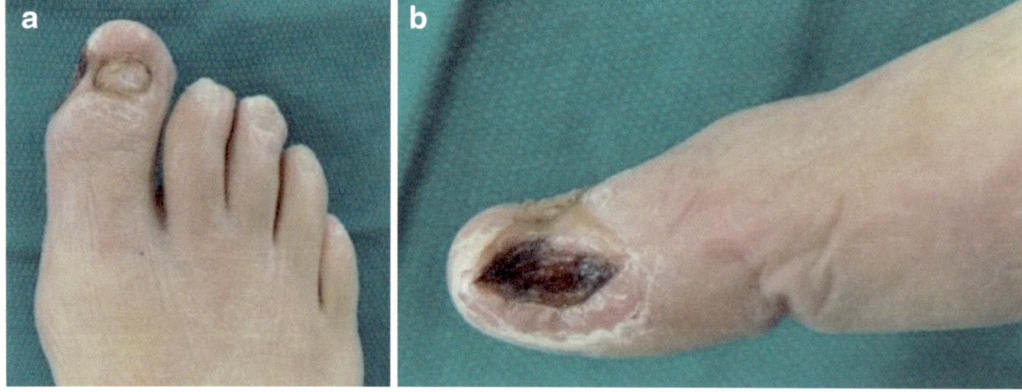

Fig. 15.26 Case 5: Stage 1 distal Symes hallux amputation. (**a**) Stage 1 surgery allowed excision of the necrotic wound shwon in Fig. 15.25b, incision and drainage of infection, and debridement and biopsy of the distal phalanx with an attempt to stabilize infection prior to definitive amputation. Staged surgery allowed vascular intervention prior to selecting the ideal level of amputation. The stage 1 procedure is commonly performed in an office-based minor procedure room. (**b**) A bone rongeur was used to resect the prominent medial condyle shown in Fig. 15.25c after wound excision and repeat prep of the wound base. (**c**) The wound was left open to drain. Note that the width of the wound was not amenable to primary closure and leaving exposed bone at the base of this wound is not very conducive to successful resolution of osteomyelitis despite long-term medical treatment

Fig. 15.27 Stage 2 distal Symes hallux amputation in case 5. (**a, b**) Clinical appearance 8 days later following vascular intervention. Note that cellulitis had resolved; however, the base of the wound was not viable

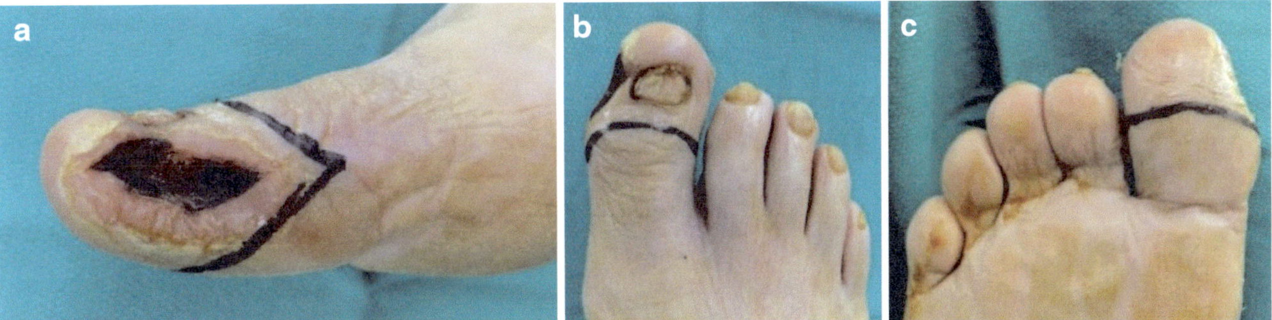

Fig. 15.28 Distal Symes hallux amputation incision plan in case 5. (**a**) Dorsal and plantar flaps were drawn fairly distal with the intent to provide coverage over the disarticulated interphalangeal joint. (**b**) The dorsal incision was made just proximal to the toenail matrix in an effort to preserve flap length but avoid regrowth of nail spicules. (**c**) The plantar flap can be longer if desired; however, a mismatch of dorsal and plantar flap lengths creates challenges at the time of closure. This same incision plan is useful for ulcers located at the distal tip of the toe

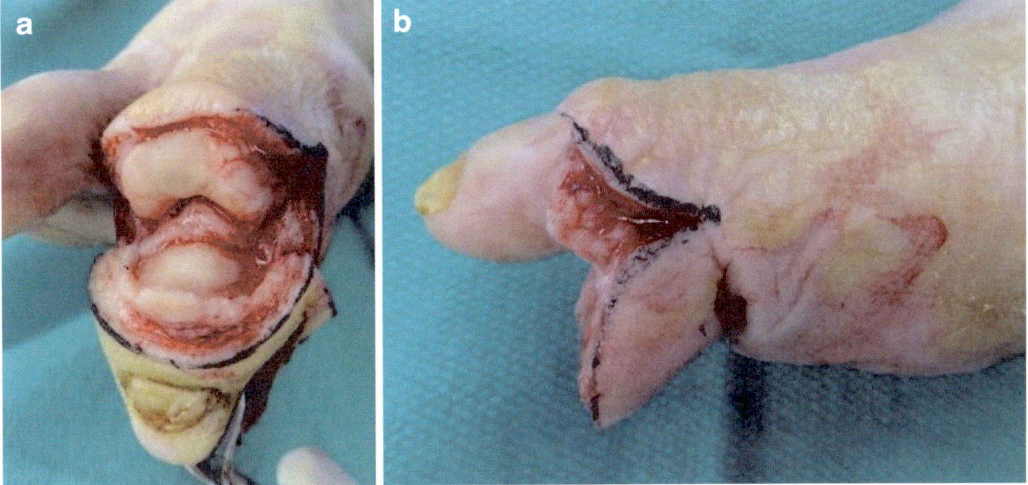

Fig. 15.29 Disarticulation through the hallux interphalangeal joint in case 5. (**a**) The dorsal incision was made directly into the interphalangeal joint allowing ease of disarticulation. (**b**) The flaps were made full thickness to preserve flap viability and durability at the weight bearing tip of the toe

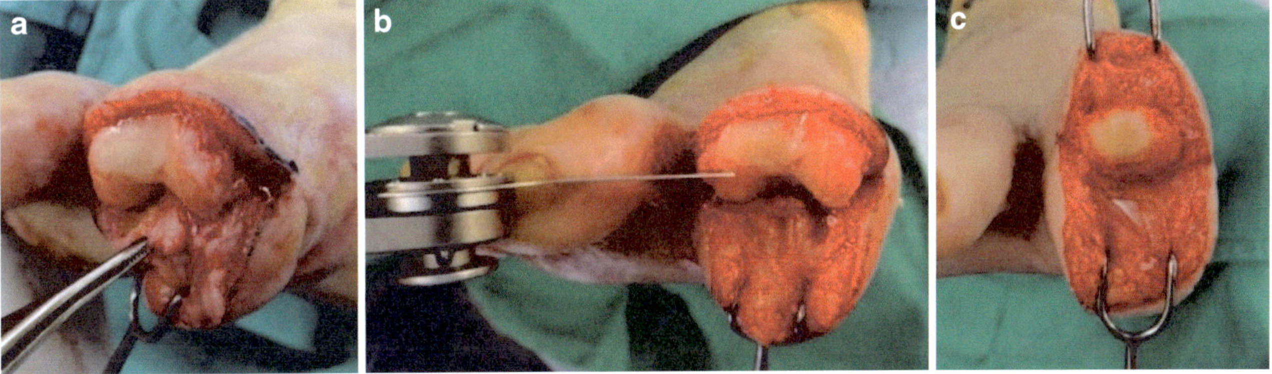

Fig. 15.30 Remodeling the head of the proximal phalanx in case 5. (**a**) The interphalangeal joint sesamoid was removed from the FHL tendon. (**b**) A bone saw was used to remodel the weight bearing surface of the head of the proximal phalanx. (**c**) The overall length of the proximal phalanx was preserved despite medial, lateral, and plantar remodeling

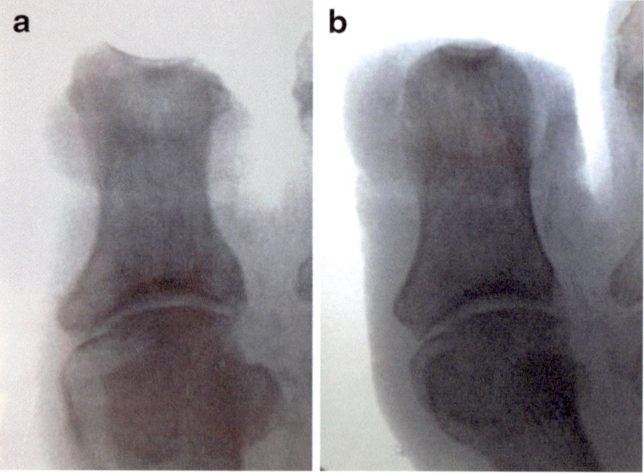

Fig. 15.31 Intraoperative radiographs to confirm the desired shape of the proximal phalanx in case 5. (**a**) Initial imaging taken after IPJ disarticulation demonstrating the irregular structure at the head of the proximal phalanx. (**b**) The remodeled head of the proximal phalanx resembled the natural tip of a distal phalanx in an attempt to recreate a new tip of the toe. Note that the entire length of the proximal phalanx is preserved with the distal Symes hallux amputation

Staged surgery is common for acute infection. Single-stage flap closure is more likely for chronic wounds versus acute soft tissue infection. Initial incision and drainage for acute infection is followed by ray amputation with possible insertion of antibiotic beads about 3 days later. The flap is raised partially, and beads are removed with a simple outpatient procedure 2 weeks later. Repeat biopsy of the proximal margin is common with this technique which involves medullary canal biopsy to preserve metatarsal length.

Complete First Ray Amputation

Complete resection of the first ray is undesirable but sometimes necessary due to recurring wounds, persistent osteomyelitis, or when surgically treating complications of extensive Heterotopic ossification from prior partial first ray amputation. An example is shown in case 9, Figs. 15.49, 15.50, 15.51, and 15.52. Preservation of at least the metatarsal base helps to maintain the insertion of

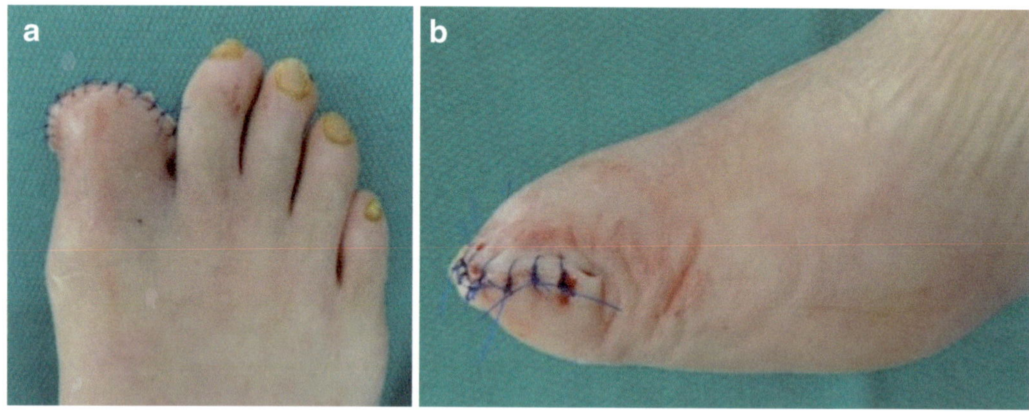

Fig. 15.32 Tension-free closure of the dorsal and plantar flaps in case 5. (**a**, **b**) Simple sutures were used to approximate the dorsal and plantar flaps without tension on the fragile tissues. Note that a relatively normal-appearing toe was preserved for both cosmetic value and postoperative function. Tip-of-toe ulcers are commonly associated with an excessively long first toe which works in favor of the distal Symes hallux amputation

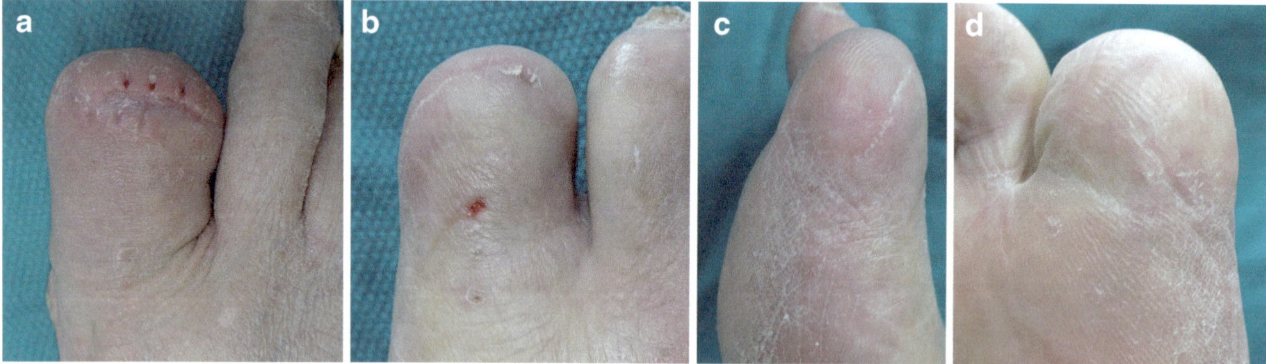

Fig. 15.33 Healing progress postoperatively at 6 weeks and 4 months postoperatively in case 5. Ischemic sores at the tip of the hallux have predictably slow healing with distal amputation. This patient underwent vascular intervention between the stage 1 and stage 2 procedures. Distal Symes hallux amputation for neuropathic ulceration often leads to a better outcome with more prompt healing of the surgical site as compared to ischemic sores. (**a**) Note complete healing at 6 weeks postoperatively and preservation of a functional hallux 4 months later (**b–d**)

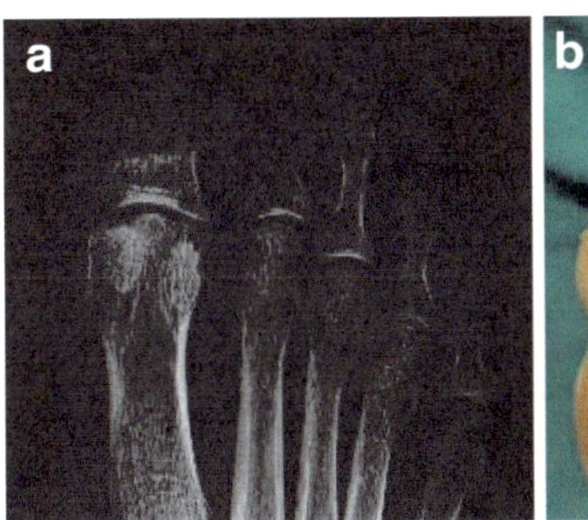
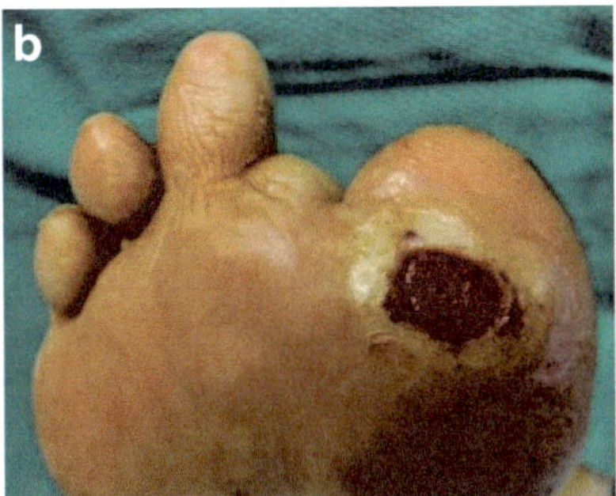
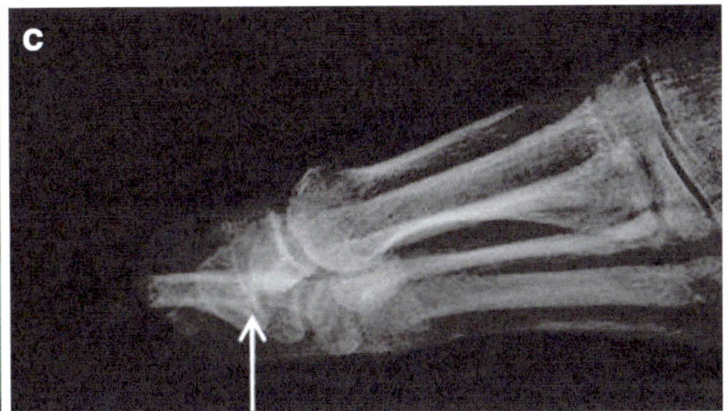

Fig. 15.34 Case 6: Partial hallux amputation. (a) Partial hallux amputation typically involves resection through the mid or proximal one third of the proximal phalanx. Clean resection with a bone saw is ideal with the intent to avoid medial, lateral, or plantar bone prominence. Preservation of a portion of the proximal phalanx avoids exposure or cross contamination of the metatarsal head, maintains position and potential function of the sesamoid bones, and preserves a more cosmetically appealing foot structure. (b) Preserving the base of the phalanx in this manner has potential disadvantages including recurrent ulceration beneath the amputation stump. (c) Postoperative lateral X-ray demonstrates plantar positioning of the stump of the proximal phalanx (*arrow*) which did lead to re-ulceration

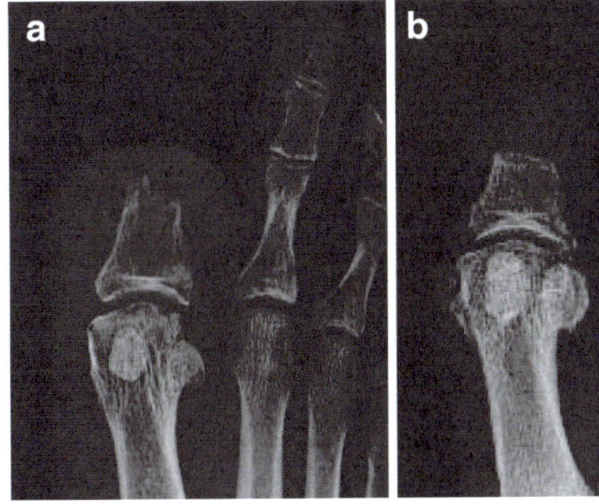
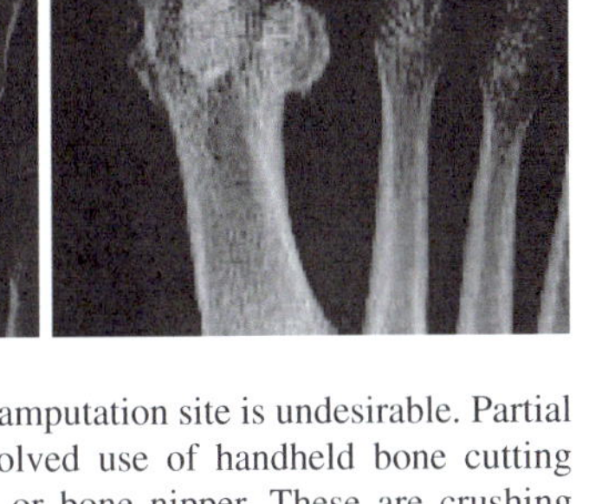

Fig. 15.35 Irregular bone at the amputation site is undesirable. Partial foot amputation historically involved use of handheld bone cutting instruments including a rongeur or bone nipper. These are crushing instruments that lead to fragmentation and (a) undesirable spikes of bone as shown here. (b) Clean resection with a bone saw is preferred in an effort to create a smooth boney contour

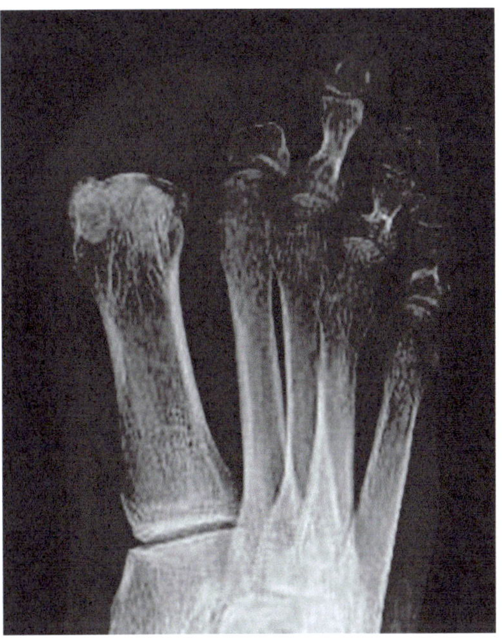

Fig. 15.36 Case 6: First metatarsal phalangeal joint disarticulation. Recurrent ulceration at the partial hallux amputation stump seen in Fig. 15.34 was treated with first MPJ disarticulation. The standard dorsal and plantar flap incision technique is typically used; however, the plantar ulcer required a dorsal only flap. The metatarsal cartilage is generally left intact to minimize propensity for cross contamination. We have not identified circumstances where cartilage preservation has been problematic. The sesamoids remain functional but may retract slightly in the proximal direction once the hallux has been removed. Second ray overload is less common when the first metatarsal head is preserved; however, recurrent ulceration under the sesamoids may require conversion to first metatarsal head resection

the tibialis anterior (TA) and peroneus longus (PL) tendons. Disarticulation at the first metatarsal cuneiform joint is useful when attempting to obtain a clean margin or when treating HO with care taken to preserve the TA and PL attachments to the medial cuneiform. Preserving the base of the first metatarsal with the expectation of long-term postoperative antibiotics may be the best plan with regard to future foot function, especially if conversion to TMA becomes necessary in the future.

Insertion of antibiotic beads and staged surgery to remodel the medial cuneiform and transfer the TA is common with complete first ray amputation. Most patients undergoing this procedure have previously undergone partial first ray amputation and removal of the base is being done in isolation due to recurrent wound breakdown or persistent osteomyelitis. Case 10 (Figs. 15.53, 15.54, 15.55, 15.56, and 15.57) demonstrates this point.

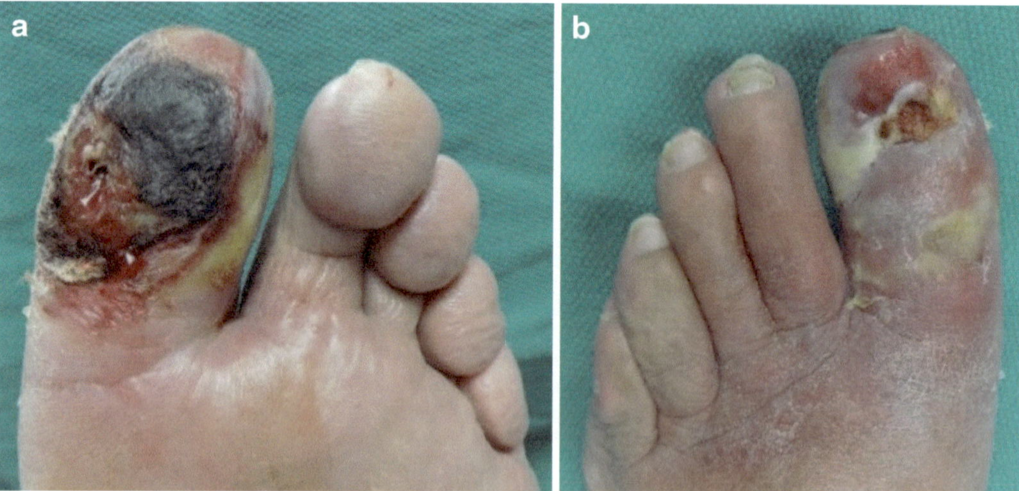

Fig. 15.37 Case 7: Traditional partial first ray amputation technique. (**a**) Widespread infection and necrosis of the hallux which started as plantar gangrene was treated with first ray amputation. (**b**) The plantar tissue had necrosed full thickness down to the bone, and widespread abscess had caused tissue compromise on the dorsum of the foot

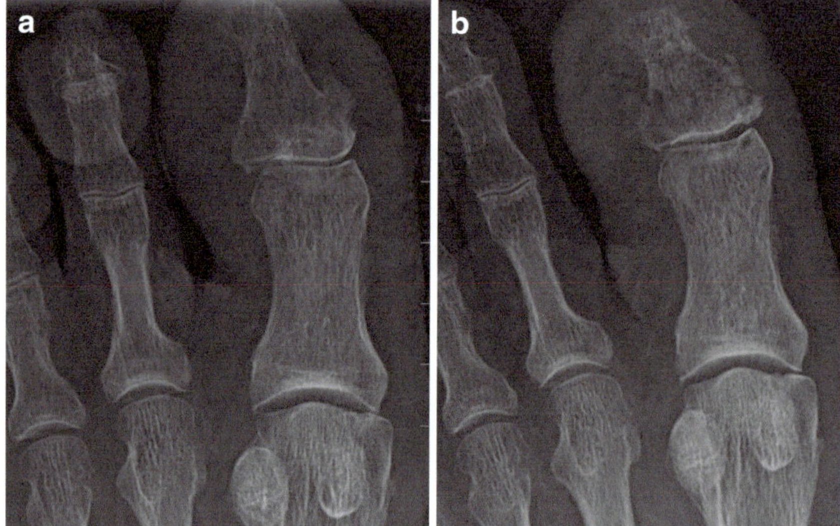

Fig. 15.38 Serial X-rays case 7. Comparison of serial X-rays may show subtle signs of osteomyelitis with cortical erosion being more common than other classic signs of osteomyelitis, especially in contiguous spread osteomyelitis. Cortical erosion is most likely to occur at the location of the ulcer which puts the radiologist at a disadvantage since they only see the X-ray. Correlation of clinical and radiographic finding is therefore optimal. (**a**) Baseline X-rays at the time of initial presentation for gangrene were helpful later when complications developed. (**b**) Radiograph 2 weeks later showed progressive erosion of the distal phalanx

Postoperative Management

Postoperative weight bearing status varies depending on procedure, level of amputation, and incorporation of flaps. All plantar flaps are kept strictly non-weight bearing for about 6 weeks following surgery. Patients are instructed to minimize activity and leg dependency in an effort to avoid excessive swelling and hematoma formation which increase the risk for flap failure. Partial toe amputation (without plantar flap) allows early weight bearing in a post-op shoe until suture removal. First ray amputation procedures are allowed minimal touchdown (heel mostly) until the incision is well healed. Sutures may be removed at 2 weeks postoperatively in healthy patients without compromised healing potential. Sutures

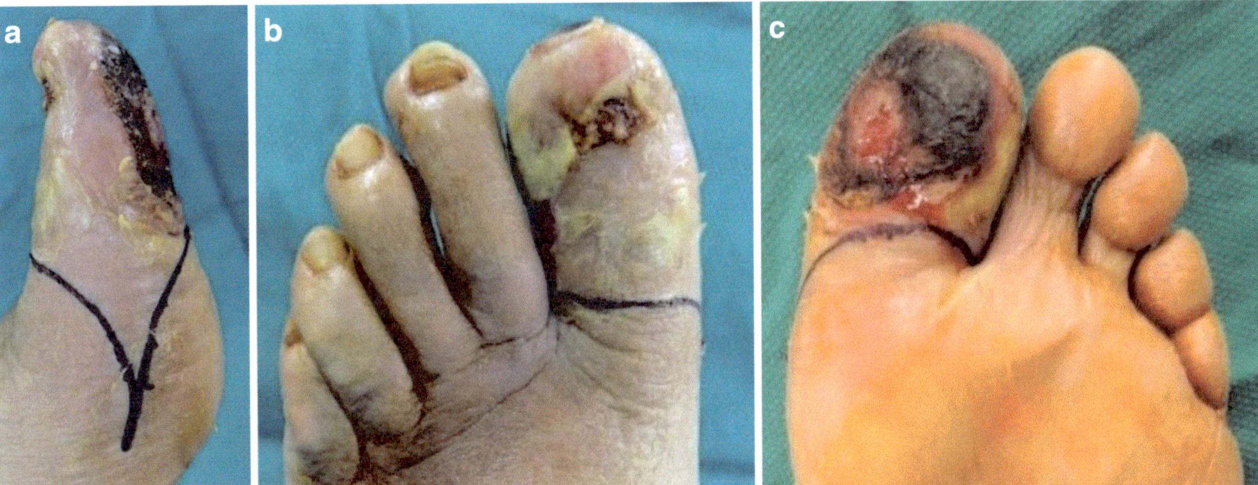

Fig. 15.39 Dorsal and plantar flap incision design for traditional partial first ray amputation in case 7. (**a**) The medial apex of the incision was midline from dorsal to plantar with a proximal run out along the metatarsal shaft. The dorsal and plantar flaps were nearly equal in length. (**b**, **c**) Transverse incisions were drawn at the proximal line of tissue demarcation at the base of the toe. The lateral apex was midline at the proximal sulcus deep within the interdigital space. The lateral apex comes to a point and is a notably fragile part of the incision with propensity for poor healing due to difficulty with making an incision between the toes. Tissue quality may also be poor between the toes due to maceration, necrosis, or callus

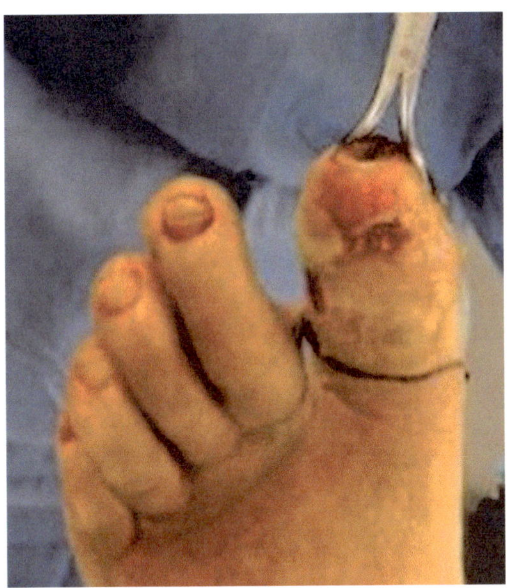

Fig. 15.40 A sharp towel clamp was placed for manipulation of the digit in case 7. Cross contamination to the proximal incision site was minimized using this no-touch technique

are commonly left in place for up to 6 weeks for those with diabetes or vascular disease where wound healing can be delayed.

Postoperative use of accommodative orthotics and orthopedic shoes will minimize the chance of recurrent or transfer ulceration. A toe box filler for the first ray defect is generally not needed and has a tendency to cause undesirable pressure and irritation at the amputation site.

Complications

As with any osteomyelitis-related surgery, complications can occur. Recurrent wounds, persistent osteomyelitis, hematoma, heterotopic ossification, and repeat amputation are common following wound and infection surgery. The surgeon and patient should expect that recovery is not predictable and that staged surgery is the norm. The pursuit of a definitive surgery often results in a more proximal amputation which leads to compromised function and ongoing problems.

Noncompliance with weight bearing restrictions is likely the primary cause of wound dehiscence. Failure to address underlying bony deformity and/or equinus deformity can lead to recurrent ulceration. Even in the best of circumstances, transfer lesions after partial first ray resection are common and sometimes unavoidable. Antibiotic therapy also carries risk of complications including renal compromise and superinfection. These risks need to be balanced against the risks associated with surgery. Timing of surgery, careful surgical technique, ideal procedure selection, optimization of vascular perfusion, eradication of infection, and postoperative compliance are the keys to success with surgical treatment of first ray osteomyelitis.

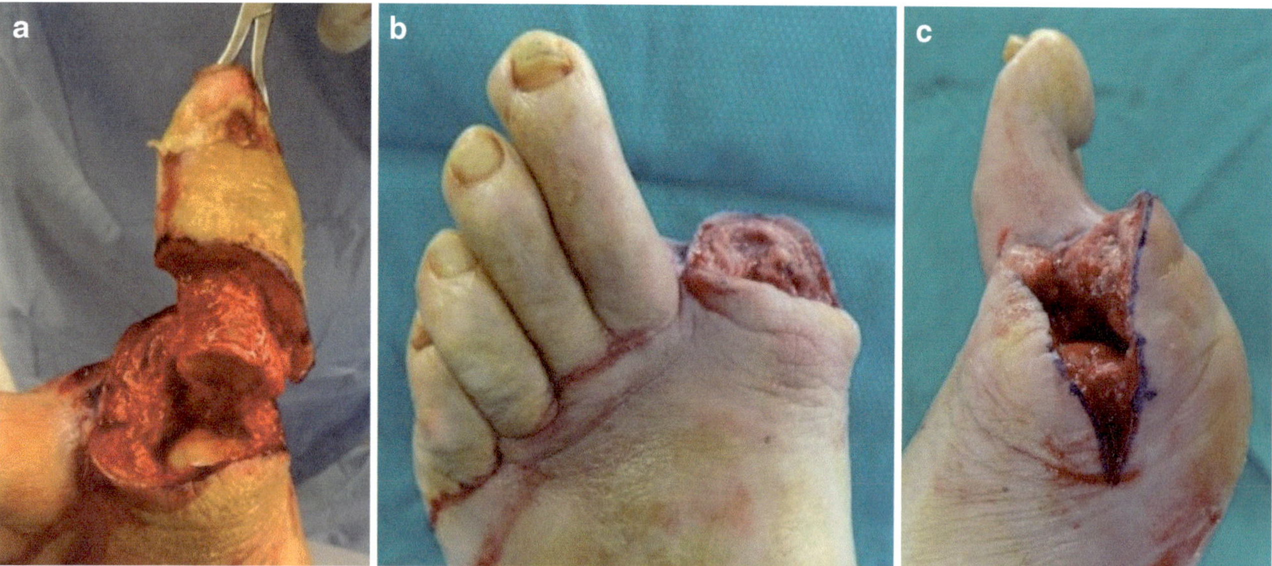

Fig. 15.41 Disarticulation at the metatarsal phalangeal joint in case 7. The dorsal and plantar flaps were incised full thickness down to bone. (**a**) The flaps were then raised with subperiosteal dissection along the proximal phalanx to the metatarsal phalangeal joint allowing disarticulation of the hallux. This created a potentially clean surgical site, and the surgeon may consider re-prepping the wound site and changing gloves. There is no attempt to perform layered dissection looking for bleeding vessels as this has the potential to compromise tissue vascularity. (**b, c**) Careful hemostasis was obtained once the hallux was removed

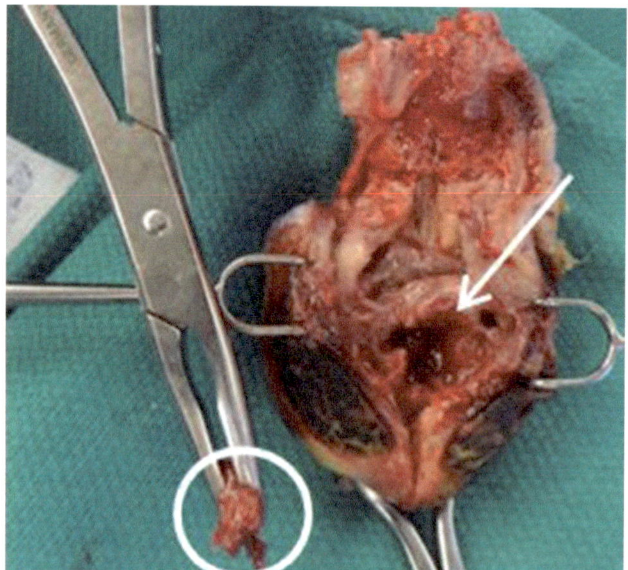

Fig. 15.42 Bone biopsy in case 7. Biopsy was taken from the digital specimen on the back table to minimize chance of cross contamination to the clean wound. The toe was split along the plantar surface to allow direct visualization of the compromised soft tissue and bone structure. Bone specimen for culture was taken from the distal phalanx using a rongeur (*circle*). While bone biopsy is the gold standard, surgical findings are also important with regard to accurate diagnosis of osteomyelitis and determination of clean margins. Note that the plantar soft tissues were necrotic down to bone (*arrow*). Operative findings should be described in the operative note including necrosis of the bone, pus within the bone, fragmentation secondary to infection, involvement of joints, depth of tissue necrosis, and proximal tissue viability. These are valuable insights with regard to the need for amputation, intraoperative decision-making regarding ideal level of amputation, and postoperative care protocol including accurate diagnosis of osteomyelitis and duration of antibiotics

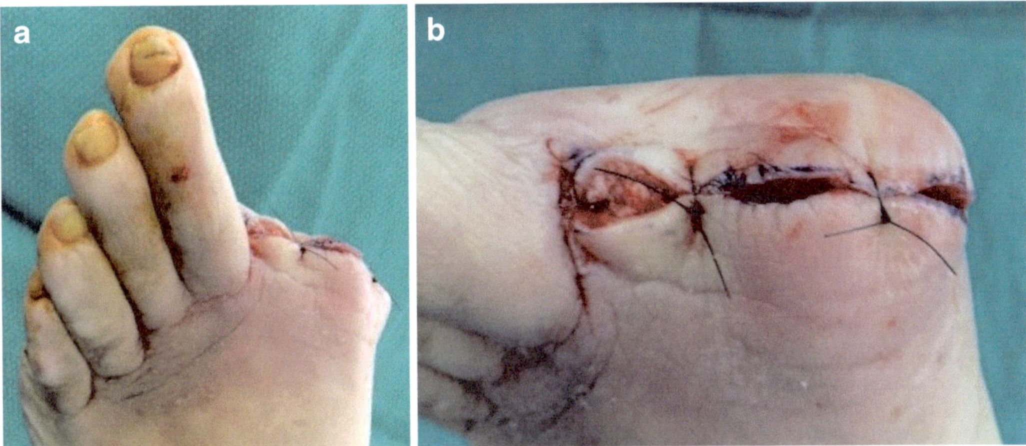

Fig. 15.43 Stage 1 first ray amputation with partial closure in case 7. Acute soft tissue infection was treated with staged surgery. (**a, b**) Several loose sutures were placed to provide temporary coverage of the first metatarsal head and maintain mild stretch on the soft tissues to minimize secondary contamination and proximal retraction of the flaps while waiting several days for the vascular intervention and the stage 2 amputation procedure

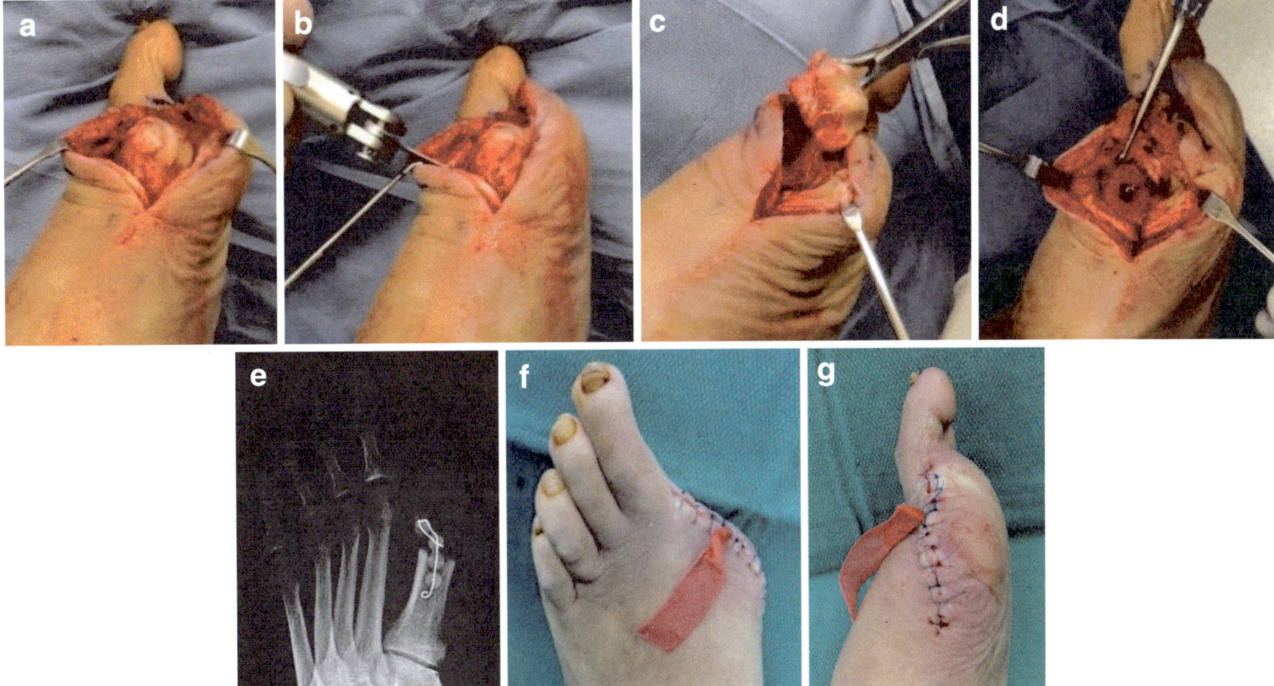

Fig. 15.44 Stage 2 partial first ray amputation in case 7. (**a**) The flaps were raised providing access to the first metatarsal shaft. (**b**) A bone saw was used for metatarsal resection at the neck of the metatarsal. (**c**) The metatarsal head was then removed with the aid of a sharp towel clamp. The medullary canal of the metatarsal shaft was then inspected for signs of infection. (**d**) Margin biopsy can be taken from within the medullary canal using a bone curette. Surgical description of bone quality at the proximal margin resection site is helpful when determining likely persistence of osteomyelitis at this level. (**e**) Antibiotic beads can be placed within the medullary canal and are removed in 2 weeks postoperatively. (**f, g**) Closure was performed with simple sutures and a drain or packing may be placed as shown here

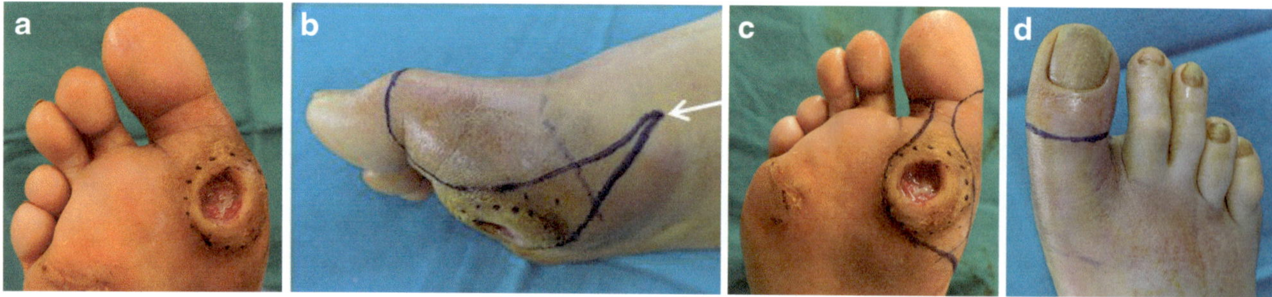

Fig. 15.45 Case 8: Partial first ray amputation with incorporation of a rotational flap. (**a**) This full thickness neuropathic ulceration at the plantar aspect of the first MPJ was not amenable to standard first ray amputation incision techniques since the plantar flap was compromised by the plantar wound defect. Our preferred first ray amputation flap technique is shown here which utilizes available tissue from the medial and dorsal aspect of the first MPJ and hallux. (**b**, **c**) Note that the proximal aspect of the incision is directed onto the medial aspect of the foot (*arrow*) which creates a curved flap and avoids an incision into the weight bearing arch. This technique is easily converted to a transmetatarsal amputation should that become necessary. (**d**) The dorsal aspect of the flap is essentially transverse and made just proximal to the interphalangeal joint of the hallux. Note how the flap closely circumscribed the ulcer and used all available tissue except the toenail and digital pulp of the toe

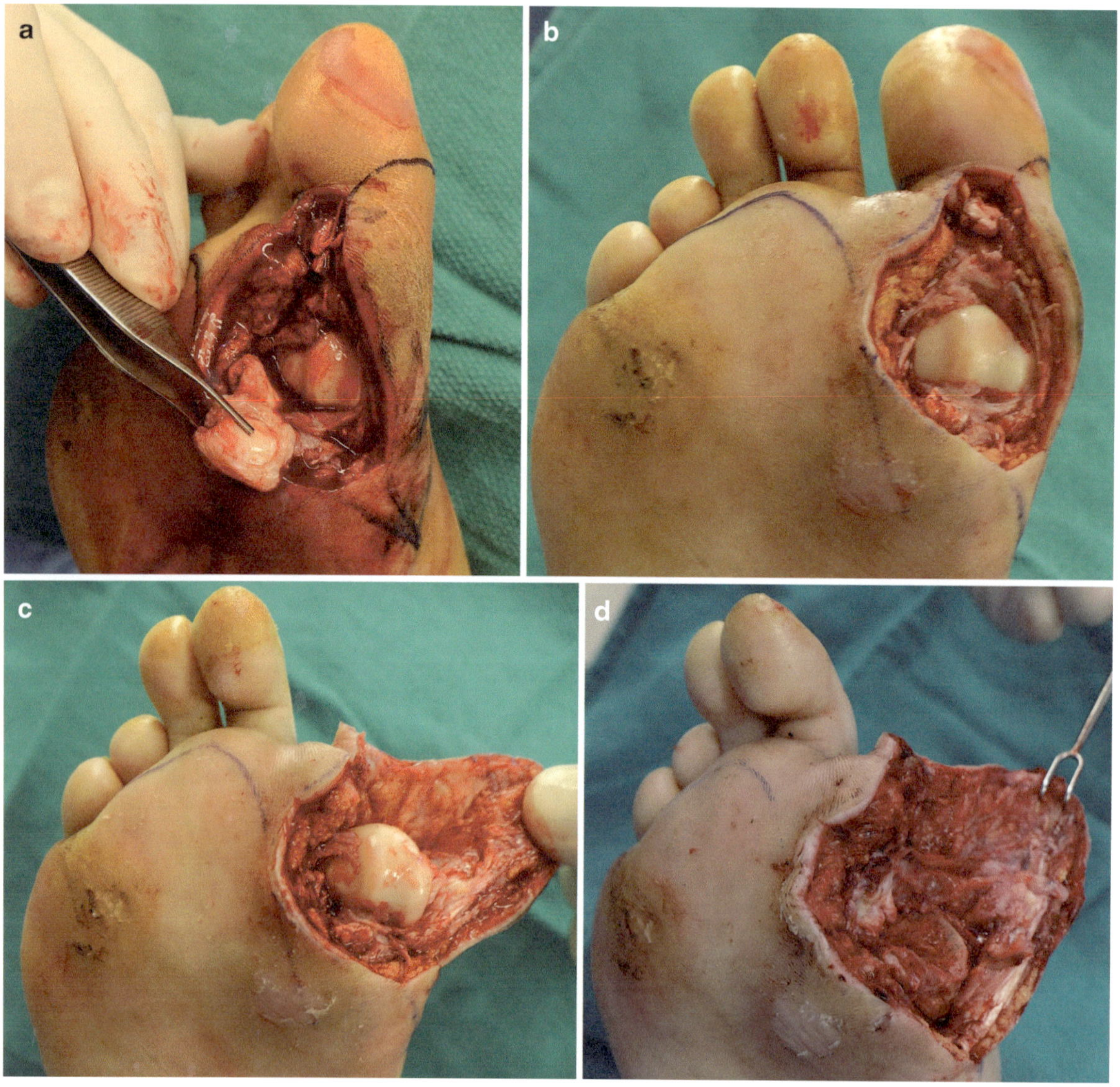

Fig. 15.46 Raising the flap followed by partial first ray amputation in case 8. The ulcer was initially excised followed by repeat wound prep and change of gloves. (**a**, **b**) The first metatarsal head was exposed after excision of the sesamoids. Sesamoid biopsy was positive for osteomyelitis. (**c**) The flap was raised off the dorsal and medial aspect of the hallux allowing MPJ disarticulation. (**d**) The level of metatarsal resection was just proximal to the native plantar tissue which avoids pressure on the flap. Note the large, vascular flap that will be rotated to cover the plantar wound defect

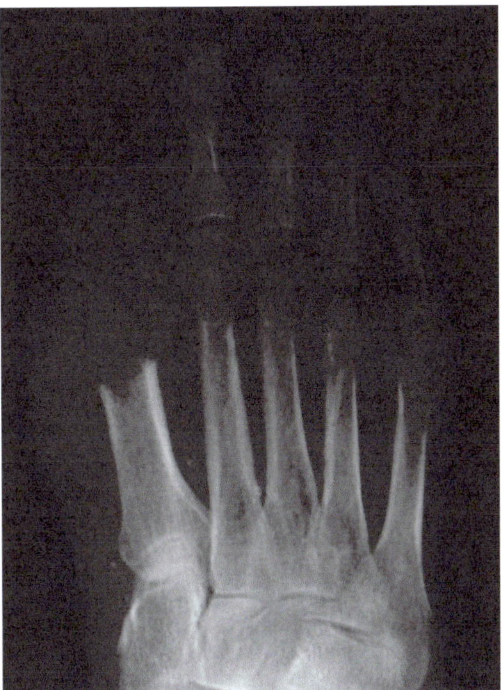

Fig. 15.47 Intraoperative imaging confirmed desired level of partial first ray resection in case 8. The flap allowed coverage at this desirable level of bone resection despite the large plantar wound. Bone preservation at this level is more conducive to medial column function and potential future conversion to transmetatarsal amputation. Metatarsal resection just proximal to the metaphyseal flare with slight medial to lateral and dorsal to plantar angulation minimizes medial and plantar prominence

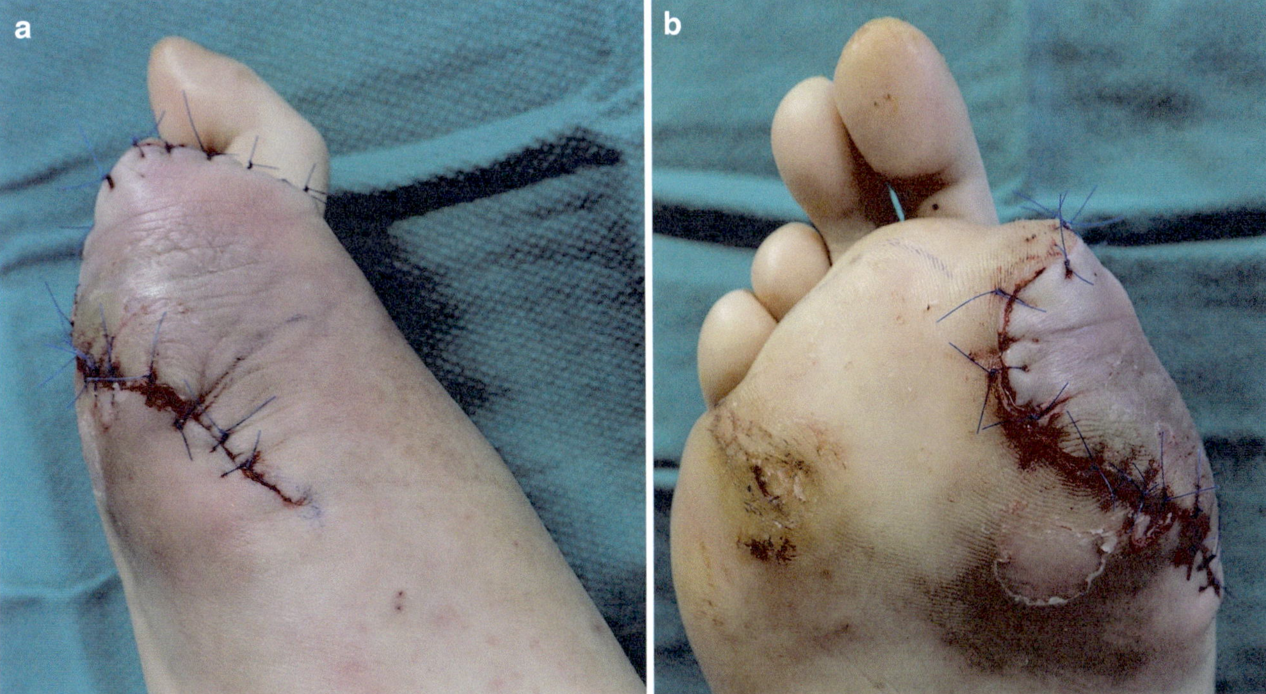

Fig. 15.48 Flap coverage of the plantar wound in case 8. (**a, b**) Simple sutures were placed to provide tension-free closure of the flap. This procedure may be performed as a single or multiple stage procedure. Raising of the flap is typically preserved until stage 2 when appropriate, otherwise the flap has a tendency to retract and become indurated if allowed to shrivel while waiting for the stage 2 procedure. A drain or sterile packing is commonly placed if there is concern for hematoma formation

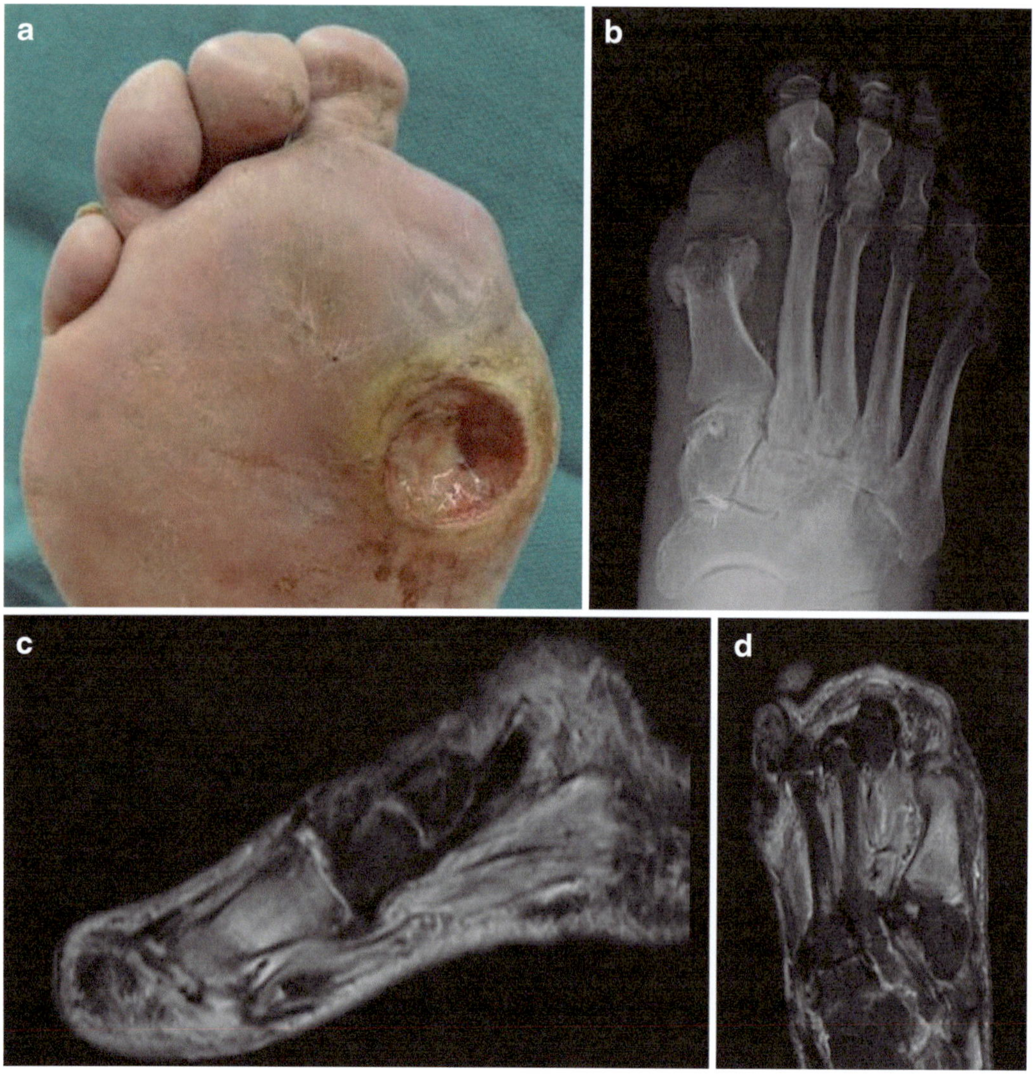

Fig. 15.49 Case 9: Near-complete first ray amputation for recurrent plantar ulceration, extensive osteomyelitis, and heterotopic ossification (HO). (**a**) Recurrent planter ulceration along the medial column was associated with extensive HO from prior partial first ray amputation involving flap closure. The recurrent ulcer was mid-metatarsal over the prominent bone. (**b**) HO is difficult to differentiate from osteomyelitis, although progressive reabsorption of the hypertrophic stump raises concern for HO with secondary osteomyelitis. (**c**, **d**) MRI suggested osteomyelitis extending to the base of the first metatarsal

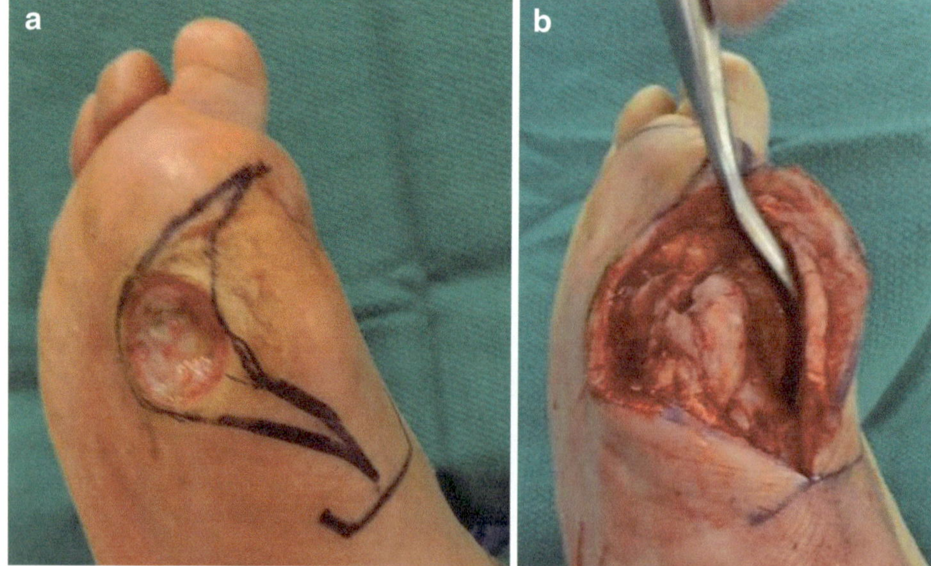

Fig. 15.50 Modified first ray amputation flap for midshaft plantar ulcer in case 9. (**a**) A dorsally based advancement flap was used which allowed excision of the large plantar wound, wide access for metatarsal resection, and immediate coverage of the defect. This ulcer would otherwise be difficult to excise and close with standard techniques. (**b**) A metatarsal elevator was used to expose proximally to the level of the metatarsal base

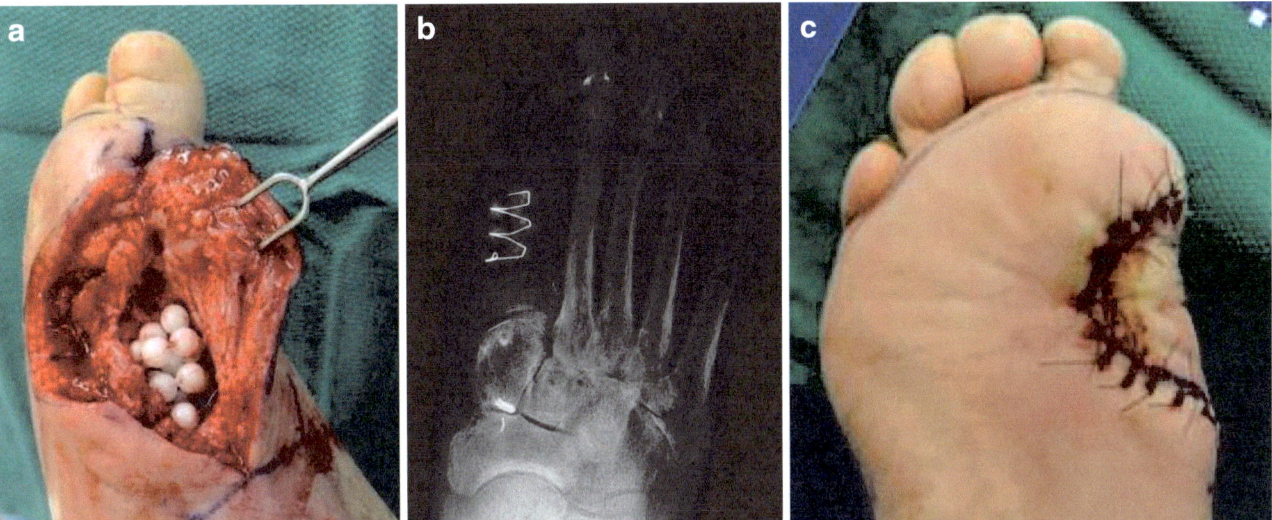

Fig. 15.51 Near-complete first ray amputation with flap closure over antibiotic beads in case 9. (**a**) Intraoperative photo with beads placed within the soft tissue pouch after metatarsal resection. (**b**) Radiograph with proximal metatarsal base preserved and implantation of coiled antibiotic bead chain. (**c**) The flap was advanced and closed primarily. Preserving the base of the metatarsal is controversial in this case since patients with known history of heterotopic ossification are likely to have recurrence. Antibiotic bead implantation allows subsequent washout which decreases the risk of heterotopic ossification by minimizing hematoma formation. This patient also received immediate post-op radiation therapy as described in Chap. 12. Inflammation on MRI does not equate to necrotic or dead bone, and the metatarsal base was viable on direct intraoperative inspection. Preservation of the base avoids disruption of the tibialis anterior and peroneus longus tendon insertions

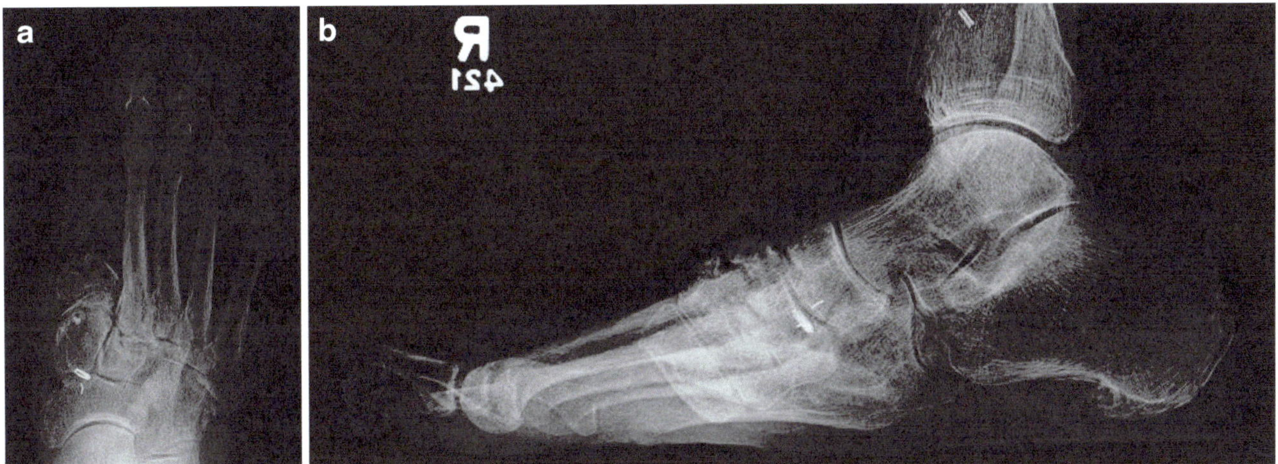

Fig. 15.52 Long-term postoperative radiographs in case 9. Weight bearing postoperative X-rays show no recurrence of HO despite a prior patient history. Foot function was compromised due to loss of the first ray with high risk of second ray overload, transfer ulceration, and midfoot charcot arthropathy

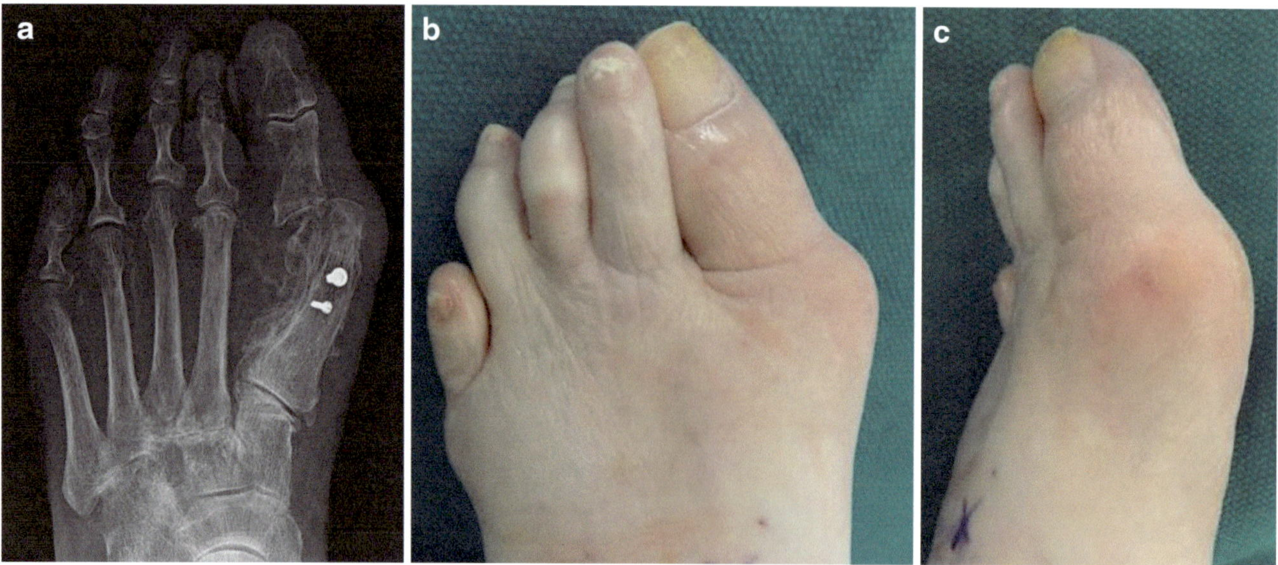

Fig. 15.53 Case 10: Extensive first ray osteomyelitis associated with recurrent hallux valgus and resultant chronic ulceration. (**a**) First MPJ dislocation following prior hallux valgus surgery. Radiographs demonstrate periosteal reaction extending to the base of the first metatarsal. This could represent heterotopic ossification from prior surgery or extensive osteomyelitis. (**b**, **c**) Clinical presentation of a chronic and painful dorsal medial ulceration over the prominent metatarsal head with recurring cellulitis

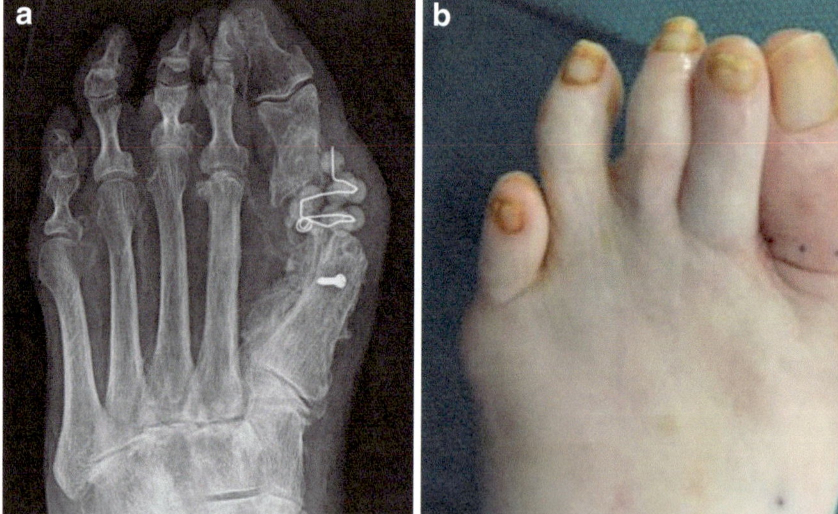

Fig. 15.54 Stage 1 procedure involved first metatarsal head resection and biopsy with placement of antibiotic beads in case 10. (**a**) Antibiotic beads functioned as a spacer and provided concentrated local delivery of antibiotics while waiting for biopsy results. Staged surgery allowed biopsy and resolution of soft tissue infection prior to definitive closure. (**b**) The first toe has been preserved at this point but will have limited function after first metatarsal head removal

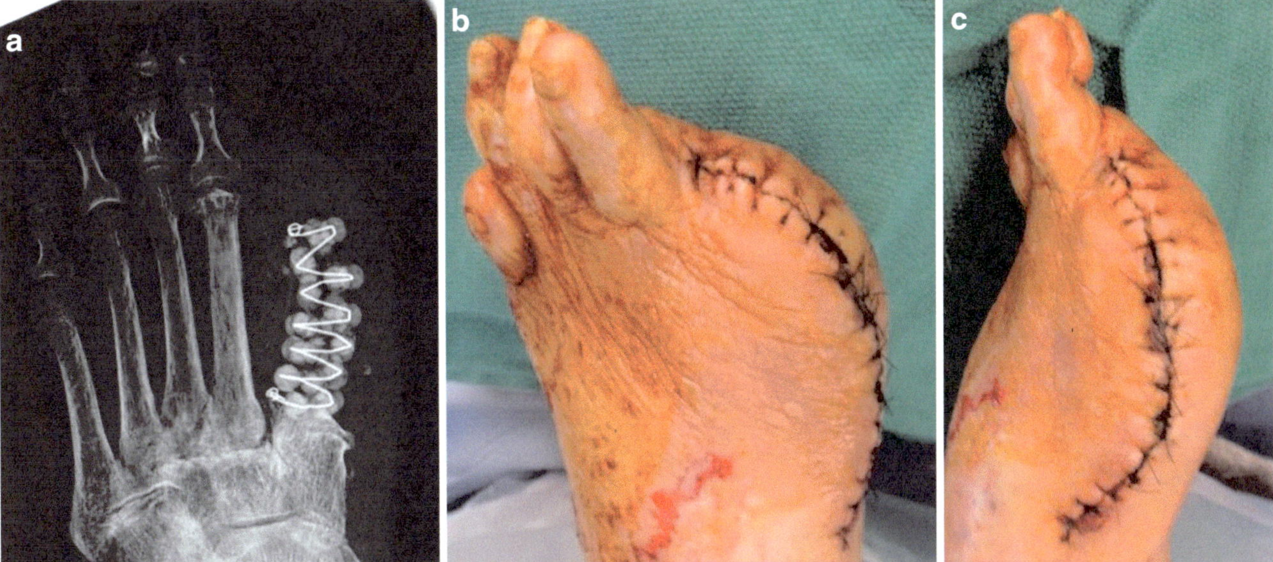

Fig. 15.55 Stage 2 and stage 3 procedures with first ray amputation in case 10. Biopsy confirmed first ray osteomyelitis. The high intermetatarsal angle would predispose to recurrent ulceration no matter the level of metatarsal resection. Proximal periostitis was suggestive of widespread osteomyelitis leading to the decision for first metatarsal cuneiform disarticulation. (**a**) A coiled antibiotic bead chain was placed within the soft tissue defect created by metatarsal removal which helped with hematoma management and local antibiotic delivery. (**b, c**) The antibiotic beads were removed 14 days later through a small distal opening of the incision

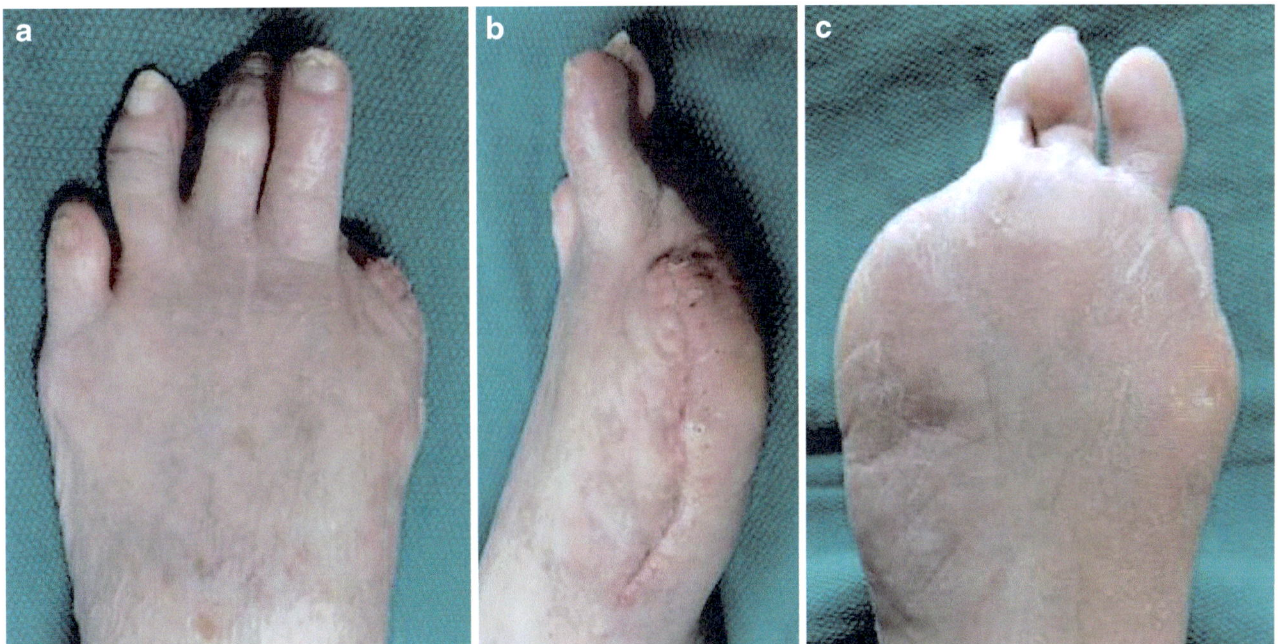

Fig. 15.56 Clinical appearance of complete first ray amputation 6 weeks after antibiotic bead removal in case 10

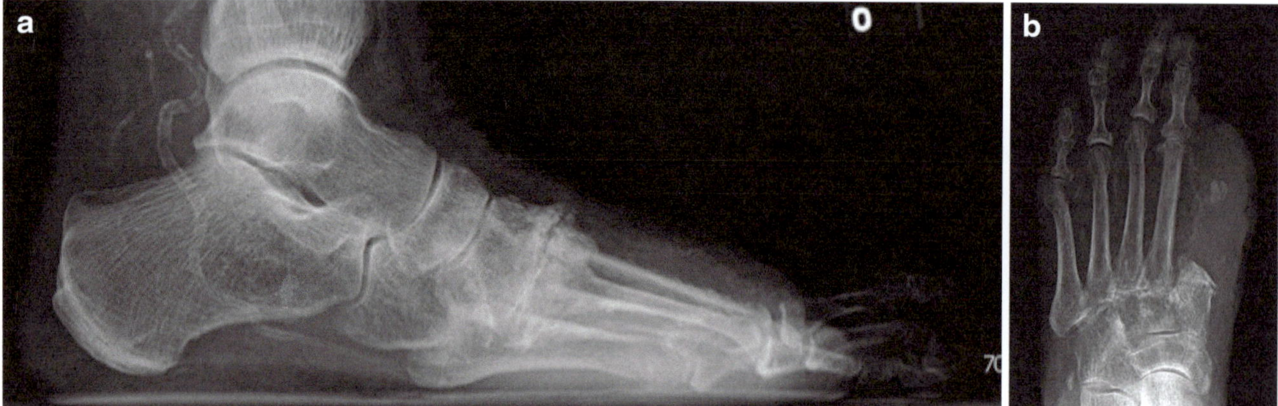

Fig. 15.57 Postoperative weight bearing radiographs in case 10. (**a**, **b**) Disarticulation at the first metatarsal cuneiform joint is not a desirable level of amputation from a structural or functional standpoint and is avoided when possible. This approach is largely reserved for revision surgery when more conservative resection has failed. Recurring heterotopic ossification can also be treated with disarticulation

Conclusion

Surgeons are always in search of definitive procedures, especially with regard to diabetic foot surgery. It is the author's opinion that first ray wound and infection surgery is not conducive to definitive procedures which is likely due to the tremendous force applied when walking. All levels of first ray amputation are prone to transfer ulceration which commonly leads to repeat surgery. A practical approach is to assume future need for revision surgery and plan accordingly regarding level of bone resection and incision design. Flap closure and staged surgery is highly amenable to this treatment approach as the flap can be raised multiple times including years later. A conservative bone resection approach that preserves structure yet corrects biomechanical issues is appropriate for complicated neuropathic wounds. The surgeon should resist the temptation to determine the level of first metatarsal resection based solely on MRI findings. Infected bone is not necessarily dead bone, and medial column function is too important to be cavalier about level of resection. Short resection has significant impact on foot stability, medial column function, second ray overload, and future conversion to transmetatarsal amputation (TMA). Incorporation of antibiotic beads and long-term antibiotics helps from this regard since metatarsal resection through the surgical neck is frequently not a surgical cure for infection of the first metatarsal. Short or complete resection of the first metatarsal is undesirable but sometimes necessary due to extensive tissue loss, heterotopic ossification, or advanced bone necrosis. The ideal procedure for a given patient should address abnormal mechanics and structural deformities and attempt to preserve the important weight bearing function of the first ray to minimize the potential for new risk factors.

References

1. Ahmed ME, Tamimi AO, Mahadi SI, Widatalla AH, Shawer MA. Hallux ulceration in diabetic patients. J Foot Ankle Surg. 2010;49:2–7.
2. Nube VL, Molyneaux L, Yue DK. Biomechanical risk factors associated with neuropathic ulceration of the hallux in people with diabetes mellitus. J Am Podiatr Med Assoc. 2006;96:189–97.
3. Boffeli TJ, Bean JK, Natwick JR. Biomechanical abnormalities and ulcers of the great toe in patients with diabetes. J Foot Ankle Surg. 2002;41:359–64.
4. Frykberg RG, Bevilacqua NJ, Habershaw G. Surgical off-loading of the diabetic foot. J Am Podiatr Med Assoc. 2010;100:369–84.
5. Frykberg RG, Zgonis T, Armstrong DG, Driver VR, Giurini JM, Kravitz SR, Landsman AS, Lavery LA, Moor JC, Schuberth JM, Wukich DK, Andersen C, Vanore JV. Diabetic foot disorders: a clinical practice guideline. J Foot Ankle Surg. 2006;45:S1–66.
6. Borkosky SL, Roukis TS. Incidence of re-amputation following partial first ray amputation associated with diabetes mellitus and peripheral sensory neuropathy: a systemic review. Diabet Foot Ankle. 2012;3.
7. Kadukammakal J. Assessment of partial first-ray resections and their tendency to progress to transmetatarsal amputations. J Am Podiatr Med Assoc. 2012;102:412–6.
8. Boffeli TJ, Hyllengren SB. Uni-lobed rotational flap for plantar hallux inter-phalangeal joint ulceration complicated by osteomyelitis. J Foot Ankle Surg. 2015. doi: 10.1053/j.jfas.2014.12.023.
9. Aragon-Sanchez J, Lazaro-Martinez JL, Pulido-Duque J, Maynar M. From the diabetic foot ulcer and beyond: how do foot infections spread in patients with diabetes? Diabet Foot Ankle. 2012;3.
10. Boffeli TJ, Collier RC. The lateral hallux stress dorsiflexion view: a case series demonstrating clinical utility in midterm hallux limitus. J Foot Ankle Surg. 2014. doi: 10.1053/j.jfas.2014.07.012.
11. Schrudde J, Petrovici V. The use of slide-swing plasty in closing skin defects: a clinical study based on 1308 cases. Plast Reconstr Surg. 1981;67(4):467–81.
12. Raspovic A. Gait characteristics of people with diabetes-related peripheral neuropathy, with and without a history of ulceration. Gait Posture. 2013;38:723–8.
13. Patry J, Belley R, Cote M, Chateau-Degat ML. Plantar pressures, plantar forces, and their influence on the pathogenesis of diabetic foot ulcers. J Am Podiatr Med Assoc. 2013;103:322–32.
14. Boffeli TJ, Pfannenstein RR, Thompson JT. Radiation therapy for recurrent heterotopic ossification prophylaxis after partial metatarsal amputation. J Foot Ankle Surg. 2015. doi: 10.1053/j.jfas.2014.07.010.
15. Boffeli TJ, Peterson MC. Rotational flap closure of first and fifth metatarsal head plantar ulcers: adjunctive procedure when performing first or fifth Ray amputation. J Foot Ankle Surg. 2013;52:263–70.

Osteomyelitis of the Central Toes

Kyle W. Abben and Troy J. Boffeli

Introduction

Phalangeal osteomyelitis of a second, third, or fourth toe typically results from contiguous spread of infection from chronic wounds associated with neuropathy or gangrene. The central toes have unique anatomy, function, deformity, and surgical procedure selection criteria and therefore are commonly treated differently than the first and fifth toes. Nonhealing ulcerations of the central toes are common in patients who have a combination of digital deformity and profound peripheral neuropathy which is mostly diabetic in nature. Digital gangrene and ischemic wounds are associated with peripheral vascular disease, and late stage onset of osteomyelitis is common once bone becomes exposed after autoamputation or when dry gangrene turns into infected wet gangrene. The central toes have minimal subcutaneous tissue covering the prominent bone and joint structures at the tip of the toe and around the interphalangeal joints which predisposes to bone infection when the soft tissue is compromised by chronic wounds, open trauma, or digital gangrene (Fig. 16.1).

Biomechanical Considerations in Neuropathic Ulceration

Digital deformities and abnormal biomechanical issues associated with central toe ulceration include hammertoe contracture, transverse plane toe deformity, hallux valgus, hallux limitus, overlapping toes, bone spurs, arthritis, excessive toe length, and ankle equinus. Deformity alone is typically not sufficient to cause ulceration, whereas the dyad of neuropathy and deformity is almost always present. Hammertoe deformity predisposes to abnormal pressure on the dorsal aspect of the proximal interphalangeal joint (PIPJ) or distal interphalangeal joint (DIPJ) as well as the distal tip of the toe near the toenail (Fig. 16.2). Dorsal ulceration is amenable to extra-depth toe box shoe therapy, while the tip of toe ulceration associated with hammertoe contracture is less easily rectified with simple shoe or insert measures. Patients with neuropathic wounds oftentimes present with chronic wounds that already have deep-seated osteomyelitis at which point conservative measures are no longer a viable option. Hammertoe contracture also creates a retrograde buckling force on the metatarsal head, which results in abnormal pressure on the plantar aspect of the metatarsophalangeal joint (MPJ). Interdigital ulceration is associated with transverse plane deformity (medial or lateral drift), hallux valgus, and overlapping toes. Arthritic interphalangeal joints (IPJs) can also become enlarged and prominent with resultant soft tissue breakdown which may ultimately lead to osteomyelitis. Isolated elongation of a central toe (commonly the second) is associated with nonhealing and recurrent tip of toe ulceration which is highly prone to osteomyelitis of the distal phalanx. An uncomplicated wound on a long toe can be rectified with proper fitting shoes, but the longest toe is commonly contracted at the tip which exacerbates the problem.

Wound Care Challenges for Central Toe Ulceration

Conservative therapy of digital ulcerations typically focuses on reducing pressure and off-loading the problematic area, as well as appropriate local wound care. Offloading is often in the form of orthotic inserts, shoes with an extra-depth toe box to allow room for the contracted toe (s), or digital pads to protect against dorsal, plantar, or interdigital pressure. These measures are especially useful for pre-ulcerative or superficial ulcerative lesions. If these conservative measures fail to aid in timely wound healing, osteomyelitis is a frequent sequelae.

K.W. Abben, D.P.M., A.A.C.F.A.S. (✉)
Jamestown Regional Medical Center, 2422 20th Street SW,
Jamestown, ND 58401, USA
e-mail: kyle.w.abben@gmail.com

T.J. Boffeli, D.P.M., F.A.C.F.A.S.
Regions Hospital/HealthPartners Institute for Education
and Research, 640 Jackson Street, St. Paul, MN 55101, USA
e-mail: troy.j.boffeli@healthpartners.com

© Springer International Publishing Switzerland 2015
T.J. Boffeli (ed.), *Osteomyelitis of the Foot and Ankle*, DOI 10.1007/978-3-319-18926-0_16

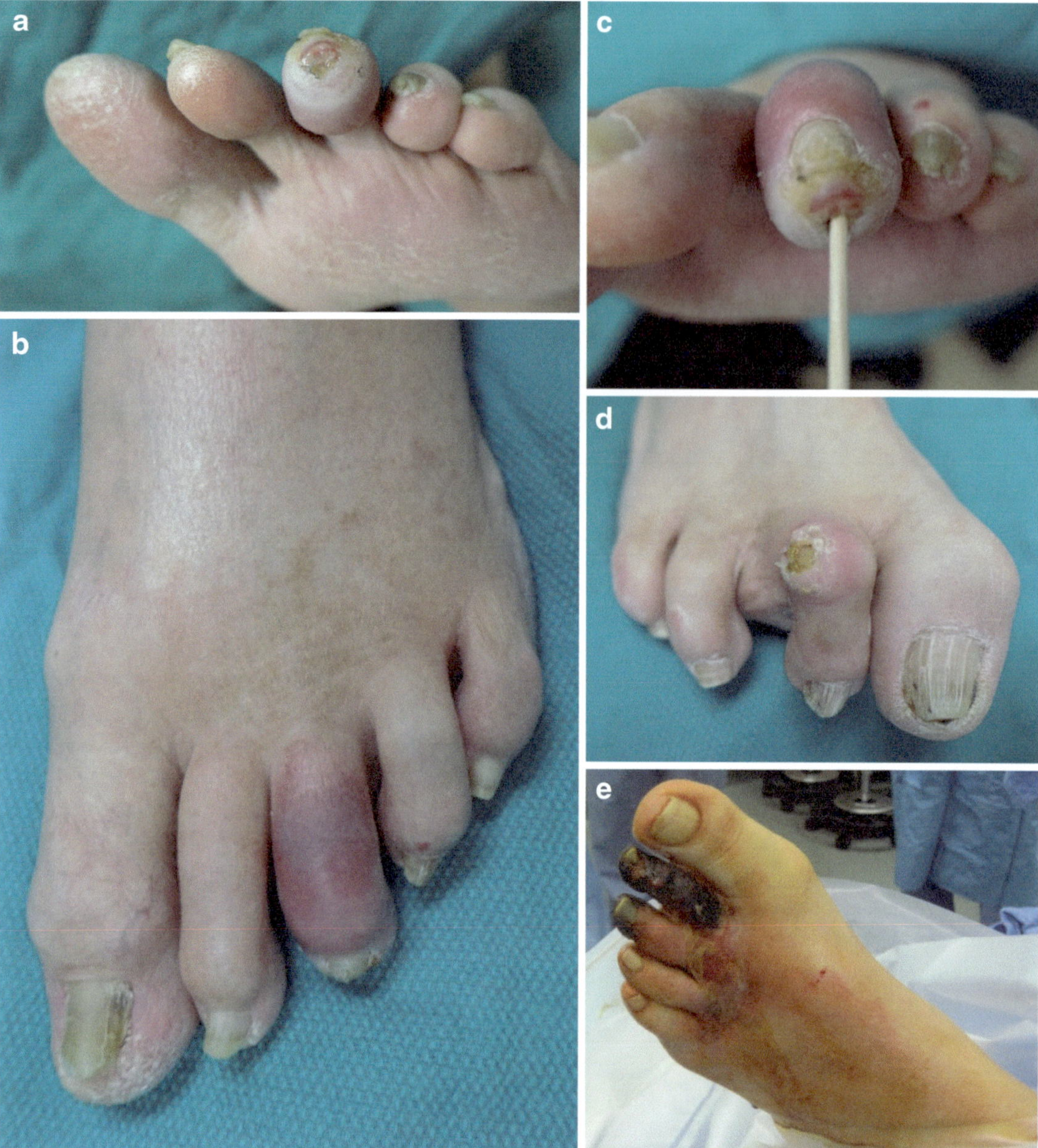

Fig. 16.1 Osteomyelitis of a central toe is typically associated with direct spread of infection from neuropathic ulcers and digital gangrene. Neuropathic ulceration at the tip of the third toe with contiguous spread of infection to the deep tissues resulted in cellulitis and osteomyelitis (**a, b**). Note how the infected wound probed deep to bone which raised suspicion for osteomyelitis at the tip of the distal phalanx (**c**). Neuropathic ulceration over prominent interphalangeal joints also leads to bone and joint infection (**d**). Osteomyelitis associated with digital gangrene is usually a late stage finding that develops secondary to infection of the surrounding tissue (**e**)

Conservative off-loading measures may not be effective if the wound is caused by digital deformity more so than ill-fitting shoes. Tip of toe ulceration associated with mallet toe deformity does not respond to longer shoes, and interdigital wounds may not resolve with wider shoes if the problem is caused by hallux valgus or an overlapping second toe. Understanding the biomechanics of neuropathic forefoot ulceration is therefore important and has significant impact when deciding on the ideal treatment plan including surgical procedure selection.

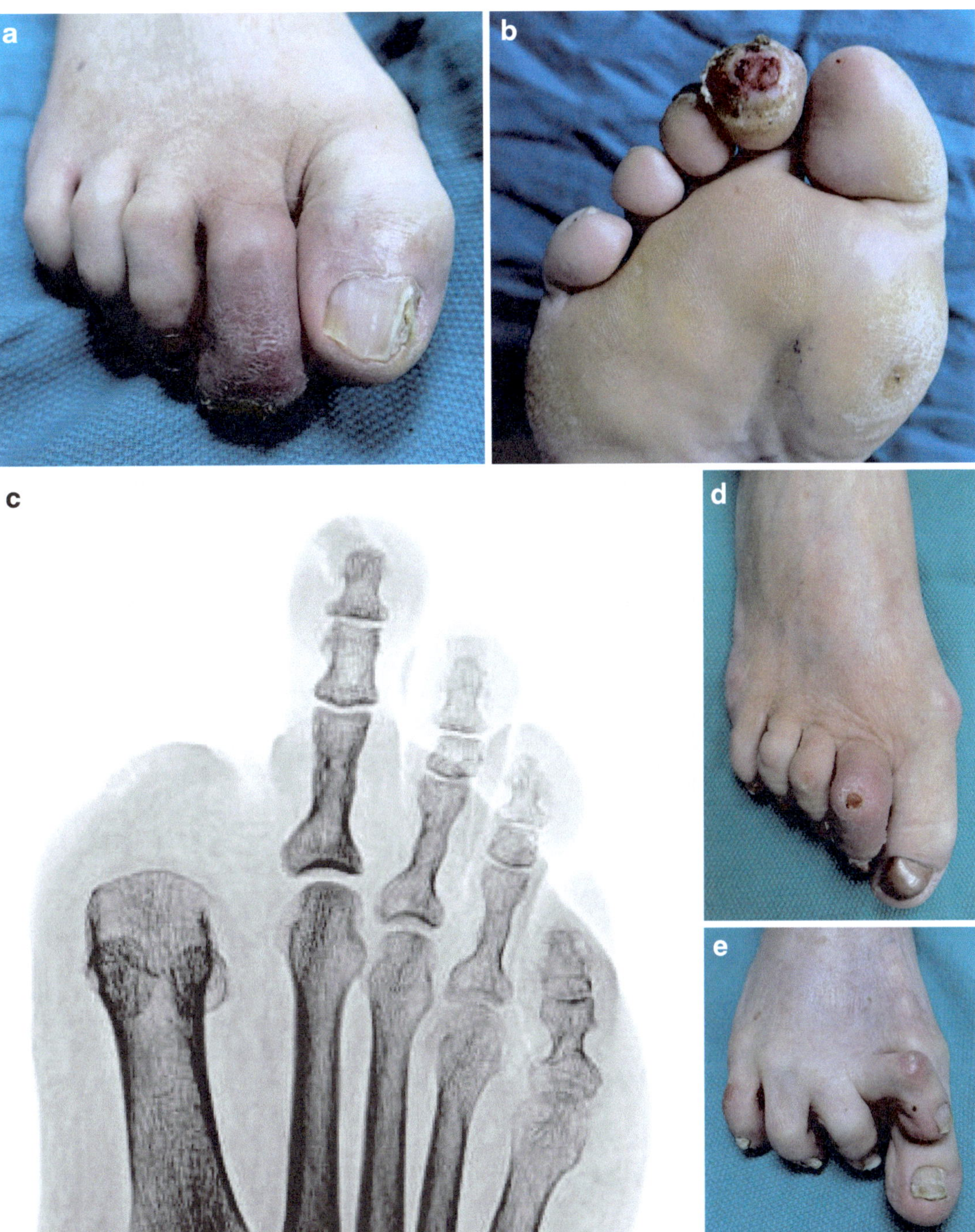

Fig. 16.2 Digital deformity predisposes to nonhealing neuropathic wounds. Neuropathic ulcers associated with digital deformity tend to be chronic and recurrent. Nonhealing sores may eventually become infected, and osteomyelitis is common in digital wounds. Long and contracted hammertoes commonly develop neuropathic ulcers at the tip of the toe (**a**, **b**). Note the classic appearance of neuropathic ulceration with callused border and healthy granulation tissue at the center of the wound. Cellulitis around the tip of the toe (**a**) with a deep wound (**b**) should raise suspicion for osteomyelitis in the distal phalanx. Excessive toe length is often created by adjacent toe amputation (**c**). Dorsal ulceration at the IPJs is associated with hammertoe contracture (**d**) and overlapping toes (**e**)

Prophylactic Surgery for Correction of Digital Deformity

Osteomyelitis of a central toe is most commonly associated with a chronic wound that has failed to heal. Early surgical intervention allows prophylactic treatment of recurrent or nonhealing ulcerations with the intent to avoid progression to contiguous spread osteomyelitis and/or acute infection requiring amputation. The central toes are very amenable to reconstructive podiatric procedures which are designed to correct structural deformity and reduce bone prominence yet maintain a functional or at least cosmetically appealing toe.

Flexor and Extensor Tenotomy for digital Ulcers Associated with Flexible Hammertoe Deformity

Distal tip of toe ulceration and dorsal ulceration at the IPJs is commonly related to flexor and extensor tendon contracture, which is accentuated during ambulation. Deformity becomes rigid with time but often remains flexible for years. Flexor tenotomy has been documented as a reliable procedure to treat tip of toe ulcerations if performed early enough in the life cycle of an ulcer before deeper structures become infected [1]. Isolated flexor tenotomy is reserved for distal tip of toe ulcerations, while dorsal PIPJ ulcerations may require both flexor and extensor tenotomy. In our practice, digital tenotomy is typically performed in the office under local anesthesia and sterile conditions (Fig. 16.3). Care must be taken to thoroughly evaluate the contracted toe preoperatively, as tenotomy may lengthen an already elongated toe resulting in increased pressure if not accommodated by longer shoes. Tip of toe ulcers associated with an elongated and contracted toe, a severely diseased toenail, and deep ulceration with potential for osteomyelitis are best treated with distal Symes amputation (discussed later in this chapter). Rigid joint contracture is typically not amendable to tenotomy and may respond better to IPJ arthroplasty.

Elective Hammertoe Surgery for Digital Ulceration

Interdigital wounds and wounds over the dorsal aspect of an IPJ are due to prominent underlying bone structures caused by prominent joints, arthritic spurs, transverse plane digital deformity, overlapping toes, and malunion of prior digital fracture (Fig. 16.4). Hallux valgus deformity also contributes to increased interdigital pressure from abutting toes. Conservative treatment, such as wound debridement, wide shoes, toe spacers, and lamb's wool, may allow healing or prevent interdigital calluses from turning into formal ulcerations. Of note, wider shoes may not solve the problem if hallux valgus is the under-lying cause of interdigital pressure (Fig. 16.5). Consideration should be given to addressing digital deformity or boney prominence when there is propensity to develop wounds around the IPJs, especially in high-risk diabetic patients. Timeliness is important as this preventive approach may allow a minor outpatient or office-based procedure before a pre-ulcerative lesion or recurrent sore becomes deep and infected.

PIPJ and DIPJ arthroplasty traditionally involves removal of the distal portion of the proximal or middle phalanx, respectively. Periarticular exostectomy with preservation of the joint is also common for interdigital wounds. Bone resection allows removal of prominent bone, relaxation of deformed joints, bone specimen for biopsy, and possible wound excision and closure. A dorsal incisional approach is typical regardless of wound location as interdigital incisions are challenging. An elliptical dorsal incision allows dorsal wound excision and primary closure, whereas interdigital wounds may be left to heal secondarily. The surgeon can also attempt to heal the ulcer preoperatively with offloading and local wound care followed by traditional hammertoe or bunion surgery once the ulcer is completely healed.

Osteomyelitis Associated with Digital Gangrene

Phalangeal osteomyelitis associated with gangrene typically develops late in the course of digital gangrene. Noninfected dry gangrene of the lesser toes is primarily treated with vascular intervention, while the affected toe is initially left alone to allow demarcation. Dry gangrene can be monitored for months while waiting to see if autoamputation is likely to occur. This process can be successful depending on restoration of digital perfusion and extent of tissue necrosis. Autoamputation ideally occurs distal to the tip of the distal phalanx which allows natural healing. Autoamputation through the IPJs results in bone and cartilage exposure which is less amenable to secondary healing. Some patients are able to granulate over the end of the bone, but osteomyelitis may eventually develop if bone remains exposed for an extended period of time. Conversion to a clean surgical site is often preferred and may simply require cutting the bone short enough that the soft tissue can finally heal over the bone.

Dry gangrene may eventually turn to infected wet gangrene as the nonviable tissue becomes necrotic and infected. Infected gangrene is commonly associated with osteomyelitis since full-thickness necrosis includes necrosis of the periosteum and joint capsule. The wait and watch approach is no longer an option once infection develops and surgical treatment is typically necessary. A surgical cure of phalangeal osteomyelitis associated with gangrene is likely to be achieved with toe, ray, or transmetatarsal amputation (TMA),

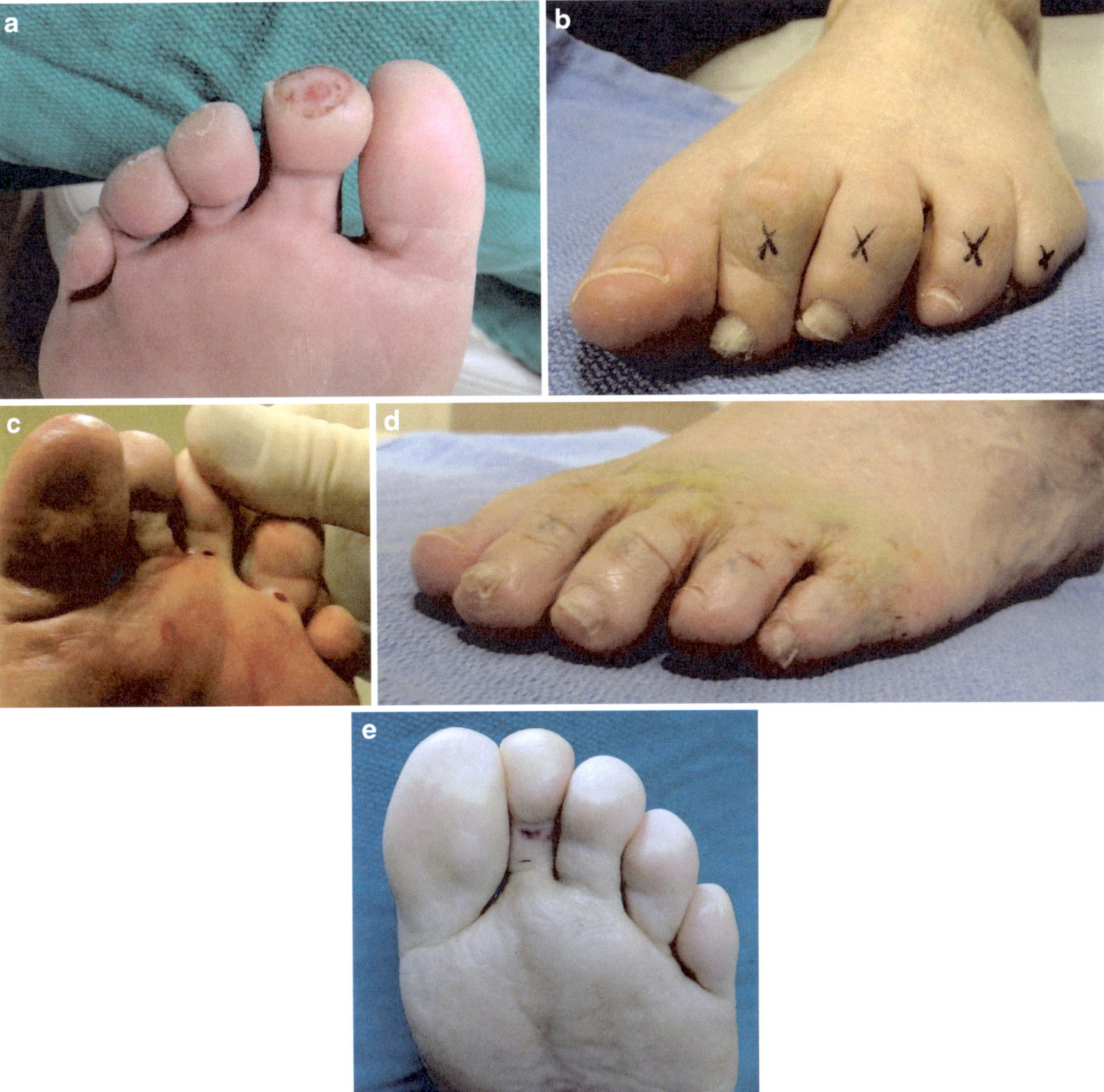

Fig. 16.3 Clinical examples of flexor tenotomy for tip of central toe ulcers associated with flexible hammertoe contracture. Digital contracture is highly correlated with tip of toe ulceration. This second toe wound was recurrent due to hammertoe contracture (**a**). Early intervention with flexor tenotomy before worsening ulceration turns to infection, and osteomyelitis is ideal under these conditions. Flexor tenotomy can be performed on one or all of the lesser toes depending on clinical findings. Note abnormal pressure on the tips of toes 2–5 with site marking for office-based tenotomy (**b**). Minimally invasive flexor tenotomy with plantar PIPJ capsulotomy was performed using a #62 blade through plantar midline incisions (**c**). Advanced DJD of the PIPJ or more complex toe deformities are be better treated with joint arthroplasty or fusion. Dorsal MPJ tenotomy and capsulotomy is common as well. Note improved toe position 1 week after tenotomy (**d**). Minimally invasive surgery allowed normal activity in a compressive bandage and surgical shoe. No sutures were needed for this transverse incision, and normal shoes and bathing are allowed 1 week after surgery. Note a fully healed transverse incision 1 week after office-based flexor tenotomy without suture on the second toe (**e**). The same procedure was performed on the third, fourth, and fifth toes 2 years prior

but healing may be compromised in comparison to patients undergoing amputation for neuropathic conditions.

Central digital gangrene can also occur due to an embolic event which is less likely to become infected or need amputation. Embolic lesions tend to be smaller and may impact multiple toes which should prompt work up to identify a cause. These lesions are more amenable to the wait and watch approach to allow demarcation and eventual healing.

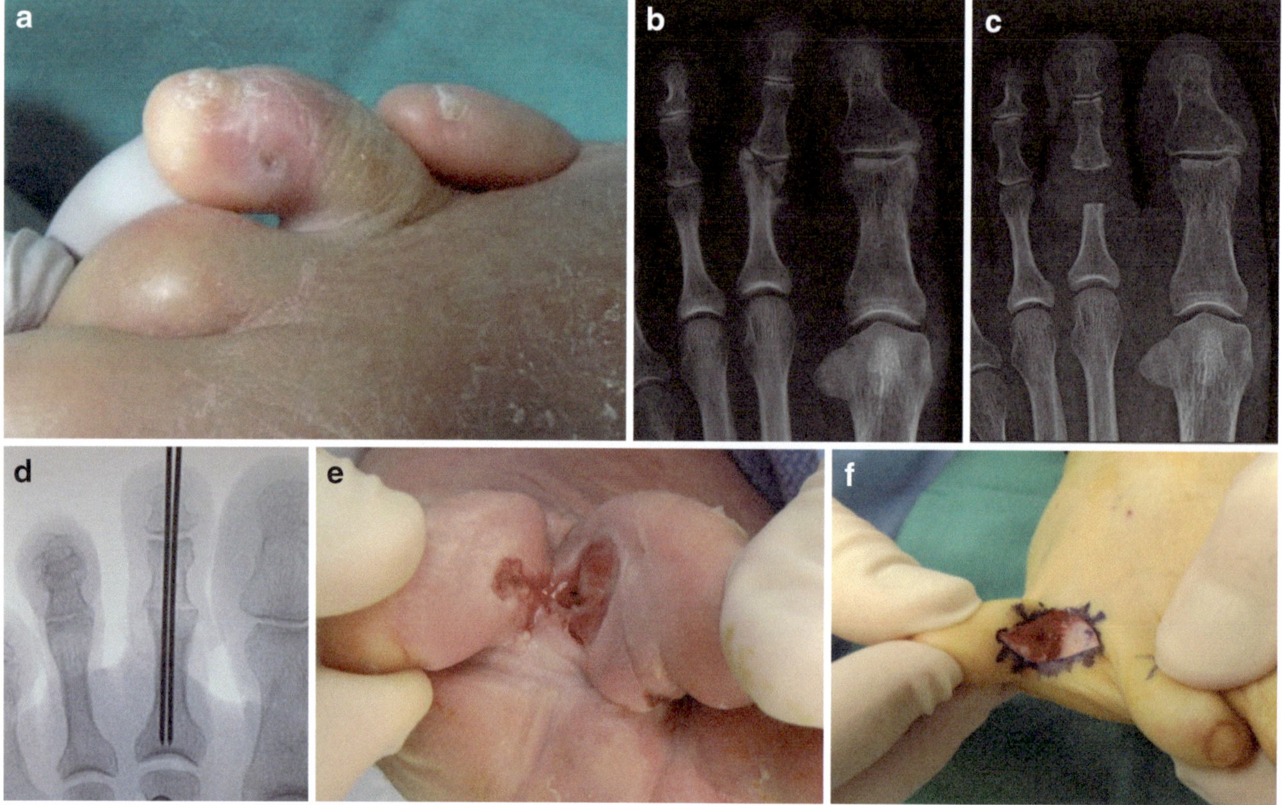

Fig. 16.4 Osteomyelitis associated with interdigital ulceration. Interdigital ulcers (**a**) commonly start as soft corns that eventually develop deep sinus tracts near prominent bone and joint structures. Note a malunited fracture at the second PIPJ with propensity for interphalangeal pressure on the adjacent toes (**b**). Bone spur resection or IPJ arthroplasty may be the most prudent prophylactic intervention for persistent sores that have failed to heal despite proper offloading and wide shoes. Arthroplasty of the PIPJ removed the prominent underlying bone and provided specimen for biopsy (**b**, **c**). Arthrodesis is less desirable with infection but is an option for uncomplicated sores (**d**). Consideration is given to arthroplasty with partial syndactylization for adjacent interdigital ulceration with poor quality tissue in the interdigital space (**e**, **f**)

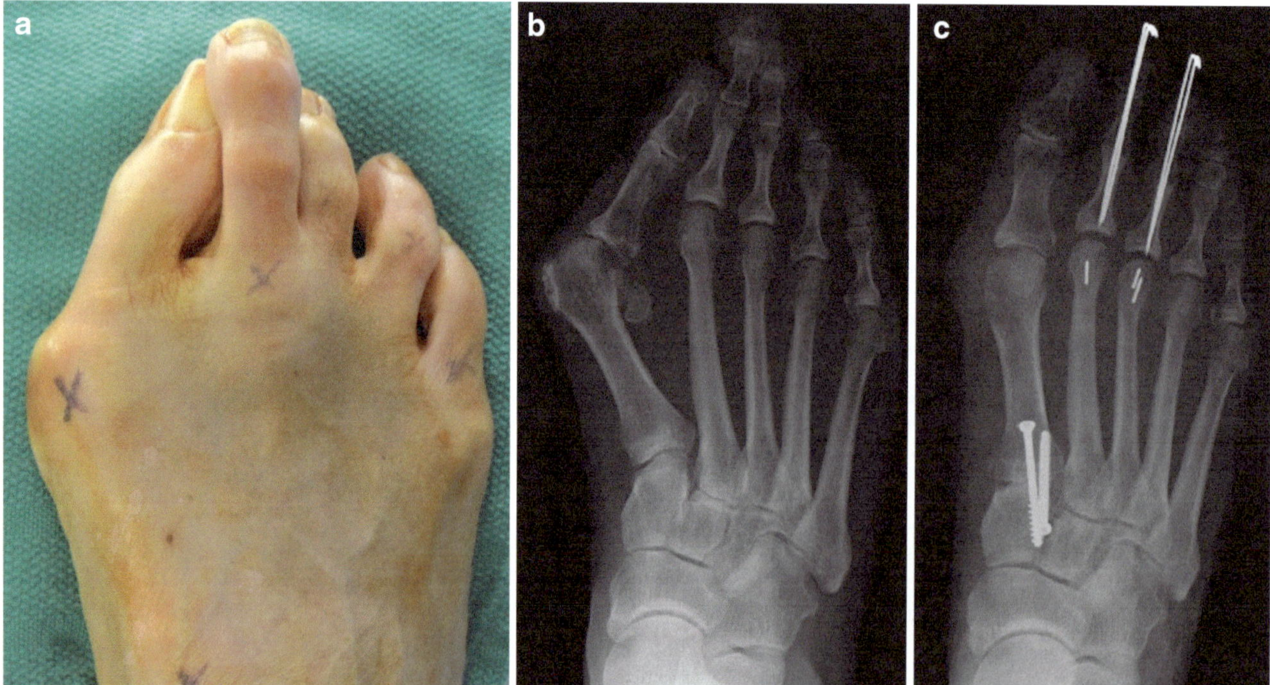

Fig. 16.5 Interdigital ulceration associated with an overlapping second toe and hallux valgus deformity. Hallux valgus deformity complicates matters with regard to ideal procedure selection for interdigital second toe ulceration (**a**, **b**). Second digital amputation may be the most prudent approach once a deep wound becomes complicated with cellulitis and osteomyelitis. Elective reconstructive procedures including bunionectomy, first MPJ or midfoot fusion, and hammertoe repair are more feasible if surgery is performed before the onset of infection (**c**)

Diagnosis of Central Digital Osteomyelitis

The diagnosis of central digital osteomyelitis requires consideration of the entire clinical picture since standard X-rays have a poor diagnostic track record. Advanced imaging is less practical for the small phalangeal bones of the central toes. Special X-ray techniques are helpful to isolate the area of concern since imaging of the involved toe may be compromised by overshadowing from adjacent toes and digital contracture (Fig. 16.6). The probe-to-bone test is particularly useful with toe ulcerations since bone is fairly close to the skin surface, though the positive predictive valve has been controversial [2, 3]. A nonhealing digital wound with deep depth or sinus tract concerning for bone or joint exposure plus clinical evidence of soft tissue infection should raise suspicion for osteomyelitis. Plain radiographs and laboratory workup combined with clinical findings are the mainstay of diagnosis at this stage, and we rarely pursue advanced imaging for central toe wounds. Bone biopsy is the next logical step which can be obtained in the process of bone debride-

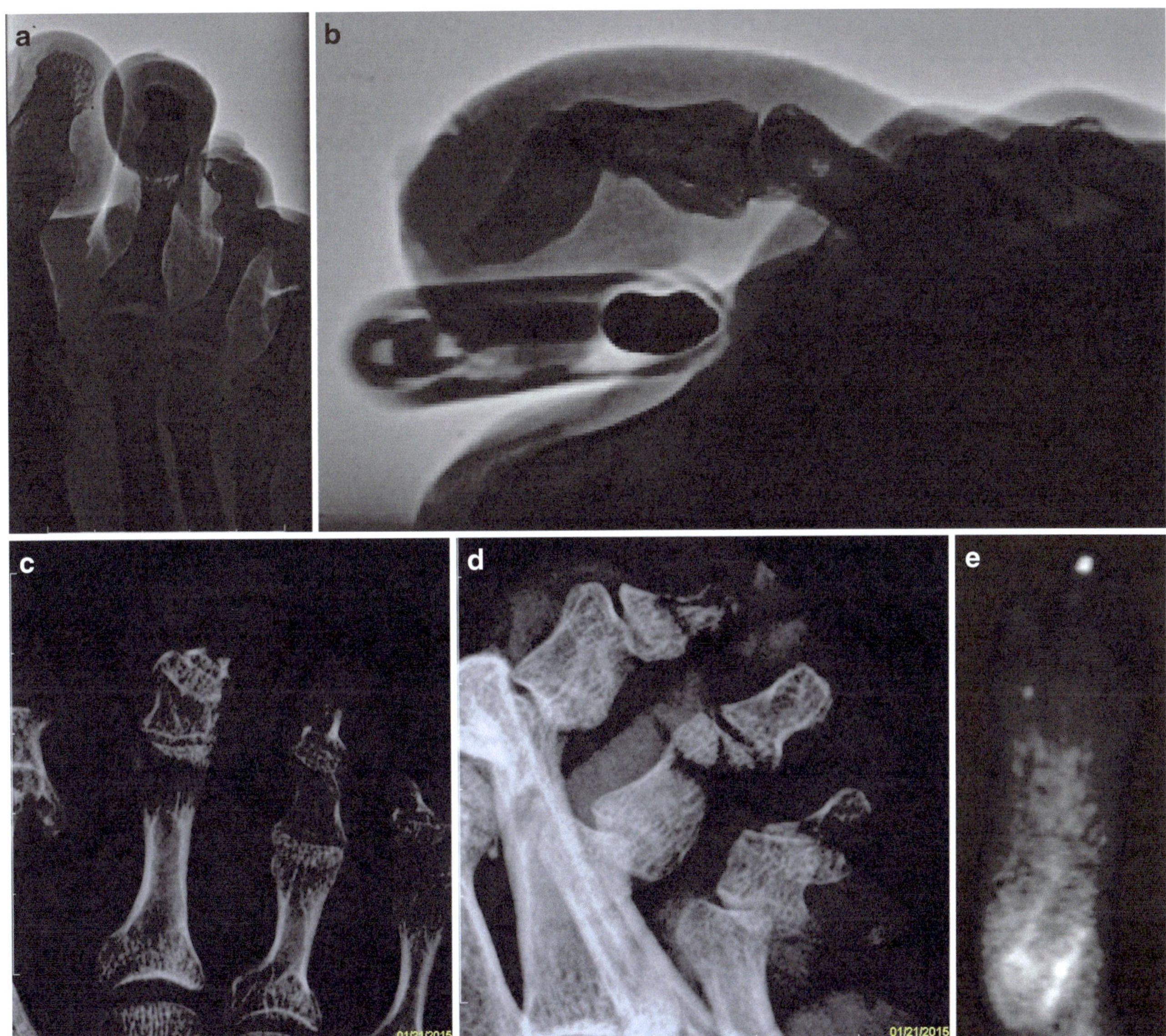

Fig. 16.6 Imaging for central toe osteomyelitis. Cortical erosion near the site of ulceration is the most common finding in osteomyelitis associated with contiguous spread of infection. Radiographic signs of osteomyelitis are not immediately visible on standard X-rays, but baseline imaging is useful to evaluate for underlying structural deformity. Other conditions may be identified on standard X-ray including arthritis, malunited fractures, and gouty arthropathy. Contracture of the distal phalanx (**a**) created imaging challenges for the tip of second toe ulcer shown in Fig. 16.2b. A raised toe view helped to isolate the tip of the distal phalanx on this lateral view (**b**). Osteomyelitis was found on biopsy despite normal X-ray findings. A different patient with erosion of the second distal phalanx correlated with location of ulceration at the tip of the toe (**c**, **d**). Comparison to the adjacent third toe distal phalanx helps to pick up early loss of cortex since the tip of the distal phalanx has a naturally occurring irregular cortical margin. Bone scan is not part of our routine work up for lesser toe infection but may be useful in certain circumstances (**e**). Note how uptake is localized to the tip of the second toe

ment, IPJ arthroplasty, tip of toe amputation, or removal of the entire toe. The decision to remove the entire toe has more to do with compromised soft tissue or severe deformity that is not amenable to reconstructive procedures which are determined by clinical exam rather than MRI or bone scan. Needle biopsy of a central toe is possible but can be challenging due to the small nature of the phalanges and close proximity of wounds to the IPJs, toenail, and vascular structures. Needle biopsy does not address digital deformity or bone prominence, and therefore open bone resection may be the most prudent method to obtain bone specimen for biopsy.

Isolated Medical Management

Cellulitis associated with digital ulceration or gangrene can be treated medically, but recurrent cellulitis should raise suspicion for underlying osteomyelitis. Isolated medical management of digital osteomyelitis has limited indications, as antibiotics do not address the underlying structural and biomechanical pathology that is responsible for the nonhealing ulcer. The open wound and exposed bone typically persist beyond the point of even long-term antibiotics, which is not conducive to successful medical therapy. Osteomyelitis of a central toe is therefore most commonly treated surgically or with a combined medical/surgical approach. The central toes are fairly amenable to wide resection of the infected bone which frequently allows a short course of oral antibiotic therapy to treat any residual soft tissue infection. Surgery can therefore be curative, avoiding potential cost and side effects of long-term parenteral antibiotics.

Surgical Management of Central Toe Infection

In our practice, phalangeal osteomyelitis is primarily treated with surgical intervention, which is supported in the literature [4, 5]. Intravenous antibiotics require adequate blood flow to the affected area, which is commonly compromised in diabetic patients with nonhealing toe ulcers. Blood flow is also compromised in areas of abscess, bone necrosis, and gangrene. Surgical treatment allows resection of diseased tissue back to a healthy margin which in turn allows a shorter but more effective course of antibiotic therapy. The primary goal of surgical management is source control of the infection, as well as eradication of infected bone all while preserving the most functional toe or foot possible. We also advocate early surgical intervention in infection cases to preserve as much soft tissue as possible for primary or flap closure. Staged surgery is common with acute infection which allows early incision and drainage of abscess, bone biopsy, medical treatment, and delayed closure.

The ideal level of central digital amputation is unique to the individual clinical situation and is based on a number of factors including extent of infection, location of the wound, and available soft tissue for closure (Fig. 16.7). A more distal level of amputation is generally preferred from a functional and cosmetic standpoint, but propensity for re-ulceration is a major consideration when dealing with complicated neuropathic ulcers. We typically disarticulate at the MPJ if there is sagittal or transverse plane deformity at the MTPJ or when osteomyelitis involves the entire proximal phalanx and attempt partial toe amputation or toe sparing arthroplasty for early infection without severe digital deformity.

Distal Symes Amputation for Tip of Toe Ulceration and Osteomyelitis of the Distal Phalanx

Nonhealing ulcerations with underlying osteomyelitis at the tip of a central toe is frequently treated with distal Symes amputation (Figs. 16.8, 16.9, 16.10, 16.11, 16.12, 16.13, 16.14, and 16.15). We prefer to perform this procedure early in the progression of the nonhealing or recurrent wound before osteomyelitis sets in; however, these patients frequently present to the office after a wound has been progressing underneath a thick callus and osteomyelitis has already begun to develop. Tip of toe wounds frequently probe to bone, and there is oftentimes concomitant nail pathology and digital contracture. Distal Symes amputation allows complete excision of the nonhealing ulceration, diseased nail, and underlying bone infection. Removal of the distal phalanx also allows release of digital contracture by removing the distal insertion of the long flexor tendon. We typically perform this procedure in the office under local anesthesia and sterile conditions. Staged open distal Symes amputation is commonly performed when cellulitis is present. This allows bone biopsy and culture prior to initiation of oral or intravenous antibiotics with the second-stage surgery performed days later (Figs. 16.16, 16.17, and 16.18). Our surgical technique presented here was originally published in the *Journal of Foot and Ankle Surgery* which provides retrospective outcome data [5].

Partial Toe Amputation Through the Proximal Phalanx

Partial toe amputation through the proximal phalanx allows the proximal portion of the toe to remain in an effort to keep the metatarsophalangeal joint complex intact, as well as to keep adjacent toes from drifting to fill in the void as commonly seen with complete digital amputation. However, dorsal contracture or transverse drift of the metatarsophalangeal

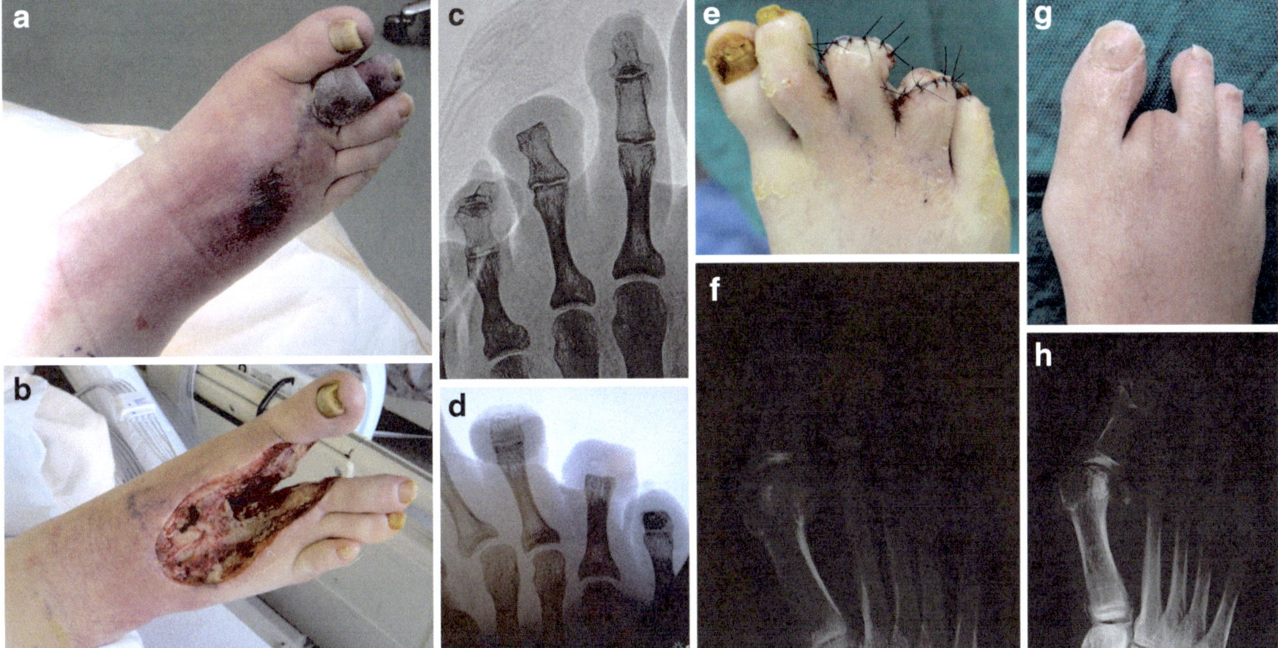

Fig. 16.7 Selection of ideal level of amputation for central toe osteomyelitis. The ideal level of amputation is largely dependent on the clinical situation for an individual patient. The extent of soft tissue infection, necrosis, and ulceration are frequently the main factors that determine level of infection. This patient required a web splitting open second ray amputation for wide spread abscess and necrosis associated with osteomyelitis (**a**, **b**). Timely diagnosis and early aggressive surgical treatment is intended to avoid this scenario which ultimately required amputation at the midfoot level. Distal Symes amputation through the DIPJ on the other hand preserves a fairly normal third toe structure (**c**). Distal Symes amputation with resection of the distal portion of the middle phalanx (**d**, **e**) on the third toe allows clean margin bone biopsy and better mobility of the flap for closure. Amputation through the fourth PIPJ (**d**, **e**) preserves part of the toe but is less commonly performed since the prominent head of the proximal phalanx may predispose to recurrent wounds from adjacent toe pressure or dorsal irritation from shoe. Amputation though the proximal phalanx is common for wounds and infection at or distal to the PIPJ. Leaving the base of the proximal phalanx helps to preserve MPJ function and may prevent drift of the adjacent toes (**f**, **g**). Progressive hallux valgus deformity following partial second toe amputation resulted in recurrent interdigital ulceration (**h**) necessitating revision surgery. Digital hammertoe contracture or transverse plane deformity at the involved MPJ is best treated with MPJ disarticulation as opposed to leaving a portion of the proximal phalanx

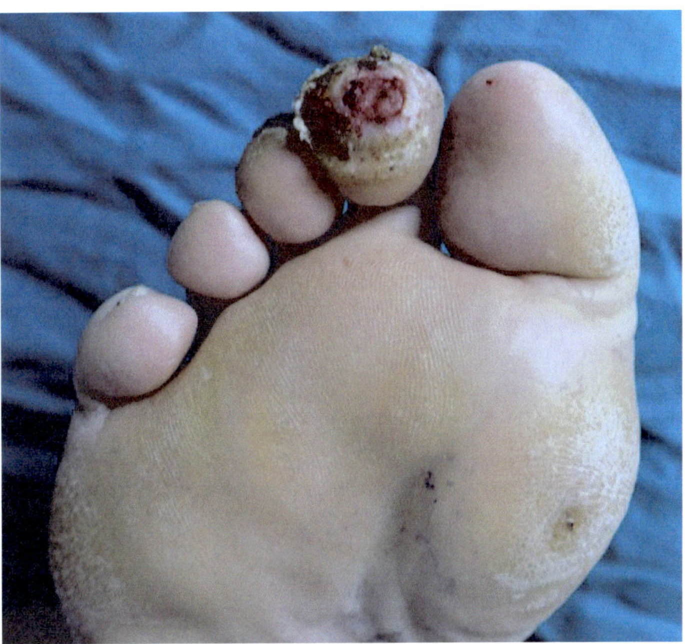

Fig. 16.8 Distal Symes amputation for tip of toe ulceration complicated by osteomyelitis of the distal phalanx. Tip of toe amputation for osteomyelitis of the distal phalanx is ideally performed early in the course of infection in an attempt to avoid loss of the entire toe. Catching the infection early avoids soft tissue necrosis and preserves the plantar soft tissue used for advancement flap closure of the wound. This relatively benign-looking chronic wound presented with dorsal toe cellulitis as shown in Fig. 16.2a, b. Osteomyelitis was suspected based on clinical appearance and positive probe to bone despite normal X-ray finding shown in Fig. 16.6a, b. Immediate surgery during the initial office visit allowed excision of the wound, resection of the distal phalanx, bone biopsy before initiation of antibiotics, permanent removal of the diseased toenail, and single-stage wound closure. Concomitant medical treatment consisted of 14 days of oral antibiotics for residual soft tissue infection

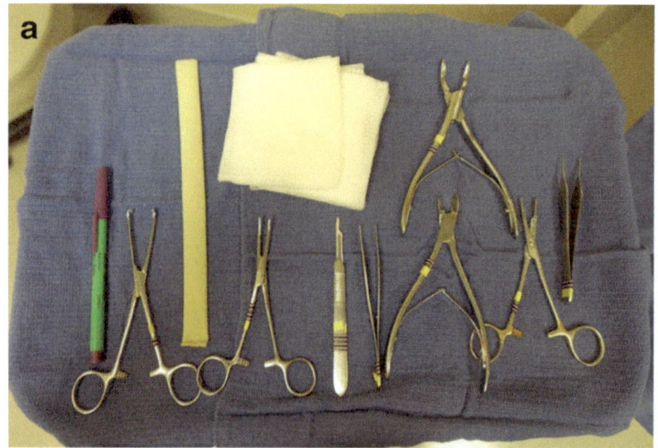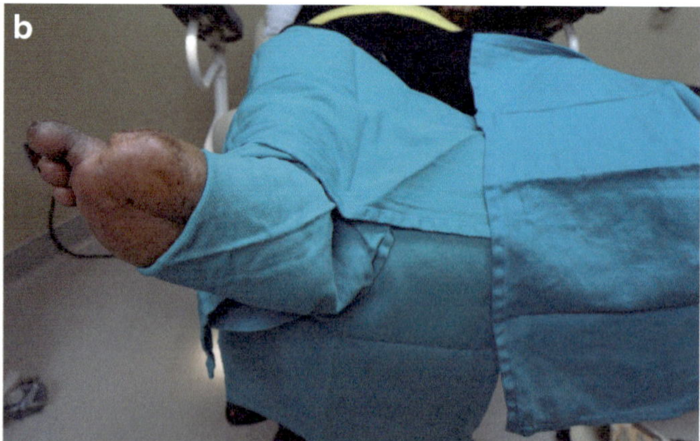

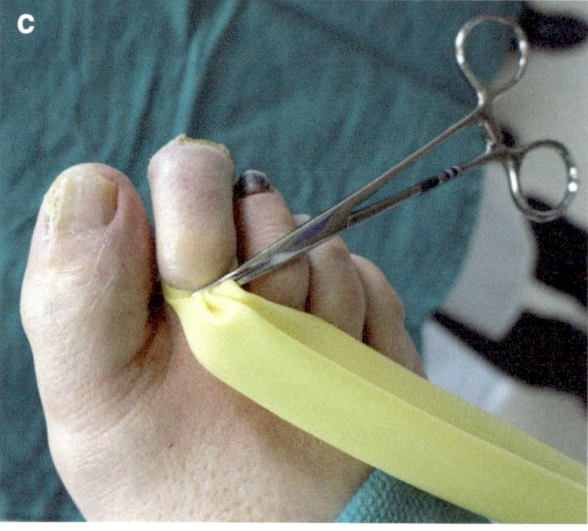

Fig. 16.9 Setup for office-based distal Symes amputation. Distal Symes amputation is typically performed in the outpatient clinic minor procedure room under sterile conditions and local anesthesia. Minimal instrumentation is required including elastic drain for digital tourniquet, hemostat, bone cutting forceps, tissue forceps, #15 scalpel, needle driver, skin suture, and rongeur (**a**). After sterile prep of the operative foot and ankle, the extremity is draped with sterile towels (**b**). Disposable drapes can also be used if desired. Hemostasis is achieved with an elastic drain tourniquet which allows the surgeon to release the tourniquet temporarily to confirm adequate hemostasis before reapplication for closure (**c**)

joint can leave a problematic digital stump, and these patients may be better served with complete digital amputation. Intact and viable soft tissue extending to the PIPJ is needed for this procedure, and final decisions regarding the level of amputation are made intraoperatively based on direct inspection of the tissue and bone (Fig. 16.19). Compromised interdigital tissue on one side of the toe associated with ulceration or gangrene can be accommodated by creating a long flap on the opposite side to cover the bone stump. Poor condition of tissue deep in the interdigital space may be best treated with MPJ disarticulation.

PIPJ Arthroplasty for Acutely Infected Dorsal Wound Associated with Hammertoe Deformity

Nonhealing ulcerations over the dorsal IPJs are commonly treated with either arthroplasty of the affected joint or partial/complete digital amputation. The PIPJ is more commonly involved due to its prominence with hammertoe deformity. The DIPJ is typically involved in mallet toe deformities and arthritis, though these are less common (Figs. 16.20 and 16.21).

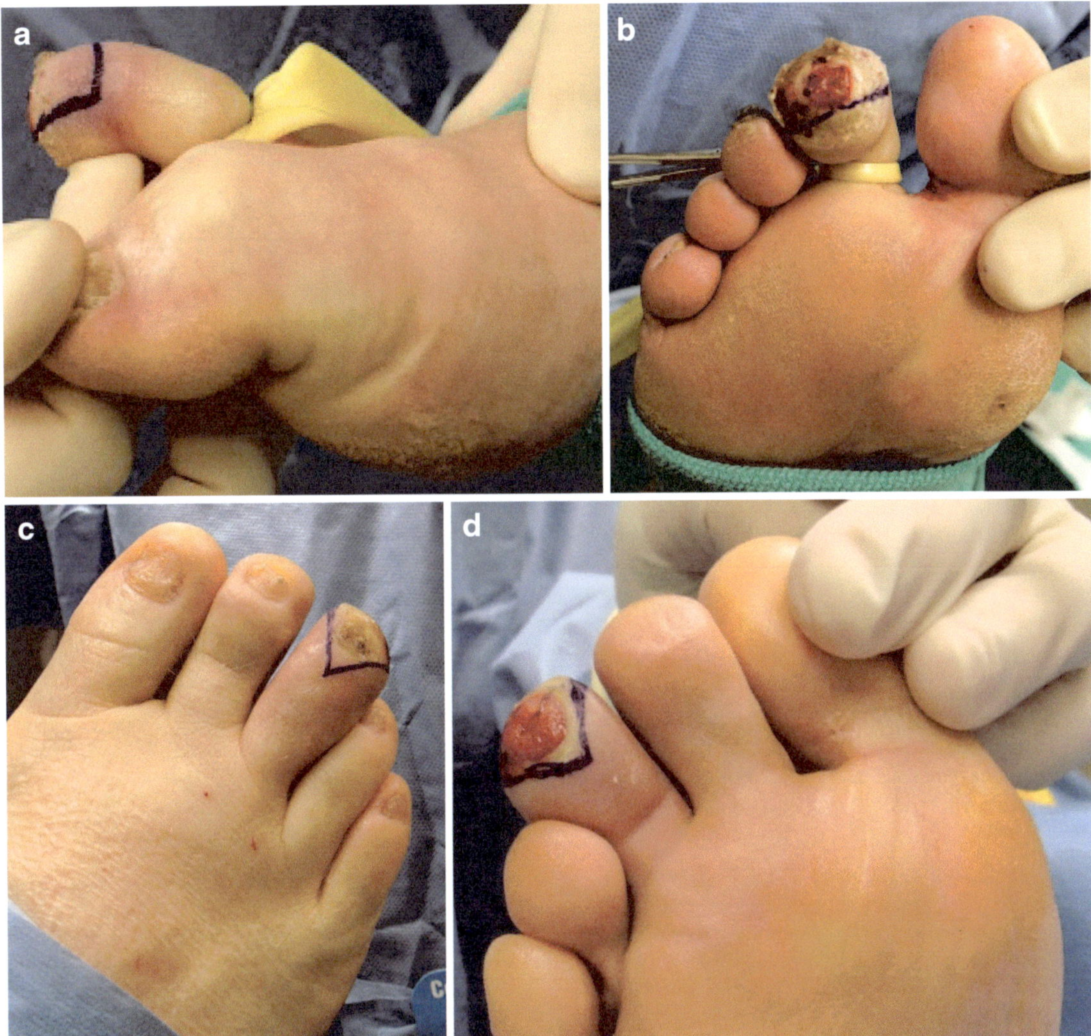

Fig. 16.10 Incision options for distal Symes amputation. Dorsal and plantar amputation flaps are ideally of equal length for digital amputation which can be difficult to achieve at the tip of the toe due to the location of the nail bed and nail matrix. Distal Symes amputation involves a plantar flap that is advanced dorsally to cover the wound defect and middle phalanx after amputation (**a**). The dorsal incision is placed transversely over the DIPJ, just proximal to the nail matrix. The plantar incision is kept close to the edge of the ulceration to preserve plantar flap length (**b**). Care is taken to completely remove the nail matrix to prevent nail regrowth postoperatively. Alternatively, medial and lateral flaps can be created (**c**, **d**). This incision design may require more proximal bone resection to accomplish wound closure and is primarily used when the plantar flap is compromised by a large wound

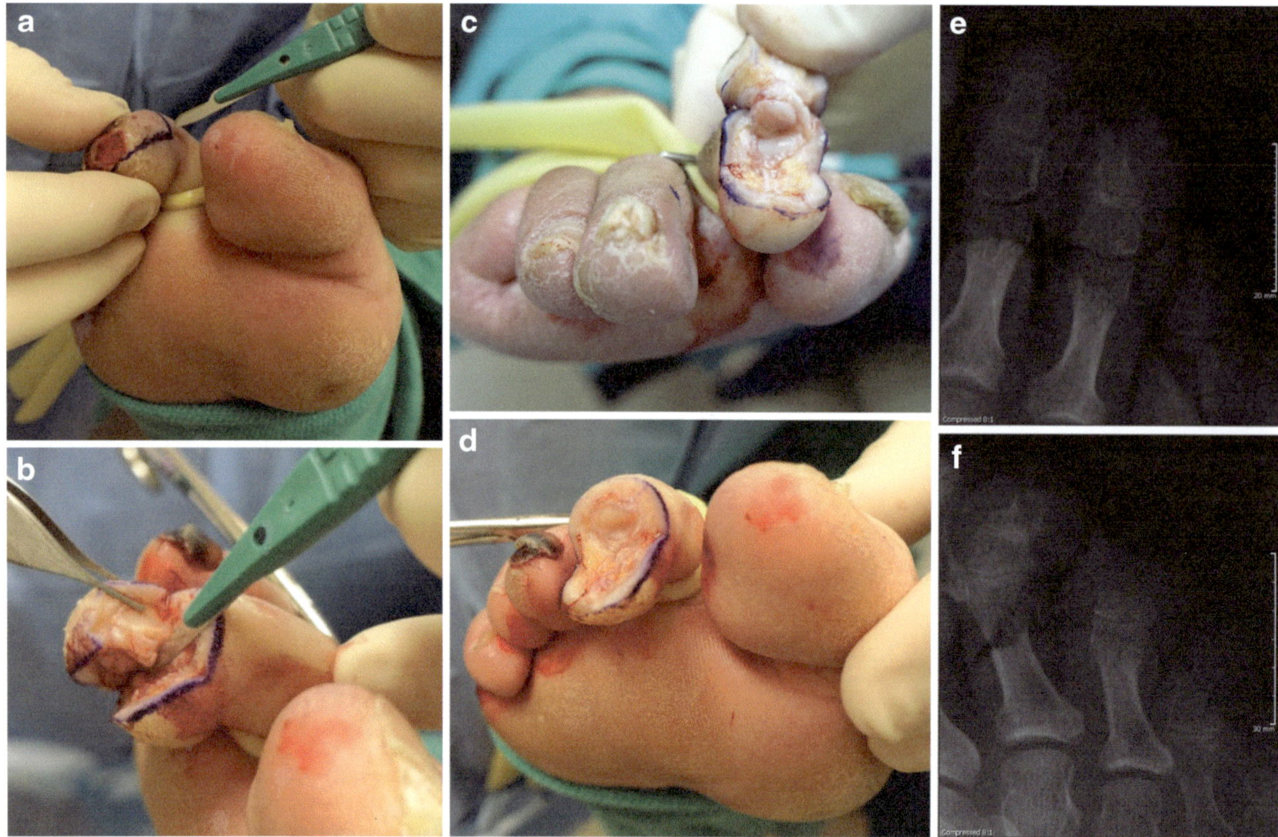

Fig. 16.11 Distal Symes amputation surgical technique. Full-depth incisions are made at 90° to the skin surface. Note that this is not a belly of the blade incision but rather the tip of the #15 blade is plunged directly to bone (**a**). This technique minimizes the chance for beveling of the incision and allows precise creation of a full-thickness plantar flap. The dorsal incision conveniently enters directly into the DIPJ which allows easy access for disarticulation. This joint is commonly arthritic and contracted which results in difficulty separating the phalanges. An alternative approach is to access the joint from the plantar direction. Cutting the long flexor tendon opens the joint in a plantar to dorsal direction allowing disarticulation of the DIPJ (**b**, **c**). The distal aspect of the middle phalanx is inspected for signs of infection which is rarely the case (**d**). The distal end of the middle phalanx can be removed if needed which improves flap mobility, provides margin biopsy, and further reduces distal pressure. Note that half of the middle phalanx remains if a portion of the middle phalanx is removed as shown on before and after X-rays of a different patient (**e**, **f**)

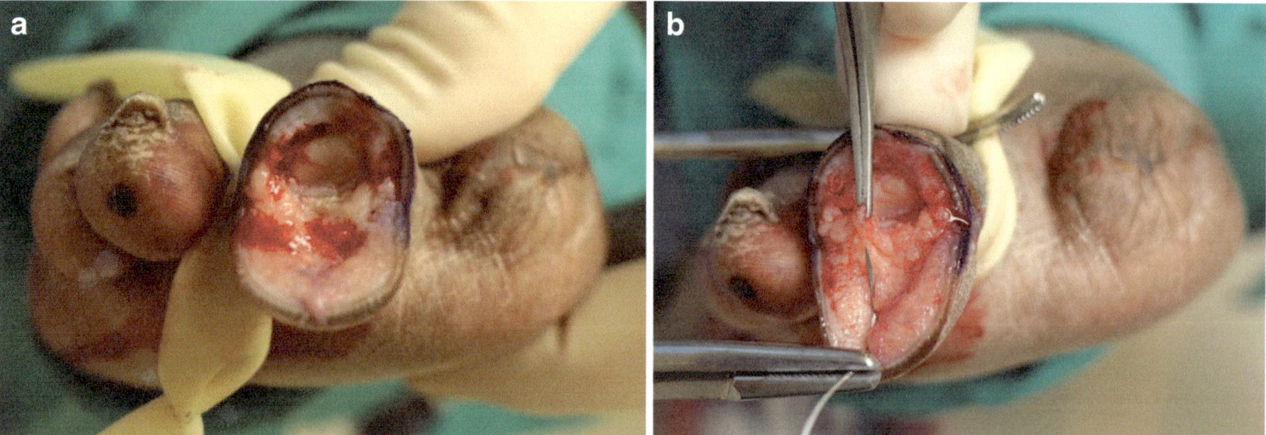

Fig. 16.12 Hemostasis with distal Symes amputation. Vascularity to the plantar flap is tenuous, and care is taken to avoid further compromise when obtaining hemostasis. Post-op bleeding is minimal due to the tamponade effect of flap rotation and skin sutures. The tourniquet is release prior to closure to check for pulsatile flow from the plantar vessels located immediately beneath the flexor tendon sheath (**a**). These plantar vessels are ideally preserved but can be tied using a stick tie technique if significant bleeding is noted (**b**). Minimal dead space remains after flap advancement and closure making extensive use of cautery counterproductive

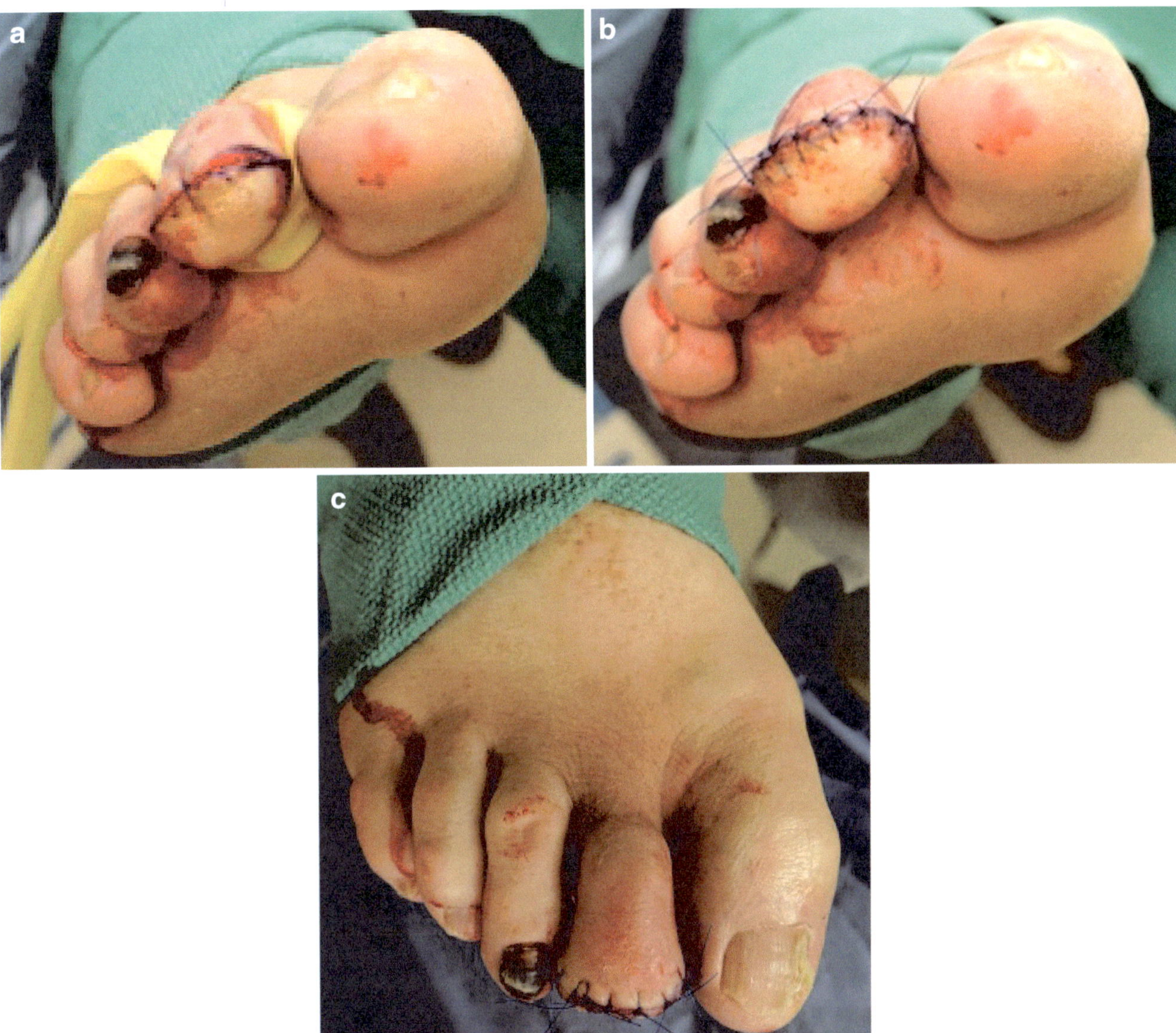

Fig. 16.13 Advancement flap closure in distal Symes amputation. The plantar flap is advanced dorsally to cover the wound defect and exposed bone. Note how one simple suture placed at the center of the flap pro- vides tension-free coverage (**a**). Additional simple sutures are then placed to provide complete closure (**b, c**)

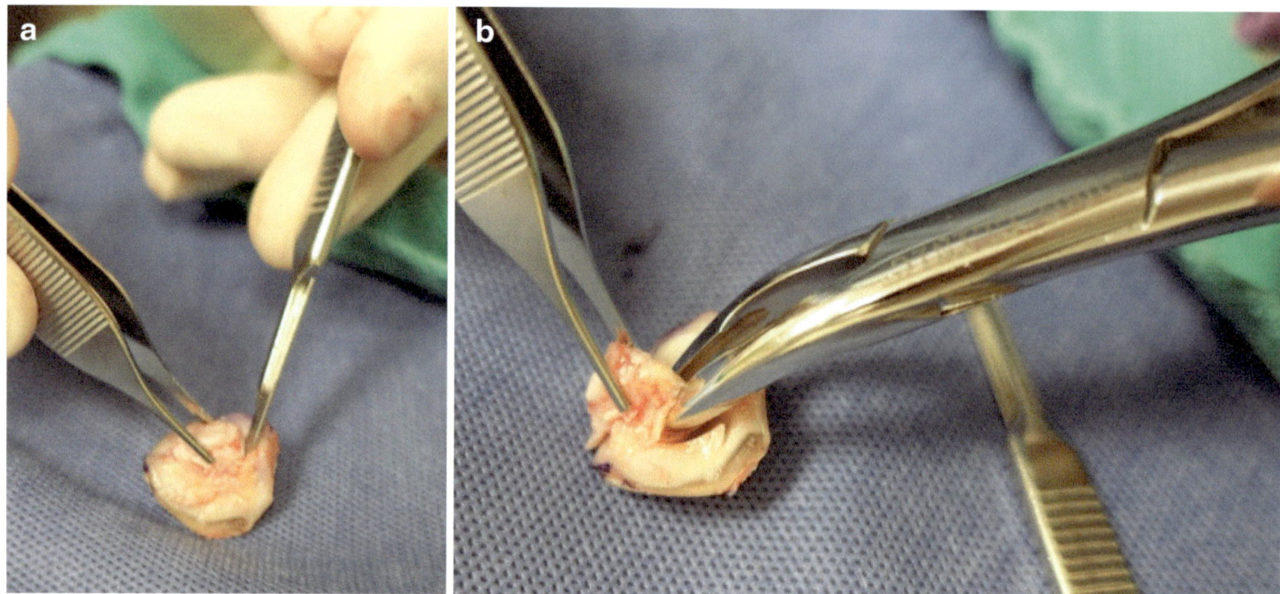

Fig. 16.14 Distal Symes amputation bone biopsy technique. An "inside-out" bone biopsy technique minimizes the risk of cross contamination from the open wound. Once the distal portion of the toe has been removed from the surgical field, it is placed on the Mayo stand for later biopsy procurement after the wound is closed. The forceps is holding the base of the distal phalanx during dissection to access the tip of the phalanx for bone culture (**a**). A rongeur was used to remove a portion of distal phalangeal bone near the ulcer location for culture (**b**). The remainder of the amputated tip, including the ulcer and residual distal phalanx, is then sent to histology in formalin. Clean margin bone biopsy can be taken from the distal aspect of the middle phalanx using a sterile bone nipper, which is sent for histological examination in formalin

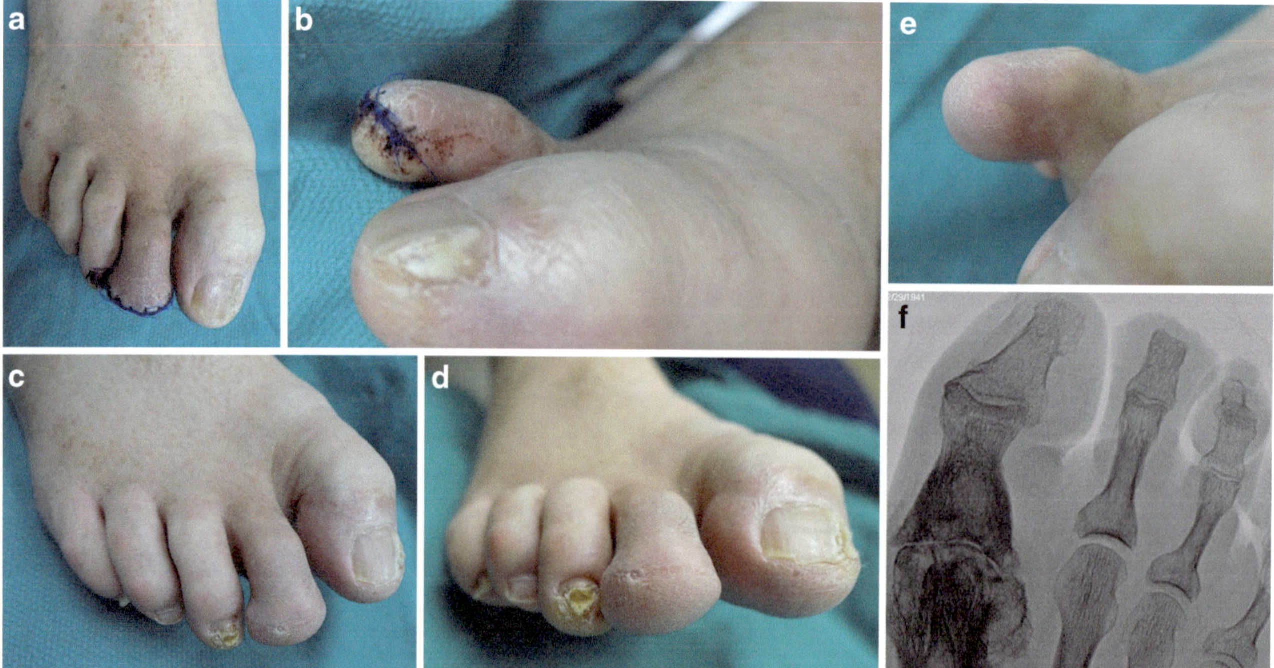

Fig. 16.15 Postoperative results following distal Symes amputation. Complete resolution of infection is shown 1 week later (**a**, **b**). Biopsy results confirmed osteomyelitis of the distal phalanx. Complete healing is shown 6 weeks later with preservation of a fairly normal-appearing toe (**c–e**). Intentional shortening of a long toe, release of the long flexor tendon, and repositioning the plantar fat pad over the distal tip are intended to decrease the risk of future breakdown. Post-op X-rays demonstrate removal of the distal phalanx (**f**). Note how this conservative procedure maintains a normal second toe length. Pre-op X-rays are shown in Fig. 16.6a, b

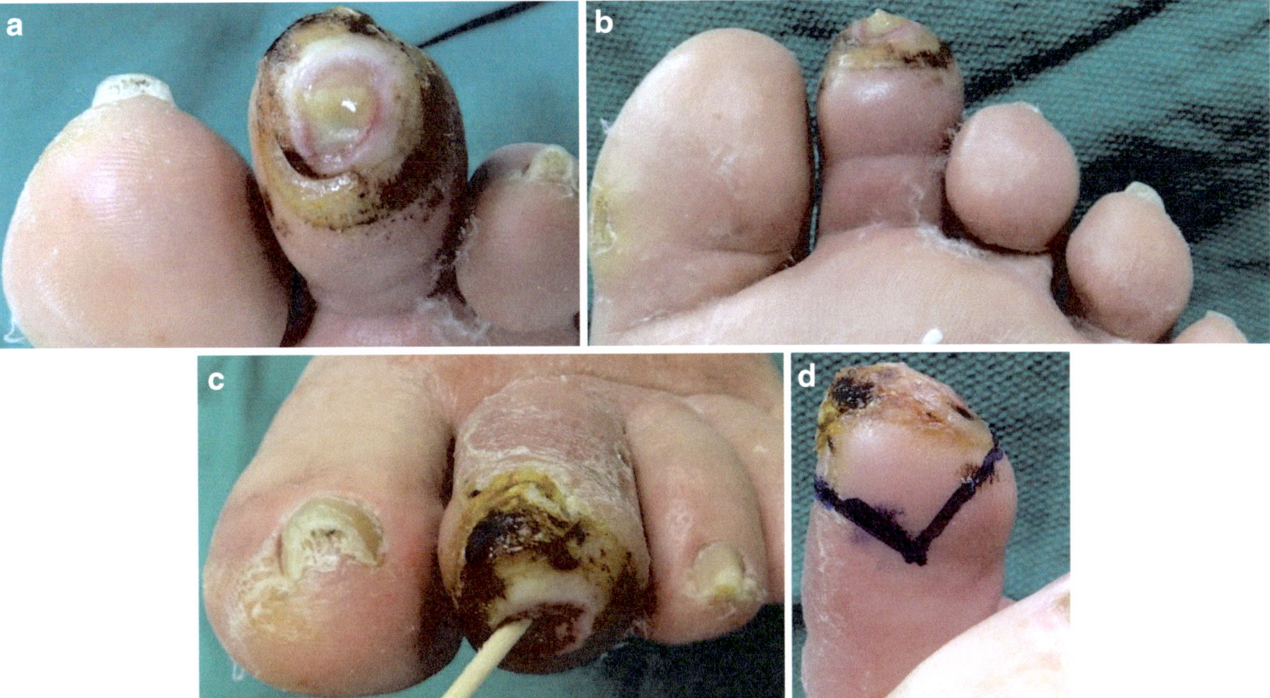

Fig. 16.16 Two-stage distal Symes amputation for acute infection. This patient presented with severe infection secondary to a tip of second toe ulcer with purulent drainage and cellulitis to the base of the toe (**a**, **b**). Probe-to-bone test revealed exposed bone at the site of infection (**c**). Treatment involved immediate open distal Symes amputation in the office followed by hospitalization and delayed revision and closure once infection had stabilized. The incision design was the same as for the elective distal Symes amputation (**d**). The stage 1 surgery was intended to remove necrotic soft tissue and bone and preserve enough tissue for eventual flap closure. The middle phalanx was left intact during the first operation to minimize cross contamination

Complete Central Toe Amputation with MPJ Disarticulation

Amputation through the MPJ and partial ray amputation to include the metatarsal head is commonly needed due to compromised soft tissue associated with infected neuropathic ulcers and gangrene. Primary closure is ideal but not always possible. Transverse and sagittal plane deformity often requires MPJ disarticulation in an effort to avoid re-ulceration over residual stump prominence commonly associated with partial toe amputation. Neuropathic patients with hallux valgus frequently develop interdigital ulceration along the medial side of the second toe due to hallux abutment. Reconstructive procedures including hammertoe repair and bunionectomy can be considered in the early stages but are not practical once infection develops. We commonly perform second toe amputation in this scenario, as patients with infected neuropathic wounds are frequently not ideal candidates for elective bunion surgery due to advanced age, poor bone quality, high risk of postoperative infection, and difficulty with postoperative weight bearing restrictions

(Figs. 16.22 and 16.23). Amputation allows immediate weight bearing, does not require correction of the adjacent toes, and allows a surgical cure for infection isolated to the phalanges. Amputation also resolves pain which is common with this condition despite underlying neuropathy.

Postoperative Care

Isolated digital procedures typically tolerate immediate weight bearing in an open-toed surgical shoe, but rest and elevation are important to avoid edema and hematoma. Digital surgery for osteomyelitis frequently provides a surgical cure for osteomyelitis, and postoperative antibiotic treatment may only be needed for any residual soft tissue infection. Bone biopsy of the affected area, clean margin biopsy, and intraoperative findings are helpful from this regard. Sutures are commonly left in place for longer than 2 weeks, as delayed healing is common in patients undergoing surgery for infected wounds. Orthopedic footwear is recommended for long-term prevention of recurrent sores.

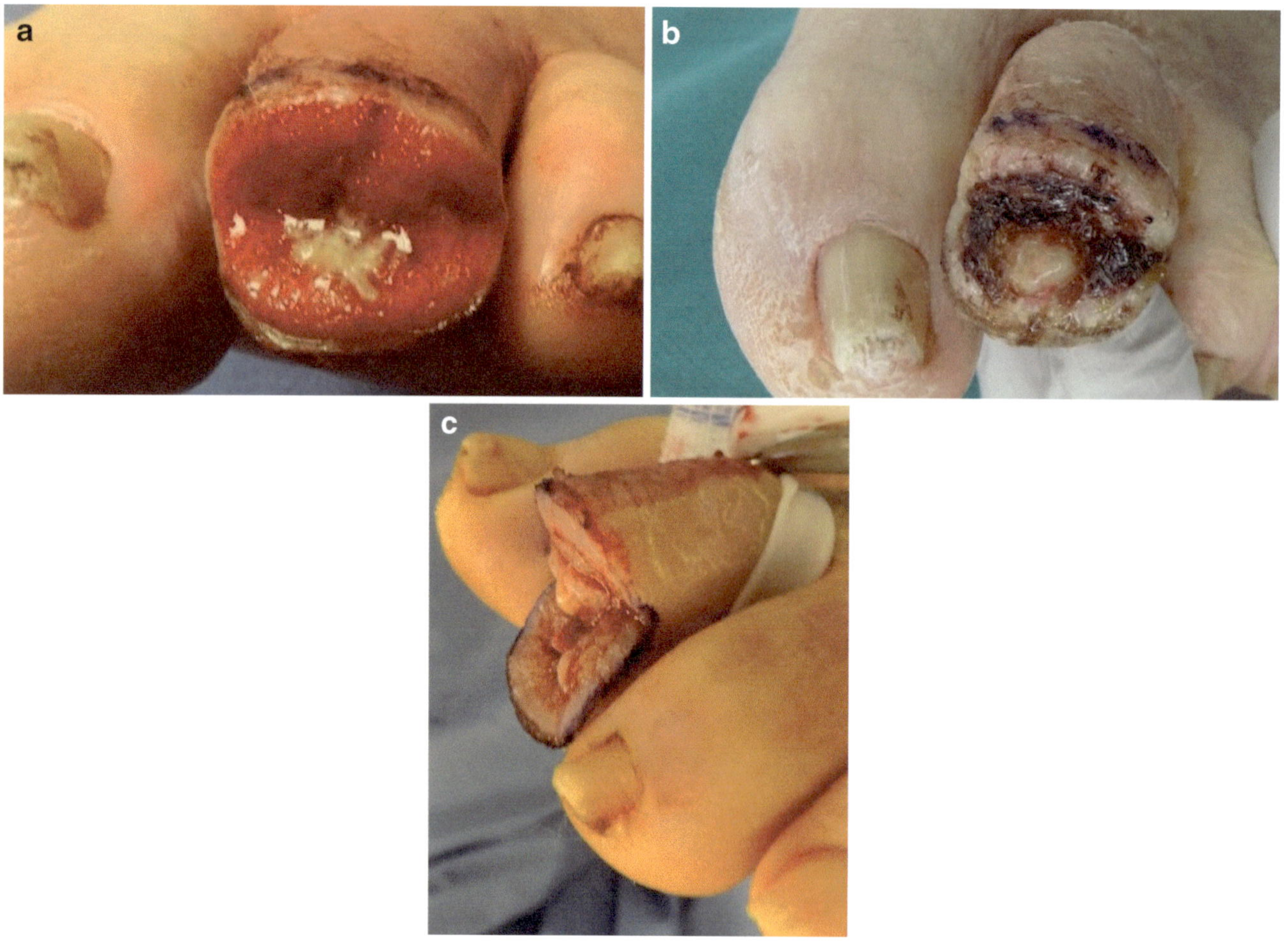

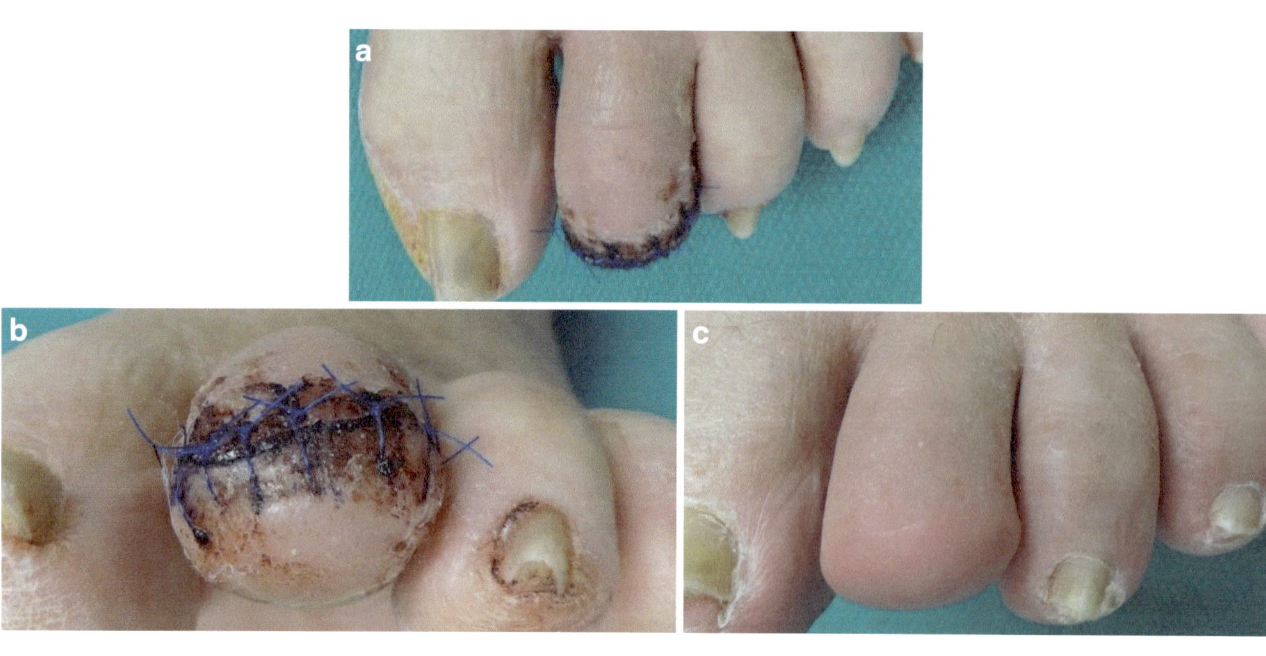

Fig. 16.17 Stage 2 distal Symes amputation with delayed closure performed 5 days later. Clinical appearance is shown 2 days after initial open amputation (**a**). Note drastic improvement of cellulitis and granulating wound bed with persistent purulence (**a**). The stage 2 procedure was performed 5 days after the initial open amputation to allow recovery of the soft tissues and resolution of the majority of infection (**b**). Conservative excision of the distal wound margins with preservation of the plantar flap identified viable tissue available for delayed closure (**c**). Clean margin bone biopsy of the middle phalanx was procured at this stage

Fig. 16.18 Clinical results with staged distal Symes amputation. Resolution of cellulitis is shown 1 week later (**a**, **b**). Complete healing with preservation of a functional toe length is shown 6 weeks later (**c**)

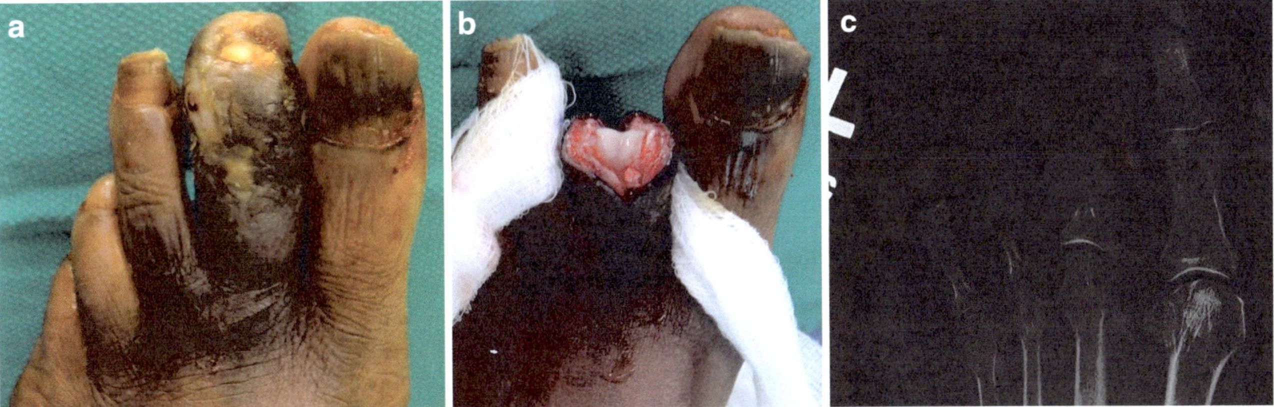

Fig. 16.19 Partial central digital amputation. Partial amputation of a central toe is an option depending on the extent of osteomyelitis and location of compromised tissue. Note that the tissue at the base of the second toe remained viable despite distal necrosis (**a**). Medial and lateral flaps were created at the line of tissue demarcation allowing PIPJ disarticulation (**b**). Note how surgical sponges were used to retract the adjacent digits during central digital amputation. The level of bone resection was determined by availability of soft tissue for primary closure. We rarely leave the distal end of the proximal phalanx due to concerns of pressure on the bulbous head. Amputation preserved a portion of the proximal phalanx which is less invasive than MPJ disarticulation and may help prevent drift of the adjacent toes (**c**)

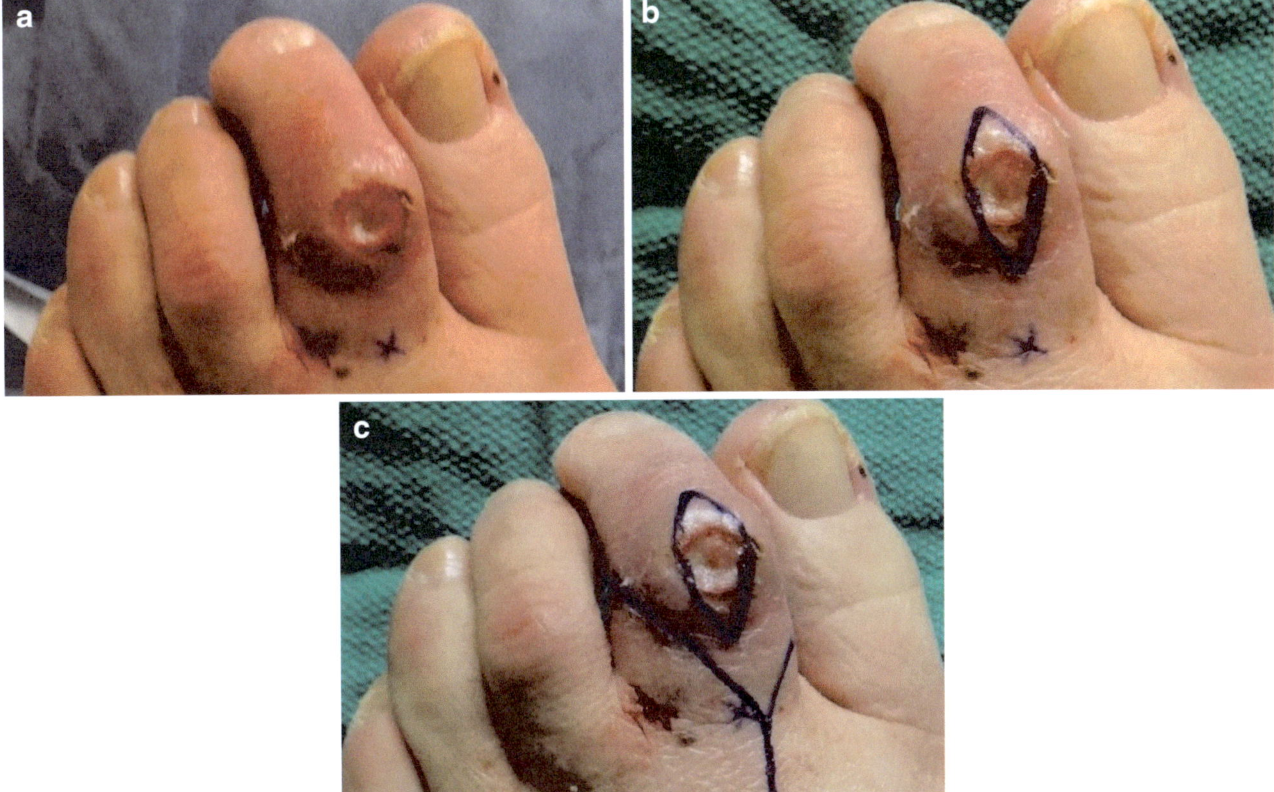

Fig. 16.20 PIPJ arthroplasty for dorsal ulceration with bone and joint infection. Pre-op appearance of dorsal PIPJ neuropathic ulceration with associated hammertoe deformity and acute infection is shown (**a**). Osteomyelitis and joint infection are fairly common with PIPJ ulcers due to the thin subcutaneous tissue on the dorsal aspect of the toes. Office-based wound excision and PIPJ arthroplasty allowed immediate incision and drainage of infection, bone biopsy, reduction of dorsal prominence, relaxation of toe contracture, and primary wound closure with several loose retention sutures (**b**). The standard toe amputation incision was drawn before the initial incision and drainage procedure which was part of the pre-op planning process to avoid compromising available flaps that may be necessary with staged surgery (**c**). Drawing future amputation incisions also allows the patient to better understand the serious nature of their condition and the surgeon's good intentions to save the toe if possible

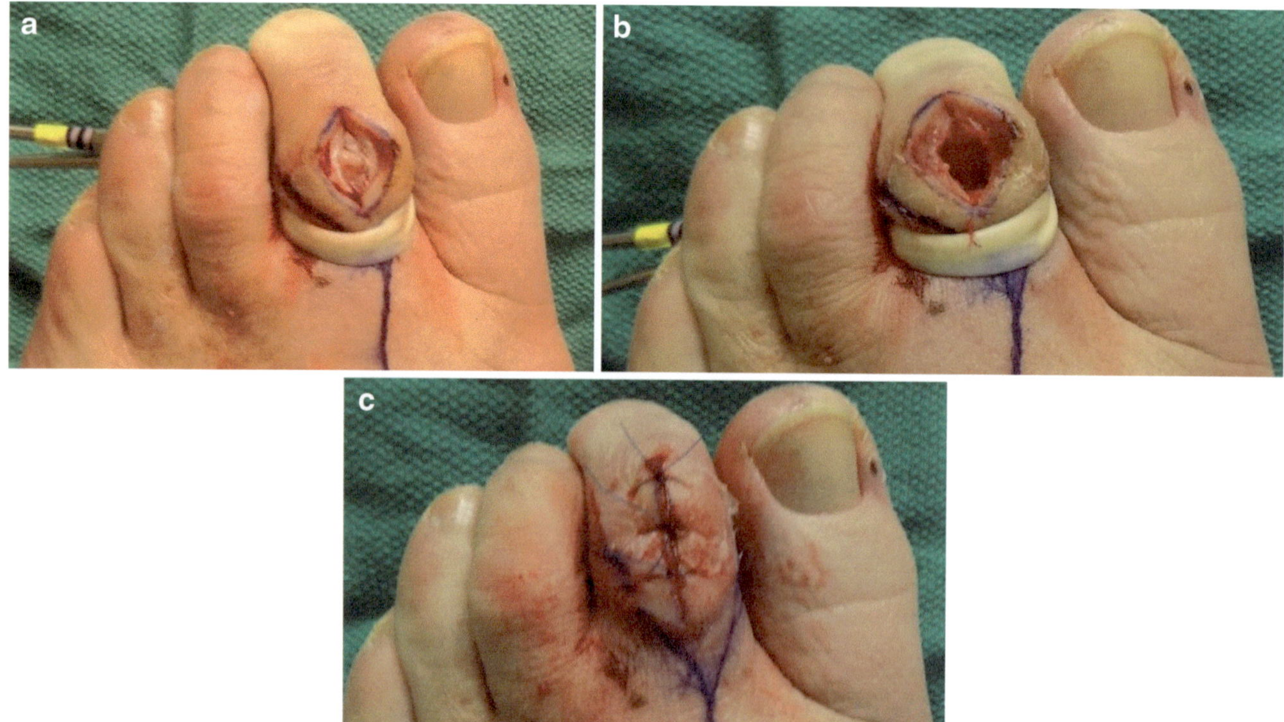

Fig. 16.21 Single-staged wound excision and PIPJ arthroplasty. A full-thickness elliptical incision was made down to bone (**a**). The head of the proximal phalanx is typically quite prominent (especially at the base of the wound), and the extensor tendon is often compromised in full-thickness wounds. Removal of the head of the proximal phalanx creates laxity in the soft tissues which allows primary closure and relaxation of toe contracture (**b**). The wound is closed when possible, but resection of the phalanx seems to stimulate robust granulation tissue allowing a previously nonhealing wound to heal by secondary intention. Wound closure involved three retention sutures in an effort to cover the bone structure yet allow drainage of infection if needed (**c**). No attempt was made to fixate the toe with intramedullary Kirschner wires due to wound and infection concerns, although there have been isolated reports in the literature of pinning digits that have undergone bone resection for osteomyelitis [4]. The head of the proximal phalanx was sent for aerobic and anaerobic culture and histology

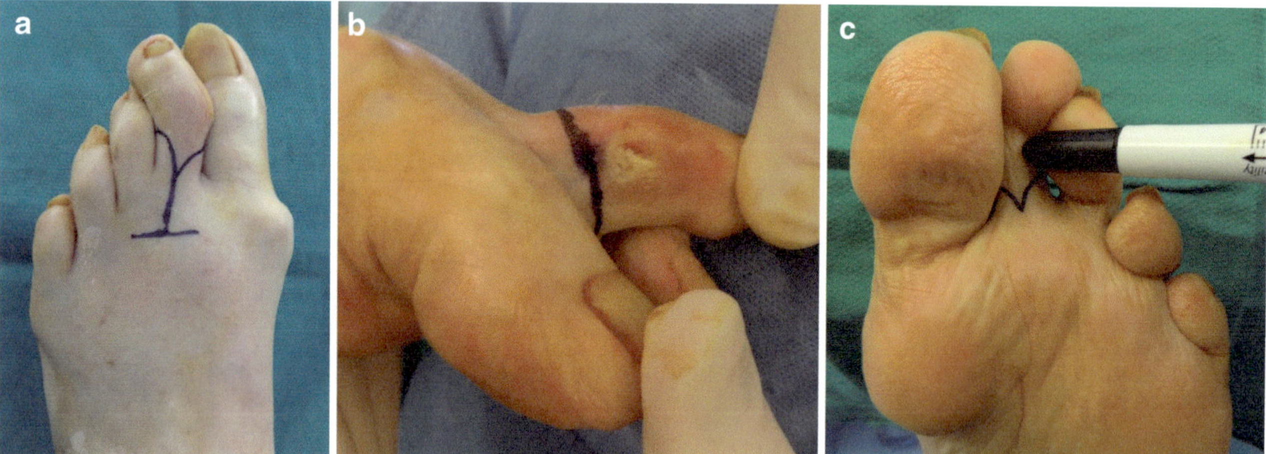

Fig. 16.22 MPJ disarticulation for complete central toe amputation. Complete toe amputation was performed due to an infected and painful interdigital PIPJ wound with joint exposure (**a, b**). This overlapping second hammertoe was complicated by hallux valgus deformity making amputation the preferred choice of procedure over PIPJ arthroplasty. The standard MPJ disarticulation incision plan creates medial and lateral flaps at the base of the toe. The dorsal incision extends proximally to access the MPJ for disarticulation (**a**). The plantar apex of the incision is specifically contained to the toe in an effort to avoid incision on the plantar weight bearing surface (**c**). The length of the medial flap was compromised by the medial ulcer (**b**) which can be accommodated by a longer lateral flap (**a**)

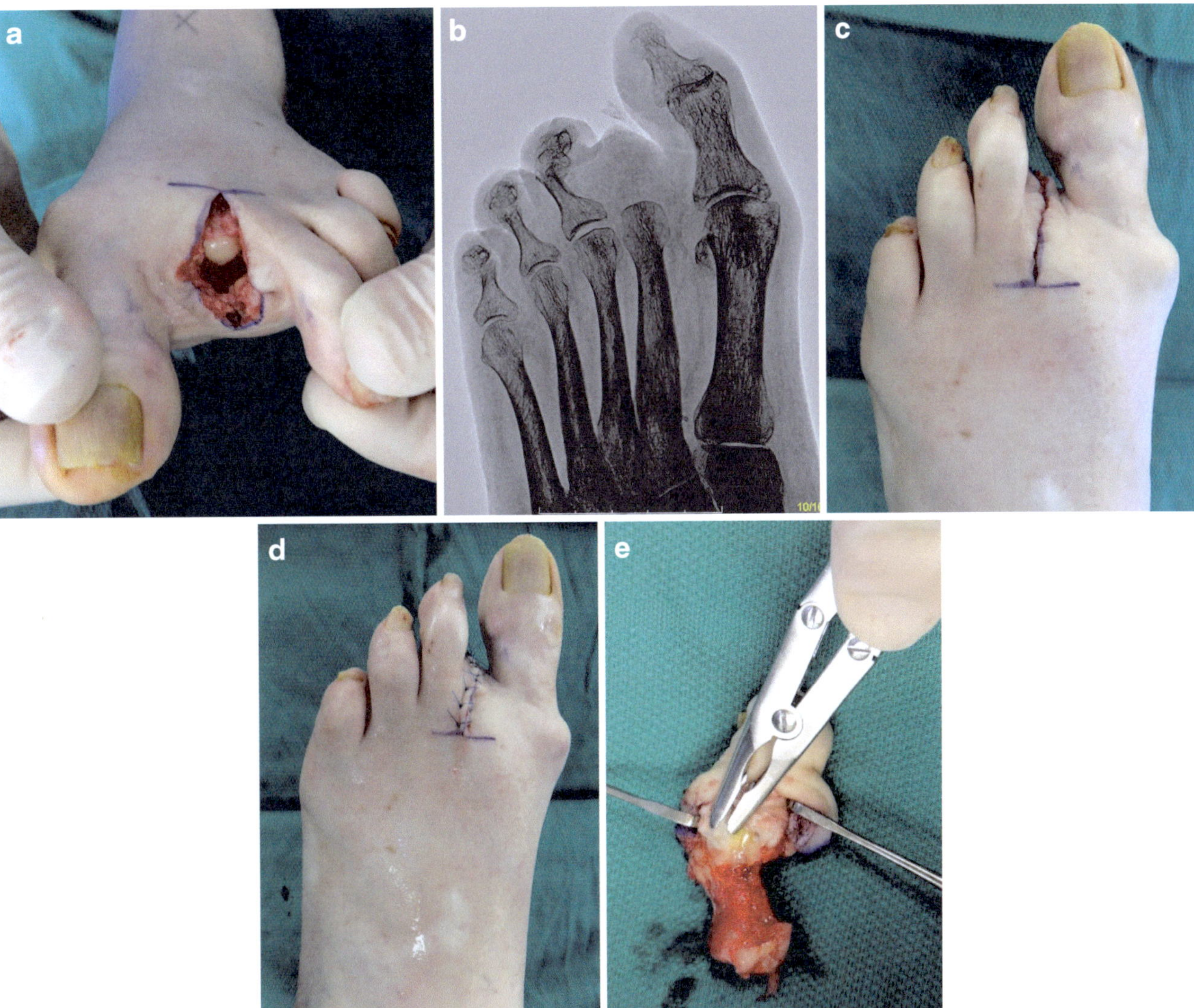

Fig. 16.23 Surgical technique for MPJ disarticulation. Amputation incisions were made directly to bone with the flaps raised full thickness to include skin, subcutaneous fat, and periosteum. MPJ disarticulation exposed the head of the metatarsal (**a**). We attempt to preserve the metatarsal head with infected digital wounds since opening the metatarsal may predispose to cross contamination (**b**). Removal of cartilage is con- troversial, but we prefer to leave the cartilage undisturbed. Note how these well-planned flaps practically fell into place (**c**). Simple sutures were placed for primary closure (**d**). Bone biopsy was taken from the PIPJ on the back table after wound closure to minimize the risk of cross contamination with the clean surgical site (**e**)

Conclusion

Osteomyelitis of a central toe is typically related to contiguous spread of infection from adjacent ulceration or gangrene. The central toes have minimal subcutaneous tissue and prominent bone structure which lead to osteomyelitis when the soft tissue becomes compromised. Digital wounds are also difficult to heal due to associated digital deformity. Advanced imaging is typically not necessary for the workup of central toe osteomyelitis as the condition is made by evaluating the entire clinical picture. Osteomyelitis of a central toe is primarily treated with surgical intervention, and medical management is an adjunctive part of the overall therapy. Consideration should be given to performing early, minimally invasive digital procedures in a clinical setting which can be preventive in an effort to avoid amputation.

References

1. Kearney TP, Hunt NA, Lavery LA. Safety and effectiveness of flexor tenotomies to heal toe ulcers in persons with diabetes. Diabetes Res Clin Pract. 2010;89(3):224–6.
2. Grayson ML, Gibbons GW, Balogh K, Levin E, Karchmer AW. Probing to bone in infected pedal ulcers. A clinical sign of underlying osteomyelitis in diabetic patients. JAMA. 1995;273(9): 721–3.
3. Lavery LA, Armstrong DG, Peters EJ, Lipsky BA. Probe-to-bone test for diagnosing diabetic foot osteomyelitis: reliable or relic? Diabetes Care. 2007;30(2):270–4.
4. Kim JY, Kim TW, Park YE, Lee YJ. Modified resection arthroplasty for infected non-healing ulcers with toe deformity in diabetic patients. Foot Ankle Int. 2008;29(5):493–7.
5. Boffeli TJ, Abben KW, Hyllengren SB. In-office distal symes lesser toe amputation—a safe, reliable, and cost-effective treatment of diabetes-related tip of toe ulcers complicated by osteomyelitis. J Foot Ankle Surg. 2014;53(6):720–6.

Troy J. Boffeli and Jonathan C. Thompson

Introduction

The development of osteomyelitis in metatarsals two, three, and four can be encountered in the setting of complicated diabetic ulcerations, infected gangrene, puncture wounds, and forefoot trauma. The presence of structural deformity, such as an elongated or plantarflexed metatarsal, hypermobile medial column, prominent metatarsal head due to retrograde forces from hammertoe contracture, previous adjacent metatarsal head resection, and ankle equinus, can increase peak ambulatory pressure on the plantar central metatarsophalangeal joints (MTPJs) leading to tissue breakdown. Such areas of pressure, while better tolerated by the general population, predispose the diabetic patient to neuropathic ulceration below the metatarsal heads that can often become complicated by osteomyelitis. Another frequent cause of lesser metatarsal head ulceration can be iatrogenic in nature, occurring after partial first ray amputation when the load previously bore by the medial column is transferred to the adjacent metatarsal heads (Fig. 17.1). This is also seen in isolated central metatarsal head resection as peak plantar ambulatory pressure is increased to adjacent metatarsals. While most common in the setting of complicated diabetic ulcerations, surgical amputation involving the central metatarsals may also be necessary in the setting of forefoot gangrene, digital infection with vascular compromise, puncture wound, and forefoot trauma.

Prevention of Central Metatarsal Osteomyelitis in Patients with Neuropathic Ulceration

When assessing the patient with a neuropathic ulceration below a central metatarsal head, recognizing the structural etiology is of the utmost importance so that any biomechanical abnormalities can be appropriately addressed. In patients with pre-ulcerative hyperkeratotic lesions or uncomplicated superficial ulceration, conservative offloading measures can be employed. Such strategies for offloading the middle column include accommodative orthoses, shoe modifications, total contact casting, traditional casting, various ankle-foot orthoses, Charcot restraint orthotic walkers (CROW), integrated prosthetic and orthotic system (IPOS) shoes, and surgical offloading measures. The total contact cast has traditionally been described as the gold standard for offloading low- to mid-grade forefoot and midfoot diabetic neuropathic ulcerations, as a 75–84 % reduction in peak plantar pressures during weight bearing has been demonstrated [1]. Oftentimes, temporary offloading strategies are beneficial in allowing an uncomplicated open wound to heal prior to undergoing preemptive surgical correction of the causative deformity in the patient without surgical contraindications. If the etiology of the ulcer is not effectively addressed with either permanent conservative or surgical methods, recurrence or persistence of the ulcer is probable. Many nonhealing neuropathic ulcers eventually become complicated, developing deep infection with abscess and osteomyelitis. Consideration should be given to pursuing early surgical intervention in an attempt to alter the course of a perpetual wound and avoid limb loss.

T.J. Boffeli, D.P.M., F.A.C.F.A.S. (✉)
Regions Hospital/HealthPartners Institute for Education and Research, 640 Jackson Street, Saint Paul, MN 55101, USA
e-mail: troy.j.boffeli@healthpartners.com

J.C. Thompson, D.P.M., M.H.A., A.A.C.F.A.S.
Mayo Clinic Health System, Orthopedic Center,
1400 Bellinger Street, Eau Claire, WI 54702, USA
e-mail: thompson.jonathan@mayo.edu

© Springer International Publishing Switzerland 2015
T.J. Boffeli (ed.), *Osteomyelitis of the Foot and Ankle*, DOI 10.1007/978-3-319-18926-0_17

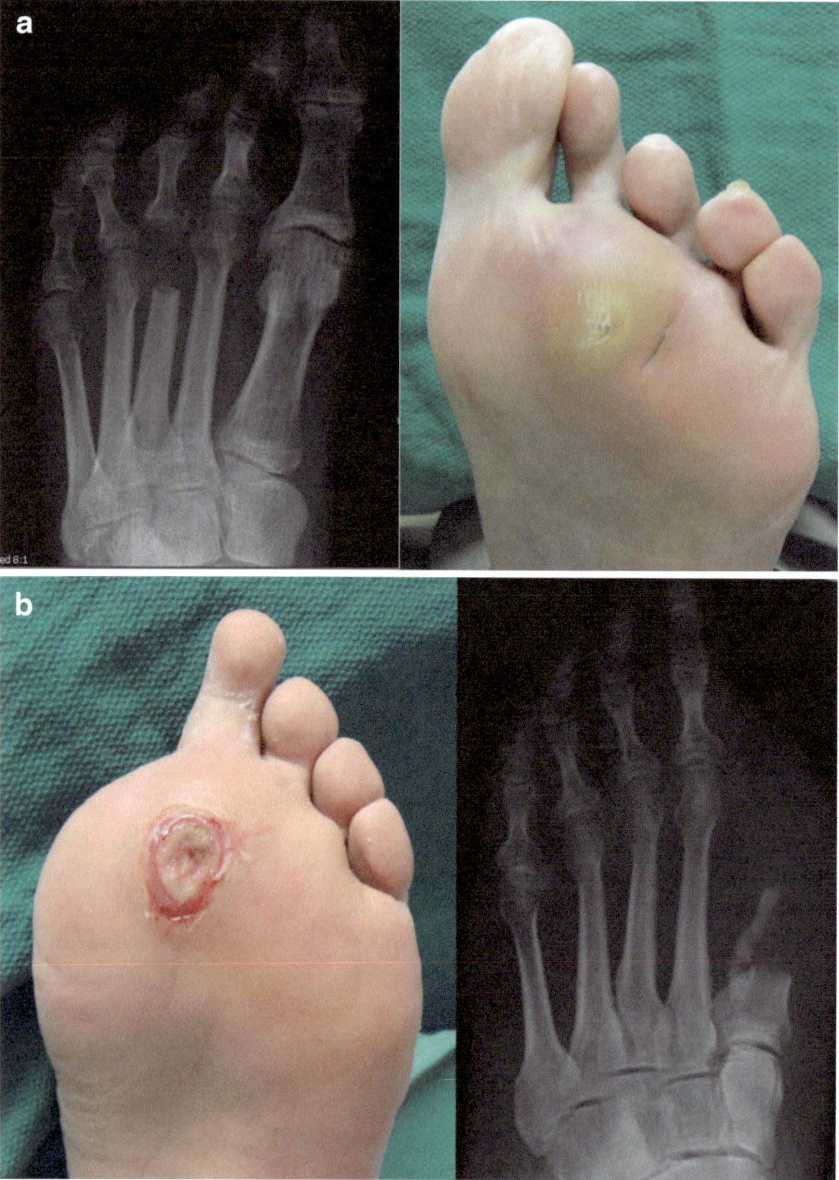

Fig. 17.1 Lesser metatarsal transfer lesions are common following partial ray resection or metatarsal head resection. Biomechanically, the metatarsal parabola is disrupted, leading to excessive peak plantar pressure below the adjacent metatarsal heads, leading to soft tissue breakdown, poor healing potential, and high likelihood of eventual infection. This is illustrated with a case exhibiting a (**a**) pre-ulcerative tranfer lesion and (**b**) a patient with full-thickness ulceration of the second ray following prior first ray amputation

Surgical Modalities for Prophylactic Correction of Structural Deformity

Central metatarsal neuropathic ulcers can be treated surgically either in a prophylactic manner prior to the development of an acute infection or in an urgent manner once infection necessitates intervention. If a contributing structural deformity is identified and relative contraindications to surgery are low, there is often value in correcting this deformity prior to the development of worsening ulcer condition and infection. For instance, ankle equinus is a common cause of plantar metatarsal head ulceration, making tendo-Achilles lengthening (TAL) or gastrocnemius recession an effective adjunct to local wound management. It is important to identify whether the gastrocnemius or gastrosoleal complex is contributory to the equinus. We tend to perform TAL for the diabetic with low activity level but profound contracture or those with recurrent sores despite prior forefoot amputation. Gastrocnemius recession is often reserved for the more active diabetic with less profound deformity to minimize the potential for developing a calcaneus gait. TAL or gastrocnemius recession can be performed in an open manner in an attempt to better control the amount of lengthening achieved provided soft tissues are amenable. Case 1 demonstrates open equinus correction to trent forefoot ulceration (Figs. 17.2, 17.3, and 17.4). The patient with profound lower extremity edema or poor skin quality with concerns for healing may be a better candidate for percutaneous lengthening. While not an absolute contraindication, the surgeon should take precautions to isolate the clean procedure site from any contaminated areas when performing tendon surgery concomitantly with open wounds or wound surgery. Staged surgery in acute infection cases is an effective means to achieve this separation. Mueller demonstrated the effectiveness of TAL on healing plantar forefoot wounds with a randomized clinical trial of patients treated with either total contact cast alone or with TAL. Two-year follow-up revealed an 81 % ulcer recurrence rate in the total contact cast cohort but a 38 % recurrence in the cast and TAL group [2].

There are many other structural deformities that may need to be addressed in a preventative manner. An elongated or plantarflexed metatarsal predisposing to plantar metatarsal head ulceration can be addressed with a metatarsal shortening osteotomy or dorsiflexory wedge osteotomy. Medial column insufficiency associated with hallux valgus deformity leading to lesser metatarsal head overloading is another common etiology. Correction of the medial column insufficiency with midfoot fusion may be necessary. Similarly, digital contracture can play a role in metatarsal head prominence, with retrograde forces from the digit causing plantar flexion of the metatarsal, which may necessitate repair of the digital deformity. The aforementioned reconstructive procedures intended for wound prophylaxis should be used with discretion as this patient population is at high risk for additional complications. Fleischli illustrated this with a reported 32 % incidence of acute Charcot neuroarthropathy following dorsiflexion metatarsal osteotomy [3]. Furthermore, elective reconstructive procedures are not typically employed if there is suspicion for infection. The wound would ideally be fully healed prior to reconstructive bone procedures requiring internal fixation, although this is not always feasible. The surgeon should use discretion when considering placing internal fixation in an area with previous ulceration and potential for subclinical osteomyelitis. Complete clinical, radiographic, and laboratory assessment to rule out low-grade infection is prudent in this situation. If concern persists in regard to performing reconstructive procedures requiring internal fixation, localized procedures such as metatarsal head resection are oftentimes effective at addressing the underlying biome-

chanical deformity. However, such endeavors should only be attempted when necessary as potential for transfer lesions or complicating heterotopic ossification (HO) can negatively affect the anticipated outcome.

Surgical Management of Central Metatarsal Infection

Surgical intervention for central metatarsal infection is common in the setting of infection spreading proximally from a digital wound or an infected neuropathic ulcer below the metatarsal head. Infection in these settings can manifest as acute soft tissue abscess, gas gangrene, acute or chronic osteomyelitis, unrelenting cellulitis with associated ulceration, or nonviable wet gangrene. Lack of viable soft tissue for primary closure of a lesser digital wound associated with proximal ulceration, necrosis, gangrene, or vascular insufficiency may necessitate surgical intervention at the metatarsal level as well. Central ray procedure options generally consist of single or multiple metatarsal head resection, partial or complete ray resection, or transmetatarsal amputation (TMA). Careful evaluation of the underlying pathomechanics, viability of surrounding soft tissues, size of the local wound defect, and extent of osteomyelitis is critical in selecting the optimal procedure.

Isolated Central Metatarsal Head Resection

Central metatarsal head resection can be an effective procedure in the setting of an isolated plantar metatarsal head ulceration. Full-thickness plantar metatarsal head ulcers with exposed bone most likely involve osteomyelitis with concomitant sepsis of the MTP joint. In the patient with a wound probing to bone and exhibiting underlying structural deformity but no acute soft tissue cellulitis or abscess, the surgeon may consider performing isolated metatarsal head resection in order to remove the infected bone and obtain bone biopsy while concomitantly addressing the underlying structural deformity. Early surgical intervention once the bone becomes exposed can limit the amount of resection required, as morbidity increases if the local soft tissues become acutely infected, raising the risk for systemic sepsis and more proximal foot amputation or limb loss.

When considering isolated metatarsal head resection, appropriate imaging modalities such as MRI are useful to evaluate for involvement of the adjacent proximal phalanx, determine the extent of proximal osteomyelitis extension in the metatarsal, and assess for associated deep abscess. Indications for isolated metatarsal head resection include osteomyelitis that appears to be contained to the metatarsal head with minimal adjacent soft tissue involvement. Metatarsal head resection can be performed under monitored

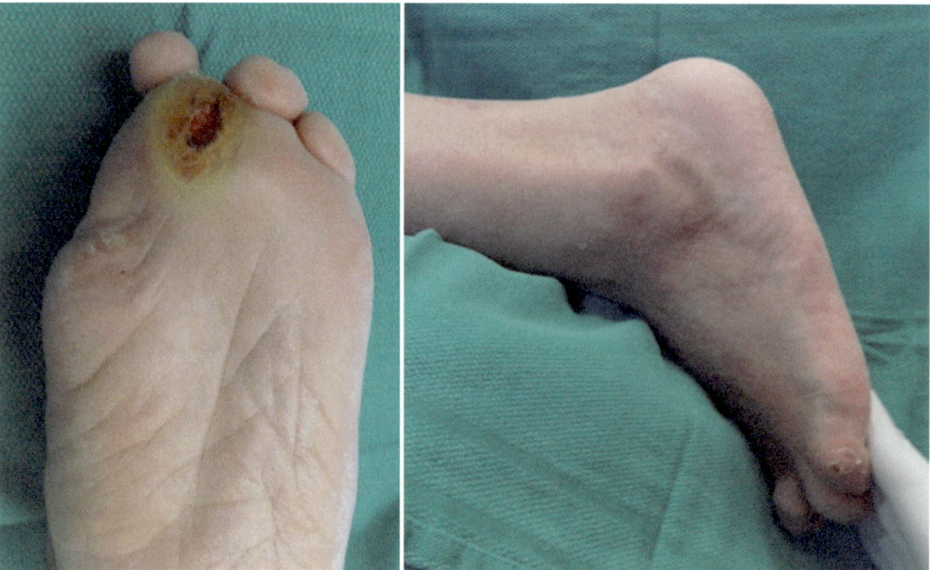

Fig. 17.2 Case 1: Nonhealing forefoot ulcers associated with ankle equinus. Limited ankle dorsiflexion is shown here with the knee in the extended position. Flexing the knee significantly improved ankle joint dorsiflexion indicating isolated gastrocnemius equinus. Ankle equinus increases peak plantar pressure to the forefoot contributing to recalcitrant neuropathic forefoot ulcers. Equinus deformity is difficult to manage conservatively and posterior lengthening is warranted

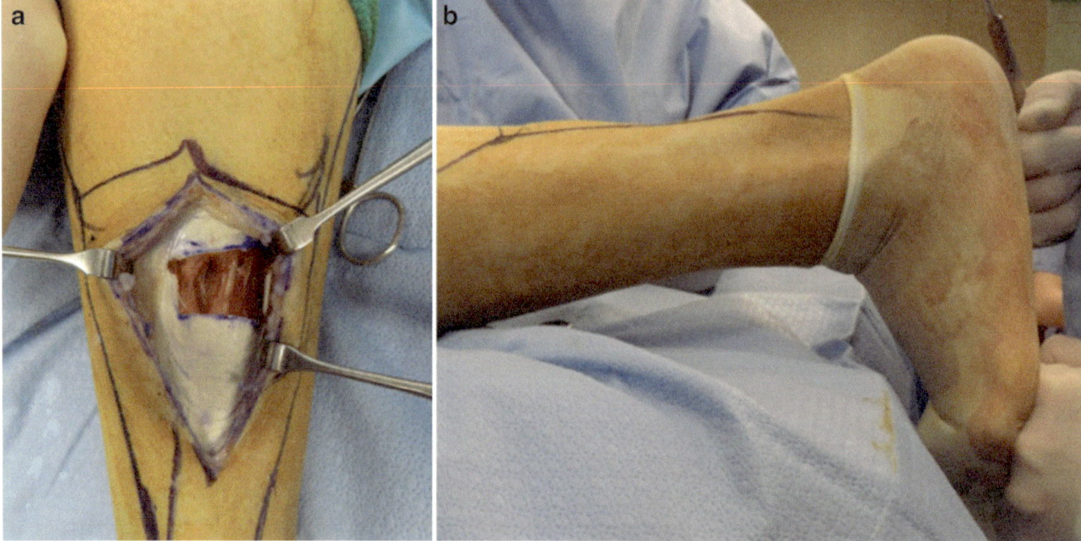

Fig. 17.3 Case 1 with open gastrocnemius recession. (**a**) We prefer gastrocnemius recession for the relatively more active diabetic patient with forefoot ulceration associated with less profound equinus deformity in an effort to minimize loss of strength and potential for development of calcaneus gait. We reserve Achilles tendon lengthening (TAL) for midfoot ulceration associated with prior midfoot amputation or Charcot arthropathy. Open gastrocnemius lengthening requires healthy soft tissues in the calf region, and uncontrolled edema is a relative contraindication since incision healing may be compromised. TAL can be performed percutaneously under these conditions. (**b**) Note that a sterile glove is placed over the prepped foot ulceration. Post lengthening ankle joint dorsiflexion is shown here with the knee extended and the foot dorsiflexed beyond 90° confirming successful release of equinus

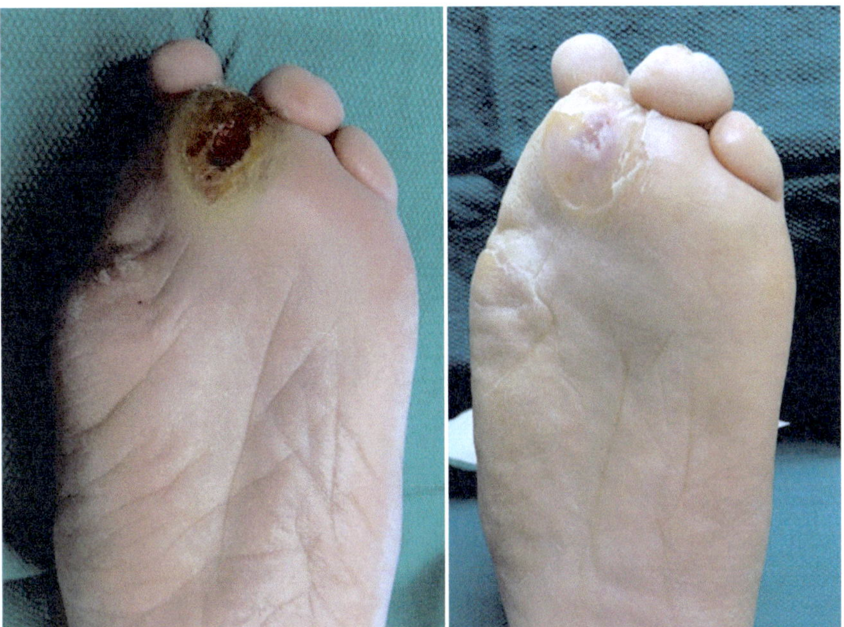

Fig. 17.4 Preop and 2-week post-op clinical appearance in case1. Once the contributory equinus deforming force is corrected, external pressure on the ulceration site is decreased. The clinical appearance pre-operatively (*left*) reveals a full-thickness ulceration that is nearly fully epithelialized by 2 weeks postoperatively (*right*)

anesthesia care with a local anesthetic block. If the plantar metatarsal head ulceration is full-thickness in nature, it is typically excised in full-thickness fashion and closed primarily (Fig. 17.5). Partial thickness ulcerations may be superficially debrided and allowed to heal secondarily. The metatarsal head can be accessed via a dorsal incision directly over the distal metatarsal as demonstrated in case 2 (Fig. 17.6 and 17.7). Alternately, if proximal extension of a plantar incision is necessary for debridement purposes, the metatarsal head could be resected through a single plantar incision. A saw is introduced into the dorsal incision and used to resect the metatarsal head immediately proximal to the metaphyseal flare. Care is taken to bevel the cut in a slightly dorsal-distal to plantar-proximal manner to avoid subsequent prominences on the weight bearing surface (Fig. 17.7). A grasping device is then used to remove the metatarsal head via a rolling motion, where the head is purchased on the medial and lateral aspects and twisted away from its periosteal attachments. The bone is inspected for clinical signs of osteomyelitis, including intraosseous purulence, medullary bone compromise, and cortical erosion. The specimen is sectioned into two pieces for microbiologic and pathologic analysis. The environment should be inspected for proximal tracking of soft tissue infection, particularly in the flexor and extensor tendon sheaths. The base of the proximal phalanx is

also evaluated to assess for signs of infection and may require associated digital amputation if phalangeal involvement appears likely. If no purulence or cellulitis is present, primary closure is performed at the time of bone resection. When feasible, primary closure is desirable in order to promote prompt healing of the soft tissue often while the patient remains on antibiotic therapy. Continued bone exposure while attempting to heal the area by secondary intention is less desirable, particularly when the wound persists beyond the duration of antibiotic therapy.

Partial Central Ray Amputation

In the setting of an infected digital ulcer with osteomyelitis or soft tissue infection extending proximally, the traditional incision for partial ray amputation is a racquet-type incision with extension of the proximal arm of the incision over the dorsum of the foot [4]. Case 3 demonstrates an extensive central ray amputation for dersol abscess (Fig. 17.8, 17.9, 17.10, and 17.11). Alternately, when performing ray amputation and excising a plantar metatarsal head ulcer, the ulcer and adjacent digit can be excised with an elliptical incision extending from the plantar forefoot to the dorsal base of the digit. The incision is made in a full-thickness manner down to the level of bone, with care being taken to incise

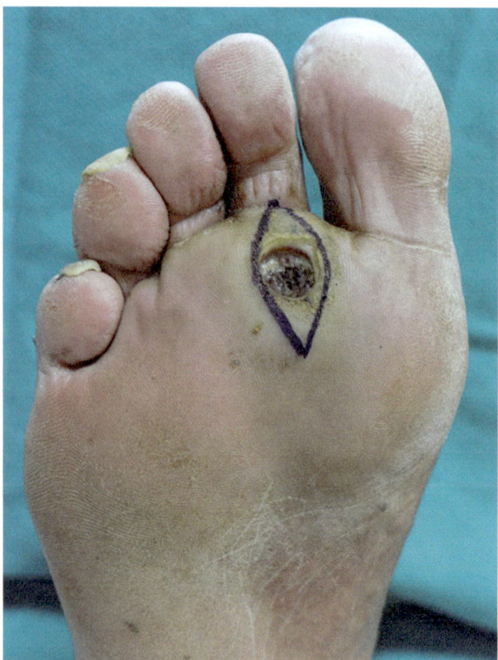

Fig. 17.5 Plantar ulcer excision may be considered. Plantar ulcer excision may not be necessary as the area will typically granulate and heal promptly once the underlying structural deformity is corrected with metatarsal head resection. However, larger full-thickness ulcers may be best treated with excision and primary closure in addition to metatarsal head resection through a dorsal incision

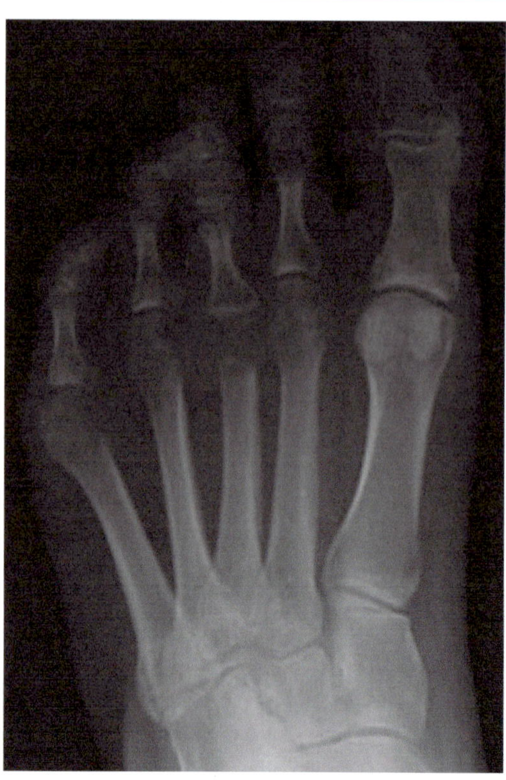

Fig. 17.7 Two-week post-op radiographic appearance in case 2. The third metatarsal head has been resected immediately proximal to the metaphyseal flare. The cut is made in a dorsal-distal to proximal-plantar orientation to avoid prominence on the weight bearing surface of the foot. Care was taken to maintain maximal metatarsal length in the event that subsequent transmetatarsal amputation would become necessary

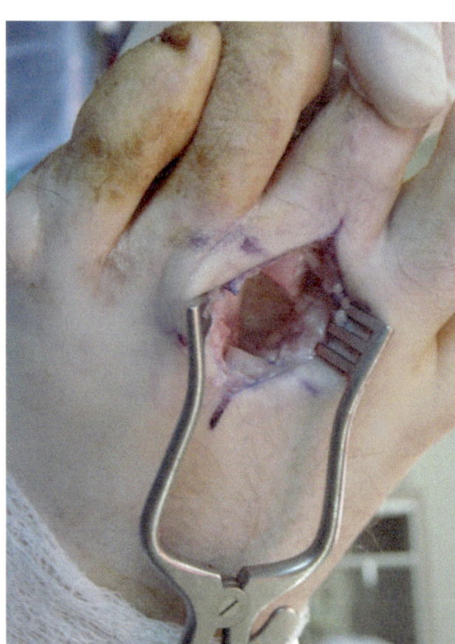

Fig. 17.6 Case 2 with dorsal incision for third metatarsal head resection. The metatarsal head is resected from a dorsal incision made directly above the distal aspect of the metatarsal. A McGlamry elevator can be used to free the metatarsal head of soft tissue attachments prior to a cut being made with a saw immediately proximal to the metaphyseal flare. The adjacent proximal phalanx base is assessed for signs of osteomyelitis this would typically warrant digital amputation as well

perpendicular to the skin. The digit is then disarticulated at the level of the metatarsophalangeal joint. The need to perform partial metatarsal resection is based on preoperative imaging and intraoperative findings, such as frankly necrotic cartilage and bone or abscess extending proximally in the flexor or extensor tendon sheaths. Thus the dorsal incision is then extended proximally along the metatarsal if necessary (Fig. 17.9). When acute soft tissue infection is present, the flexor and extensor tendon sheaths and fascial planes should be investigated for proximal extension of the infection and incised as necessary for effective debridement. The ideal level for central metatarsal resection is the neck, which is immediately proximal to the metaphyseal flare. The periosteum is raised circumferentially around the metatarsal shaft, with care being taken to avoid excessive stripping of the periosteal layer as this can increase the possibility of developing subsequent heterotopic bone growth at the resection site. The bone is then cut with a sagittal saw in a slightly beveled manner from dorsal-distal to proximal-plantar to avoid prominence on the plantar weight bearing surface. While avoiding unnecessary dissection between the metatarsals, the distal bone fragment is then excised. The metatarsal fragment is

Partial Central Ray Resection

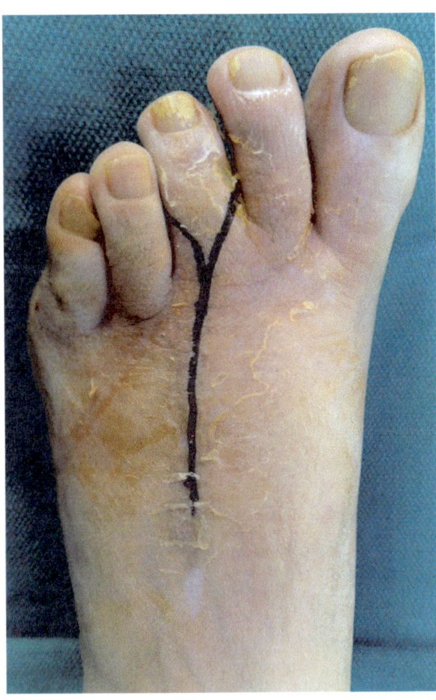

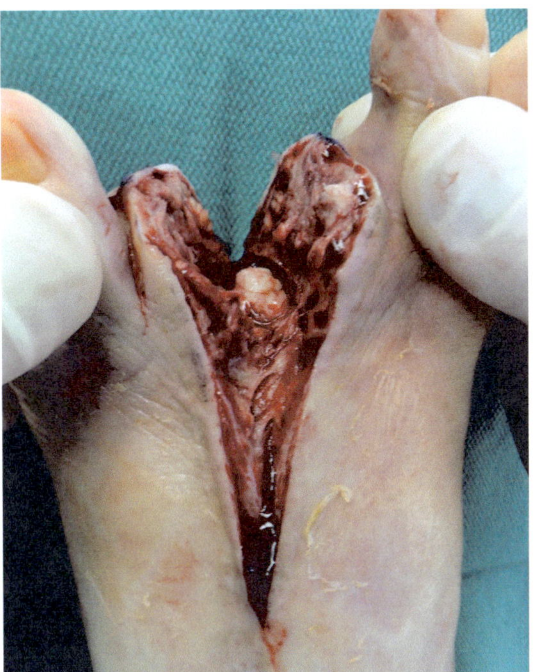

Fig. 17.8 Case 3: third ray amputation. The traditional central ray amputation incision consists of a racquet-type incision with care being taken to create medial and lateral digital flaps for closure of the interdigital defect. The handle of the racquet extends across the dorsal forefoot as shown here for access to the metatarsal and the proximal extension was required for drainage of abscess and soft tissue gas. The dorsal incisional approach avoids a plantar weight bearing surgical wound. The handle of the racquet can extend plantarly which allows wound excision and primary closure if indicated. Larger and full depth nonhealing wounds may be best excised and closed primarily although the plantar wound will typically granulate and heal promptly once the source of abnormal pressure is removed via metatarsal head resection

Fig. 17.9 Proximal extension of incision for drainage of abscess in case 3. A full-thickness incision is carried proximally on the dorsal aspect of the foot if partial metatarsal amputation is deemed necessary. This is contingent on the appearance of the metatarsal head after disarticulating at the MTPJ and whether there is proximal extension of abscess. The incision shown here required more proximal extension than is typically necessary due to proximal soft tissue emphysema involvement requiring debridement. The metatarsal head is then resected immediately proximal to the metaphyseal flare in a dorsal-distal to plantar-proximal fashion with a saw. The head is sectioned for a pathology and microbiology specimen

sectioned for microbiologic and pathologic analysis, which allows the surgeon to assess viability of the medullary canal and cortical bone. The intramedullary canal of the remaining metatarsal shaft is also evaluated to assess the clinical appearance of the retained bone. A separate proximal margin pathology specimen can be obtained to help determine the route and duration of antibiotic therapy. Oftentimes, this proximal margin specimen can be obtained by curettage of the exposed medullary canal in an attempt to preserve cortical bone length in the event that transmetatarsal amputation would be necessary in the future (Figs. 17.10).

Proximal Metatarsal Amputation

While the ideal level for central metatarsal resection is typically at the neck immediately proximal to the metaphyseal flare, resection through the mid-shaft or base of the metatarsal may infrequently be necessary based on the extent of

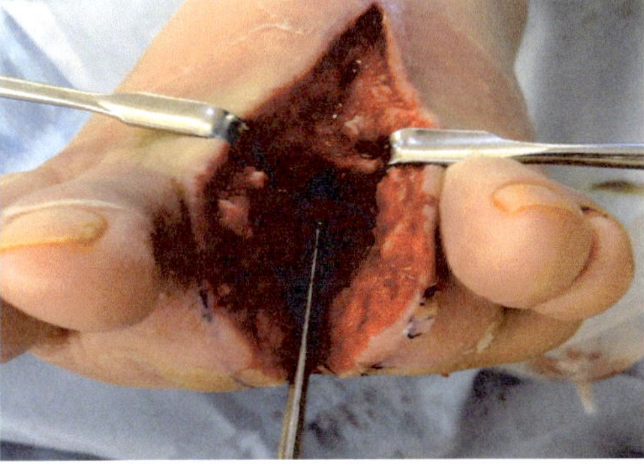

Fig. 17.10 Proximal margin bone specimen obtained with curette in case 3. A separate proximal margin pathology specimen can be obtained to help determine the route and duration of antibiotic therapy. This is frequently obtained in the final staged surgery prior to delayed primary closure. Oftentimes, this proximal margin specimen can be obtained by curettage of the remaining medullary canal in an attempt to preserve cortical bone length in the event that subsequent transmetatarsal amputation would become necessary

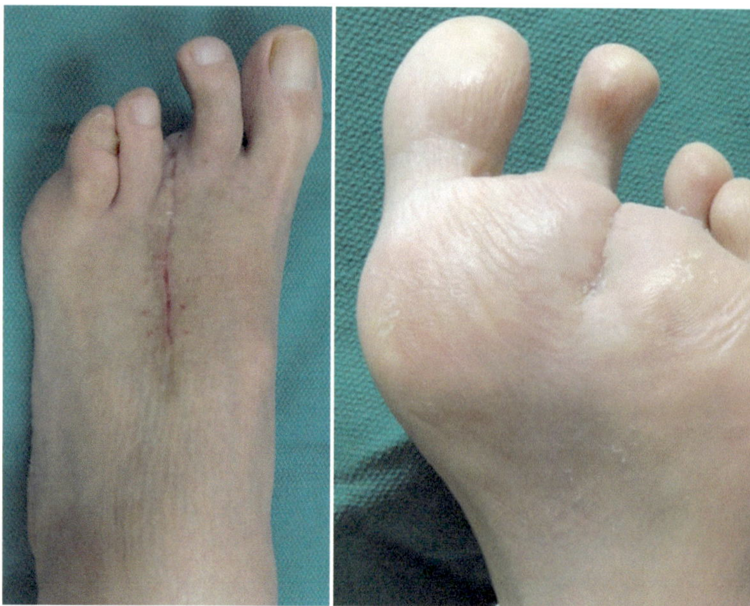

Fig. 17.11 Six-week post-op clinical appearance in case 3. Sutures are typically left in for 4–6 weeks depending on the progression of healing. Once the surgical site is fully healed, the patient should be placed into an accommodative orthosis to avoid the development of transfer lesions on adjacent metatarsal heads

proximal involvement of infection or complicating heterotopic ossification. Osteomyelitis can spread proximally along the metatarsal shaft via the periosteum or medullary canal, which may be identifiable preoperatively on radiograph or MRI or intraoperatively on direct inspection. While bone can be resected at the mid-shaft or base of the metatarsal, disarticulation at the tarsometatarsal joint is not ideal and often not practical as it requires dissection of important midfoot ligaments and can potentially destabilize adjacent metatarsals throughout the transverse arch. Thus the central metatarsal base is typically retained to act as a spacer, even if residual infection is felt to persist in the base. One option in this setting is to perform conservative resection through the mid-shaft of the metatarsal without obtaining a clean margin from osteomyelitis (Fig. 17.12). The exposed medullary canal can be curetted to remove spreading infection within the canal while maintaining the solid cortical shell, which may be useful for maintaining an effective parabola in the event of subsequent TMA. Alternately, amputation can be performed through the metatarsal base while retaining a portion of it for stability purposes. Due to the likelihood of residual osteomyelitis persisting after resection, antibiotic beads can be placed into the resection site for local elution of antibiotics as an adjunct to ongoing parenteral therapy. The antibiotic beads are left in place for about 2 weeks. Repeat irrigation and debridement with proximal margin biopsy are often performed during the subsequent bead removal procedure. An alternative minimally invasive approach can be utilized when osteomyelitis has spread to the proximal metatarsal but no adjacent soft tissue abscess persists. A minimally invasive two-incision method was utilized in case 4 (Fig. 17.13, 17.14, and 17.15) with a small incision being made over both the distal forefoot and the proximal metatarsal. The metatarsal was resected through the base using a proximal incision, freed of soft tissue attachments using an elevator, and removed from the distal incision. Residual dead space can be managed with a drain or antibiotic bead application.

Conversion to Transmetatarsal Amputation and Panmetatarsal Head Resection

Transmetatarsal amputation or panmetatarsal head resection may become necessary at some point in the course of treating a patient with single or multiple previous digital amputation or metatarsal head resection in order to provide the patient with the most functional outcome while decreasing potential for repeat ulceration [5]. Case 5 demonstrates our

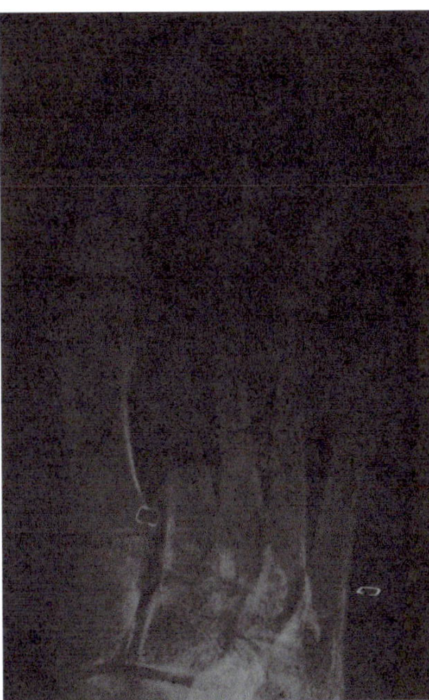

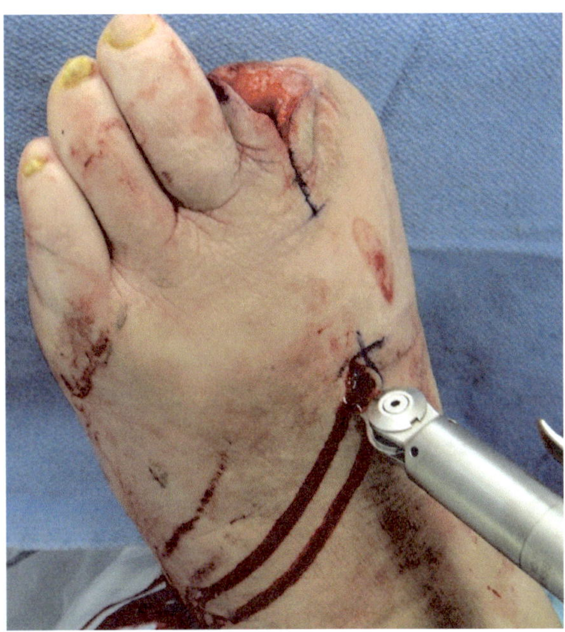

Fig. 17.12 Mid-shaft metatarsal amputation. The metatarsal can be resected through the mid-shaft when contiguous spread of infection advances into the proximal metatarsal. Care is taken to preserve metatarsal length when possible as this affects the ability to maintain a congruous metatarsal parabola in the event subsequent transmetatarsal amputation becomes necessary

Fig. 17.13 Case 4: Proximal metatarsal resection through accessory incision. This two-incision technique can be considered in the setting of proximal extension of osteomyelitis without adjacent soft tissue abscess. The proximal aspect of the metatarsal can be resected through a separate incision and removed through a smaller distal ray amputation incision

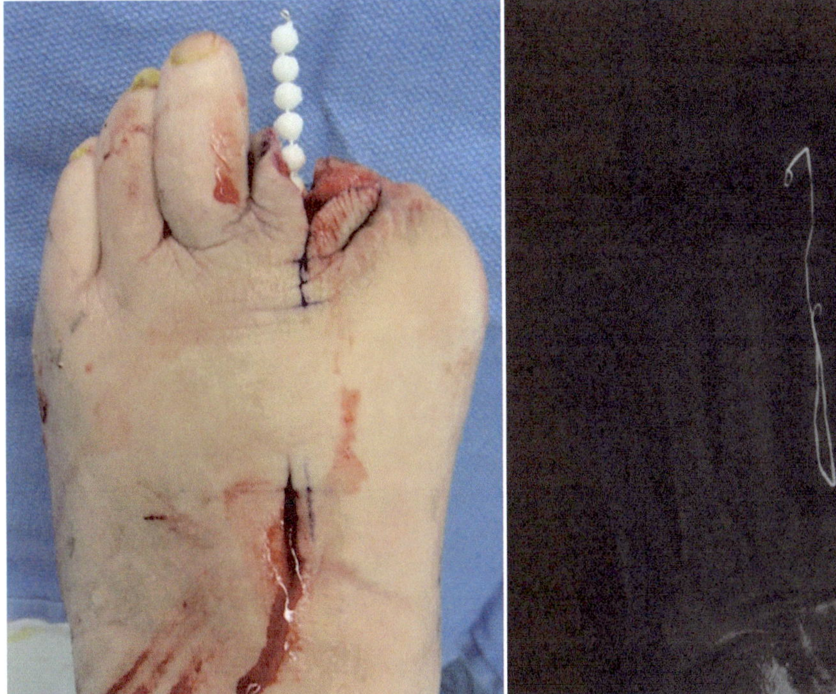

Fig. 17.14 Staged surgery for dead space management in case 4. The potential for hematoma formation can be minimized by utilizing a staged surgical approach with antibiotic bead application or applying a drain. Antibiotic beads are typically left in place for 2 weeks prior to removal

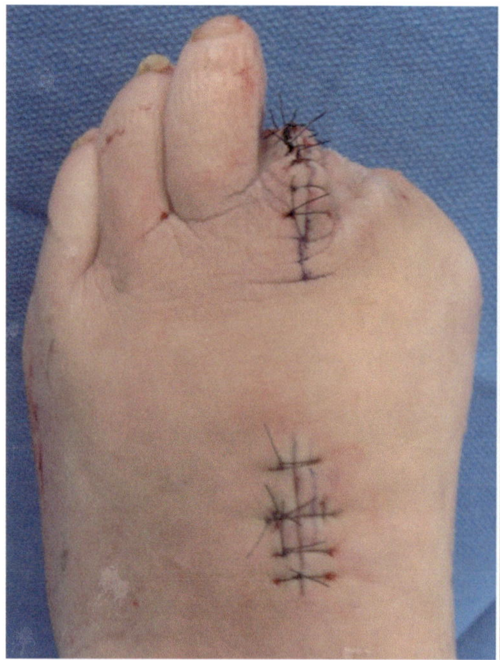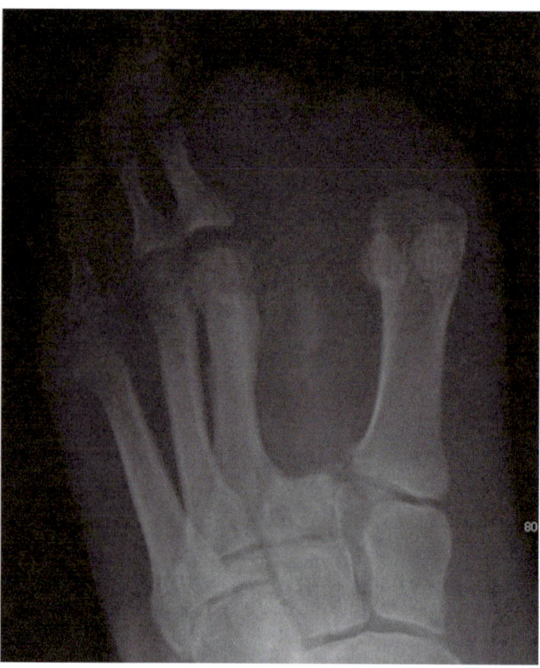

Fig. 17.15 Clinical and rediographic appearance in case 4 two weeks after antibiotic bead removal. The postoperatively clinical appearance displays that two separate incisions in this setting minimize the extent of soft tissue dissection required to perform proximal metatarsal amputation

technique for plantor flap panmetatarsal head resection (Fig. 17.16, 17.17, 17.18, and 17.19. These procedures are routinely considered in revision surgery after partial first ray resection with subsequent transfer lesion of the second metatarsal head requiring excision. This can be a relatively common occurrence, as some investigators have found a re-ulceration rate as high as 69 % after partial first ray resection [6]. If the second metatarsal head is resected in isolation, the third, fourth, and fifth metatarsal heads become increasingly predisposed to transfer ulcers and subsequent osteomyelitis. Thus we often prefer either panmetatarsal head or transmetatarsal amputation in situations where both partial first metatarsal and either partial second or third metatarsal heads have previously been resected. This will also be considered when two adjacent lesser metatarsal heads have been removed. Panmetatarsal head and transmetatarsal amputation reestablish a functional parabola and minimize the potential for transfer lesions. Panmetatarsal head resection may be considered when osteomyelitis does not involve the proximal phalanx and the digits are not severely contracted or deformed, thus being at lower risk of subsequent digital ulceration (Fig. 17.17). In the standard patient population undergoing repeat partial foot amputation, the remaining digits are often at high risk for complicating ulcerations due to contracture, thickening, dystrophic toenails, and poor interdigital skin quality. Thus patients with these findings are often better served with transmetatarsal amputation. Transmetatarsal amputation is often a more definitive procedure in terms of reestablishing an effective metatarsal parabola for weight bearing while removing largely nonfunctional digits. For further reading on transmetatarsal amputations, see Chapter 19.

Staged Surgical Approach

Management of acute infection involving the central rays commonly requires a staged surgical approach. It is not unusual for an infection to require two or three surgeries with serial debridement before being amenable to closure. Staged surgery allows concomitant soft tissue cellulitis to improve or resolve on antibiotics after evacuating the foci of infected bone and tissue. The region is allowed to drain, which can help to resolve the infection and prevent hematoma formation. The patient with persistent cellulitis or abscess with elevated laboratory values not improving clinically may require additional surgical debridement without closure every couple days while remaining inpatient. Once cellulitis has resolved or significantly improved and no gross signs of infection are present, final debridement, bone biopsy, and delayed primary closure can be performed. During this surgery, a proximal margin pathology specimen can be obtained from a previously

Transmetatarsal Amputation Versus Panmetatarsal Head Resection for Transfer Ulcer After Partial First Ray Resection

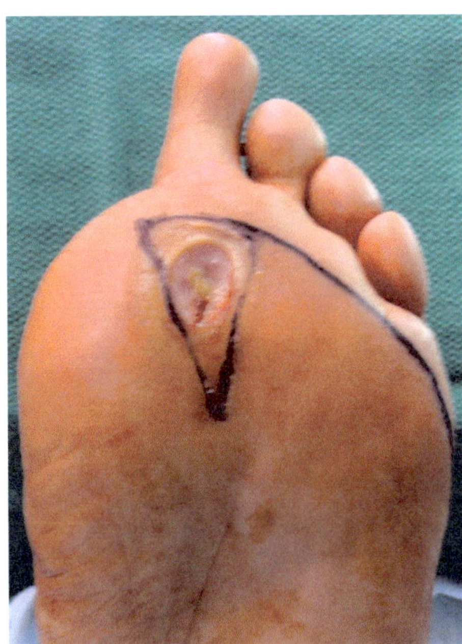

Fig. 17.16 Case 5: Plantar flap panmetatarsal head resection. Panmetatarsal head resection can be considered in the patient with second ray transfer lesion associated with prior first ray amputation. Advantages over transmetatarsal amputation are sparing the lesser digits for cosmesis and footwear functionality. The condition of the digits is one of the main factors in determining procedure selection. *Republished with permission of the Journal of Foot and Ankle Surgery* [5]

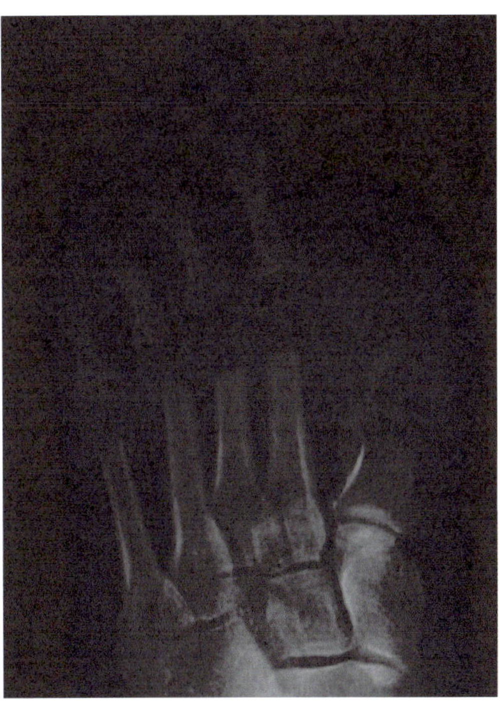

Fig. 17.18 Case 5: Postoperative X-rays showing level of metatarsal head resection. The metatarsal heads are resected immediately proximal to the metaphyseal flare through the plantar incision. Even though the digits are retained, care is taken to maintain a congruous metatarsal parabola for maximal functionality. Preoperative X-ray are shown in Fig 17.1b with prior short first ray amputation

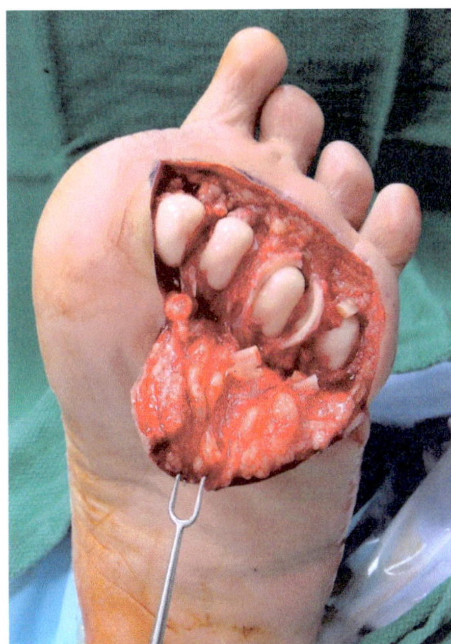

Fig. 17.17 Raising the plantar rotational flap in case 5. A local plantar rotational flap is raised in full-thickness fashion. The plantar plate apparatus and flexor tendons are excised from the flap as long as their removal does not compromise viability. A minimal-touch technique is used on the flap to avoid unnecessary compromise

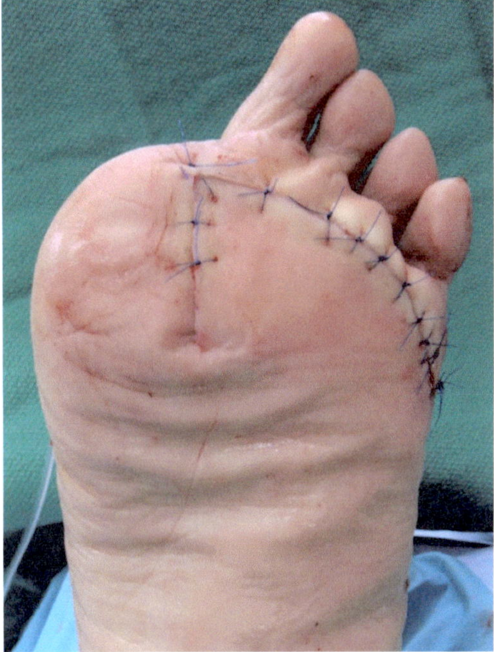

Fig. 17.19 Plantar flap closure in case 5. The plantar flap is advanced medially to allow for primary closure of the soft tissue deficit. In the event of future complications, this flap easily converts to a plantar rotational flap transmetatarsal amputation

resected metatarsal, which assists in determining whether residual osteomyelitis persists and dictates the duration and route of antibiotic therapy. A repeat culture specimen may also be necessary at this time if the culture from the initial surgery exhibited many organisms that confound the ability to narrow the antibiotic spectrum. Furthermore, staged surgery assists in reducing the potential for HO at the resection site that can increase complications such as re-ulceration. HO likely occurs when osteoprogenitor cell-containing hematoma derived from the metatarsal medullary canal extravasates into the adjacent soft tissues and leads to this undesired bone formation [7]. Staged surgery minimizes the potential for HO-causing hematoma by decreasing the potential for bleeding at the surgical site during serial debridements and evacuating previously formed hematoma. For further reading on heterotopic ossification, see Chapter 12.

In the patient whose clinical and laboratory findings fail to improve despite serial debridements, consideration should be given to the potential for inadequate initial resection or additional foci of infection that have not effectively been addressed. Staged surgery may not be necessary in the setting of an infection that does not exhibit associated cellulitis and when the entirety of the infection can be fully resected during the primary procedure. However, given the complicated nature of lower extremity infections with potential for negative local and systemic sequelae, a low threshold should exist for managing these patients with a staged surgical approach.

Conclusion

The central forefoot can often become complicated by osteomyelitis in a number of settings. When due to structure-related ulceration, both prophylactic conservative and surgical offloading measures should be considered in attempts to resolve the ulcer before osteomyelitic development. Surgical management of osteomyelitis should be aimed at sufficient surgical resection using biomechanically sound principles to minimize the potential for recurrence. Staged surgery is typically necessary to effectively address the complicated nature of these infections. During the primary surgery, consideration should be given to potential revision options such as transmetatarsal amputation to avoid compromising those options should they become necessary in the future.

References

1. Birke JA, Sims Jr DS, Buford WL. Walking casts: effect on plantar foot pressures. J Rehabil Res Dev. 1985;22(3):18–22.
2. Mueller MJ, Sinacore DR, Hastings MK, et al. Effect of Achilles tendon lengthening on neuropathic plantar ulcers: a randomized clinical trial. J Bone Joint Surg. 2003;85-A(8):1436–45.
3. Fleischili JE, Anderson RB, Hodges DW. Dorsiflexion metatarsal osteotomy for treatment of recalcitrant diabetic neuropathic ulcers. Foot Ankle Int. 1999;20:80–5.
4. Boffeli TJ, Thompson JC. Partial foot amputations for salvage of the diabetic lower extremity. Clin Podiatr Med Surg. 2014;31:103–26.
5. Boffeli TB, Reinking RR. Plantar rotational flap technique for pan-metatarsal head resection and transmetatarsal amputation: a revision approach for second metatarsal head transfer ulcers in patients with previous partial first ray amputation. J Foot Ankle Surg. 2014;53:96–100.
6. Borkosky SL, Roukis TS. Incidence of repeat amputation after partial first ray amputation associated with diabetes mellitus and peripheral neuropathy: an 11-year review. J Foot Ankle Surg. 2013;52:335–8.
7. Boffeli TJ, Pfannenstein RR, Thompson JC. Radiation therapy for recurrent heterotopic ossification following partial metatarsal ray resection. J Foot Ankle Surg. 2015;54:345–9.

Fifth Ray Osteomyelitis

18

Troy J. Boffeli, Jessica A. Tabatt, and Kyle W. Abben

Introduction

Osteomyelitis of the fifth ray may involve one or more of the fifth toe phalanges, the fifth metatarsal, or the cuboid. Bone infection along the lateral column of the foot is largely associated with contiguous spread of infection from adjacent neuropathic ulcers, decubitus ulcers, and gangrene. Osteomyelitis associated with hematogenous spread and direct inoculation of bone from a puncture wound or open fracture is less common at this location. Ulcers along the lateral column frequently lead to osteomyelitis and joint infection due to the relatively thin nature of the local tissue and prominence of underlying bone and joint structures. Gangrene that extends proximally beyond the tip of the fifth toe is not very amenable to auto-amputation, with osteomyelitis being common once bone becomes exposed or when dead tissue becomes infected. Lateral column decubitus ulcers around the fifth metatarsal head or base are generally associated with plantar flexion and inversion contracture deformity of the foot and ankle, which is common in stroke and other neurologic conditions associated with spasticity. Neuropathic ulcers at the lateral column are frequently associated with musculoskeletal deformities like hammertoe contracture, tailor's bunion deformity, cavovarus foot structure,

and metatarsus adductus. The combination of neuropathy, minimal subcutaneous tissue, and underlying deformity leads to nonhealing wounds that frequently become complicated by underlying bone infection.

Successful treatment of osteomyelitis under these conditions is highly dependent on resolution of not only bone infection but also the wound deficit and associated mechanical deformity. Antibiotic therapy alone is not likely to be effective if the bone remains exposed and prominent or if a complicated wound persists at the conclusion of medical treatment. A combination of medical and surgical treatment is therefore warranted for most cases of fifth ray osteomyelitis. There is sparse literature that addresses surgical management of ulcerations specifically at the fifth ray. The primary author's ideal surgical treatment plan is based on the size and location of the ulceration along the fifth ray, the extent of anticipated osteomyelitis, and structural abnormalities as detailed in Fig. 18.1. Consideration is also given to local perfusion and the quality of the surrounding soft tissues which may be necrotic from gangrene or infection. The surgical goals are to remove dead and prominent bone, obtain bone biopsy, close the wound when possible, and achieve biomechanical balance in an effort to limit future breakdown and subsequent amputation. A staged surgical approach is commonly employed in an effort to achieve these complex goals. In our experience, the fifth toe and metatarsal head can be removed with little consequence to weight bearing function of the foot or ability to wear shoes. More proximal resection of the fifth metatarsal has greater impact to foot function and stability and is avoided when possible. A substantial effort is therefore warranted to preserve at least 50 % of the metatarsal in partial fifth ray amputation. This chapter will focus on surgical treatment strategies for fifth ray osteomyelitis with emphasis on patient selection for partial or complete fifth ray amputation. This includes biomechanical implications, surgical technique, flap design principles, and staging protocols which allow use of implantable antibiotic beads and delayed tendon balancing.

T.J. Boffeli, D.P.M., F.A.C.F.A.S. (✉)
Regions Hospital/HealthPartners Institute for Education and Research, 640 Jackson Street, St. Paul, MN 55101, USA
e-mail: troy.j.boffeli@healthpartners.com

J.A. Tabatt, D.P.M.
Essentia Health St. Joseph's Brainerd Clinic,
2024 South 6th Street, Brainerd, MN 56401, USA
e-mail: jatabatt@gmail.com

K.W. Abben, D.P.M., A.A.C.F.A.S.
Jamestown Regional Medical Center,
2422 20th Street SW, Jamestown, ND 58401, USA
e-mail: kyle.w.abben@gmail.com

© Springer International Publishing Switzerland 2015
T.J. Boffeli (ed.), *Osteomyelitis of the Foot and Ankle*, DOI 10.1007/978-3-319-18926-0_18

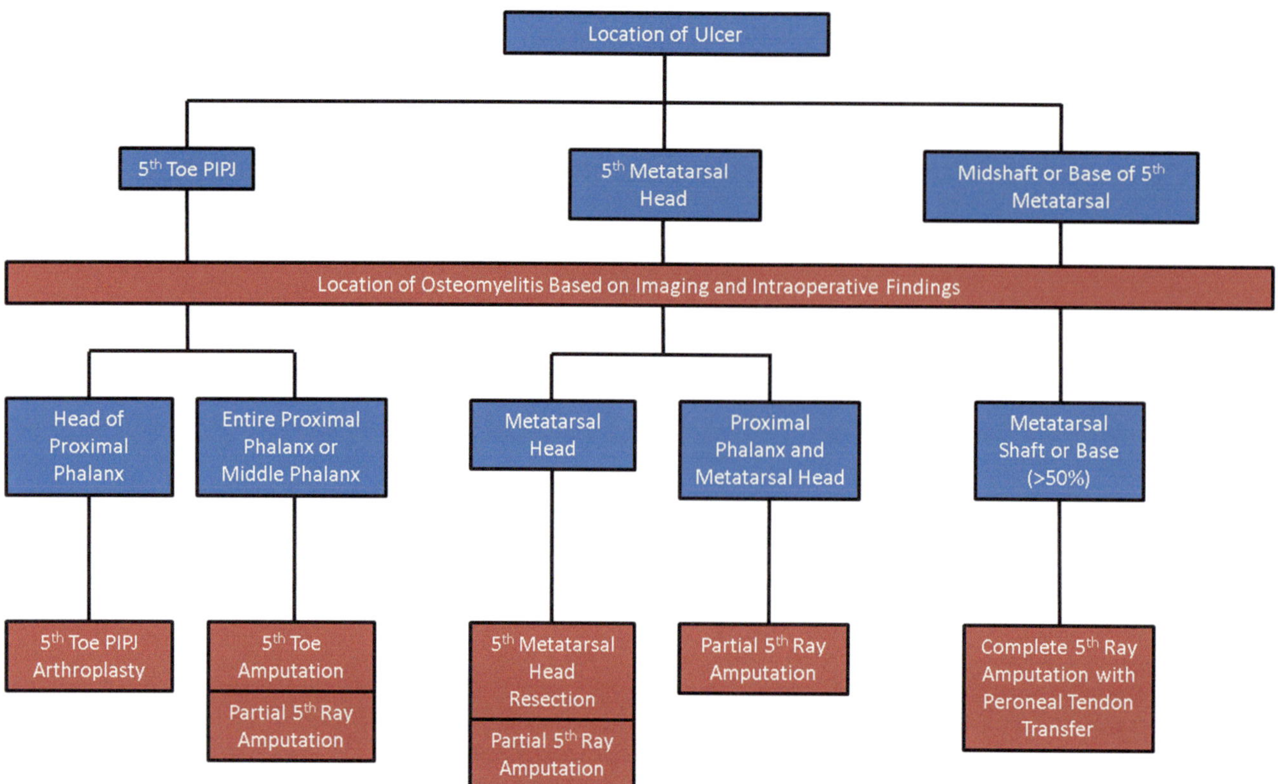

Fig. 18.1 Flow diagram to assist with procedure selection for infected fifth ray ulcerations with suspicion of osteomyelitis. Ideal procedure selection for fifth ray osteomyelitis is based on underlying deformity, location of the ulceration, and extent of osteomyelitis. Consideration is also given to circulation and the quality of the surrounding soft tissues which may be necrotic from gangrene or infection

Ulceration and Osteomyelitis of the Fifth Toe

Partial fifth ray amputation is common for fifth ray osteomyelitis but early intervention with traditional podiatric reconstructive procedures can also be effective at achieving the surgical goals while avoiding amputation. A study by Faglia demonstrated that internal pedal amputations, such as phalanx and metatarsal head resection, is a feasible alternative to ray or toe amputation when appropriate [1]. Osteomyelitis of the fifth toe is generally associated with contiguous spread of infection from adjacent ulceration or gangrene. In the absence of an open wound, the clinician should look for other causes of suspicious radiographic finding including gout, trauma, or degenerative arthritis. Fifth toe ulcers are typically caused by repetitive pressure over prominent bone associated with hammertoe deformity, bone spurs, heloma molle, and arthritis (Fig. 18.2). Neuropathy plays a large but not exclusive role as many of these wounds are chronically painful. Hammertoe deformity or exostosis can lead to prominent bone at the interphalangeal joints (IPJ), which can cause a sinus tract or ulceration leading to osteomyelitis. In general, partial toe amputation, distal Syme's amputation,

and metatarsophalangeal joint (MPJ) disarticulation are less common on the fifth toe compared to the other toes due to concern for continued lateral prominence that would lead to shoe rubbing and future wound breakdown.

Proximal Interphalangeal Joint Arthroplasty

Fifth toe PIPJ arthroplasty is useful for dorsal, lateral, and medial PIPJ ulcerations associated with osteomyelitis that is isolated to the head of the proximal phalanx. This conservative surgical approach can effectively treat osteomyelitis of the head of the proximal phalanx by excising the wound and infected bone as well as correcting digital deformity which further reduces the risk of recurrent ulceration. The standard PIPJ arthroplasty technique can be utilized with a dorsal linear approach, but a modified ulcer excision plan is best for cases involving ulceration (Fig. 18.3). Prophylactic PIPJ arthroplasty prior to the onset of osteomyelitis is useful for nonhealing or recurrent PIPJ wounds. Resection of the head of the proximal phalanx also provides a specimen for bone biopsy and relaxes the surrounding tissues to allow primary closure of small wound defects.

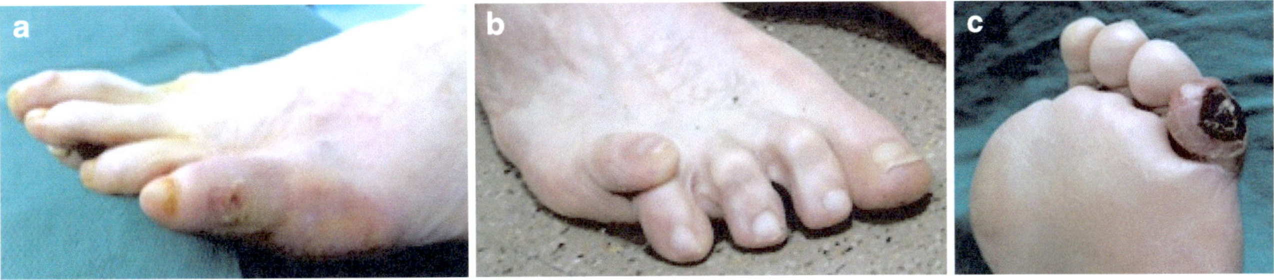

Fig. 18.2 Conditions leading to fifth toe osteomyelitis. (**a**) Neuropathic ulcers overlying the fifth proximal interphalangeal joint (PIPJ) are a common cause of fifth toe osteomyelitis. (**b**) Structural deformities like overlapping or underlapping digital deformities, hammertoe contrac- ture, DJD, and malunited fractures predispose to tissue breakdown and nonhealing wounds on the medial, lateral, and dorsal aspects of the PIPJ. (**c**) Contiguous spread of infection from digital gangrene is also common

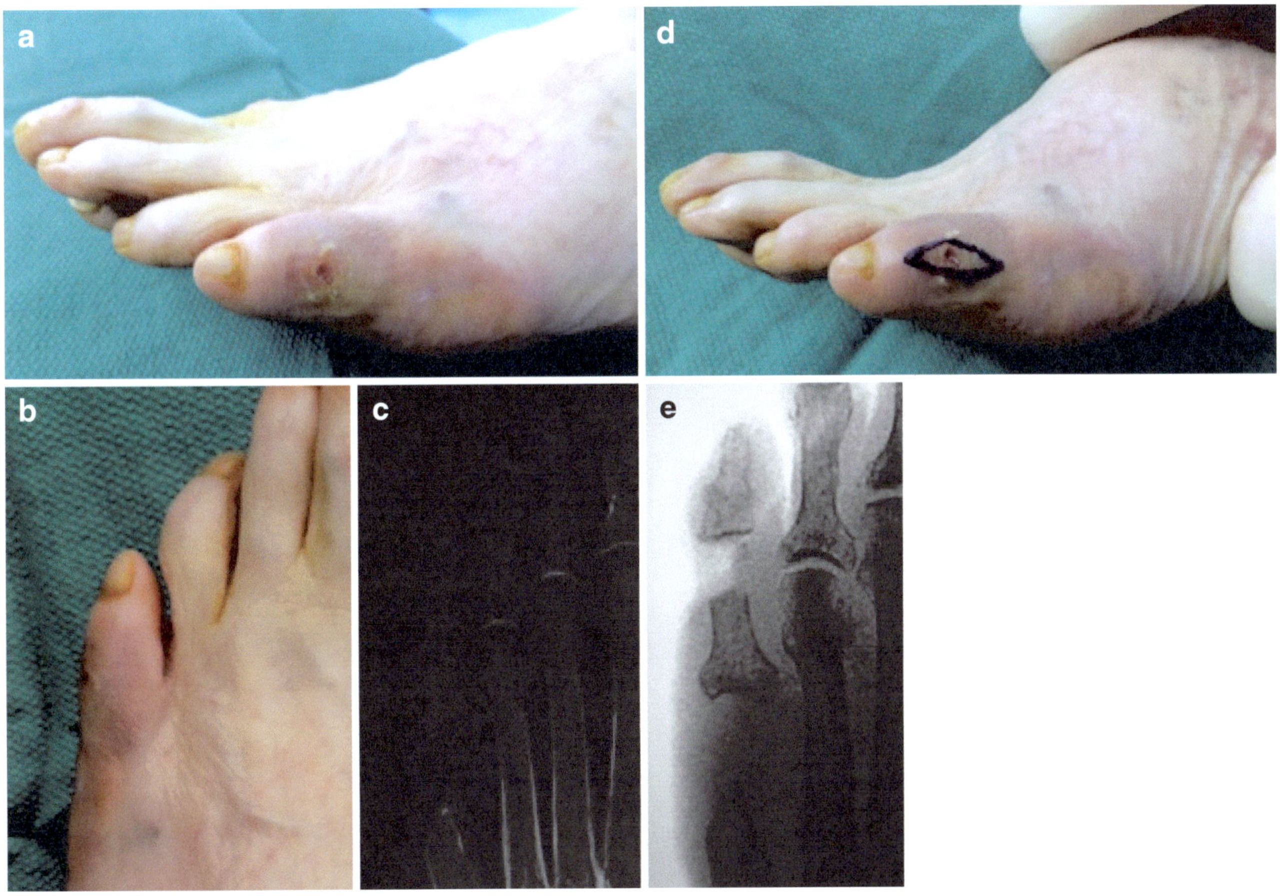

Fig. 18.3 Fifth toe arthroplasty for infected proximal interphalan- geal joint ulcer. (**a–c**) Early intervention for a painful wound with recurring cellulitis, positive probe to bone test, and relatively nor- mal X-ray findings allowed arthroplasty instead of amputation for osteomyelitis. The patient had prior fifth metatarsal head resection for similar wound complications. (**d**, **e**) Elliptical excision of the ulcer and arthroplasty of the proximal interphalangeal joint allowed primary closure of the chronic wound. Removal of the head of the proximal phalanx eliminated the prominent bone and provided spec- imen for biopsy

Fourth and Fifth Digital Syndactylization

Syndactylization of the fourth and fifth toes is useful for persistent interdigital ulcers and ulcerated deep interspace heloma molle (Fig. 18.4). This is a cosmetically appealing alternative to amputation allowing concomitant wound excision, PIPJ arthroplasty, and primary wound closure. Another indication for syndactylization is fifth digital instability after arthroplasty requiring excessive bone loss. Wide resection of the proximal phalanx increases the

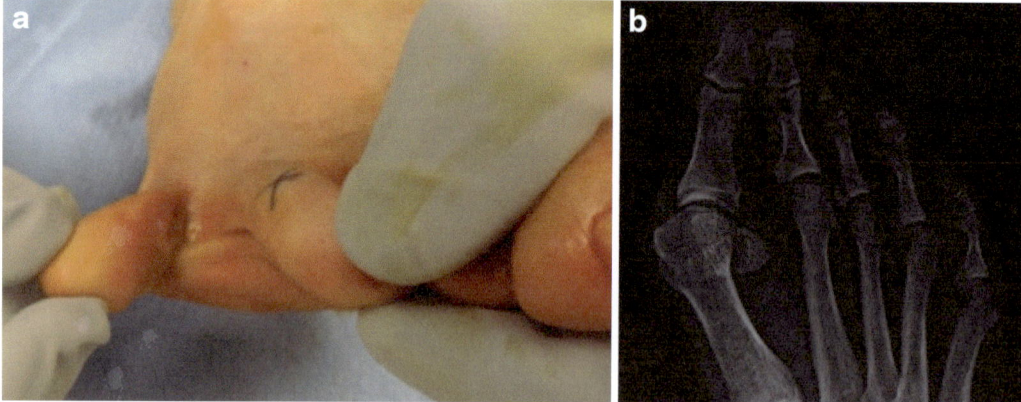

Fig. 18.4 Partial syndactylization and fifth proximal interphalangeal joint (PIPJ) arthroplasty for interdigital ulceration complicated by osteomyelitis. (**a**) Fourth interspace chronic callus predisposed to periodic interdigital ulceration resulting in fifth toe osteomyelitis and PIPJ sepsis. The tissue deep in the interdigital space is commonly abnormal with maceration and scar tissue formation from longstanding heloma molle. (**b**) Preoperative X-ray demonstrated pressure of the head of the fifth proximal phalanx on the fourth metatarsal head. Early intervention with a reconstructive approach prior to tissue necrosis allowed excision of the ulcer, resection of the head of the fifth proximal phalanx, and partial syndactylization of the fourth and fifth toes

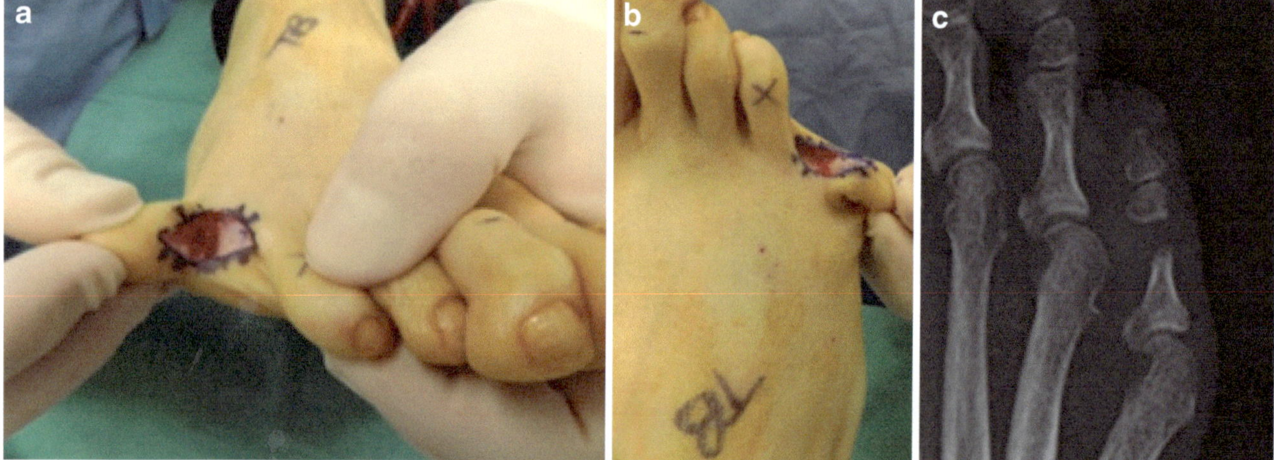

Fig. 18.5 Partial syndactylization technique. (**a**) The partial syndactylization technique confines interdigital wound excision to the deep aspect of the interdigital space with the intent to preserve more normal looking toes as compared to complete syndactylization. The wound was excised with careful attention to preserve the dorsal and plantar digital neurovascular structures. (**b**) Disarticulation of the fifth proximal interphalangeal joint provided exposure for arthroplasty. (**c**) The head of the proximal phalanx was removed which served as biopsy specimen and also reduced pressure on the fourth metatarsal head

chance of a flail toe without proper stabilization. The goal of partial syndactylization is to preserve a more normal toe appearance yet remove abnormal tissue deep in the interdigital space. A transverse elliptical incision extends along the bases of the fourth and fifth toes which removes both the ulcer and macerated tissue between the toes (Fig. 18.5). This approach allows direct access to the head of the proximal phalanx, which is resected with a bone-cutting forceps. The lateral aspect of the fourth toe and medial aspect of the fifth toe are then approximated closing the interdigital wound primarily. Suture removal may be difficult in the interdigital space making absorbable sutures ideal (Fig. 18.6).

Fifth Toe Amputation

Osteomyelitis that encompasses the entire proximal phalanx or involves both the proximal and middle phalanges is ideally treated with complete fifth toe or partial fifth ray amputation (Fig. 18.7). The majority of patients with osteomyelitis of the fifth toe are treated with fifth ray amputation despite the fifth

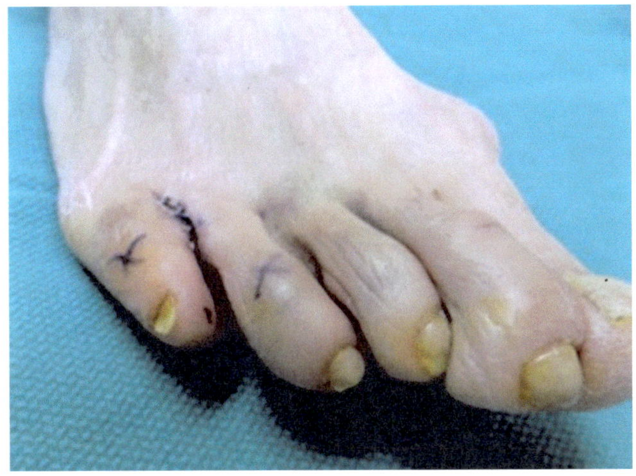

Fig. 18.6 Clinical results after partial syndactylization. Two week postoperative clinical appearance after partial syndactylization and proximal interphalangeal joint arthroplasty. Suture removal may be difficult in the interdigital space making absorbable sutures beneficial. Note how the fourth and fifth toes look relatively normal despite lack of the deep interdigital space. Early intervention allowed early diagnosis of osteomyelitis which in turn translated to minimally invasive treatment. This procedure also eliminated the chronic interdigital corn and ulcer that was painful

metatarsal being uninvolved. Leaving the fifth metatarsal head may predispose to plantar or lateral prominence and recurrent ulceration depending on bone structure. Removal of the metatarsal head also creates laxity in the soft tissues allowing primary closure of extensive soft tissue defects. One unique approach to preserve the metatarsal head involves a trap door digital fillet flap that utilizes intact dorsal tissue to cover a plantar defect or lateral tissue to cover an interspace defect (Figs. 18.8, 18.9, 18.10, and 18.11).

Fifth Metatarsal Phalangeal Joint Ulceration and Osteomyelitis

Infection around the fifth MPJ is most commonly associated with plantar or lateral fifth metatarsal head neuropathic ulceration but also occurs due to soft tissue infection spreading proximally from the fifth toe wounds or gangrene. Partial fifth ray amputation is a common surgical treatment option while complete fifth ray amputation is avoided when possible. A variety of incision plans including flap closure are available and are dictated by the size and location of the wound defect.

Fifth Metatarsal Head Resection

Early diagnosis of fifth metatarsal head osteomyelitis or early intervention for nonhealing or recurrent neuropathic

ulceration can be treated with isolated fifth metatarsal head resection (Fig. 18.12). This internal offloading technique allows plantar or lateral wounds to heal promptly and minimizes the chance of recurrence. Armstrong demonstrated that patients who received a fifth metatarsal head resection to treat plantar ulcerations had a lower reulceration rate as compared to those in a conservative treatment group [2]. There is risk of transfer ulceration to the fourth metatarsal head, but in our experience, this appears to be less common after fifth metatarsal head resection as compared to isolated removal of other metatarsal heads.

Traditional Partial Fifth Ray Amputation

The traditional approach to partial fifth ray amputation involves a standard tennis racket incision consisting of dorsal and plantar soft tissue flaps with midline proximal extension along the lateral border of the foot (Fig. 18.13). This incision approach works well for fifth toe infection and for lateral metatarsal head ulceration, since the ulceration is located within the tissue to be excised. A partial thickness plantar ulceration is also amenable to this approach since the wound should heal secondarily once the infected and prominent metatarsal head is removed. Traditional dorsal and plantar flaps are also easily converted to a transmetatarsal amputation (TMA) if necessary. Extensive tissue loss or full thickness plantar ulcerations typically require alternative incision techniques which are discussed next.

Partial Fifth Ray Amputation with Rotational Flap Closure of a Plantar Fifth MPJ Wound

A full thickness plantar ulceration at the fifth MPJ is not easily amenable to the traditional partial fifth ray amputation incision technique since the wound compromises the plantar flap. A rotational flap can be utilized to cover a large plantar wound defect with the caveat that the dorsal and lateral soft tissues at the base of the toe and MPJ remain healthy and viable (Figs. 18.14, 18.15, 18.16, and 18.17) [3]. A staged approach is possible if abscess or cellulitis is present. Stage 1 involves excision of the ulceration and debridement and biopsy of the fifth metatarsal head. Stage 2 involves raising the flap, amputation of the fifth toe, fifth metatarsal resection, and flap closure of the wound. An alternative staged technique involves open amputation with preservation of the flap using several loose sutures to maintain stretch and provide temporary coverage during stage 1. Stage 2 is performed several days later which involves washout, clean margin bone biopsy, and final flap closure.

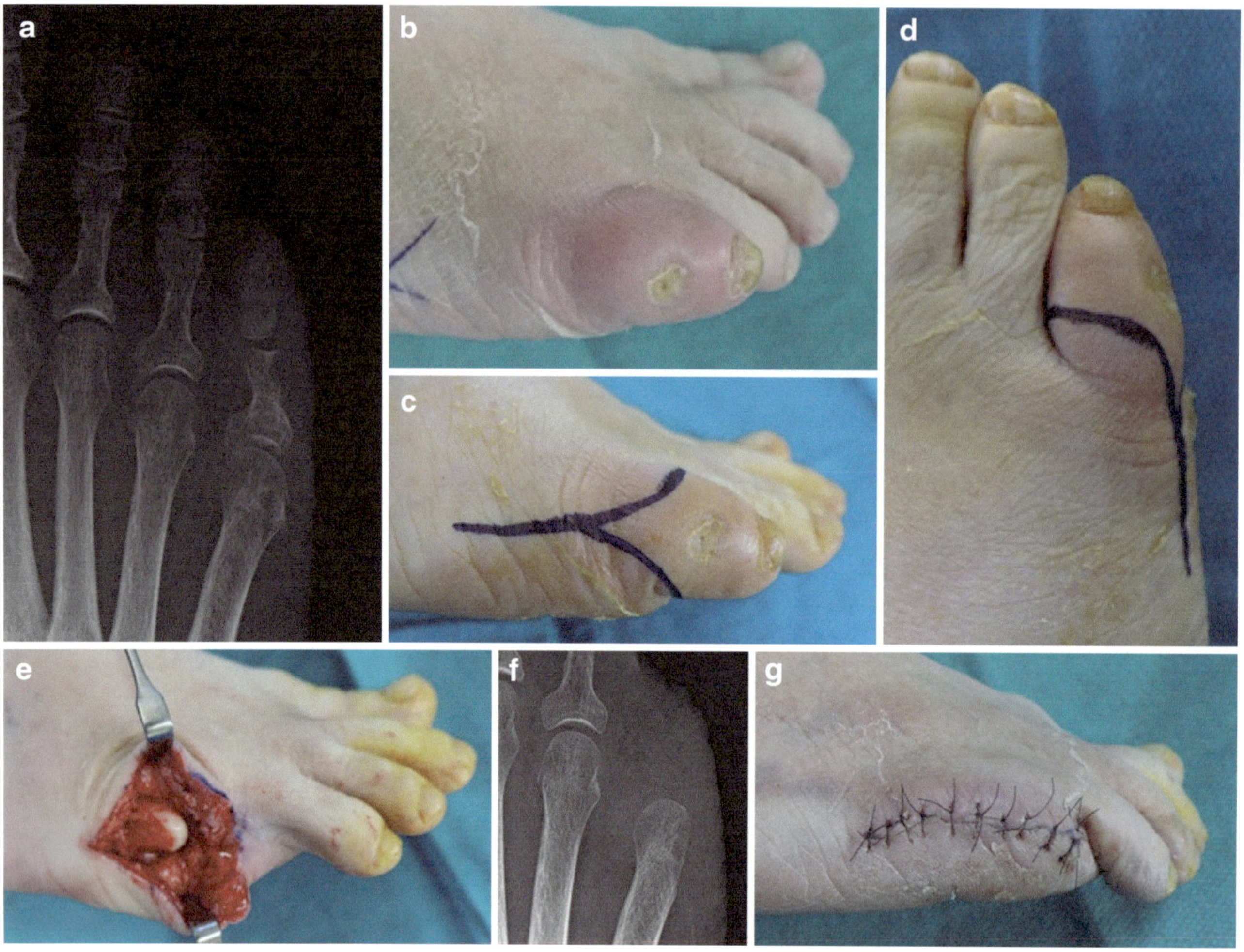

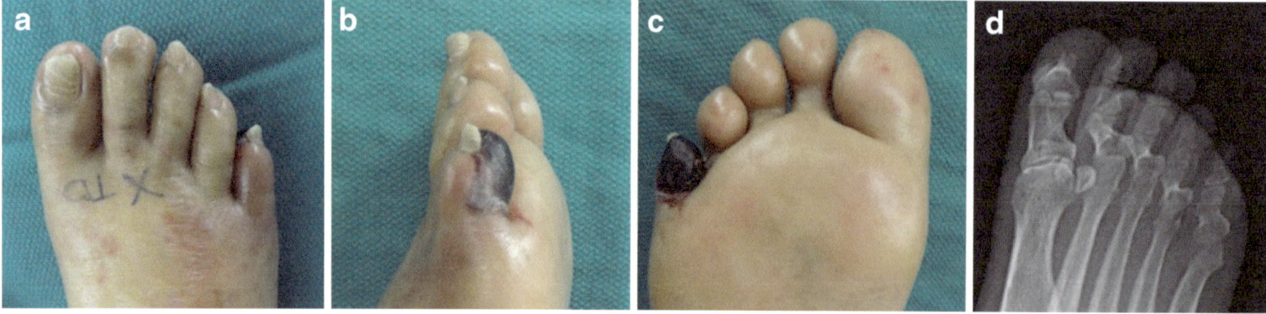

Fig. 18.7 Fifth toe amputation. (**a**, **b**) Proximal interphalangeal joint osteomyelitis involving both the middle and proximal phalanges is typically treated with complete fifth toe or partial fifth ray amputation. (**c**, **d**) A standard tennis racket incision with dorsal and plantar flaps was utilized for the amputation. (**e**, **f**) Note that the lateral head of the fifth metatarsal was remodeled which provided clean margin biopsy and reduced lateral prominence. (**g**) Primary wound closure with simple sutures allowed prompt healing with resolution of infection 5 days later. Confirmation of a clean bone margin allowed a short course of oral antibiotics

Fig. 18.8 Isolated fifth toe amputation with dorsal trap door digital fillet flap. (**a–d**) Digital gangrene commonly results in soft tissue infection and eventually osteomyelitis. Full thickness gangrene compromised the plantar tissue making primary closure with isolated fifth toe or fifth ray amputation challenging. Note that the dorsal tissue is not gangrenous but is compromised by infection and vascular insufficiency

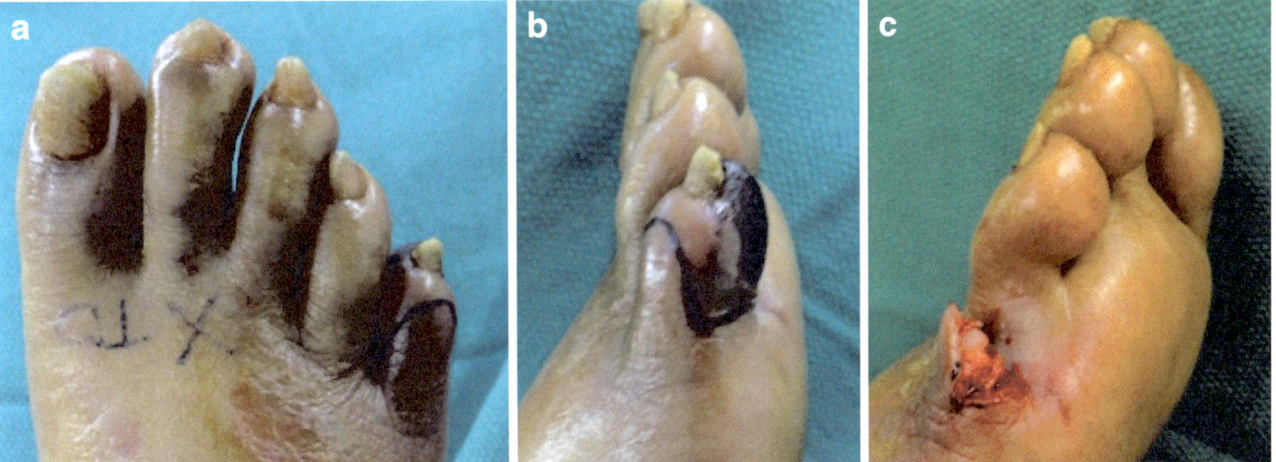

Fig. 18.9 Trap door digital fillet flap technique. (**a, b**) A fishmouth type incision was made around the infected and gangrenous tissue. The dorsal flap of tissue was preserved to allow primary closure with fifth toe amputation. Note how the dorsal flap technique does not allow easy access for fifth metatarsal head resection although the lateral apex of the incision (**b**) could be extended proximally. (**c**) The flap was raised full thickness off the proximal phalanx to preserve flap viability

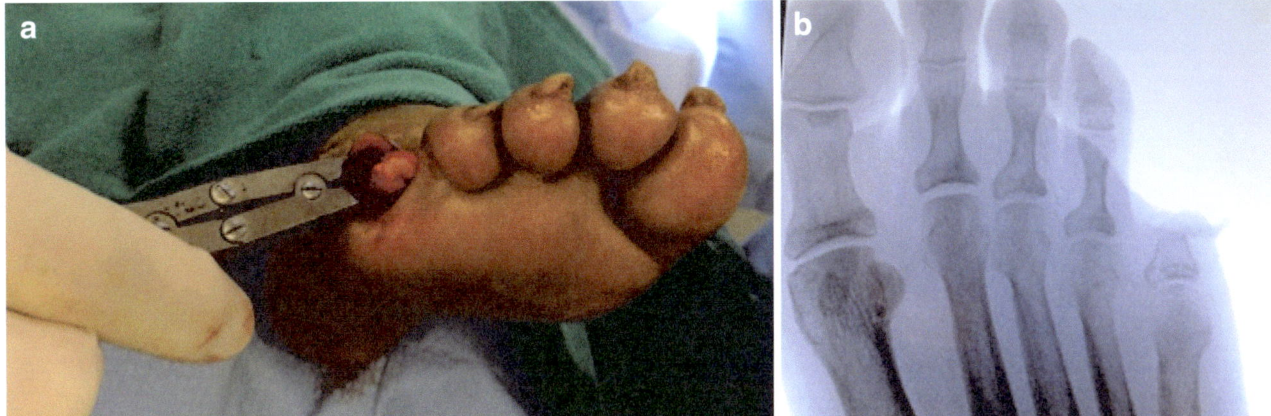

Fig. 18.10 Bone resection for partial fifth toe amputation. (**a, b**) Toe amputation was performed through the base of the proximal phalanx. Ray amputation is typically at the neck of the fifth metatarsal although partial or complete fifth toe amputation is an option under special circumstances including gangrene. This patient had compromised vascularity and poor health status which lead to this "less is more" approach. There is potential for shoe pressure along the lateral aspect of the fifth digital stump

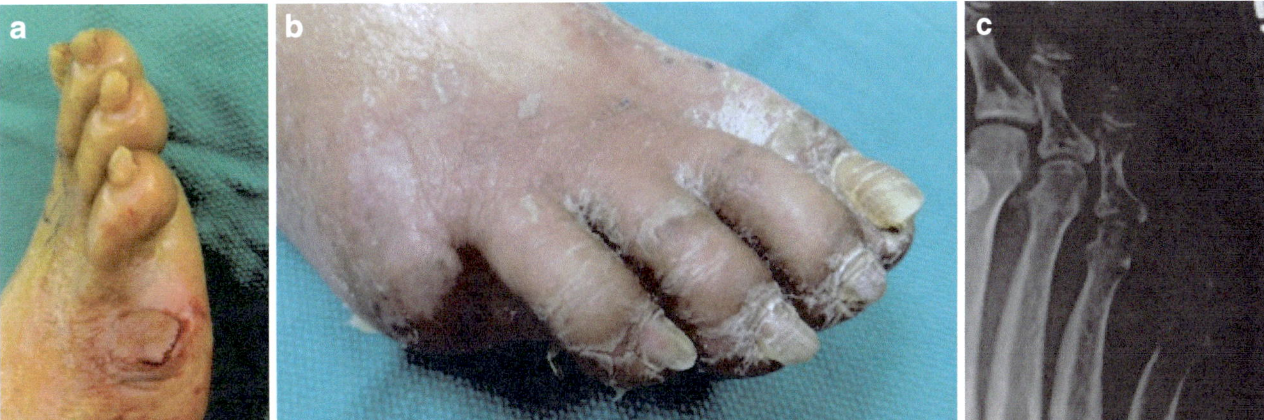

Fig. 18.11 Healed trap door digital fillet flap. (**a**) The trap door flap was closed to cover the soft tissue defect. Note that the compromised plantar tissue was entirely unavailable for contribution to wound coverage which necessitated this advanced plastic surgical technique. (**b, c**) Healing of the trap door flap at 6 weeks without recurrent soft tissue or bone infection

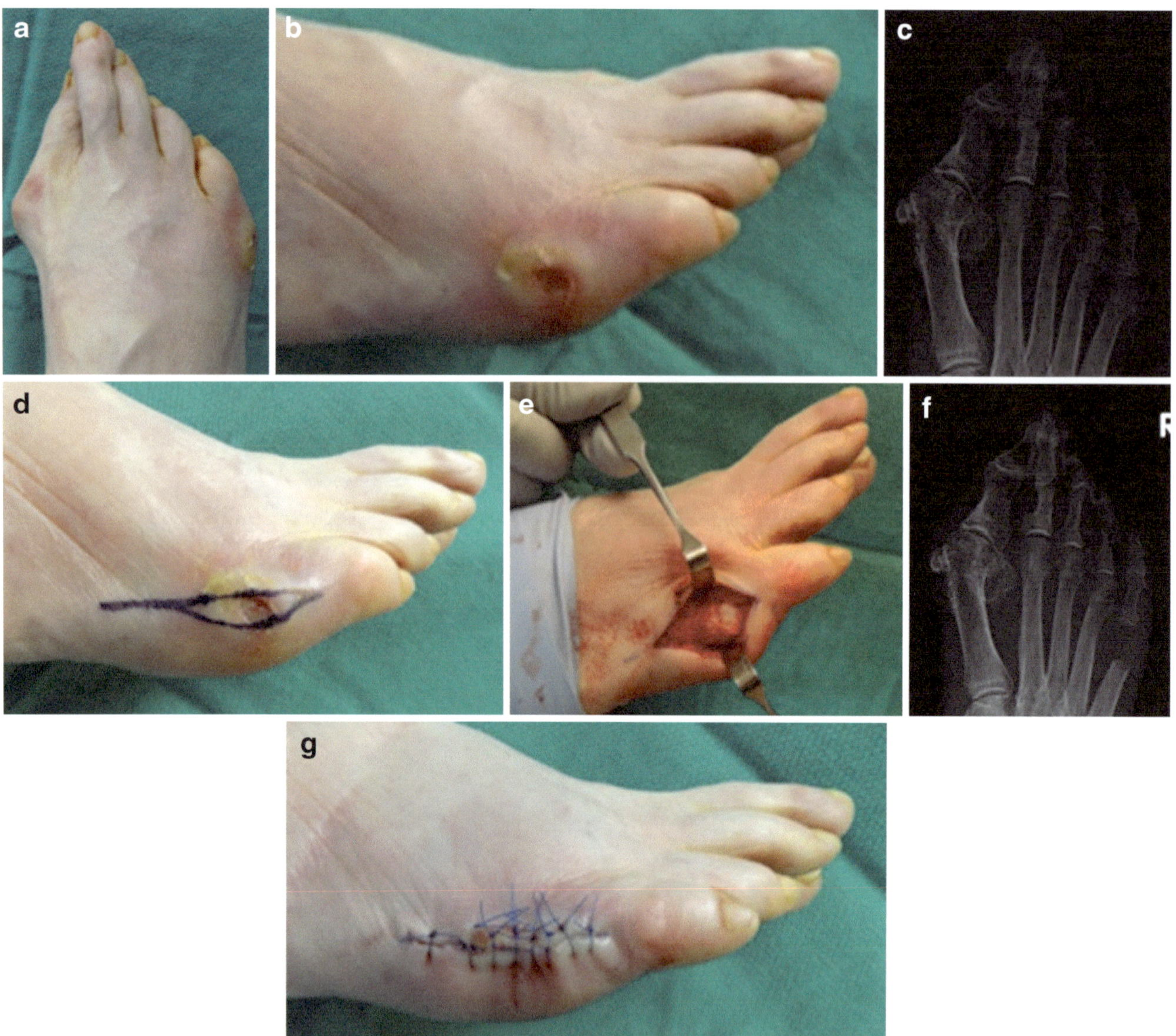

Fig. 18.12 Fifth metatarsal head resection. (**a–c**) Tailor's bunion deformity predisposed to neuropathic ulceration over the lateral aspect of the fifth metatarsal head. Early intervention at the first sign of local cellulitis and bone exposure allowed fifth metatarsal head resection rather than partial ray amputation. (**d, e**) Elliptical excision of the ulcer with proximal runout allowed exposure for metatarsal head resection. (**f**) Resection of the metatarsal head not only removed the bony prominence, but allowed for bone biopsy and (**g**) primary wound closure

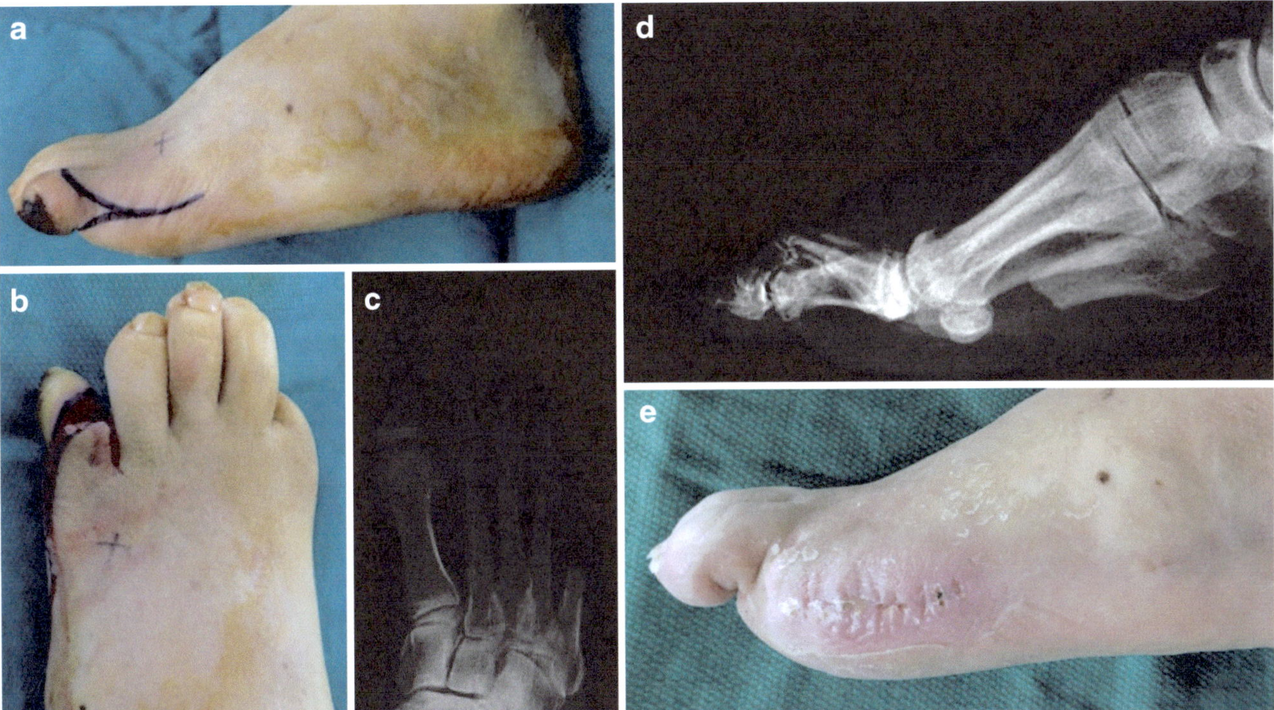

Fig. 18.13 Traditional partial fifth ray amputation technique with demonstration of tennis racket incision. (**a**) Note that the proximal extension was midline along the lateral aspect of the foot which created matching dorsal and plantar flaps. (**b**) A dorsal flap of tissue from the fifth toe was preserved to allow tension free closure. (**c**, **d**) Postoperative X-rays showing the desired angle and location of metatarsal resection just proximal to the metaphyseal flare. Bone resection was performed with a saw with the intent to avoid plantar and lateral prominence. (**e**) Healing at 3 weeks postoperatively

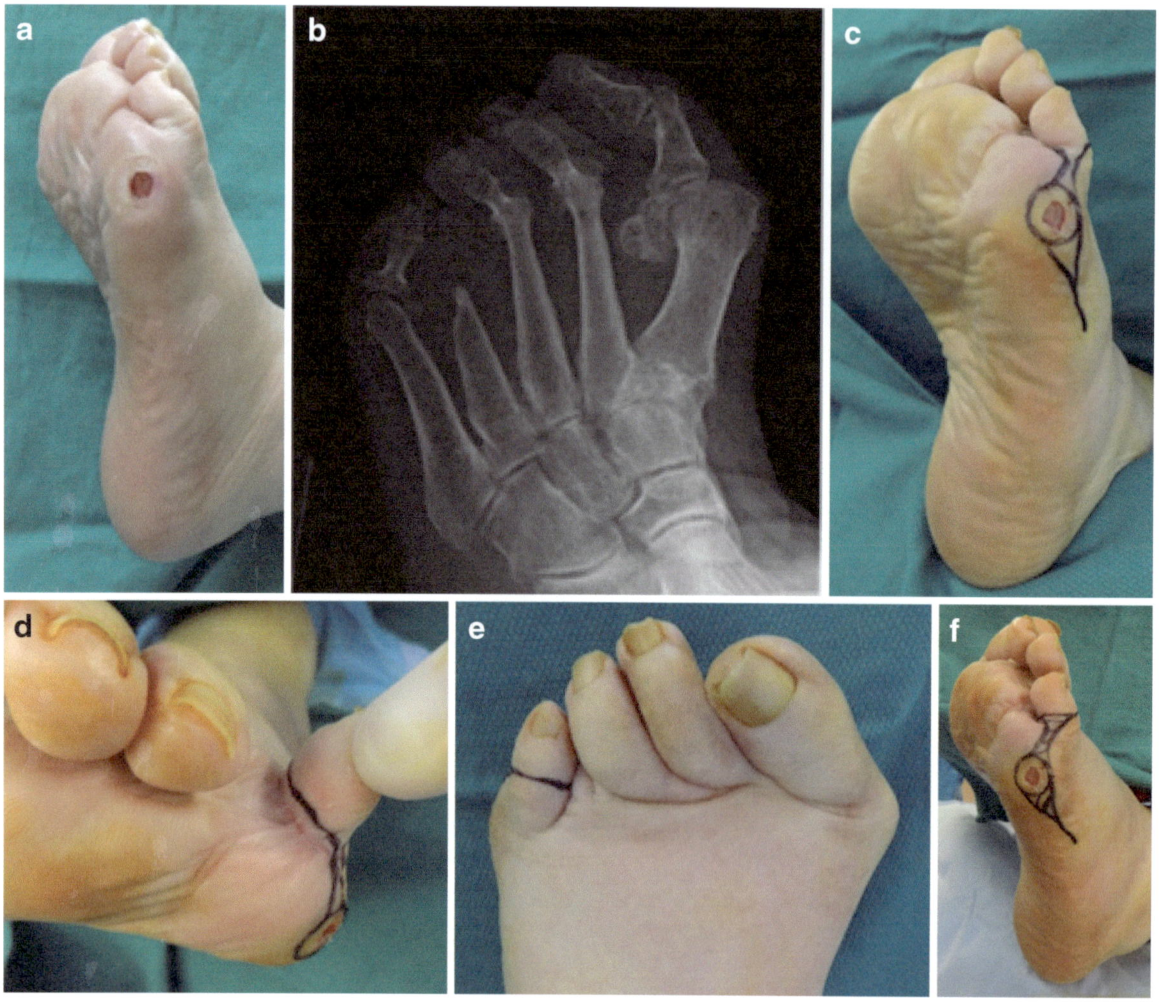

Fig. 18.14 Partial fifth ray amputation with rotational flap for plantar ulceration. (**a**) Preoperative photo demonstrating a chronic plantar fifth metatarsal head ulceration with undermining and exposure of the bone and joint. (**b**) X-ray shows predisposing factors including tailors bunion deformity, fifth digital contracture, and prior fourth ray amputation. (**c–e**) Flap design incorporating the healthy dorsal and lateral tissues with plan for ulcer excision with removal of the undermined wound margin. Note how the incision is carried onto the (**d**) medial aspect of the fifth toe within the interdigital space and the (**e**) transverse nature of the dorsal digital incision. This flap design is easily converted to transmetatarsal amputation should that become necessary later. (**f**) The tissue to be discarded is marked here to show how nearly all available tissue is used to provide tension free wound closure

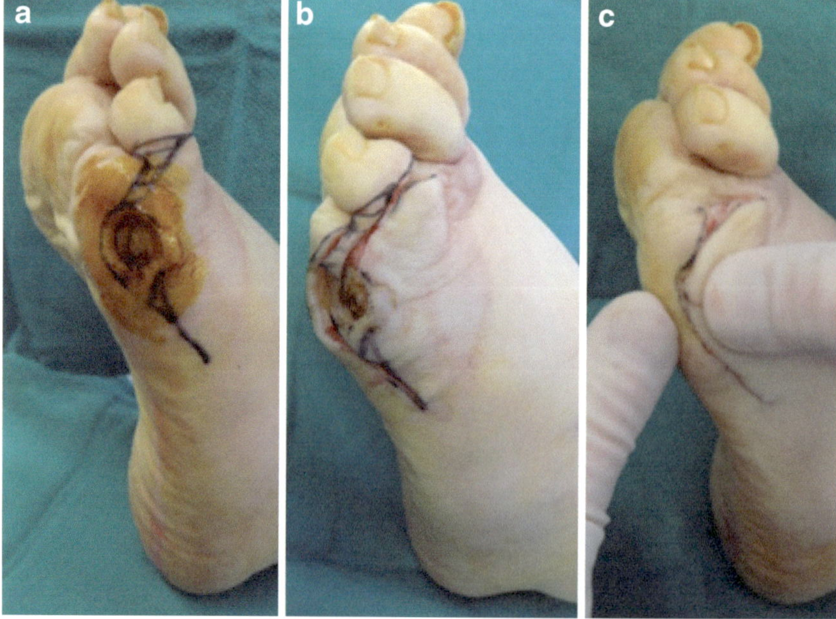

Fig. 18.15 Raising the fifth ray amputation flap. (**a**) The ulcer was excised followed by re-prepping of the wound site prior to raising the flap. (**b**) The flap was raised full thickness utilizing atraumatic technique and the tip of the toe was removed. (**c**) Note potential flap coverage even before resection of the proximal phalanx or metatarsal head

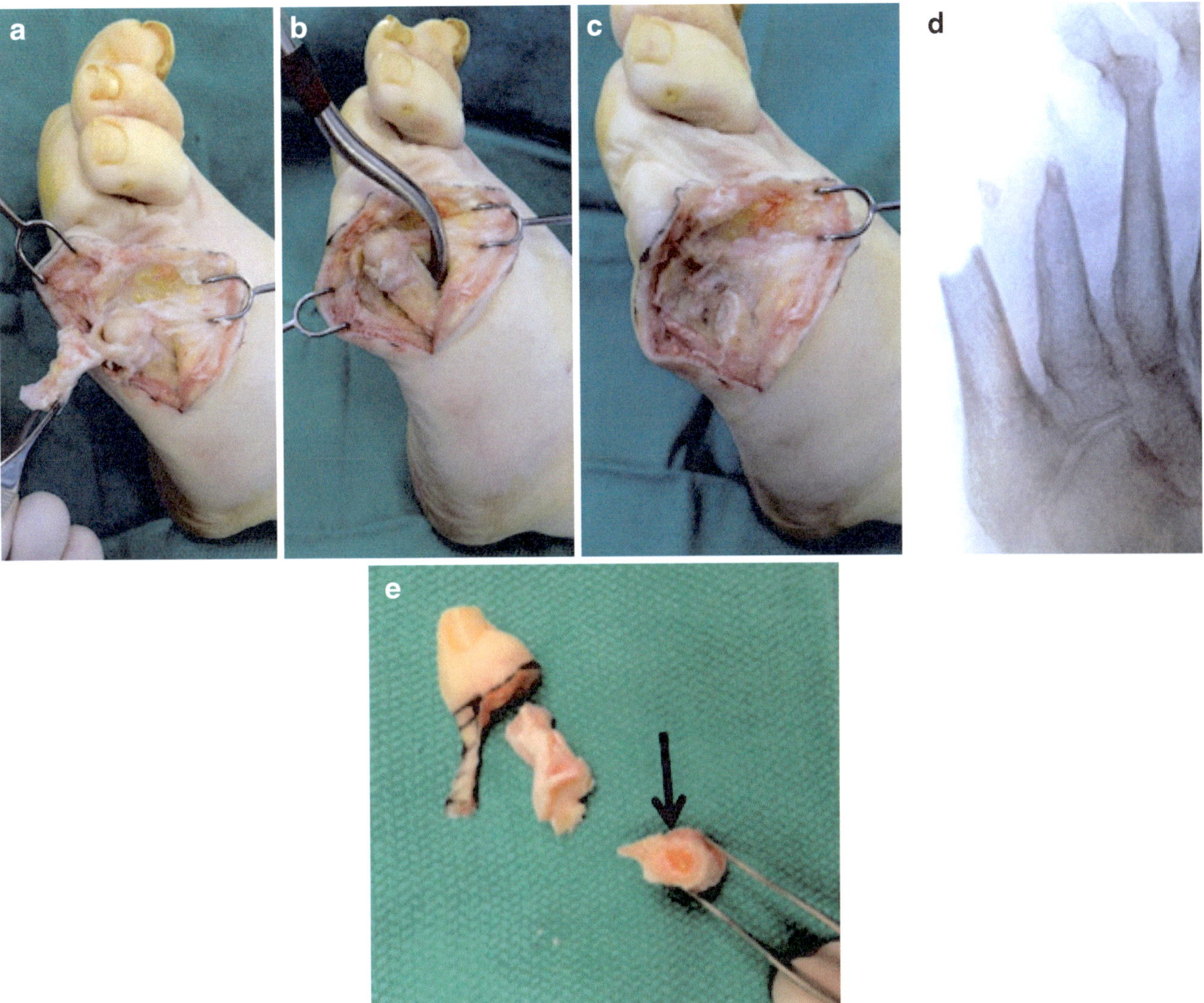

Fig. 18.16 Fifth metatarsal head resection. (**a**, **b**) The fifth toe was disarticulated at the metatarsophalangeal joint, and limited elevation of the periosteum was performed at the fifth metatarsal neck. (**c**) Clean bone resection involved the use of a power saw. (**d**) Intraoperative radiograph shows heterotopic ossification (HO) at the previous partial fourth ray amputation stump therefore HO prophylaxis was ordered postoperatively as described in Chap. 12. (**e**) Bone cultures were obtained from the metatarsal head. Inspection of the medullary canal of the metatarsal confirmed healthy bone and likely clean margin (*arrow*)

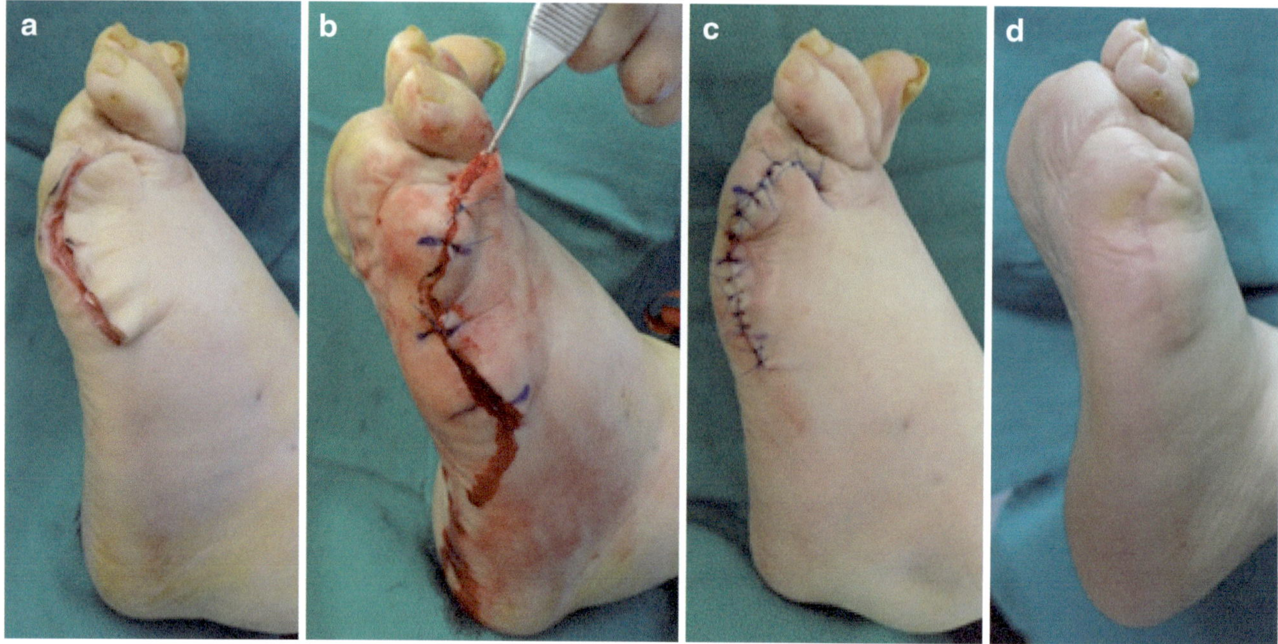

Fig. 18.17 Flap closure of the plantar wound. (**a**) The flap provided adequate coverage of the defect in this relaxed position. (**b**) The tourniquet was released to assess tissue viability and hemostasis. Remodeling of the distal apex was performed after partial closure to remove a dog ear. (**c**) Tension free flap closure with simple sutures. (**d**) Ten weeks postoperatively with healed flap

Digital Fillet Flap Partial Fifth Ray Amputation

A digital fillet flap can be incorporated into partial fifth ray amputation when there is extensive compromise of the plantar and interdigital soft tissues (Figs. 18.18, 18.19, 18.20, and 18.21). This flap is more fragile than the previously described flap as the digital tissue is thin and circulation can be compromised. Staged surgery is common, with this technique. Stage 1 involves raising a flap which is created using viable tissue on lateral and dorsal fifth toe and metatarsal head region (Fig. 18.18). The fifth toe and metatarsal head are resected and bone biopsy is obtained for definitive diagnosis of osteomyelitis. The flap is then rotated achieving partial closure with retention sutures (Fig. 18.19). Preliminary sutures allow partial coverage over an otherwise exposed fourth MPJ and maintains slight stretch on the flap to avoid shrinkage until the stage 2 procedure several days later. The stage 2 procedure involves raising the original flap followed by washout and debridement of the wound bed. Clean margin bone biopsy is commonly performed. The flap is remodeled to fit the size of the wound after debridement of nonviable tissue. The flap is again rotated into position and sutured without tension (Fig. 18.20). Depending on the size of the original defect, complete closure may not be possible and a portion of the wound may be left to heal by secondary intention.

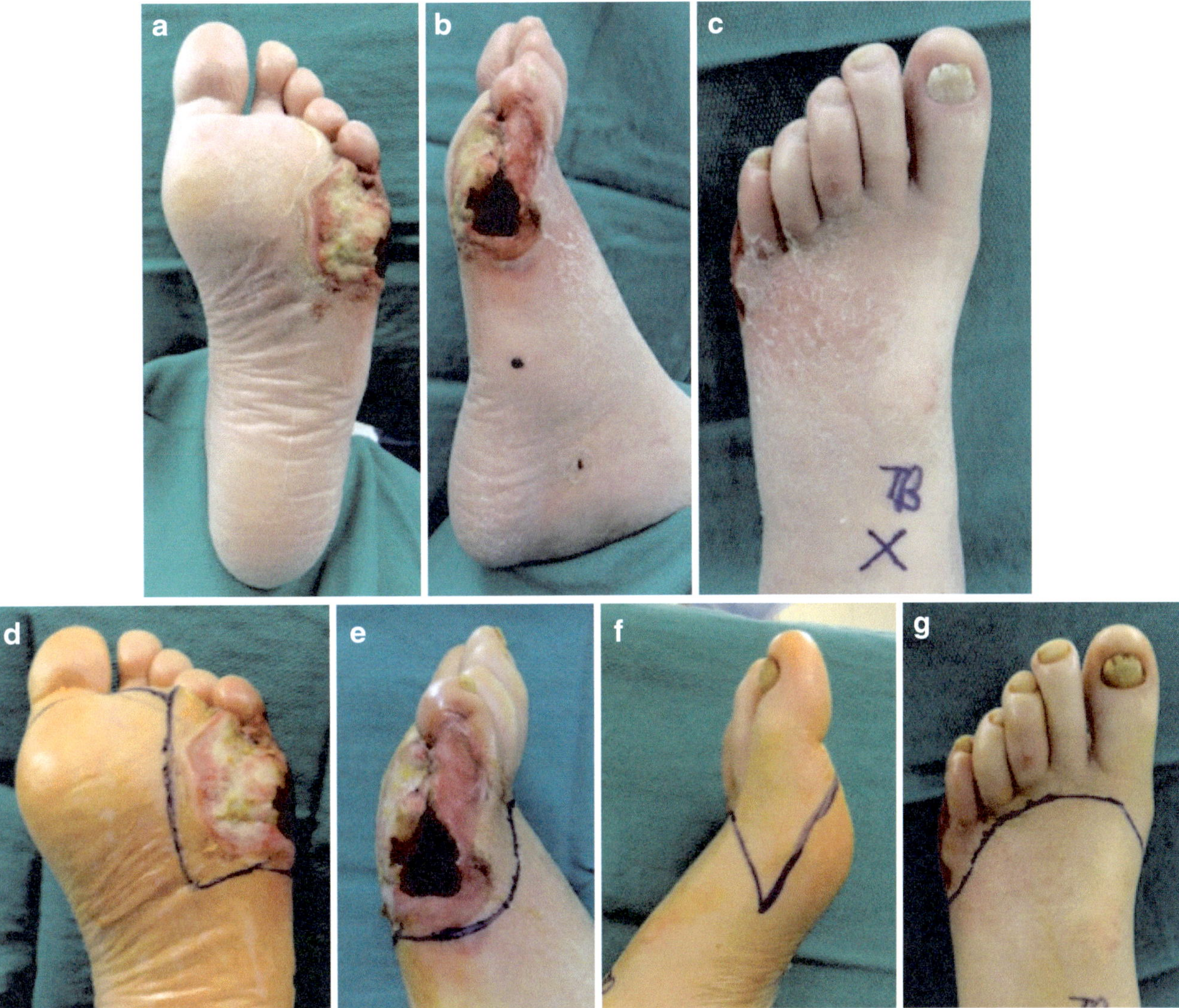

Fig. 18.18 Fifth ray amputation for infected gangrene with fifth digital fillet flap. (**a–c**) Compromised plantar and lateral soft tissues created substantial challenges regarding fifth ray amputation. Early onset of soft tissue infection and underlying osteomyelitis of the fifth metatarsal phalangeal joint necessitated surgical treatment. Transmetatarsal amputation (TMA) is likely under these circumstances yet the plantar soft tissue defect also compromised TMA closure options. (**d–g**) The medial plantar artery angiosome rotational flap TMA is an option for this condition as described in Chap. 19. Our initial attempt was to contain the amputation to the fifth ray although future revision amputation options were drawn prior to fifth ray amputation. This helps to ensure that revision options are not compromised by the initial procedure

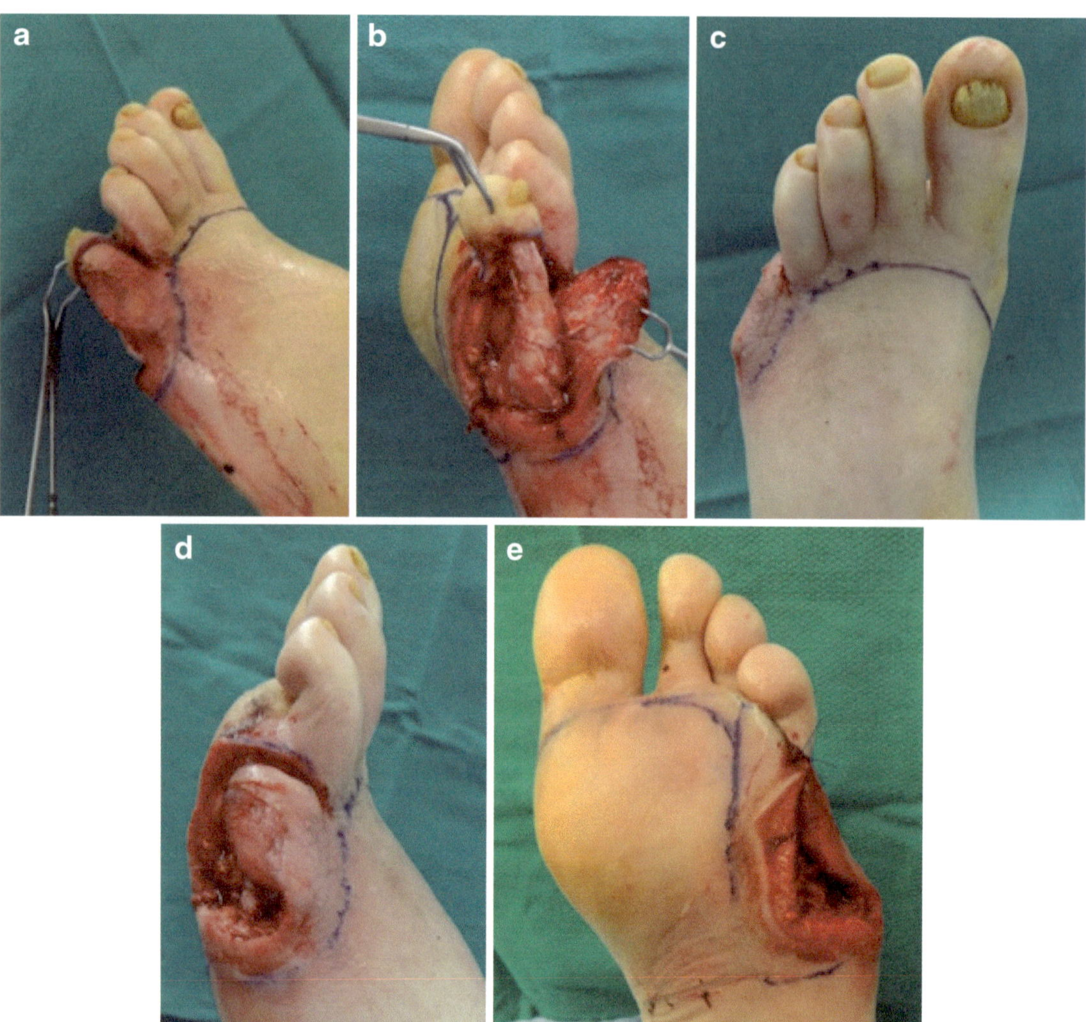

Fig. 18.19 Stage 1 partial fifth ray amputation with fifth digital fillet flap. (**a**, **b**) The dorsal digital fillet flap was preserved during stage 1 open amputation. Note how the flap utilized all available tissue from the fifth toe. The flap was raised from just behind the toenail and extended to the fifth metatarsal neck. The fifth toe phalanges were skeletalized preserving a full thickness flap with intact vascularity. Disarticulation through the metatarsophalangeal joint allowed access for fifth metatarsal head resection. (**c**–**e**) The flap provided only partial coverage at the conclusion of the stage 1 procedure. The operation was performed acutely at the time of initial presentation and several sutures were placed to maintain length of the flap. Shriveling of the flap is otherwise common and creates a situation where future coverage will be compromised

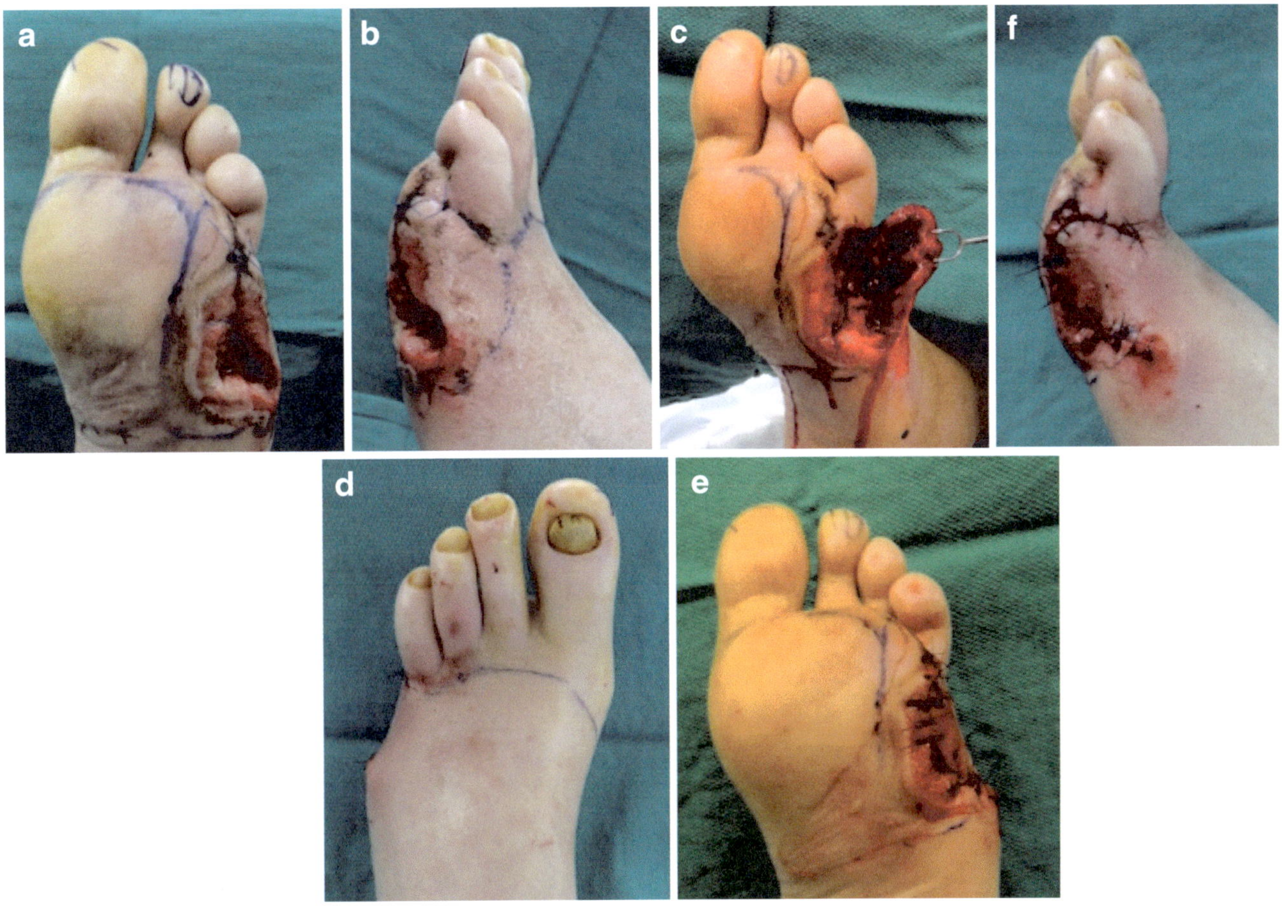

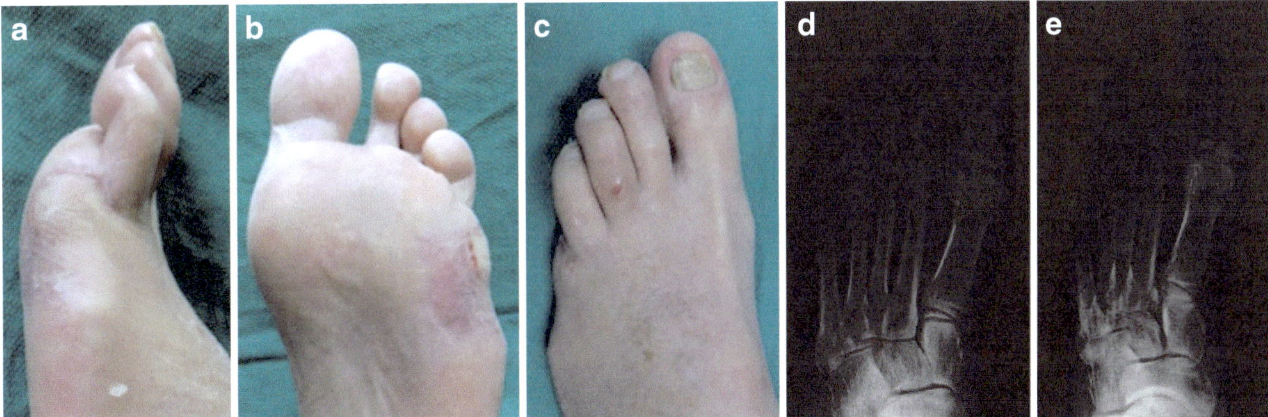

Fig. 18.20 Stage 2 partial fifth ray amputation with fifth digital fillet flap. (**a–c**) The stage 2 procedure involved raising of the flap, hematoma washout, repeat debridement and biopsy of the fifth metatarsal shaft, and flap closure. Note how the soft tissues had recovered from infection 3 days postoperatively while hematoma was seen beneath the flap. (**d–f**) The flap was advanced, rotated, and used to cover the plantar and lateral soft tissue defect. Note how the seemingly small digital flap provided coverage of a large wound. The plantar lateral portion of the flap and adjacent tissue margin was compromised by the large neuropathic ulcer. This tissue remained viable and was necessary to provide coverage of the underlying bone structure. Persistent bone exposure postoperatively commonly leads to recurrent or ongoing osteomyelitis and eventual revision with shorter amputation

Fig. 18.21 Healing progress 6 weeks after fifth ray amputation with fifth digital fillet flap. (**a–c**) Complete healing of the digital fillet flap at 6 weeks postoperatively. Failure to preserve the fillet flap would have made successful amputation at this level improbable. (**d, e**) Preoperative and 6 week postoperative radiographs demonstrate a desirable level of fifth ray amputation despite extensive soft tissue deficit

Complete Fifth Ray Amputation with Delayed Peroneal Tendon Transfer

Neuropathic ulcerations located at the base of the fifth metatarsal or over a prominent mid metatarsal stump from prior partial ray resection are often complicated by osteomyelitis. Preserving the fifth metatarsal base is important from a biomechanical standpoint but not always possible with large wound defects associated with bone exposure and osteomyelitis. Cavus foot structure is the dominant deformity present in this patient population, and patients with concomitant metatarsus adductus pose additional challenges. Charcot arthropathy can lead to lateral column ulceration with an underlying bony prominence that should be addressed in order for successful wound healing [4]. Our preference is to treat this condition aggressively to allow resection of infected bone yet maintain biomechanical balance of the foot through tendon balancing procedures. Our goal is to limit future breakdown and subsequent amputation yet preserve function of the foot. Treatment commonly involves staged complete fifth ray amputation with initial antibiotic bead insertion and delayed peroneal tendon transfer [5]. While this protocol is intended for patients with osteomyelitis at the midshaft or base of the metatarsal, we also consider this procedure if greater than 50 % of the fifth metatarsal shaft needs to be resected as wound recurrence is common when only the base of the fifth metatarsal is preserved (Fig. 18.22).

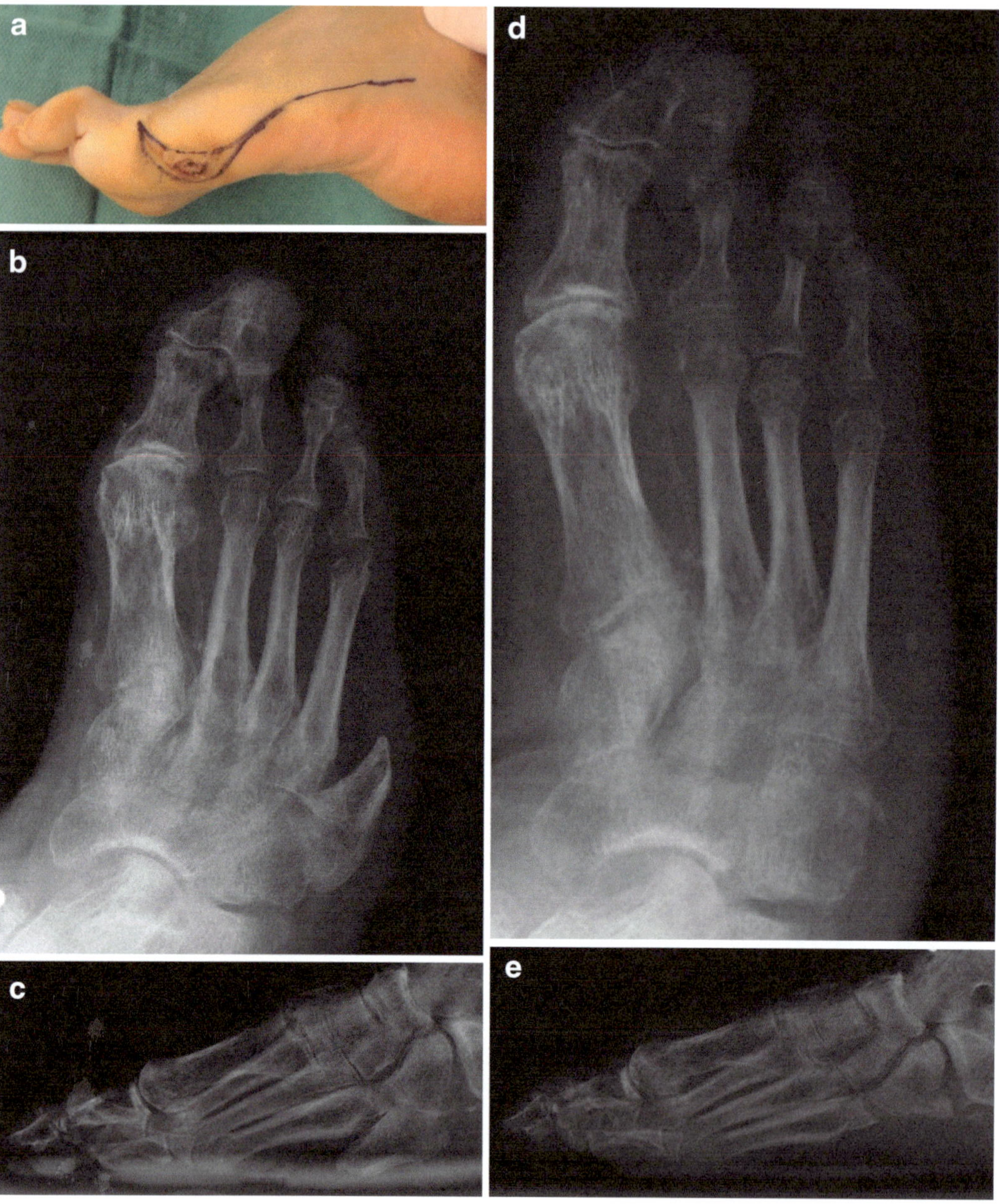

Fig. 18.22 In general, complete fifth ray amputation is avoided when possible. (**a**) Indications primarily involve recurrent midshaft ulceration following partial fifth ray amputation, when more than 50 % of the metatarsal needs to be resected due to extensive osteomyelitis, or with metatarsal base osteomyelitis associated with midfoot ulceration. (**b**, **c**) Preoperative X-rays of a patient with recurrent ulceration despite partial fifth ray amputation. Note that <50 % of the metatarsal remains with residual bone prominence. (**d**, **e**) Postoperative X-rays showing complete fifth ray resection

Complete Fifth Ray Amputation: Stage 1 Procedure

The incision design is based on the location of the wound defect which may be located at the fifth metatarsal head, midshaft, or base. Metatarsal base wounds are typically plantar lateral, but direct lateral or direct plantar wounds may occur (Fig. 18.23). If the fifth digit is present, it is removed through a standard "tennis-racquet" incision, which will allow primary closure distally (Fig. 18.13). After proximal dissection, the peroneus tertius and brevis tendons are completely removed from the fifth metatarsal base (Fig. 18.25). Surgeons tend to be hesitant regarding removal of the fifth metatarsal base due to the loss of insertion of the peroneus brevis tendon, which leads to a largely unopposed posterior tibial tendon. However, the second stage of this surgical protocol involves tendon balancing of the foot, which addresses this

concern. The entire fifth metatarsal is then removed and bone biopsy is taken from the area near the ulceration (Fig. 18.25). Next, a string of antibiotic-impregnated polymethyl methacrylate beads is placed within the void created by the absence of the fifth metatarsal (Fig. 18.26). No drain is placed, as the antibiotic beads require some degree of hematoma for proper elution of the antibiotic into the surrounding tissues. The second stage procedure is scheduled about 14 days later.

Complete Fifth Ray Amputation: Stage 2 Procedure

The second stage of this surgical protocol involves removal of the antibiotic beads, remodeling of the cuboid, and peroneal tendon transfer (Figs. 18.27, 18.28, 18.29, 18.30, 18.31, and 18.32). Typically, the peroneus longus (PL) tendon is

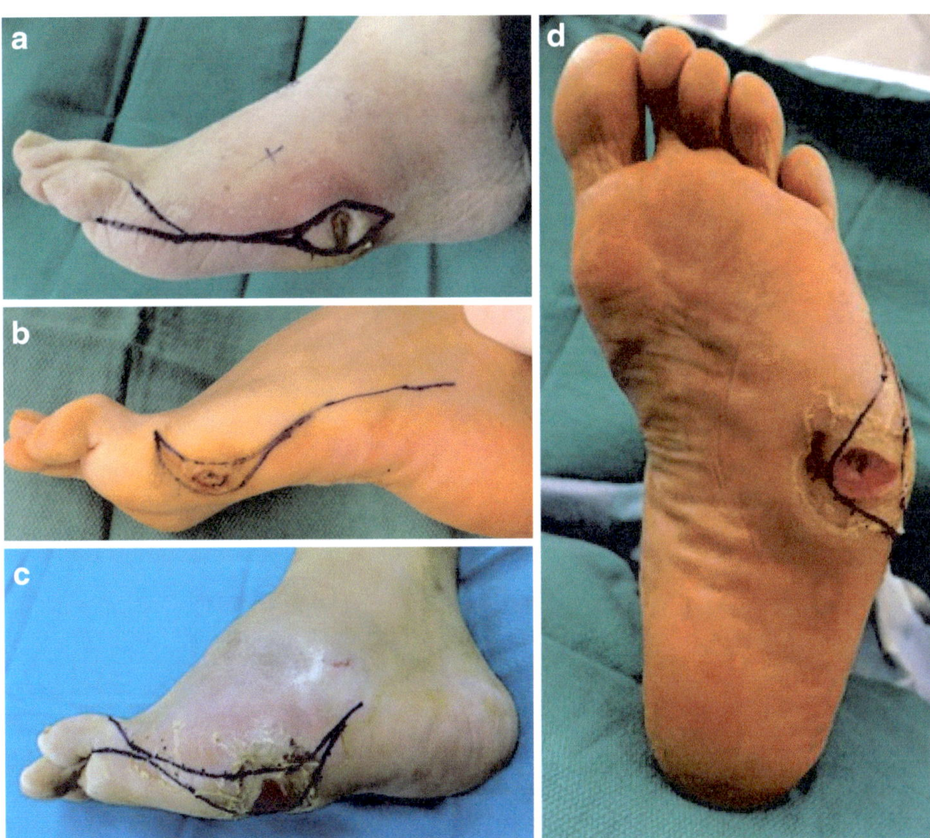

Fig. 18.23 Stage 1 incision planning for complete fifth ray amputation. Incisions are designed to completely excise the ulceration and create a proper fitting flap for immediate closure. A tennis racket incision is used to incorporate fifth toe amputation. Lateral midfoot ulcers can be quite large and flap closure can be challenging, however, a significant amount of tissue laxity is created once the entire fifth metatarsal has been removed. (**a**) This direct lateral fifth metatarsal base wound location was associated with metatarsus adductus. Fifth metatarsal base ulcerations prove challenging as isolated fifth metatarsal base excision is not practical. (**b**) Flap design similar to the fifth ray amputation flap (Fig. 18.14) is incorporated for plantar wounds at the fifth metatarsal head and midshaft locations following prior partial fifth ray amputation. (**c**, **d**) Plantar lateral midfoot ulcers are commonly associated with Charcot deformity. Note how the incision will allow advancement of the dorsal lateral tissues to provide immediate wound coverage after fifth ray amputation

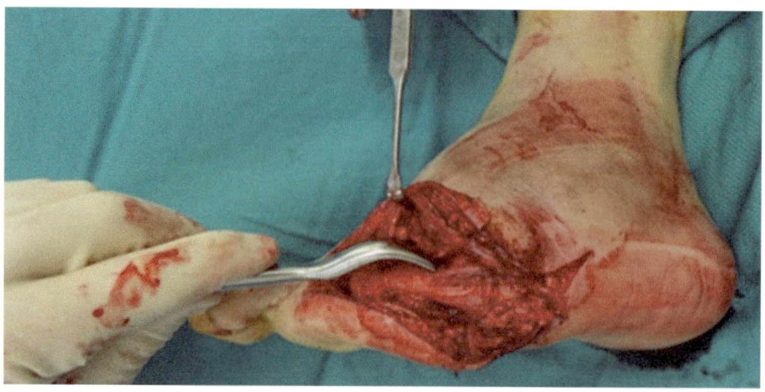

Fig. 18.24 Fifth metatarsal dissection. Preoperative photos are shown in Fig. 18.23c and d. After disarticulation of the fifth digit, subperiosteal dissection was continued proximally to the base of the fifth metatarsal, raising the dorsal flap full thickness. This is typically done with a metatarsal elevator, which minimizes trauma to neurovascular structures in the intermetatarsal space

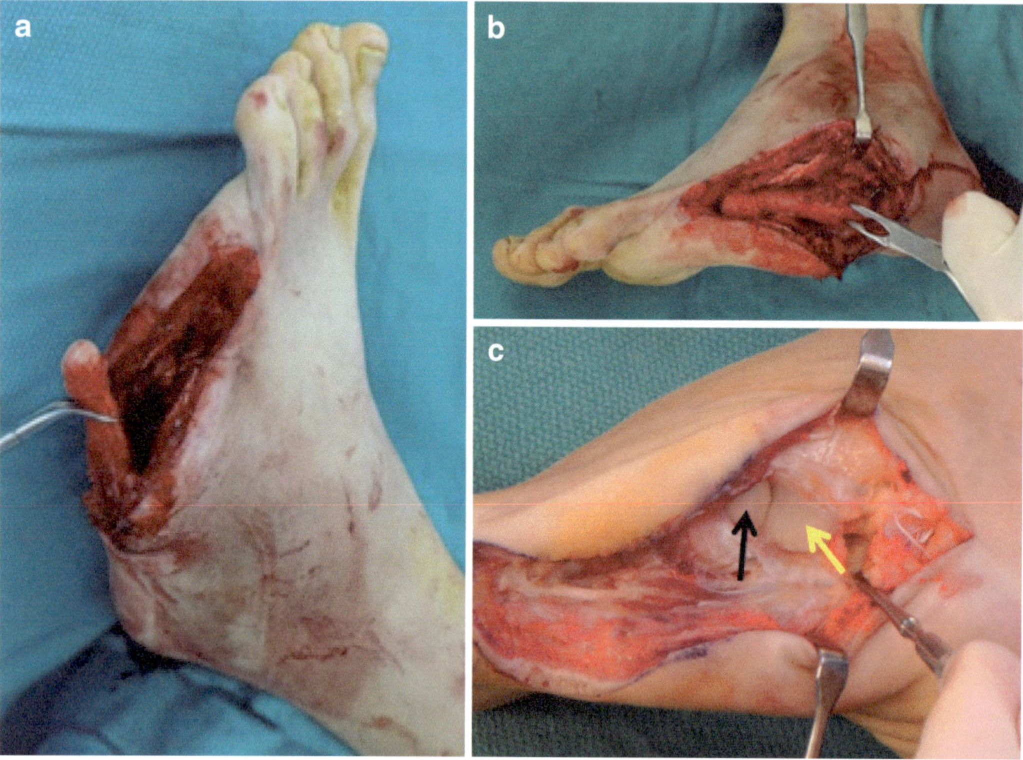

Fig. 18.25 Removal of the fifth metatarsal. (**a**) The fifth metatarsal is then pulled laterally with a penetrating towel clamp and the strong ligaments attaching the fifth metatarsal base to the cuboid and fourth metatarsal are released. The peroneus tertius and brevis tendons are then completely removed from the fifth metatarsal base. (**b**) Bone biopsy is taken from near the area of the ulceration. (**c**) Care is taken to avoid disruption of the cuboid (*yellow arrow*) or fourth metatarsal (*black arrow*) during the stage 1 procedure to minimize risk of cross contamination. Careful hemostasis is then achieved prior to antibiotic bead placement

transferred into the cuboid, as the length of the peroneus brevis (PB) tendon is frequently inadequate. There is biomechanical benefit to PL transfer as release of the PL from the first ray insertion allows the first ray to elevate, which is desirable in patients with concomitant lateral column ulceration and cavoadductus deformity. This in turn reduces lateral pressure, which helps prevent future plantar-lateral breakdown.

The antibiotic bead chain is removed through the proximal one third of the previous surgical incision (Fig. 18.27). The incision is then lengthened proximally, and the PL tendon is identified, transected, and transferred into the cuboid under anatomic tension (Figs. 18.28, 18.29, and 18.30). The PB can then be attached in a side-by-side fashion to the newly transferred PL tendon, which will augment eversion strength postoperatively. Strict non-weight bearing for 6 weeks after the second stage procedure is important to allow tendon healing. Achilles tendon lengthening and posterior tibial tendon lengthening are common during the stage 2 procedure depending on underlying contracture, foot structure, and expected function of the peroneal tendons (Fig. 18.33).

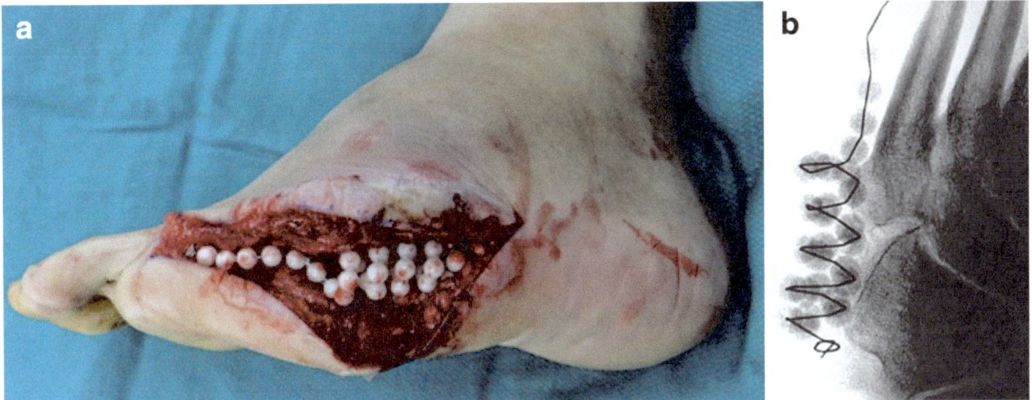

Fig. 18.26 Antibiotic bead placement. (**a**) A string of polymethyl methacrylate antibiotic beads were placed within the void created by the absence of the fifth metatarsal. The periosteal layer was closed with absorbable sutures over the antibiotic beads, which creates a bead pouch. Skin was closed with simple sutures under minimal tension. (**b**) Postoperative stage 1 X-ray demonstrating antibiotic bead placement

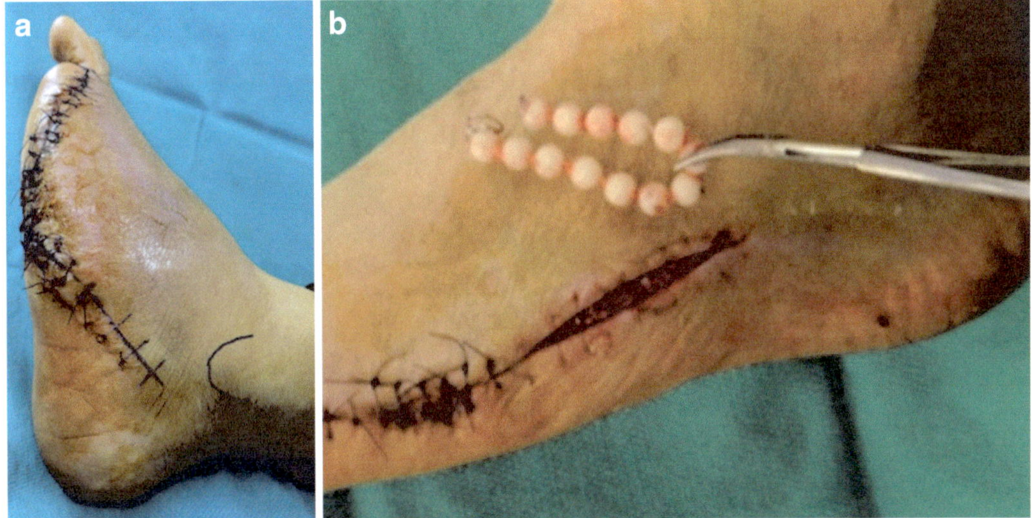

Fig. 18.27 Stage 2 surgery 14 days later with antibiotic bead removal and delayed tendon transfer. The proximal one third of the previous surgical incision was opened allowing antibiotic bead removal. The distal sutures remain intact and undisturbed. The surgery site and bead pouch were curetted and irrigated to remove hematoma. The incision is extended proximally to allow exposure of the cuboid and peroneal tendons

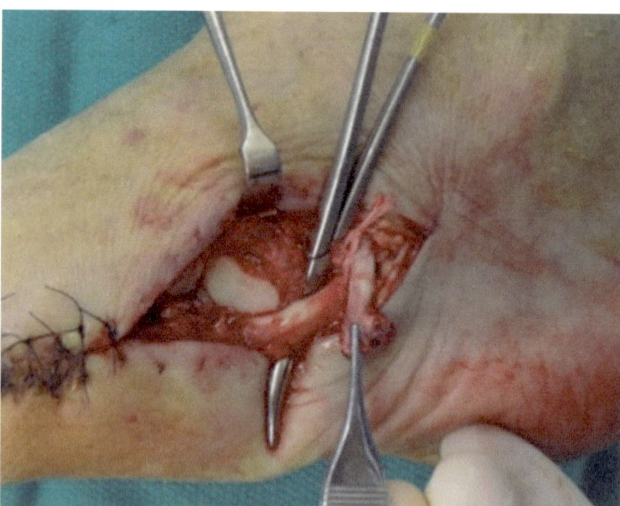

Fig. 18.28 Peroneal tendon transfer to the cuboid. (**a**) The peroneus longus tendon was then identified (*over hemostat*) and cut deep into the arch along the plantar portion of the cuboid. Note that the brevis tendon (*in forceps*) was easily found and minimally retracted after removal from the fifth metatarsal base during stage 1 surgery 2 weeks prior. This step allows intentional elevation of the first ray which is desirable with loss of the lateral column. The distal portion of the insertional fibers of the peroneus brevis are often thin and frayed after dissection from the metatarsal base and may be abnormal in cases where the wound and infection was located at the metatarsal base

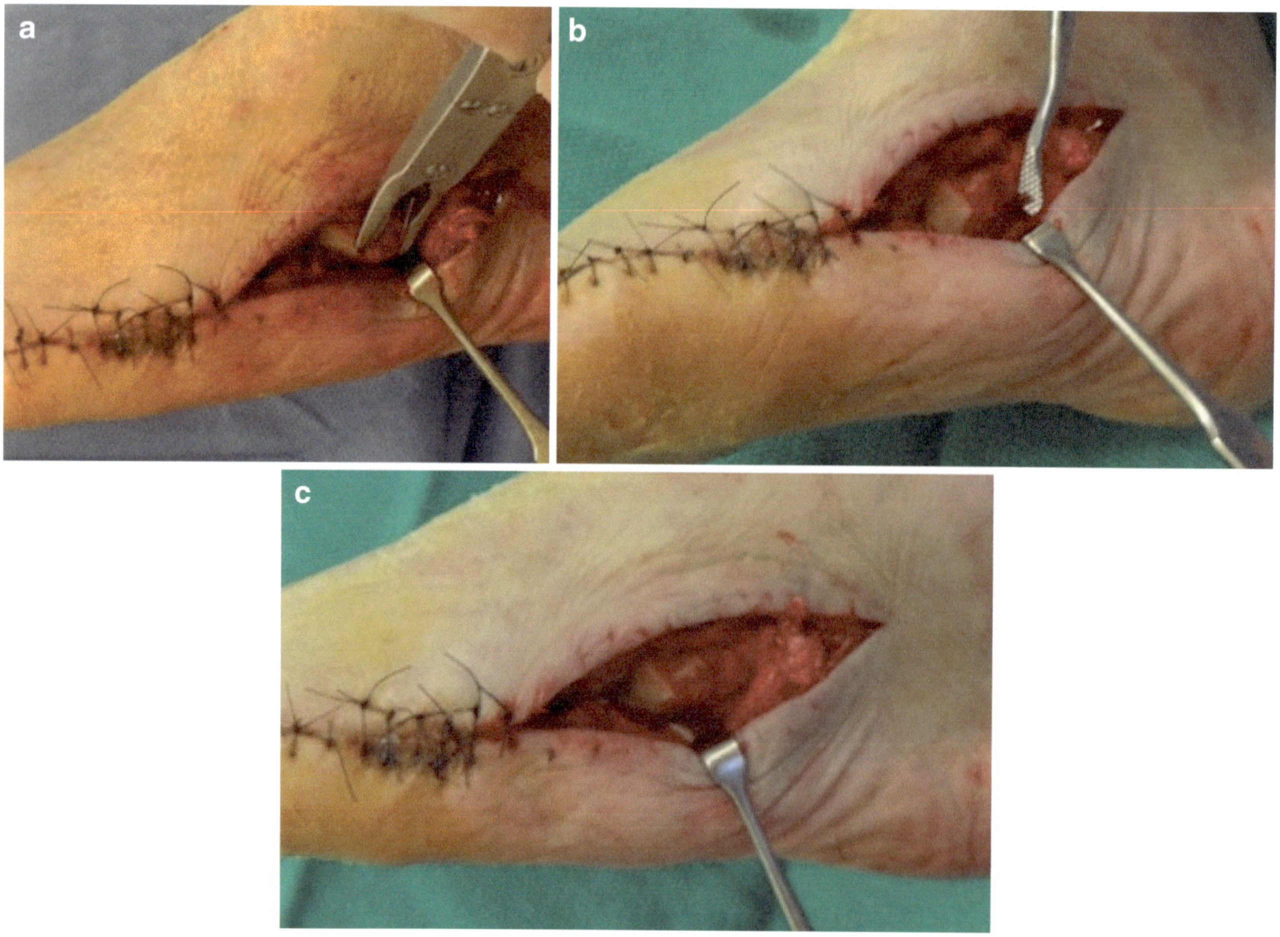

Fig. 18.29 Cuboid remodeling. The lateral and plantar prominences at the distal aspect of the cuboid were then remodeled with (**a**) a ronguer and (**b**) power rasp. (**c**) The goal is to remove the cuboid flair at the distal aspect of the groove for the peroneus longus. Bone procured from cuboid remodeling can be sent for clean margin bone biopsy, which will help guide the duration of antibiotic therapy

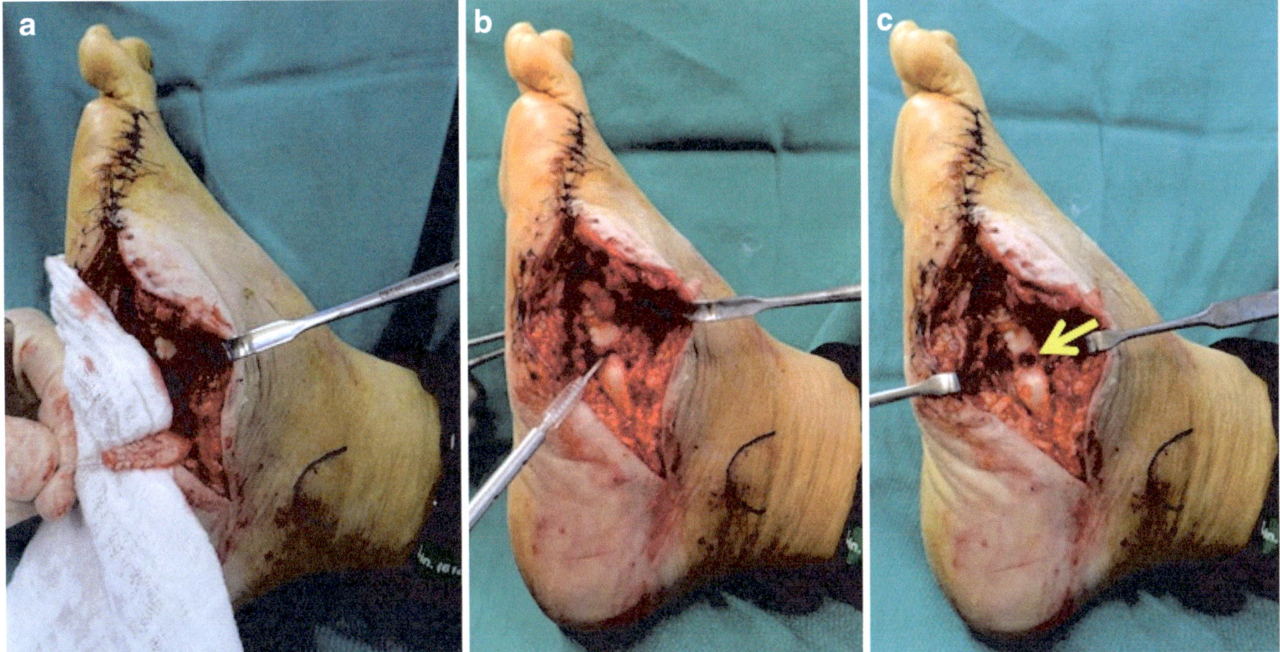

Fig. 18.30 Peroneal tendon transfer. (**a**) The peroneus longus tendon was prepared for transfer using braided composite suture. The tendon sutures were then passed from lateral to medial through a drill hole in the cuboid and out the medial portion of the foot using Kirschner wires followed by long Keith needles. This allows the prepared distal portion of the longus tendon to be pulled into the cuboid and held at anatomic tension during (**b**) insertion of an absorbable anchor. Soft tissue anchors can be used at the surgeon's discretion, but the ideal anchor material would be compatible with future MRI, should that become necessary. (**c**) The transferred tendon is shown buried in the cuboid (*yellow arrow*). The peroneus brevis tendon can then be attached in a side-by-side fashion to the newly transferred longus tendon

Fig. 18.31 Wound Closure and postoperative X-rays. (**a**) The proximal wound was again closed primarily with simple sutures. (**b**, **c**) Postoperative X-rays demonstrate that there is no longer a plantar and lateral prominence from the fifth metatarsal base. Preservation of functional eversion through peroneal tendon transfer is critical to avoid progressive inversion deformity, especially since lateral column ulcers are common with cavus foot deformity and metatarsus adductus. Note how the medial column is elevated following peroneus longus tenotomy and transfer to the cuboid despite prior cavus foot structure

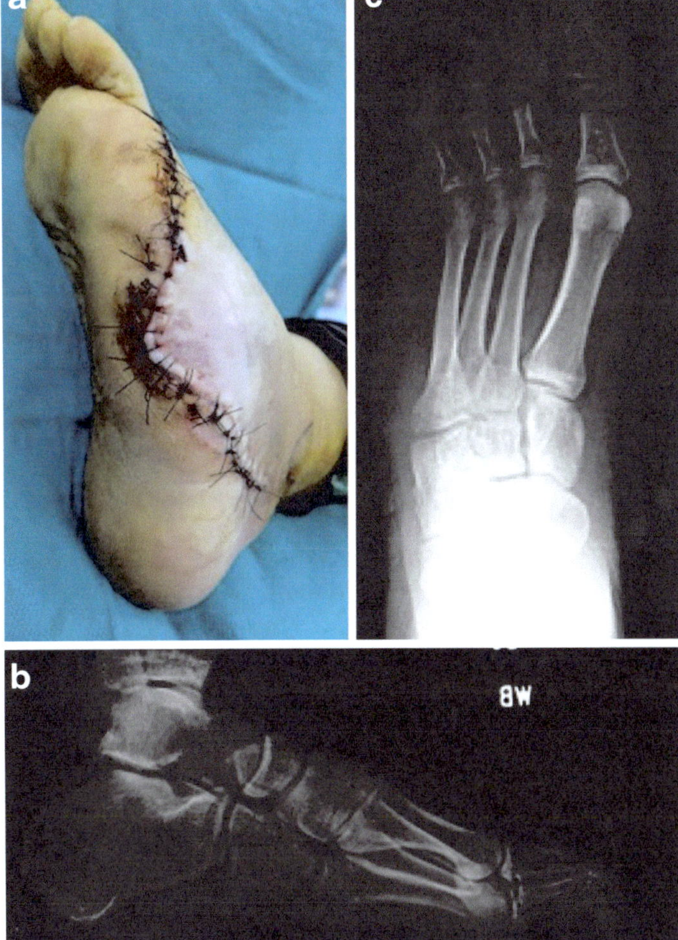

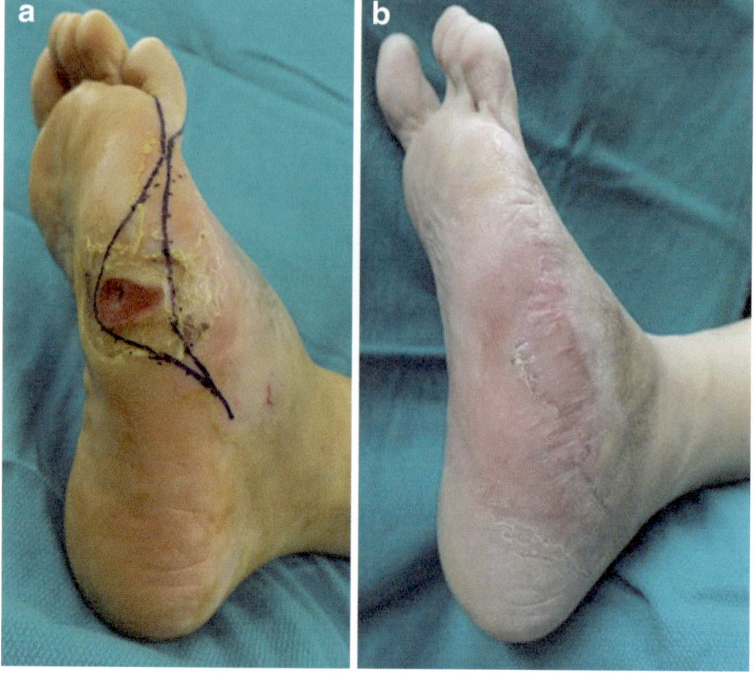

Fig. 18.32 (**a**) Preoperative appearance of plantar neuropathic ulceration. (**b**) Healed incision 6 weeks after antibiotic bead removal and peroneal transfer in complete fifth ray excision

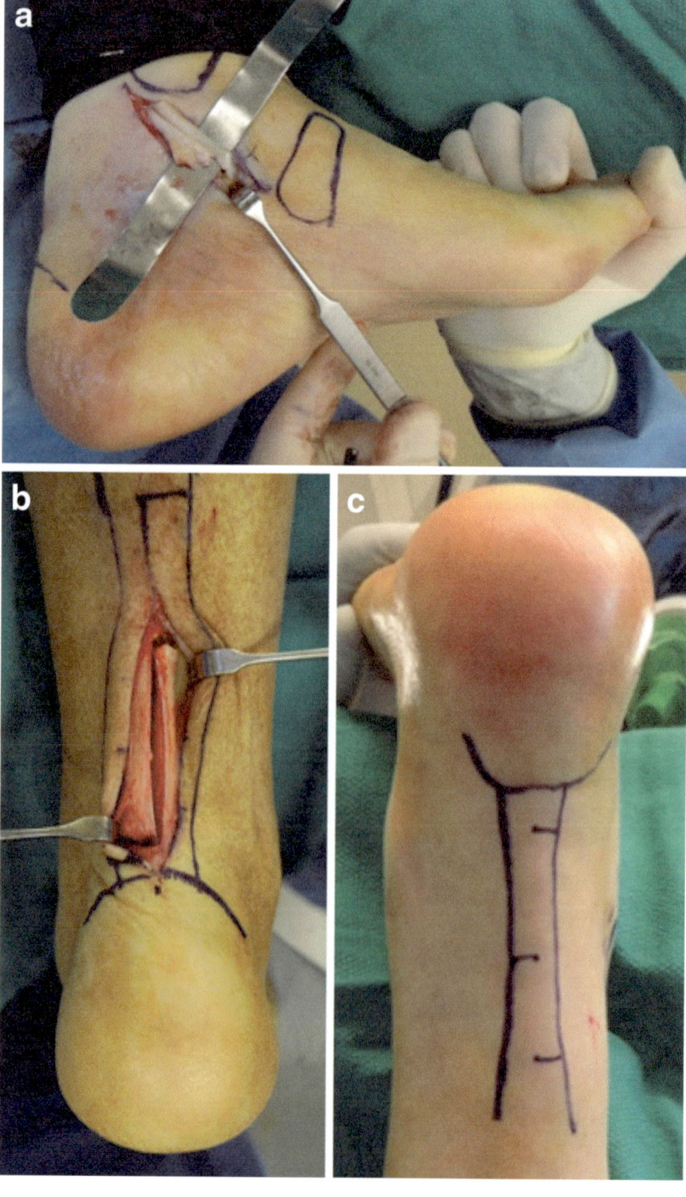

Fig. 18.33 Soft tissue balancing procedures to address loss of the lateral column. (**a**) Posterior tibial tendon "Z" lengthening plus (**b**) open "Z" tendoachilles lengthening (TAL) or (**c**) percutaneous triple hemi-section TAL are commonly incorporated to decrease inversion and equinus deformities, respectively. Tendon balancing procedures are typically performed during the stage 2 procedure or can be delayed until complete resolution of the lateral column wound issues

Conclusion

Successful treatment of osteomyelitis of the fifth ray is dependent on resolution of not only bone infection but also the wound deficit and associated mechanical deformity. The ideal surgical treatment plan is based on the size and location of the ulceration along the fifth ray, the condition of surrounding soft tissues, the extent of anticipated osteomyelitis, and structural abnormalities as described in Fig. 18.1. Various surgical procedures are available for ulcerations at each level of the fifth ray to accomplish our surgical goals including removal of grossly infected and prominent bone, bone biopsy procurement, wound closure when possible, correction of structural deformity, and improved biomechanical balance of the foot in an effort to limit future breakdown and subsequent amputation. Significant effort is made to avoid complete fifth ray amputation although this technique is useful in cases of complicated osteomyelitis located at the midshaft or base of the fifth metatarsal.

References

1. Faglia E, Clerici G, Caminiti M, Curci V, Somalvico F. Feasibility and effectiveness of internal pedal amputation of phalanx or metatarsal head in diabetic patients with forefoot osteomyelitis. J Foot Ankle Surg. 2012;51:593–8.
2. Armstrong DG, Rosales MA, Gashi A. Efficacy of fifth metatarsal head resection for treatment of chronic diabetic foot ulceration. J Am Podiatr Med Assoc. 2005;95(4):353–6.
3. Boffeli TJ, Peterson MC. Rotational flap closure of first and fifth metatarsal head plantar ulcers: adjunctive procedure when performing first or fifth ray amputation. J Foot Ankle Surg. 2013;52:263–70.
4. Rosenblum BI, Chrzan JS, Giurini JM, Habershaw GM, Miller LB. Neuropathic ulcerations plantar to the lateral column in patients with charcot foot deformity: a flexible approach to limb salvage. J Foot Ankle Surg. 1997;36(5):360–3.
5. Boffeli TJ, Abben KW. Complete fifth ray amputation with peroneal tendon transfer–a staged surgical protocol. J Foot Ankle Surg. 2012;51:696–701.

Transmetatarsal and Lisfranc Amputation

19

Troy J. Boffeli and Brett J. Waverly

Introduction

Midfoot amputation procedures including transmetatarsal and Lisfranc tarsometatarsal amputation are common and effective treatments of both osteomyelitis and gangrene of the forefoot that is not amenable to individual toe or ray amputation. In addition, when infection of the cuneiforms or cuboid is present, a combination of a Lisfranc amputation, conservative tarsal bone resection, flap coverage of midfoot wounds, and postoperative antibiotic therapy can be successful. Metatarsal osteomyelitis is most often associated with diabetes-related neuropathic ulcerations, but infection associated with gangrene or open trauma can also lead to a limb-threatening bone infection. Many diabetic patients undergoing transmetatarsal and Lisfranc amputation have previously undergone bone resection procedures or partial ray amputations in an attempt to avoid more proximal amputation yet continue to suffer from recurrent wound breakdown, gangrene, and osteomyelitis. Midfoot amputation is ideally contained at the transmetatarsal level in an effort to optimize foot function, although a Lisfranc level amputation may be necessary for extensive forefoot gangrene or midfoot wounds with metatarsal base or limited tarsal bone osteomyelitis [1, 2].

Transmetatarsal amputation (TMA) preserves a relatively functional and durable foot that is suitable for ambulation in slightly modified footwear. A well-planned TMA procedure can be a definitive treatment for recurrent neuropathic wound complications associated with osteomyelitis, forefoot deformity, and past surgery [1]. In contrast, a Lisfranc level amputation further compromises the functional lever arm of the foot and results in the loss of several important musculoten-

dinous structures including the tibialis anterior, peroneus brevis, and possibly the peroneus longus tendons [3, 4]. The short nature of a Lisfranc amputation stump and the resultant muscle imbalance including foot drop and posterior muscle contracture typically result in the need for a rigid ankle foot orthotic (AFO) in an effort to optimize foot function. The Lisfranc amputee is prone to lateral column breakdown beneath the cuboid due to overpowering of the posterior tibial and Achilles tendons and the inherent midfoot arch bony structure that places more weight on the cuboid than the cuneiforms [3, 4]. Tendon balancing procedures such as Achilles and posterior tibial tendon lengthening are more frequently needed with a Lisfranc amputation as compared to TMA [5]. The ideal level of foot amputation is ultimately decided on an individual patient basis with consideration given to the extent and location of osteomyelitis, size, and location of the wound defect, presence of gangrene or vascular compromise, prior amputation procedures, age and activity level of the patient, and underlying structural abnormalities. Cellulitis or underlying abscess can significantly compromise tissue viability, and staged surgery is routinely performed to allow resolution of soft tissue infection prior to definitive amputation and wound closure.

A principle goal when considering the ideal level of amputation, as demonstrated in Fig. 19.1, is to achieve coverage of the underlying bone structure with viable and durable soft tissue which promotes prompt healing, allows successful treatment of osteomyelitis with decreased risk of recontamination, and minimizes the likelihood of recurrent wounds [6, 7]. The metatarsal or tarsal bones can be cut short if needed to allow soft tissue coverage although excessive loss of bone structure may further compromise foot function. Incorporation of rotational flaps allows for immediate closure of large or proximal wound defects.

Careful attention to surgical principles specifically designed to optimize healing, preserve foot function, and avoid recurrent wound breakdown is the focus of our TMA and Lisfranc amputation protocols, which are presented in this chapter. The traditional TMA surgical procedure and

T.J. Boffeli, D.P.M., F.A.C.F.A.S. (✉) • B.J. Waverly, D.P.M.
Regions Hospital/HealthPartners Institute for Education and Research, 640 Jackson Street, St. Paul, MN 55101, USA
e-mail: Troy.J.Boffeli@healthpartners.com;
Brett.J.Waverly@healthpartners.com

© Springer International Publishing Switzerland 2015
T.J. Boffeli (ed.), *Osteomyelitis of the Foot and Ankle*, DOI 10.1007/978-3-319-18926-0_19

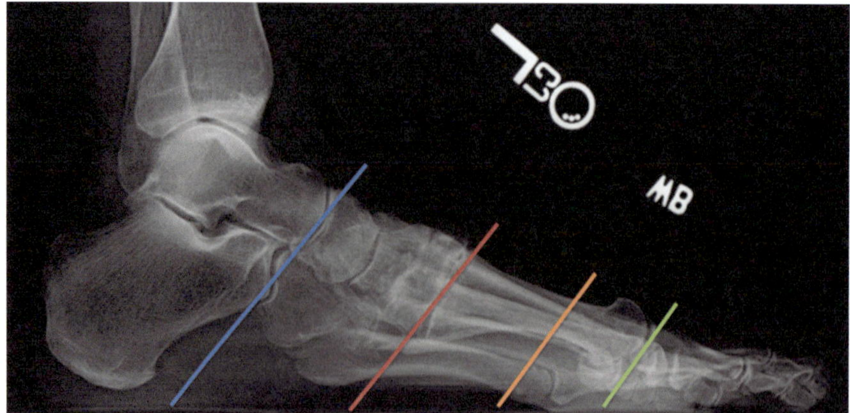

Fig. 19.1 Levels of foot amputation. Digital amputation (*green line*), transmetatarsal amputation (*orange line*), Lisfranc (tarsometatarsal) amputation (*red line*), and Chopart's amputation (*blue line*)

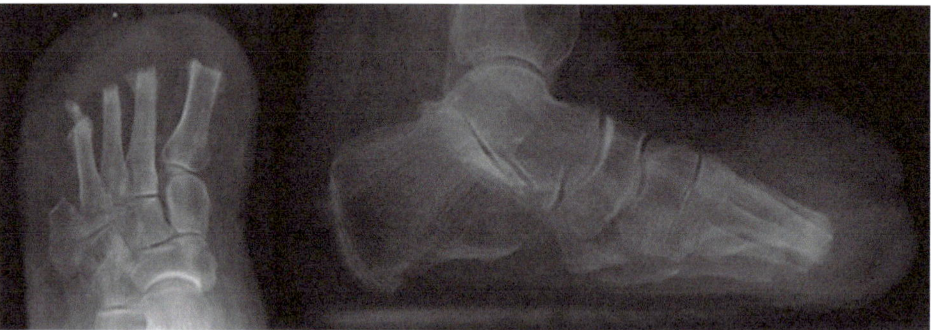

Fig. 19.2 Heterotopic ossification (HO) following transmetatarsal amputation (TMA). AP and lateral radiographs with noted HO formation to the distal metatarsal amputation stumps following TMA increase the risk of recurrent forefoot ulceration. Note massive swelling of the forefoot on the lateral view which is commonly seen with heterotopic bone formation

incision plan continues to be the desired approach for patients with neuropathic forefoot ulcers associated with metatarsal osteomyelitis and for gangrene that is isolated to the digits that is not amenable to isolated ray procedures. Incorporation of advanced podiatric, plastic, and vascular surgical approaches allows success with TMA and Lisfranc amputation for more proximal wounds and infection that would otherwise require leg amputation.

Transmetatarsal Amputation

The obvious biomechanical consequence associated with a TMA is shortening of the lever arm of the foot which impacts balance, gait, and posterior muscle group function. Care is taken to recreate a natural metatarsal parabola while attempting to preserve a functional metatarsal length when possible. Many patients undergoing TMA have pathologic mechanics due to prior surgery, digital deformity, degenerative arthritis, or neuropathic fracture which is often the reason for recurrent wounds and persistent infection. The TMA procedure is intended to improve the mechanics of this pathologic foot type which goes against the commonly held belief that partial foot amputation makes the foot more prone to problems. The ideal zone of resection is at the metatarsal neck just proximal to the metaphyseal flare. Leaving the distal metaphyseal flare predisposes the foot to recurrent tissue breakdown, since the flare is pronounced on the plantar aspect. This diaphyseal level of resection is also preferred since metaphyseal bone resection may encourage heterotopic ossification (HO) (Fig. 19.2) as described in Chap. 17 [8]. Excessive metatarsal shortening should be avoided although the extent and location of open wounds or gangrene ultimately dictate location of metatarsal resection in an effort to transect the metatarsals short enough to achieve soft tissue coverage. Rotational flaps are beneficial in this regard, which are incorporated to provide soft tissue coverage without excessive bone resection. The anticipated extent of osteomyelitis based on preoperative imaging and direct surgical inspection also influences the ideal level of bone resection. A TMA is not expected to produce a clean bone margin in cases of metatarsal osteomyelitis. A metatarsal preservation approach is preferred which combines selective bone debridement with medical treatment of residual osteomyelitis in an effort to maintain optimal postoperative foot function. Advanced surgical techniques including medullary reaming, staged resection, and insertion of antibiotic cement also supports achievement of a clinical cure of metatarsal osteomyelitis without excessive surgical resection.

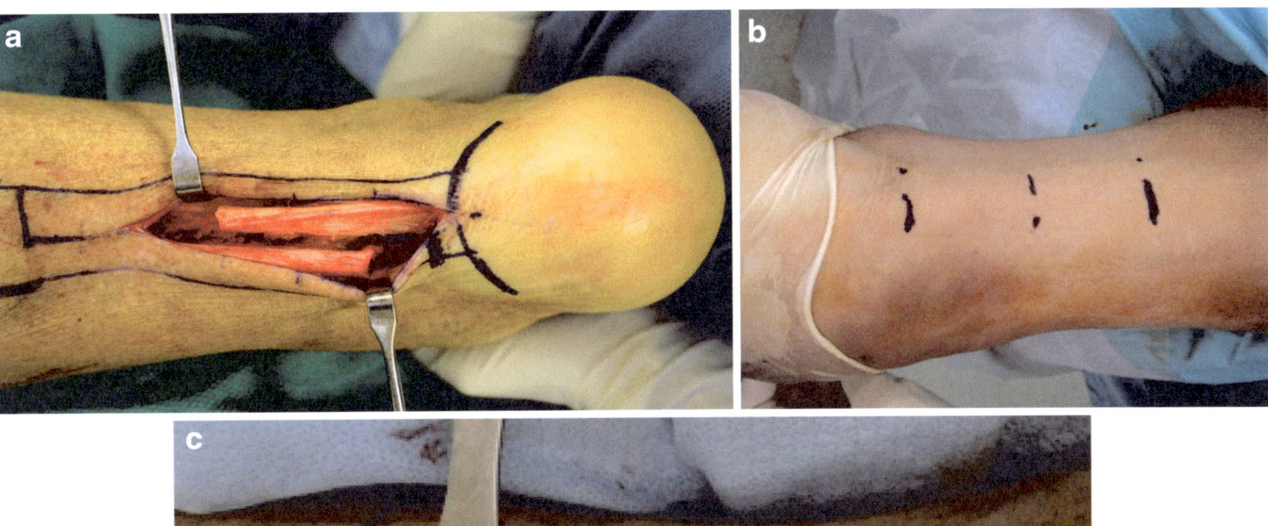

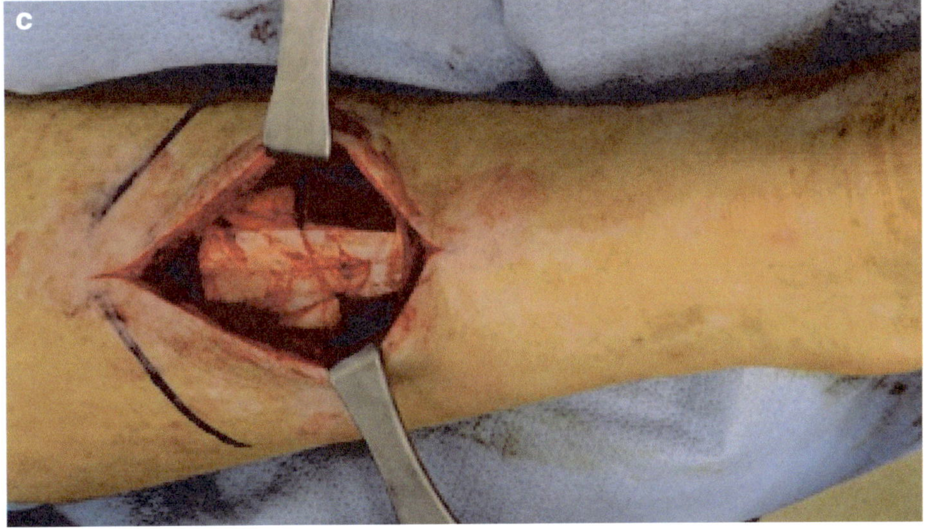

Fig. 19.3 Posterior muscle group lengthening for ankle equinus. (**a**) Open tendo-Achilles lengthening (TAL) is the most effective and controlled method to address gastroc-soleal equinus deformity. Note aggressive open lengthening which allows direct suture repair to avoid over lengthening or retraction while healing. (**b**) Percutaneous triple hemi-section TAL is desired when the soft tissue is not as amenable to open procedures. The percutaneous technique does not allow suture repair of the lengthened tendon which may result in overcorrection of the equinus deformity but has less risk of wound healing problems and is more conducive to surgery in the supine position. (**c**) Open gastrocnemius recession is indicated for patients with equinus deformity isolated to the gastrocnemius. Skin healing is generally improved at the mid-calf level although chronic edema may compromise healing of calf incisions

The outlook for gangrene-related TMA is not as optimistic when compared to osteomyelitis associated with neuropathic ulceration, due to compromised healing potential associated with vascular disease. There is less concern for osteomyelitis with gangrene although dead tissue frequently becomes infected while waiting for demarcation of gangrene. There is a fine line between allowing forefoot gangrene to demarcate and letting dry gangrene turn into infected wet gangrene. A close "wait and watch" approach is reasonable, yet waiting too long is counterproductive as vascular compromise and infection are a dangerous combination. Vascular intervention is common during this waiting period which is ideally performed prior to TMA. Antibiotics are only needed if infection is suspected or confirmed. Once healed, the gangrene-related TMA stump tends to remain durable without the tendency for recurrent ulceration unless there is concomitant peripheral neuropathy or residual deformity.

Posterior muscle group contracture or ankle equinus is a common cause of recurrent ulceration after TMA. Moore and Jolly noted that the gastrocnemius and soleus have little opposition once the extensor hallucis longus and extensor digitorum longus have been eliminated and only the tibialis anterior remains to provide dorsiflexion [9]. Many patients with neuropathic ulcers leading to TMA have preexisting equinus, which will need to be addressed if TMA is to be successful. Tendo-Achilles lengthening (TAL) or gastrocnemius recession may be performed concomitantly or after complete healing of the TMA site depending on the clinical situation (Fig. 19.3). There is risk of cross-contamination from the infected or contaminated amputation site when clean and dirty procedures are performed in the same setting;

however, this is rare due to the effectiveness of isolating the surgical sites. The authors' preference is to delay the Achilles lengthening procedure to see if it is necessary once the patient is ambulatory. One benefit of delayed posterior lengthening is the ability to rehabilitate and ambulate during the initial 6 weeks of tendon healing without risk of harm to the healing amputation site. Trying to maintain ankle dorsiflexion after concomitant TMA and TAL procedures is difficult as posterior splints can cause pressure sores on the posterior heel or plantar foot. Profound equinus contracture after TMA is more common when open guillotine TMA procedures are left to heal secondarily over the course of many months. Prolonged non-weight bearing with this approach almost assures equinus contracture. Primary closure and flap coverage of the amputation site allows prompt healing and timely return to full ambulation at about 6 weeks postoperative which is the best method to avoid equinus contracture.

Standard Transmetatarsal Amputation Procedure

The TMA procedure is typically performed under general anesthesia although intravenous sedation with an ankle block is also possible, especially in patients with neuropathy. An ankle tourniquet may be used to minimize blood loss in patients with neuropathic ulcers who frequently have robust vascular supply. The procedure is performed wet in patients with compromised circulation to ensure that viable tissue margins are achieved. The tourniquet is released prior to closure to ensure hemostasis and to assess vascularity at the level of resection. An atraumatic surgical technique is critical including use of skin hooks to manipulate the dorsal and plantar flaps. Skin incisions are made directly to bone with no attempt to undermine the tissue planes looking for blood vessels or nerves. The metatarsophalangeal joint (MPJ) capsules, sesamoids, and plantar plates are removed in an effort to minimize the chance of HO formation and to decrease the bulk of the plantar flap. The plantar flap is otherwise maintained at full thickness to maximize vascularity and protect against forces of weight bearing. Periosteal elevation at the metatarsal neck is limited to the area of bone resection which also minimizes the likelihood of HO formation. Larger bleeding vessels are tied and use of electrocautery is selective in an effort to preserve tissue viability.

The traditional TMA approach utilizes a transverse fish mouth-type incision creating dorsal and plantar flaps (Figs. 19.4 and 19.5). The plantar flap is typically longer and thicker than the dorsal flap which creates unmatched flaps at the time of closure. The dorsal incision is made just behind the sulcus of the toes which is 1–2 cm distal to the location of metatarsal bone resection. The plantar incision is made

more distally to ensure coverage. The incisions are altered accordingly if the local tissue is compromised by poor circulation, gangrene, or neuropathic ulceration. The medial and lateral apices of the incision are placed at the midway point from dorsal to plantar and midway along the first and fifth metatarsal shafts, respectively. The initial incision is made perpendicular to the skin surface using a #10 blade. A 90° plunge-cut technique is used with the entire incision made directly down to bone in an effort to maintain full-thickness flaps and to avoid beveling of the incision (Fig. 19.6). The dorsal flap is not actually raised, but rather retracted proximally to gain access to the metatarsal necks. The periosteum is then cut medially, laterally, and dorsally over the neck of each individual metatarsal. A metatarsal elevator is then used to minimally elevate the periosteum to allow access for metatarsal resection using a bone saw (Fig. 19.7). This ensures that the distal perforating inter-metatarsal vessels remain intact while avoiding excessive inter-metatarsal dissection. The periosteum distal to the metatarsal neck is left attached to the metatarsal head to be removed with the forefoot in an effort to minimize the risk of HO formation.

The metatarsals are transected proximal to the metaphyseal flare with a power bone saw while maintaining the innate metatarsal parabola (Fig. 19.7). The first and second metatarsals are cut at approximately the same length while the remaining metatarsals taper gently in the lateral direction. The metatarsals should be cut with a longer dorsal shelf compared to the plantar edge to avoid plantar prominence. The first and fifth metatarsals should be beveled more medially and laterally, respectively, to avoid problems with shoe pressure. Penetrating towel clamps are then placed medially and laterally through the digits to allow manipulation with a no-touch technique while raising the plantar flap. The toes and metatarsal heads are detached as one unit from the plantar flap (Fig. 19.8). The first metatarsal sesamoid apparatus and lesser metatarsal phalangeal joint plantar plates are then carefully dissected and removed from the plantar flap to decrease bulk and expose the underlying vascular tissue that will contribute to healing. This method seems to provide maximum flap viability with the least amount of operative trauma.

It is imperative to ensure that no bony prominences remain on the metatarsal stumps as this increases the propensity for future wound breakdown. Bone-cutting or bone-crushing forceps are avoided in favor of a power bone saw to minimize splintering which promotes HO formation and irregular bone surfaces [8]. Direct palpation of the metatarsal stumps and intraoperative imaging confirms the desired result. Thorough irrigation is used to wash away any bone debris. Bone is then procured for pathologic biopsy and culture. The optimal location of biopsy specimen is based on the location of the open wound and findings of preoperative

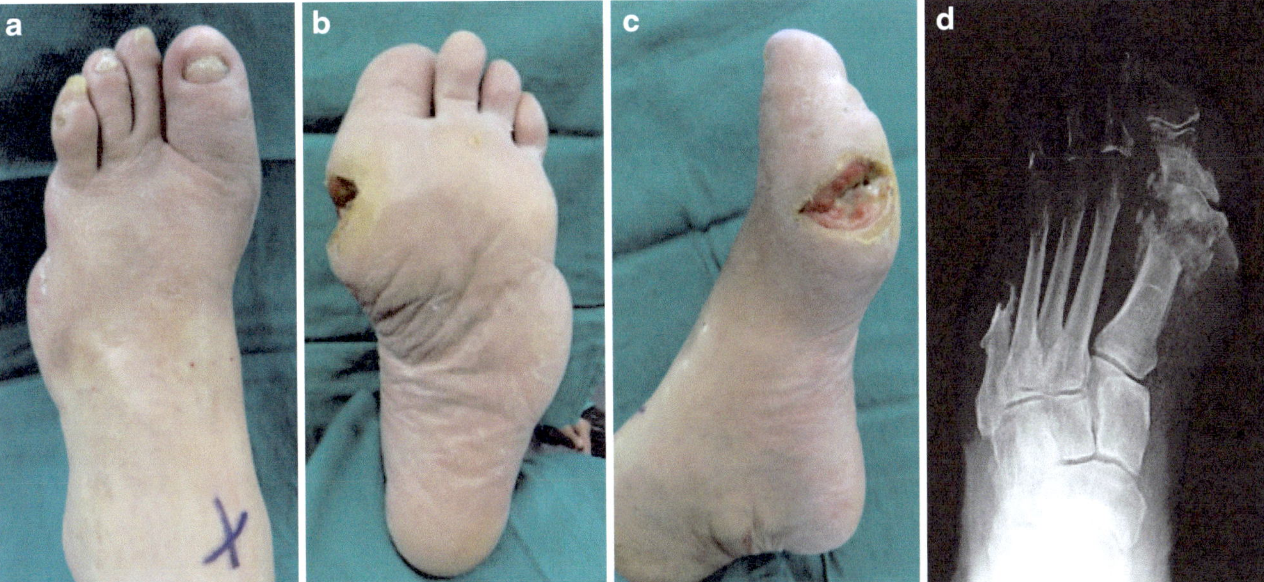

Fig. 19.4 Patient selection criteria for standard transmetatarsal amputation technique. Case demonstrating recurrent first ray ulcer complicated by extensive osteomyelitis and prior fifth ray amputation. A large plantar medial neuropathic wound with bone exposure and first metatarsal phalangeal osteomyelitis was treated with transmetatarsal amputation (TMA). The traditional TMA incision design requires viable dorsal and plantar tissue flaps. The medial wound location seen here allowed excision with the traditional TMA approach, while plantar wounds and extensive forefoot gangrene may necessitate either a shorter level of amputation or advanced plastic surgical techniques including rotational flaps

imaging (Fig. 19.9). A clean margin biopsy can be sent for evaluation of residual osteomyelitis, especially in digital osteomyelitis. Margin biopsy frequently involves curettage of an exposed medullary canal in order to preserve length of the metatarsal shaft, or a section of bone can be procured when remodeling the metatarsal stumps to achieve the proper metatarsal parabola. Biopsy from the discarded phalanges is taken on the back table after wound closure to minimize the chance of cross-contamination if the pathology and cultures are not obtained directly from the surgical site. A metatarsal head specimen is also common, depending on location of preoperative wounds and suspected location of osteomyelitis.

Note that electrocautery has not been used up to this point in the operation. The tourniquet is released if being used. Larger bleeding vessels are tied with absorbable suture ties during dissection or prior to closure. The cautery is then used sparingly for selective hemostasis. A closed suction drain may be used depending on circulation, residual bleeding, perioperative anticoagulation status, and anticipated dead space.

Interrupted skin sutures are used to close the wound as deep sutures are not typically needed or desired (Fig. 19.10). A no-touch suture technique is used to allow minimal handling of the dorsal and plantar flaps. Hash marks are helpful to preplan flap approximation with the expectation that slight puckering will occur due to the plantar flap being longer and broader than the dorsal flap. A surgical case is detailed in Figs. 19.4, 19.5, 19.6, 19.7, 19.8, 19.9, 19.10, and 19.11.

Lisfranc (Tarsometatarsal) Amputation

Compared to TMA, Lisfranc amputation is a less desirable level of amputation with regard to weight bearing function, resistance to recurrent wounds, and longevity of the stump (Fig. 19.12) [3, 4]. Lisfranc amputation is generally indicated for midfoot wounds with associated osteomyelitis in the proximal metatarsals, extensive forefoot gangrene, frostbite, and mangling injuries of the forefoot (Fig. 19.13). Extensive heterotopic ossification (HO) from prior metatarsal resection may also warrant Lisfranc disarticulation in an attempt to limit HO formation after revision surgery which is discussed in Chap. 17. Caution should be taken before proceeding with this procedure because the native biomechanics of the foot are greatly altered which may need to be addressed at the time of surgery. Disarticulation of the first metatarsal from the medial cuneiform joint may result in complete loss of tibialis anterior (TA) and peroneus longus (PL) tendon insertions depending on the need to remodel the plantar aspect of the medial cuneiform. Disarticulation of the fifth metatarsal from the cuboid results in complete loss of the peroneus brevis (PB) tendon insertion. Loss of TA function leads to foot drop and equinus contracture, while loss of PL and PB function leads to unopposed inversion through the tibialis posterior tendon. An attempt should be made to preserve or transfer these tendons at the time of amputation when possible.

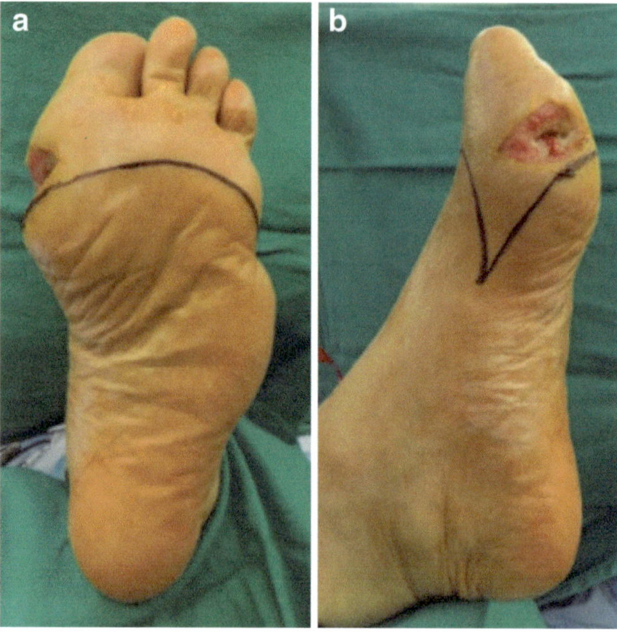

Fig. 19.5 Traditional transmetatarsal amputation (TMA) incision design. Dorsal and plantar TMA flaps were drawn with the medial and lateral apices about midpoint from dorsal to plantar and midway along the first and fifth metatarsals, respectively. This patient required a slightly shorter than typical TMA due to prior fifth ray amputation and first ray osteomyelitis. Wound location also impacts the level of bone resection

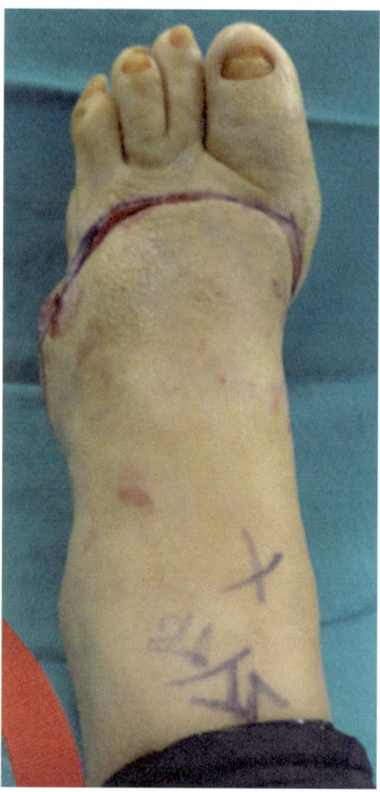

Fig. 19.6 Transmetatarsal amputation incision technique. The incision technique for midfoot amputation involves dorsal and plantar incisions made directly to bone with cuts made at 90° to the skin surface. No attempt is made to undermine the tissues searching for bleeding vessels during the initial incision as this may compromise viability of the flap

Tendon balancing may be performed concomitantly or after complete healing of the amputation site depending on the clinical situation. Achilles tendon lengthening (Fig. 19.3) is almost always necessary with Lisfranc amputation, while posterior tibial tendon lengthening is indicated for loss of peroneal tendon function or progressive inversion deformity (Fig. 19.14).

Standard Lisfranc Amputation Procedure

Similar to TMA, the Lisfranc amputation procedure is traditionally performed through a transverse fish mouth-type incision creating dorsal and plantar flaps. The plantar flap is quite thick due to the bulk of soft tissue, including thick muscle tissue in the mid-arch (Fig. 19.15). While beneficial for healing and stump durability, flap thickness limits the mobility of the flap when attempting to advance the flap around the remodeled tarsal bones. The plantar flap needs to be relatively long for this reason. The dorsal flap on the other hand is thin which creates challenges at the time of dorsal to plantar flap approximation. The dorsal incision is made transversely over the proximal shaft of the metatarsals, roughly 2 cm distal to the tarsometatarsal joint [3, 4]. The plantar incision is made more distally compared to the dorsal incision. The incisions are altered accordingly if the local tissue

is compromised by poor circulation, soft tissue defects, gangrene, or neuropathic ulceration. The medial and lateral apices are placed near the middle of the medial cuneiform and cuboid, respectively, about midway from dorsal to plantar. The incisions are made perpendicular to the skin surface. A 90° incision technique is used with the entire incision made directly to bone. Penetrating towel clamps are placed on the medial and lateral aspects of the forefoot to allow manipulation during dissection (Fig. 19.16). The base of the second metatarsal is cut even with the medial and lateral cuneiforms using a bone saw which allows a smooth transition along the distal aspect of the tarsal bones (Fig. 19.17). The peroneus brevis tendon can be identified and tagged for transfer. The entire forefoot is then disarticulated at the tarsometatarsal level and removed as one unit.

The leading edge of the tarsal bones should be rounded dorsally and plantarly to remove bony prominences, especially along the cuboid just distal to the transverse groove for the PL tendon (Fig. 19.17). A clean margin tarsal bone biopsy can be procured in this manner. Care is taken to preserve the TA and PL insertions on the medial cuneiform if possible. Adjunctive tendon procedures can be performed after disarticulation of the

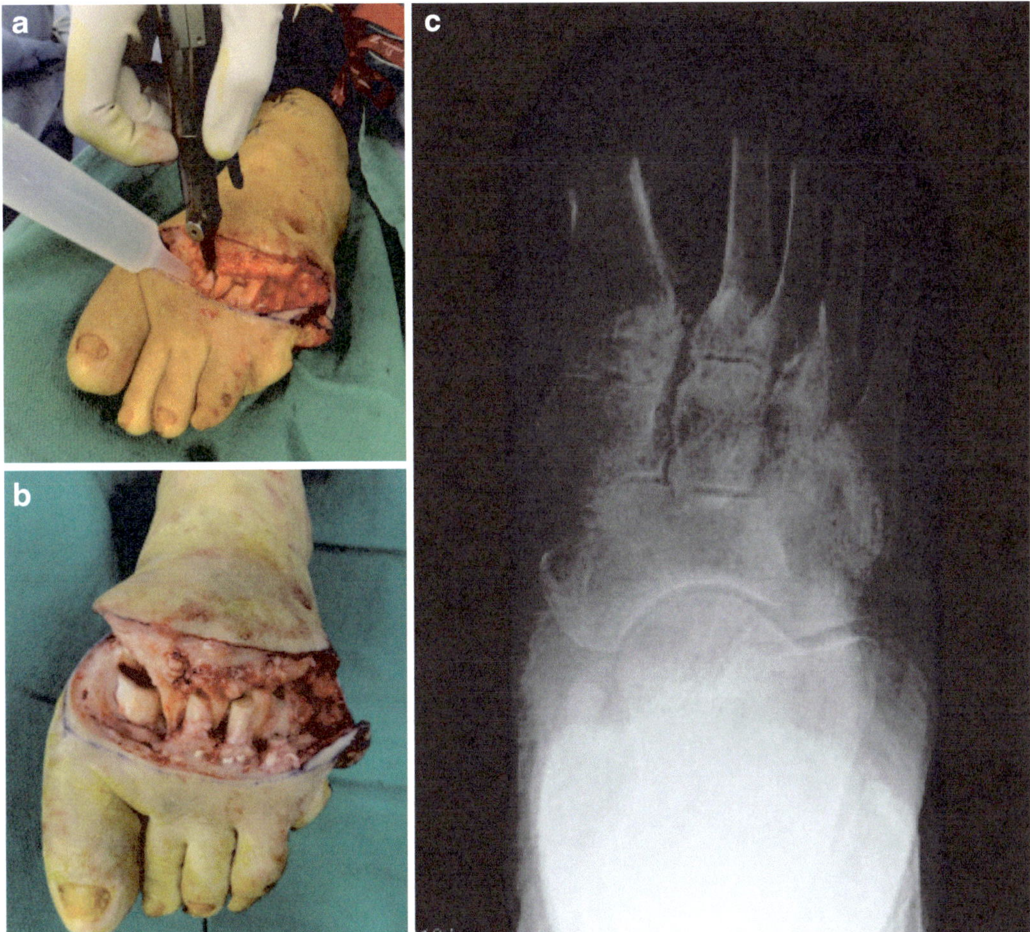

Fig. 19.7 Traditional transmetatarsal amputation with metatarsal resection performed to recreate a normal metatarsal parabola utilizing a bone saw. Irrigation was used to cool the saw and wash away bone dust in an effort to minimize risk of heterotopic bone formation. Note that minimal periosteal elevation or raising of the dorsal flap was performed for this same reason. Intraoperative imaging was used to confirm the desired level of metatarsal resection and recreation of a functional metatarsal parabola

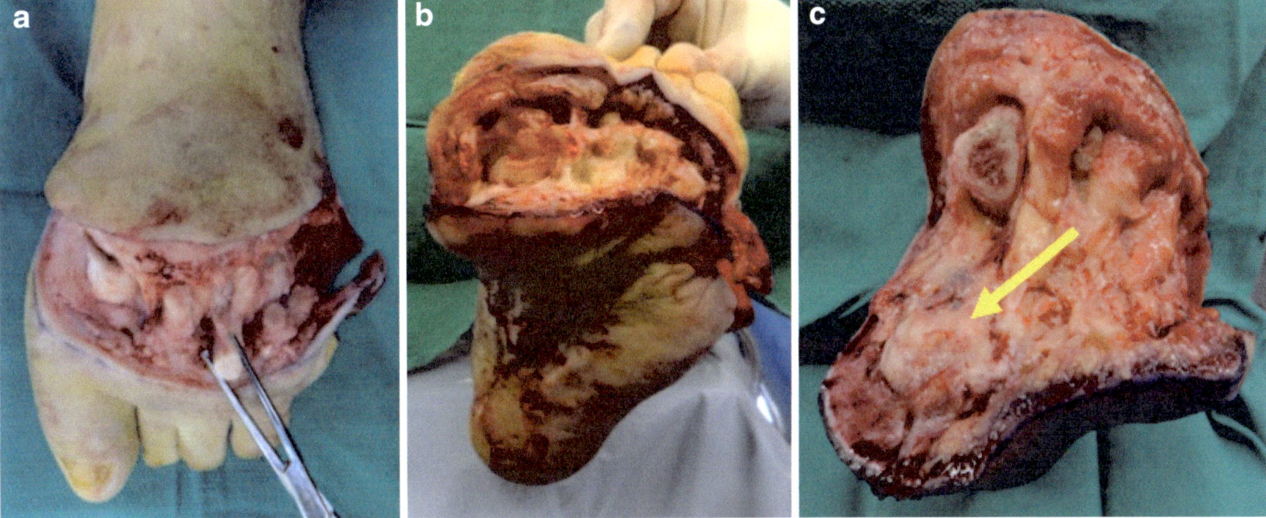

Fig. 19.8 Disarticulation of forefoot in TMA. The forefoot is disarticulated while maintaining full thickness of the plantar flap. The first ray sesamoids (*yellow arrow*) and lesser metatarsophalangeal joint plantar plates remain within the plantar flap upon disarticulation of the forefoot. These structures were then carefully dissected and removed which helps to preserve a full-thickness and well-vascularized plantar flap

forefoot when appropriate. Concern for residual infection may necessitate staged surgery for tarsal bone remodeling and tendon balancing in an effort to minimize the chance of spreading infection to more proximal structures. Disarticulation is an effective way to provide a clinical cure for osteomyelitis when performed under these guidelines.

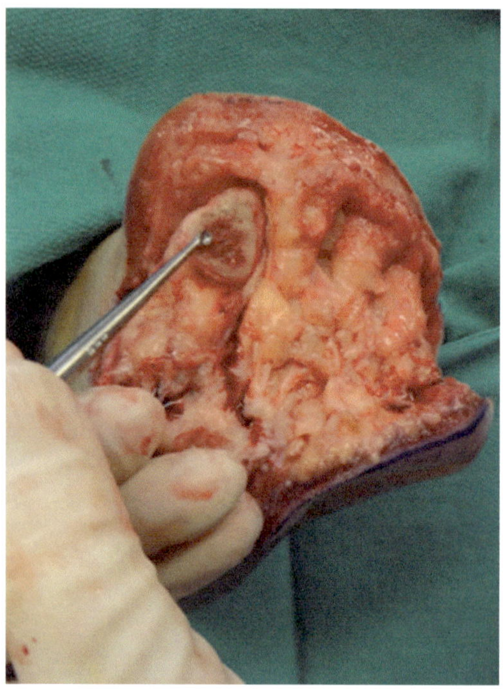

Fig. 19.9 A curette was used to procure a proximal margin biopsy from within the first metatarsal medullary canal following TMA. Direct visualization of the cortical and medullary bone provides important information regarding extent of infection and should be discussed in the operative report when relevant

Minimal electrocautery has been used throughout the procedure at this point. The tourniquet is released if used to allow evaluation of soft tissue viability and identify bleeding vessels. Absorbable suture ties are used on larger bleeding vessels. The electrocautery is then used sparingly for selective hemostasis. A closed suction drain may or may not be used depending on the potential for hematoma formation and anticipated dead space after closure.

The flaps are remodeled to ensure osseous coverage and complete closure of the wound. Interrupted skin sutures are used to close the wound. Deep sutures are not typically needed or desired.

Back table bone biopsy and culture for osteomyelitis should be performed at this time, if not obtained directly from the surgical wound prior to resection. Location of bone biopsy depends on the location of open wounds and preoperative imaging results. A surgical case demonstrating incision design, disarticulation technique, and cuboid remodeling is shown in Figs. 19.15, 19.16, 19.17, and 19.18.

Incorporating Flaps into Midfoot Amputation Procedures

The opportunity to contain amputation at the midfoot level is frequently compromised by dorsal or plantar soft tissue defects associated with neuropathic ulceration, gangrene, necrosis secondary to infection, or open wounds from recent infection surgery. This scenario typically leads to more proximal amputation including Chopart's amputation or below knee amputation. Incorporation of rotational and advancement flaps allows immediate closure despite large soft tissue defects in an effort to achieve a more distal level

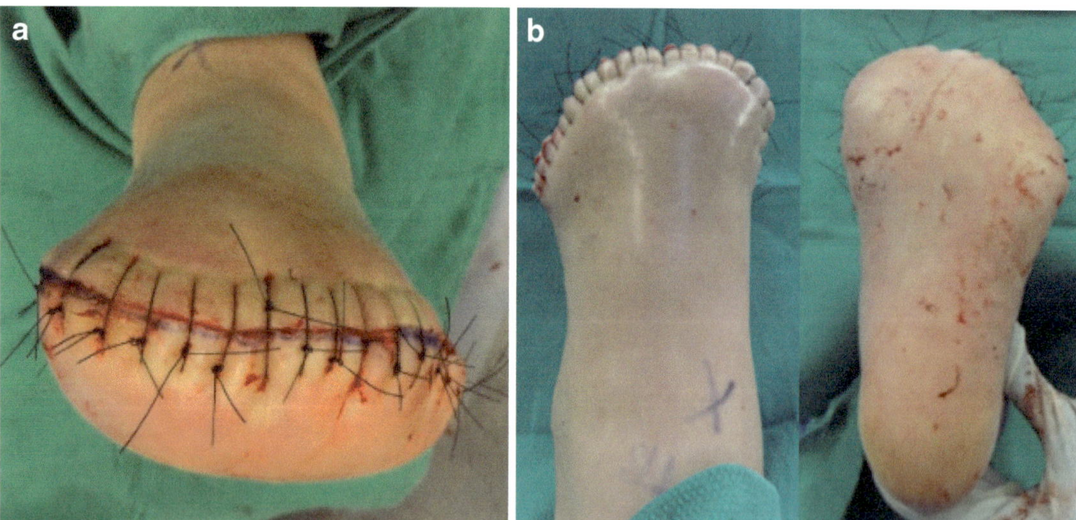

Fig. 19.10 Simple sutures were used to close the transmetatarsal amputation flaps

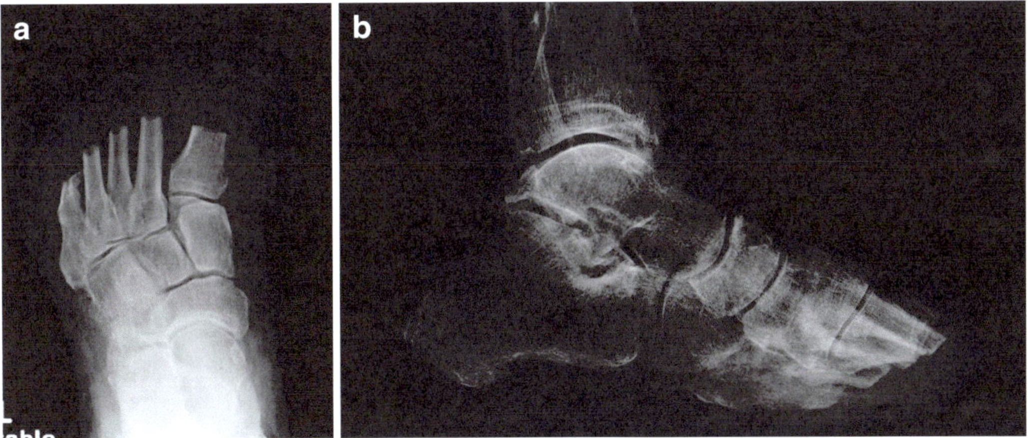

Fig. 19.11 Standard TMA postoperative radiographs. Postoperative imaging confirmed recreation of the desired metatarsal parabola. An immediate postoperative image is shown. (**a**) A gentle taper on the medial and lateral sides minimizes the likelihood of recurrent breakdown of the amputation site. (**b**) Lateral imaging confirmed tapered metatarsal resection to minimize the risk of plantar prominence

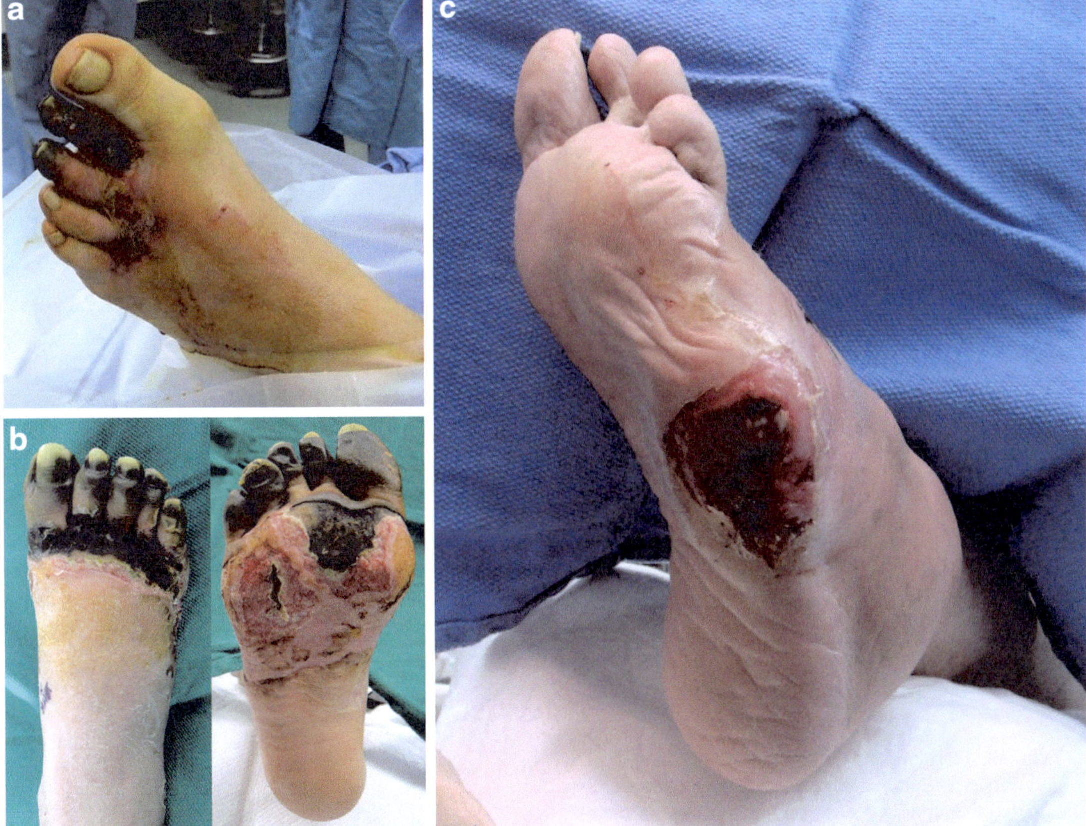

Fig. 19.12 Indications for Lisfranc amputation. (**a**) Forefoot gangrene with secondary infection, (**b**) extensive tissue necrosis from frostbite, and (**c**) midfoot ulceration with underlying osteomyelitis

of amputation [10]. Ideal flap design is based on angiosome anatomy, three-dimensional areas of soft tissue sourced by a specific blood vessel, with the medial and lateral plantar artery angiosomes being most useful [11, 12]. The medial plantar artery angiosome (MPAA) supplies the instep on the plantar medial foot. The lateral plantar artery angiosome (LPAA) is more robust and supplies the majority of the plantar foot extending from the distal heel to the entire forefoot [11]. Inline flow to the target vessel is important to ensure that the angiosome has adequate vascularity which

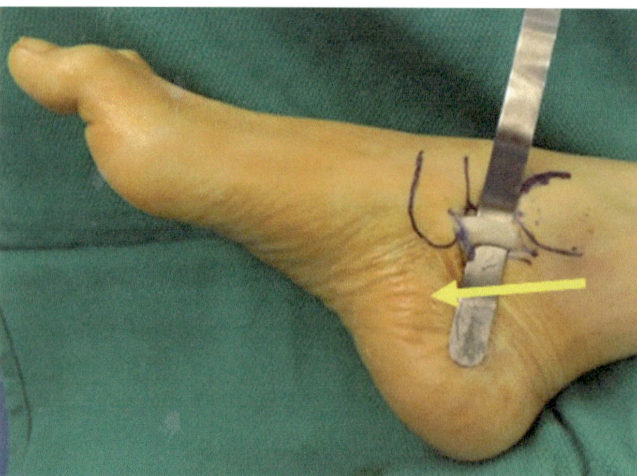

Fig. 19.13 Posterior tibial (PT) tendon open Z-lengthening. Tendon balancing beyond TAL is common with Lisfranc amputation more so than TMA. Open Z-lengthening of the PT tendon is shown with incision made from the tip of the medial malleolus toward the navicular tuberosity. The *arrow* indicates the divergence of the tibial nerve and posterior tibialis artery from the posterior tibialis tendon making this incision location safe

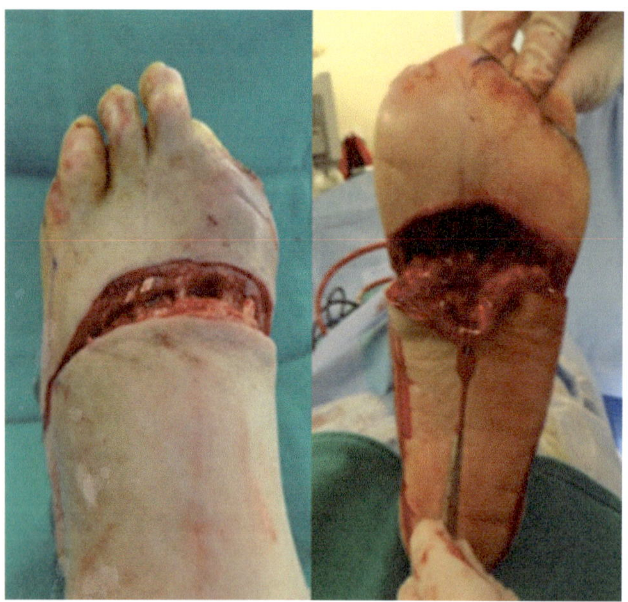

Fig. 19.14 Traditional Lisfranc amputation. Incision planning is similar to TMA with dorsal and plantar fish mouth incision design. This case represents failed first and second ray amputation due to vascular compromise of the forefoot. Incisions are made more proximal than with TMA. Full-thickness dorsal and plantar incisions are made directly down to bone

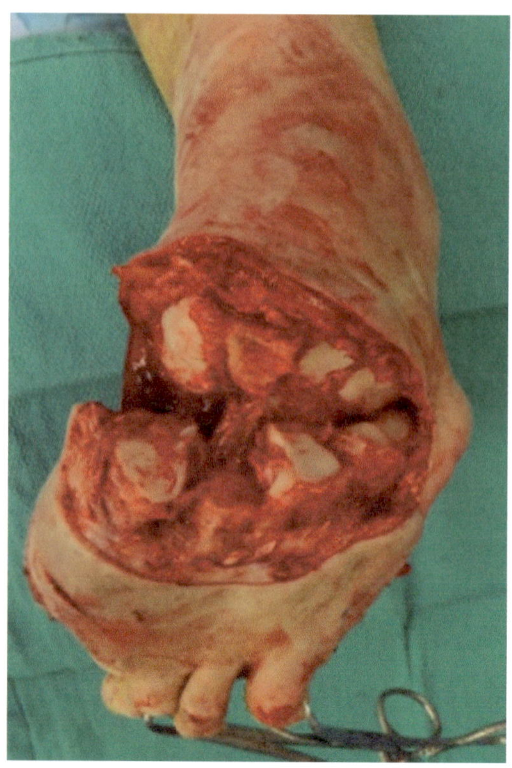

Fig. 19.15 Disarticulation through the tarsometatarsal joints allows removal of the entire forefoot. Note exposed cancellous bone after resection through the second metatarsal base even with the medial and lateral cuneiforms

Lateral Plantar Artery Angiosome Flap TMA and Lisfranc Amputation

The LPAA is more extensive than the MPAA which allows for a more extensive flap to cover soft tissue defects around the first and second MPJs or midfoot defects near the first metatarsal cuneiform joint. The LPAA flap can also cover dorsal soft tissue defects. Flap technique is detailed in Figs. 19.19, 19.20, 19.21, 19.22, 19.23, 19.24, 19.25, 19.26, and 19.27. The pivot point of the flap is made near the mid-arch, and the distal extent of the dorsal and plantar flaps are drawn more distal than with traditional TMA incisions to achieve better coverage. Rotation of the LPAA flap essentially shortens the distal reach of the flap necessitating contribution from the dorsal soft tissues. The initial incision is made full depth to completely excise the wound. The surgical site is then re-prepped prior to raising the flap and proceeding with midfoot amputation.

The LPAA flap is raised full thickness off the plantar aspect of the metatarsals. Dissection in the mid-arch is performed carefully to avoid injury to the lateral plantar artery. The proximal perforating vessels are preserved when possible in the event that retrograde flow is helpful to flap survival. A transverse dorsal incision is then made at the base of the toes.

may require advanced communication with the vascular interventionalist. Dependence on retrograde flow from the perforating peroneal or dorsalis pedis artery to the medial or lateral plantar artery is not likely sufficient under these circumstances since raising the flap compromises the intermetatarsal perforating arteries.

Fig. 19.16 Remodeling of the tarsal bones in Lisfranc amputation. The cuboid and medial cuneiform are particularly prominent after tarsometatarsal disarticulation. The amputation stump is remodeled with a bone saw or rongeur to avoid pressure points when walking or wearing shoes. Care is taken to preserve the TA and PL insertion on the plantar aspect of the medial cuneiform if possible. Note how the distal aspect of the plantar cuboid has been remodeled (*arrow*)

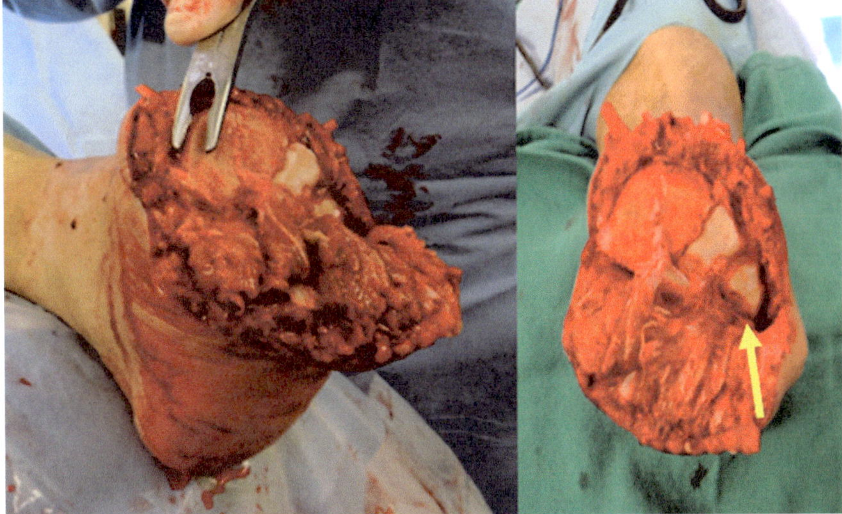

Fig. 19.17 Immediate postoperative radiographs following Lisfranc disarticulation. These non-weight bearing radiographs demonstrate significant compromise to foot structure and function. Amputation at this level is avoided when possible, but may be necessary based on compromise of the forefoot soft tissues or bone associated with gangrene, infection, wounds, frostbite or mangling injuries

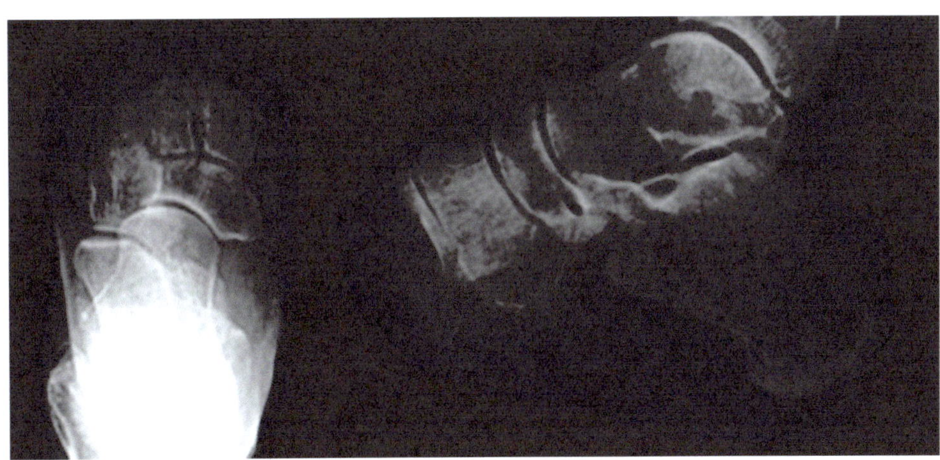

Fig. 19.18 Medial necrosis of the forefoot necessitating LPAA rotational flap TMA. (**a**, **b**)Wet gangrene with extensive necrosis of the soft tissue beneath the first metatarsal head. Note that the lateral half of the plantar forefoot remained largely viable. Below knee amputation is a common outcome for this condition, but advanced techniques incorporating staged surgery, lateral plantar artery angiosome rotational flap, and vascular intervention may allow partial limb salvage at the TMA level

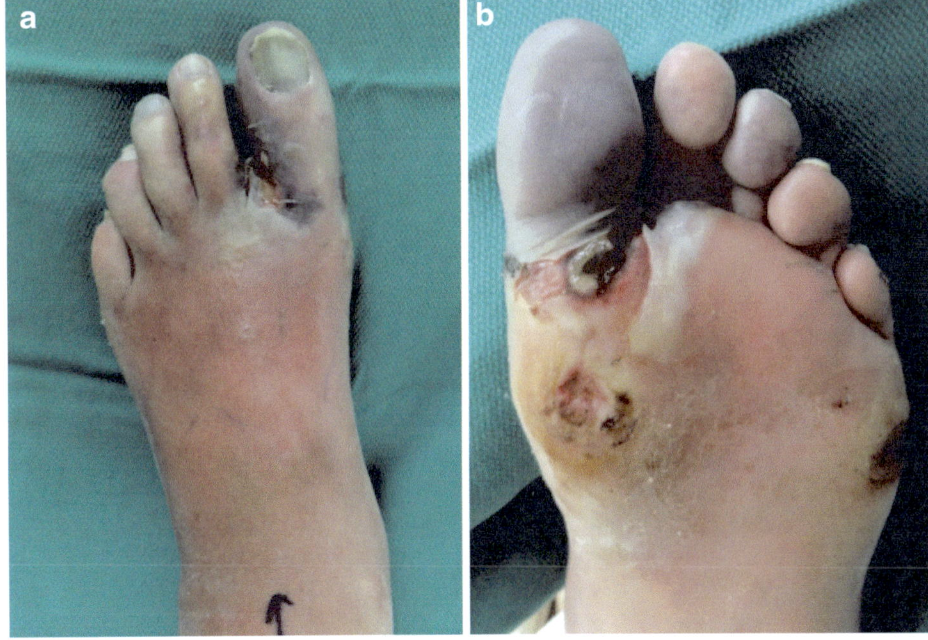

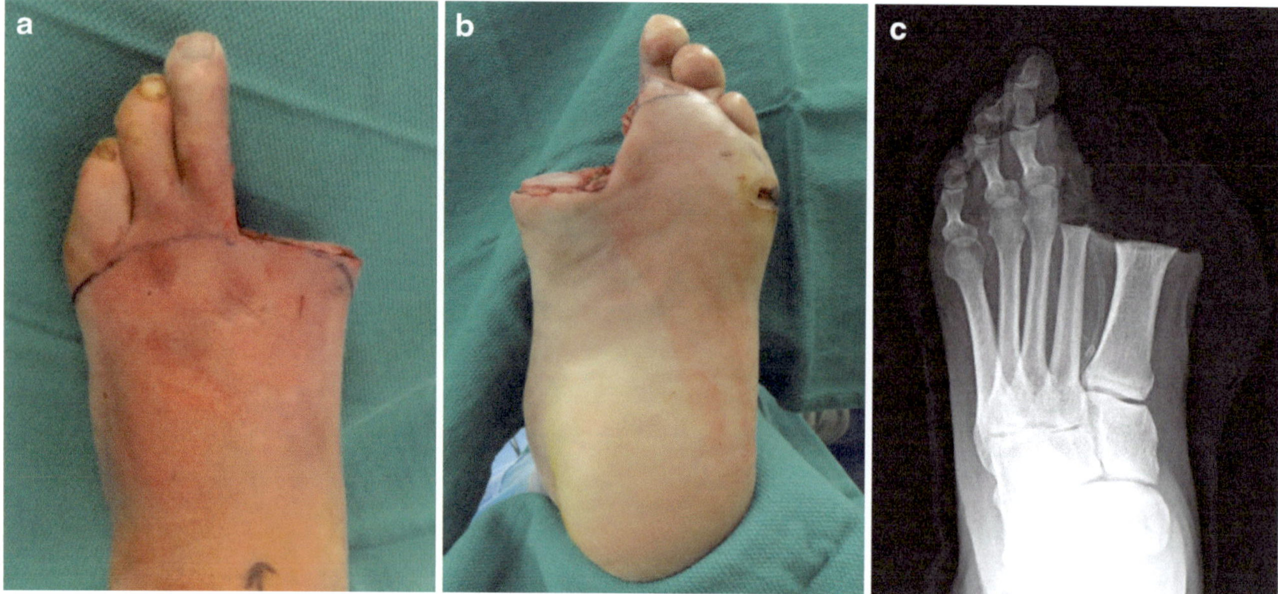

Fig. 19.19 Stage 1 surgery for LPAA rotational flap TMA involved resection of grossly necrotic tissue with a significant attempt to preserve the plantar lateral flap. (**a**, **b**) The eventual TMA incision lines including the plantar lateral flap were drawn prior to initial open amputation. (**c**) Metatarsal resection was performed in line with the incision with the anticipation of future remodeling at the time of conversion to TMA. Leaving the distal metaphyseal flare is not desirable

Fig. 19.20 Stage 2 surgery for LPAA rotational flap TMA. Stage 2 surgery was delayed 7 days to allow for demarcation of the forefoot and vascular intervention. (**a**, **b**) Note that the prior level of resection had turned black including the third toe

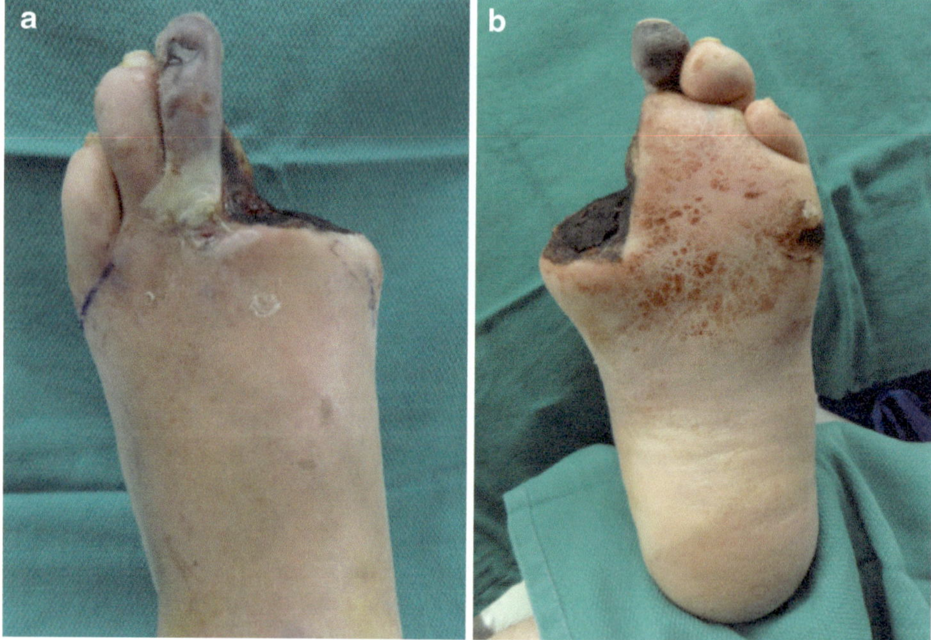

The dorsal flap is raised in a similar fashion again preserving the proximal perforating vessels. Bone resection proximal to the mid metatarsal area allows slightly shorter than typical TMA in an effort to enhance rotation of the flap and coverage of the medial soft tissue defect. Lisfranc amputation is more likely when the wound defect is located at the base of the first metatarsal, which is common with arch collapse associated with Charcot arthropathy. The LPAA flap is then rotated

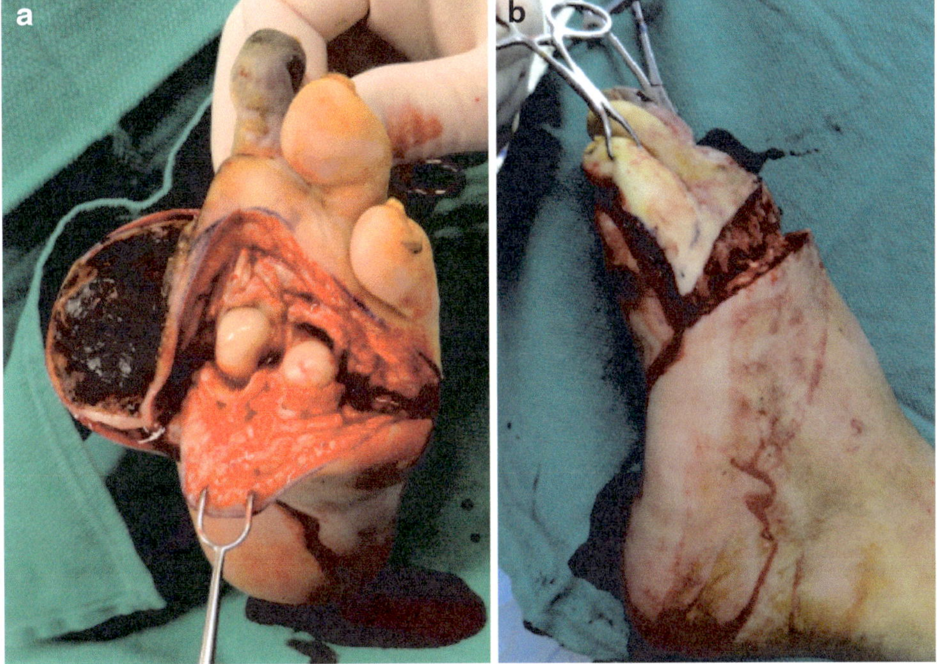

Fig. 19.21 Raising the LPAA rotational flap. The plantar flap was raised as part of the stage 2 TMA procedure. Note that the plantar soft tissues appeared viable and minimal dorsal tissue was available for soft tissue coverage

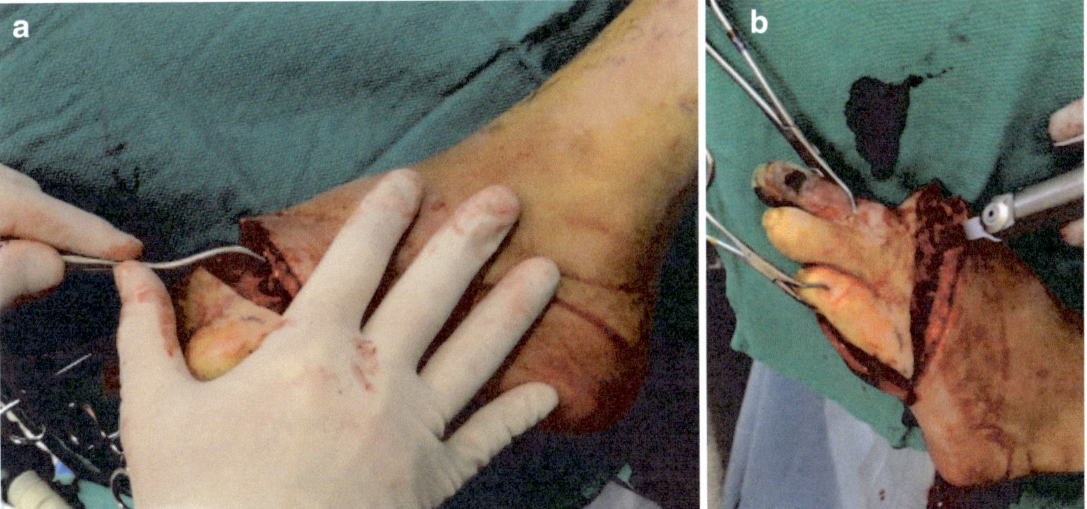

Fig. 19.22 Forefoot resection in LPAA rotational flap TMA. (**a**) The dorsal flap was raised minimally along each individual metatarsal with a metatarsal elevator. (**b**) A bone saw was then used to resect the metatarsals just proximal to the dorsal flap

in the medial direction allowing complete coverage of the plantar defect. Initial sutures begin at the plantar pivot point or apex closing the medial arch aspect of the incision. Simple sutures are then continued wrapping from medial to lateral achieving equal gap between each suture. A suction drain is commonly placed.

Medial Plantar Artery Angiosome Flap TMA and Lisfranc Amputation

A similar technique is used for the MPAA flap which allows coverage of lateral column forefoot and midfoot wounds. The same pivot point approach is utilized keeping in mind

Fig. 19.23 Intraoperative assessment of LPAA flap viability. Note that the flap will need to cover the entire wound defect without contribution from dorsal tissue

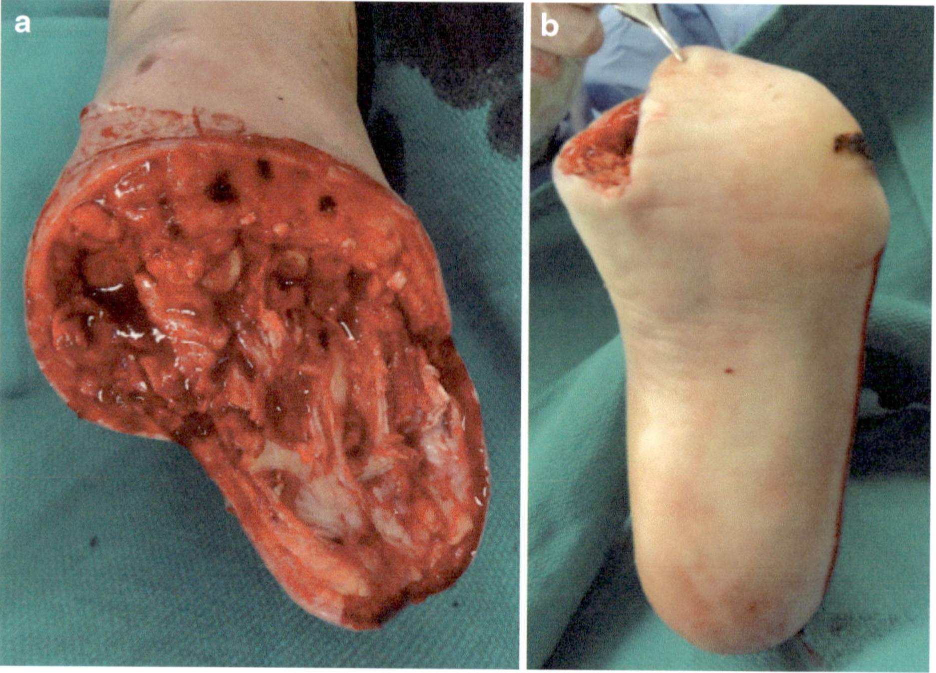

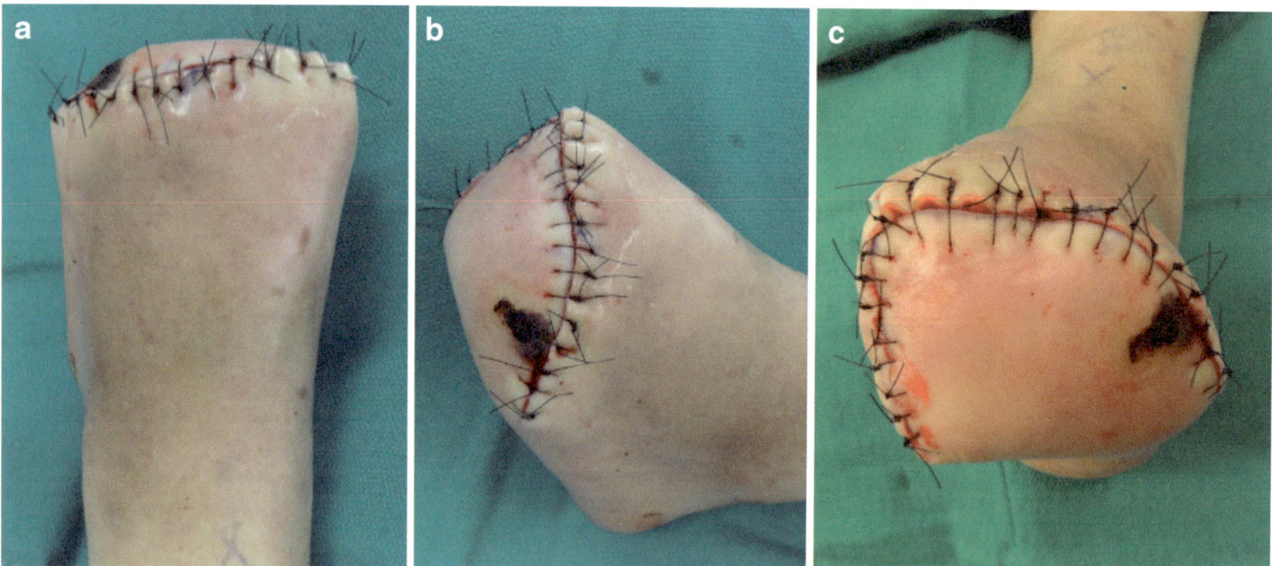

Fig. 19.24 The LPAA rotational flap was rotated and sutured in place. Note that the residual lateral wound was partial thickness and therefore not excised from the flap

that the MPAA is not as extensive as the LPAA. A portion of the MPAA flap typically involves part of the LPAA which is possible due to choke vessels. Choke vessels act as a pathway from one angiosome to another and provide indirect vascular supply in the event that the main arterial supply becomes compromised or under ischemic conditions. Choke vessels become patent 4–10 days following an ischemic event (such as surgery) in the neighboring angiosome [11, 12]. The lateral column is prone to large neuropathic ulcers at the fifth metatarsal base with concomitant inversion deformity or cavus foot structure as detailed in Figs. 19.28, 19.29, 19.30, 19.31, 19.32, and 19.33. An example of a medial plantar artery angiosome flap being utilized in Lisfranc amputation is shown in Figs. 19.33, 19.34, 19.35, 19.36, 19.37, and 19.38.

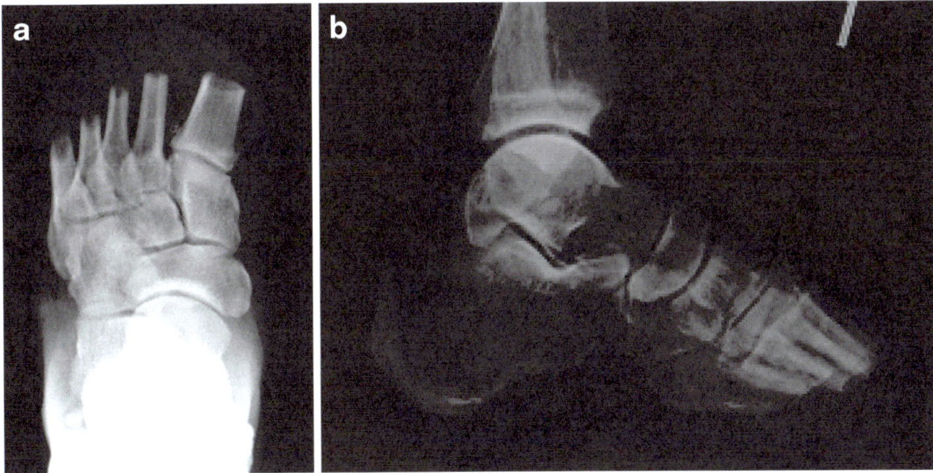

Fig. 19.25 Postoperative radiographs of LPAA rotational flap TMA. (**a**, **b**) AP and lateral radiographs showing short transmetatarsal resection typically required for LPAA rotational flap TMA

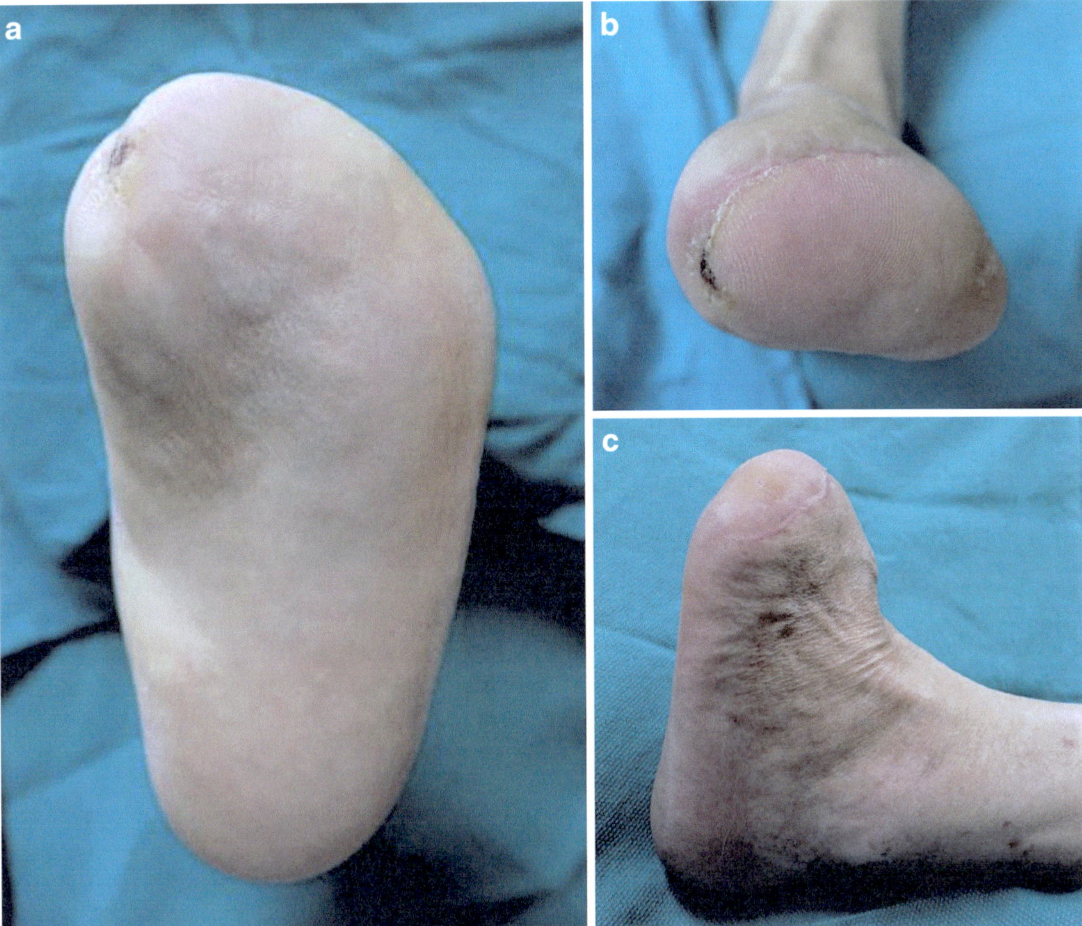

Fig. 19.26 Postoperative result with LPAA rotational flap TMA. (**a**, **b**, **c**) Clinical images at 8 months following transmetatarsal amputation with lateral plantar artery angiosome rotational flap

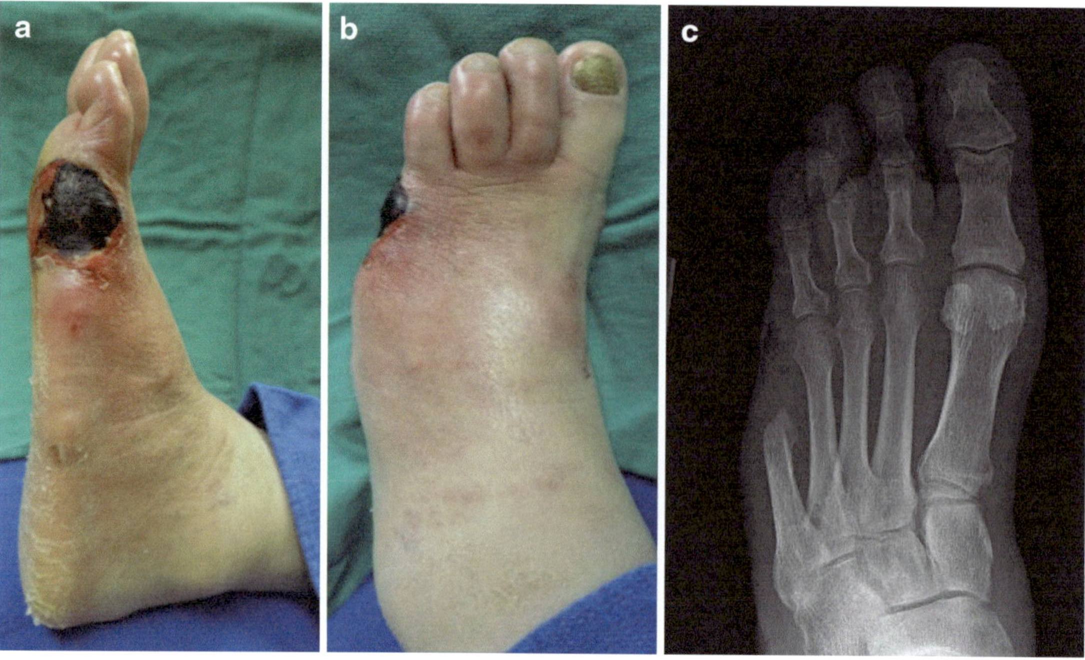

Fig. 19.27 (**a**, **b**) Plantar lateral forefoot gas gangrene treated with staged MPAA rotational flap TMA. Partial fifth ray amputation was performed 6 months prior. (**c**) AP radiograph demonstrates soft emphysema lateral to the fourth ray and osseous changes to the fourth metatarsal head. Based on clinical and radiographic finding, a diagnosis of gas gangrene and osteomyelitis was made requiring emergent open partial foot amputation

V to T Flap Midfoot Amputation

Central metatarsal soft tissue defects present unique challenges when planning midfoot amputation flaps (Fig. 19.39). These are generally on the plantar surface but dorsal defects may be associated with recent open central ray amputation. The plantar V to T flap TMA procedure works well in this circumstance as discussed in Figs. 19.40, 19.41, 19.42, 19.43, 19.44, and 19.45. The plantar V to T flap TMA incorporates adjacent LPAA and MPAA flaps to create one plantar flap. This technique is useful in patients with large central metatarsal head neuropathic ulcers [12].

Baseball Flap Midfoot Amputation Technique

Creativity is the key when dealing with massive tissue loss associated with gangrene or frostbite. Frostbite tends to be more amenable to partial foot salvage and flap techniques since the circulation to the surviving tissue is typically normal which may not be the case with gangrene caused by vascular disease. A unique flap technique, which we refer to as the "baseball flap" midfoot amputation, is shown in Figs. 19.45, 19.46, and 19.47. Combined medial and lateral soft tissue necrosis created significant challenges when attempting partial foot amputation. Piecing together available tissue flaps is much like puzzle work. The surgeon has the luxury of making the puzzle pieces to the desired shape and size but the disadvantage of limited tissue for closure. The combination of MPAA and dorsalis pedis artery angiosome (DPAA) flaps were used to provide coverage of large soft tissue defects. The long MPAA flap essentially rotated in the lateral direction covering the large lateral column defect. The DPAA was then trimmed to fit the defect across the dorsal foot. Short metatarsal resection was necessary which allowed the flaps to cover more surface area. This also provided a surgical cure for distal infection including osteomyelitis. Preoperative vascular assessment and intervention as indicated may improve the odds of success. Immediate or delayed tendon balancing may be necessary including Achilles lengthening, posterior tibial tendon lengthening, and peroneal tendon transfer.

Postoperative Care

Strict non-weight bearing for the initial 6 weeks following midfoot amputation is critical to allow progressive healing. Excessive swelling, hematoma, tension on the sutured wound, and bacterial contamination all predispose to failure with high risk for conversion to leg amputation. Clean margin biopsy and intraoperative inspection of tissue and bone helps to determine if residual infection is present which dictates length of postoperative antibiotic treatment. The rate of

Fig. 19.28 Staged surgery for MPAA rotational flap TMA. (**a**, **b**, **c**) The stage 1 procedure involved resection of grossly necrotic tissue with significant attempt to preserve the medial plantar artery angiosome for eventual flap closure of the lateral wound. (**d**, **e**) The future transmetatarsal amputation (TMA) incision lines including the plantar medial flap were drawn prior to initial open amputation. Metatarsal resection was performed in line with the incision with the anticipation of future remodeling at the time of conversion to TMA

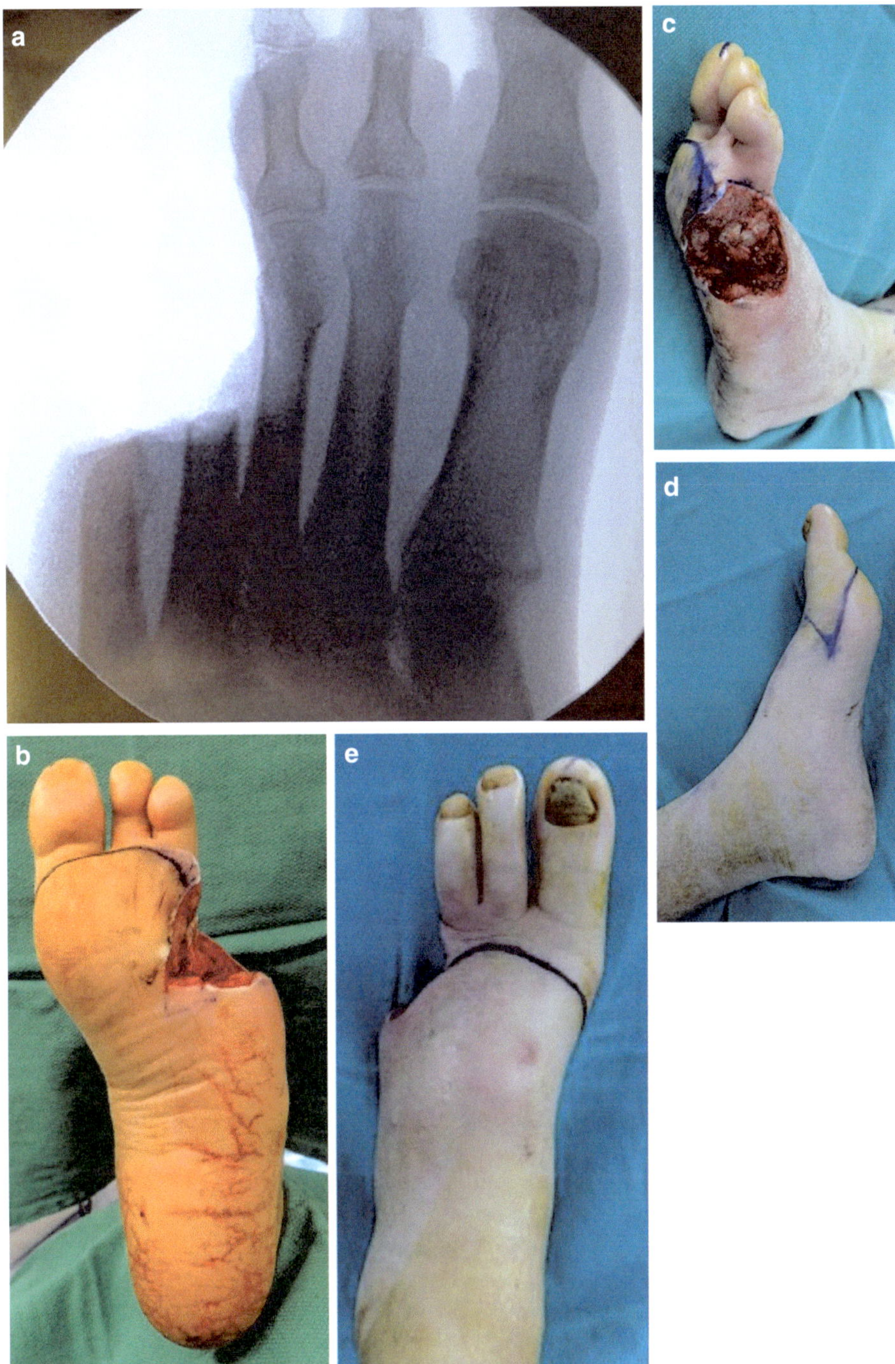

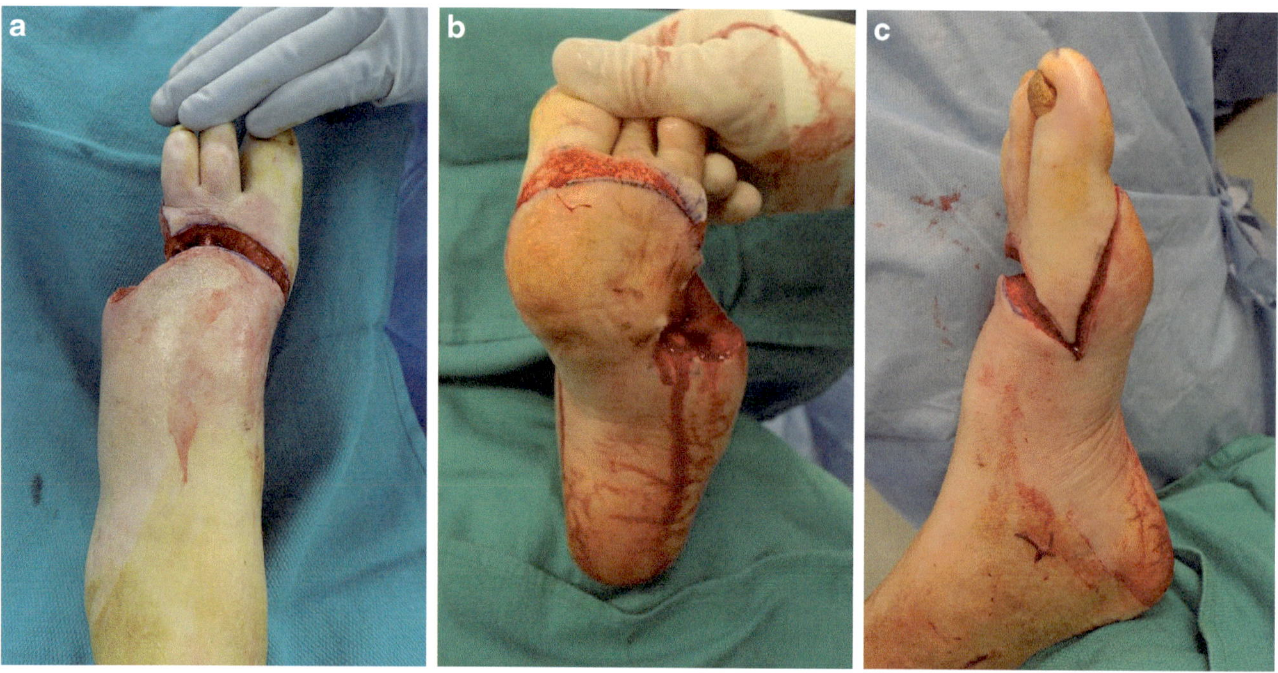

Fig. 19.29 Incision planning for MPAA rotational flap TMA. Stage 2 surgery was performed 3 days later. Incisions were made directly to bone following the preplanned flap incision design

residual osteomyelitis was found to be up to 40 % after TMA putting greater emphasis on appropriate antibiotic treatment and procedure selection [10].

Sutures should remain in place until complete skin healing, which is often delayed in the diabetic population or when vascular disease is present. It is common to leave sutures in place for 4–6 weeks in midfoot amputation. It has been the author's observation that patients are more likely to remain non-weight bearing while sutures are left in place and walking seems to commence as soon as sutures are removed.

Orthopedic shoes with a custom insert that incorporates a toe-box filler are used once the TMA site heals. A custom AFO is commonly used to improve function with Lisfranc amputation due to the short nature of the stump or potential for foot drop or posteromedial contracture. Recurrent wounds are frequently reported and ongoing preventative care after healing is necessary [13, 14].

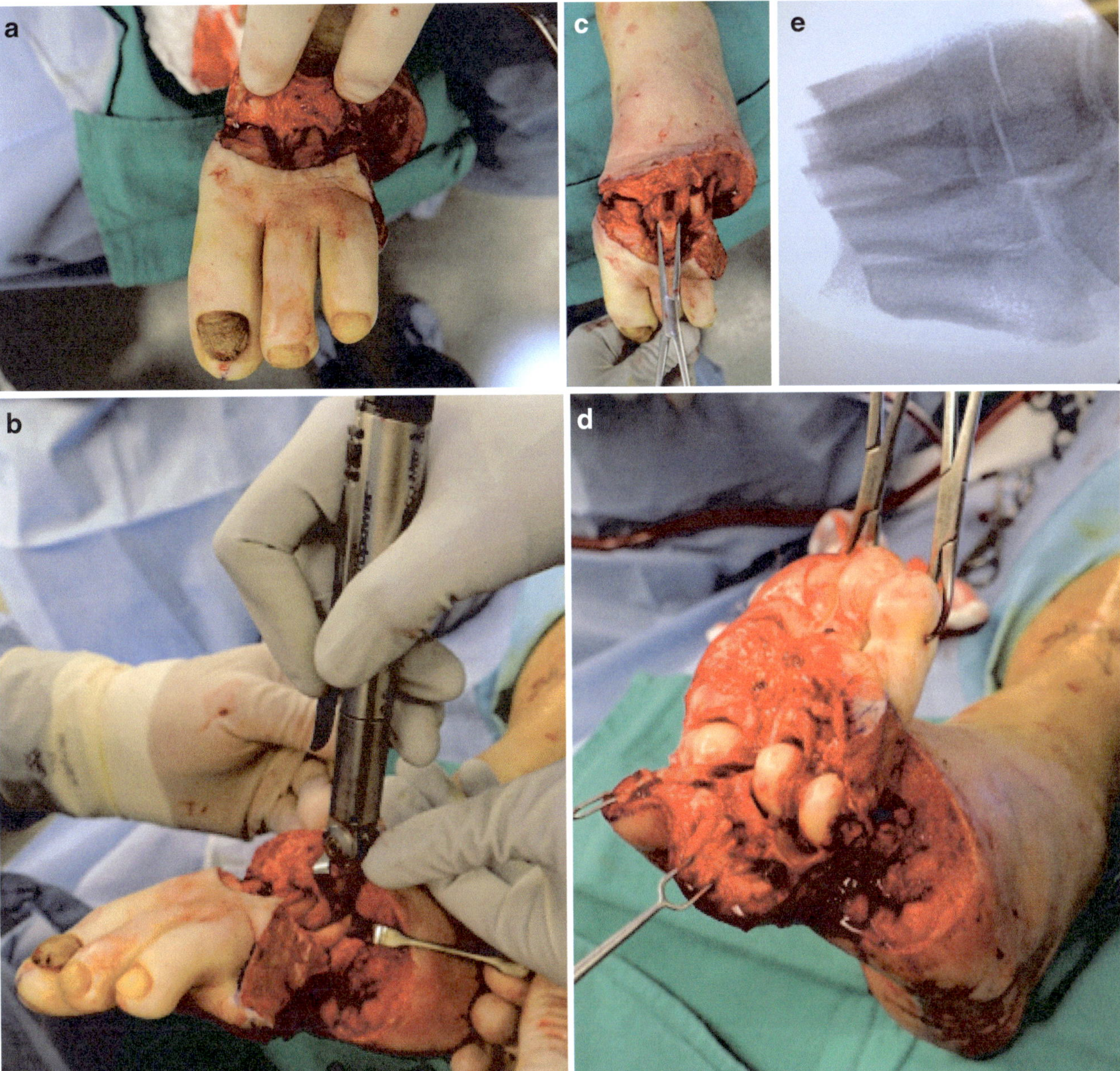

Fig. 19.30 Intraoperative flap creation for MPAA rotational flap TMA. (a) The dorsal flap was raised minimally along each individual metatarsal with a metatarsal elevator. (b) A bone saw was then used to resect the metatarsals shorter than the dorsal flap. (c) The metatarsal heads were carefully raised to prevent violation of the plantar flap. (d) The plantar flap was released from the toes which were removed as one unit. (e) Intraoperative imaging was used to assess length and contour of the amputation stump

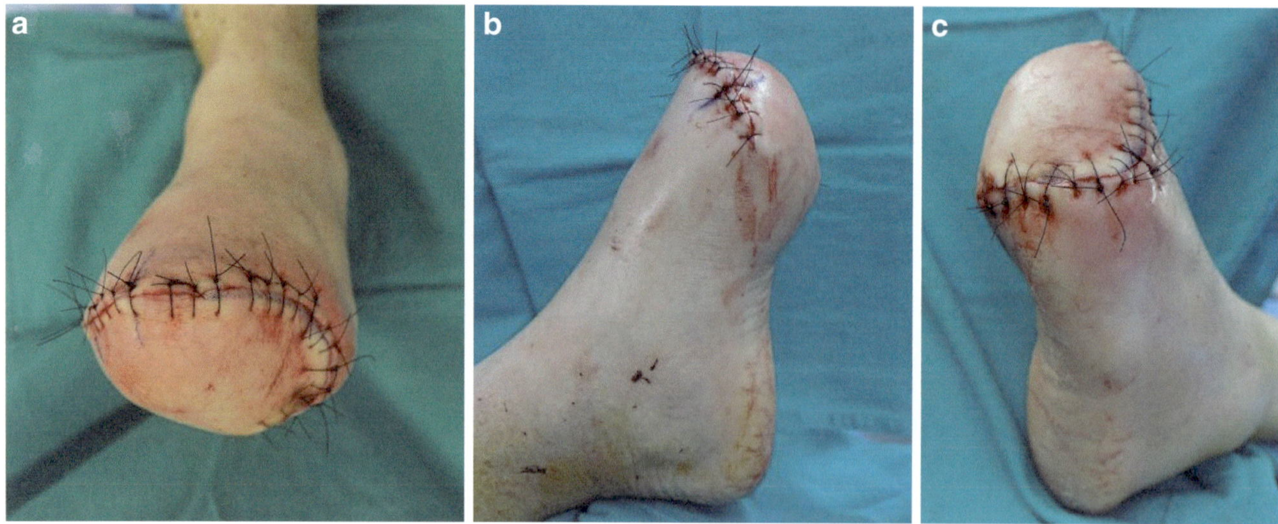

Fig. 19.31 The MPAA rotational flap was rotated and sutured in place

Fig. 19.32 Postoperative radiographs of MPAA rotational flap TMA showing the desired transmetatarsal level of amputation despite gas gangrene

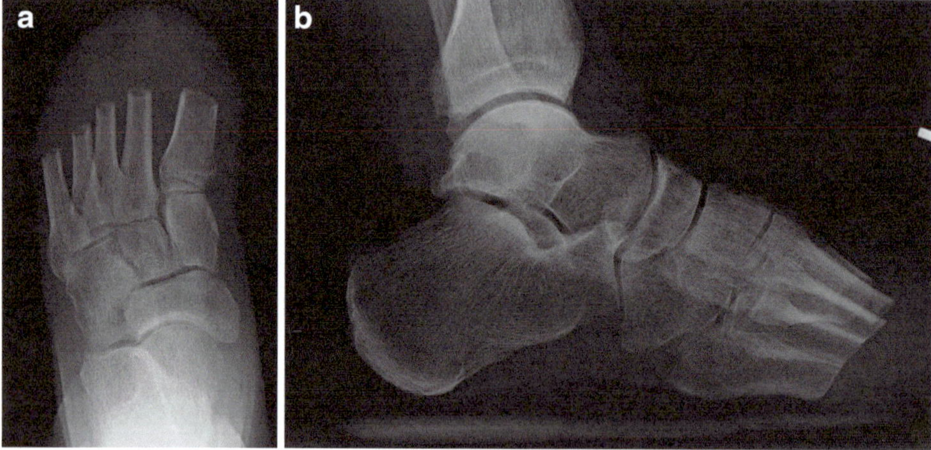

Fig. 19.33 MPAA rotational flap Lisfranc amputation. Charcot related plantar lateral midfoot wound complicated by gross instability and osteomyelitis of the cuboid and lateral metatarsal bases. Incision plan shown here allows excision of the wound and use of a rotational flap incorporating the medial plantar artery angiosome (MPAA) for a Lisfranc amputation. The MPAA primarily covers the non-weight bearing portion of the medial arch while the flap drawn here incorporates a fairly substantial portion of the lateral plantar artery angiosome. Careful dissection when raising the flap may preserve a portion of the lateral plantar artery although the extensive nature of wound excision may compromise this vessel. Opening of choke vessels between angiosoms allows the surgeon wide variation when planning flaps

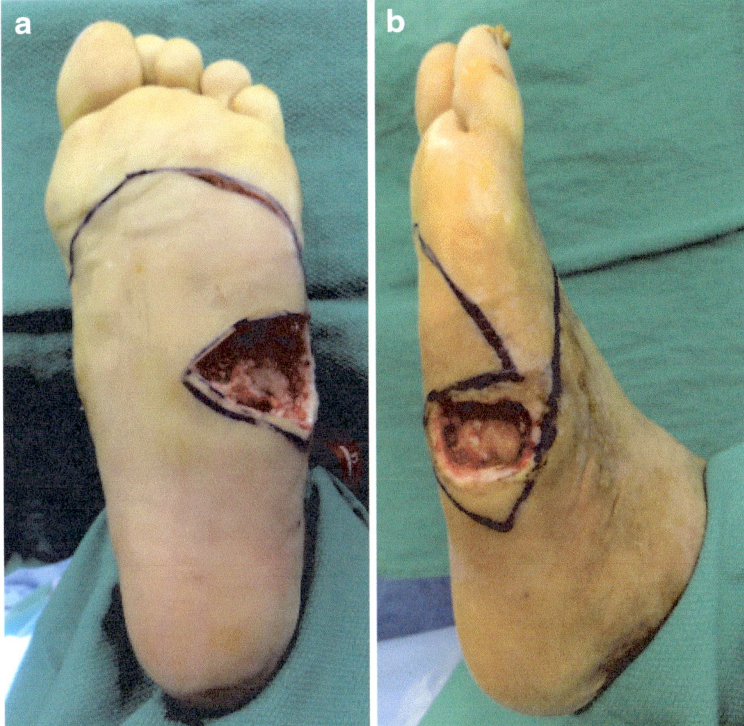

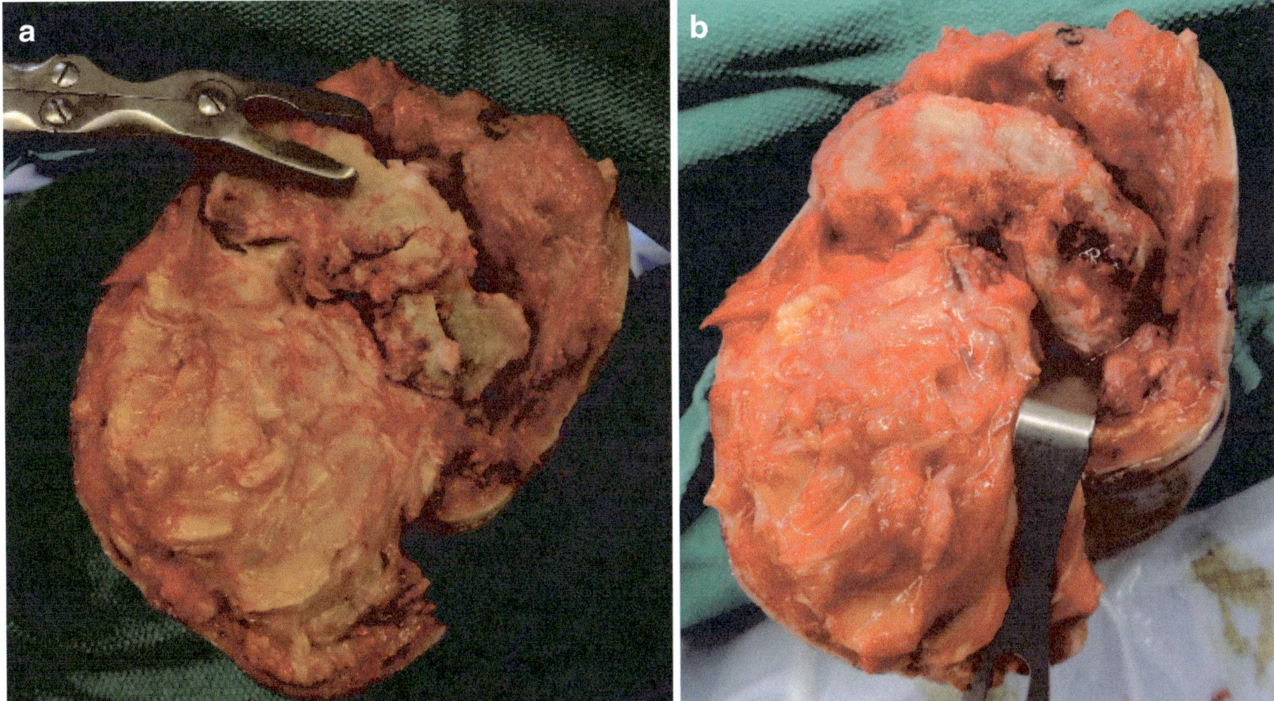

Fig. 19.34 Bone remodeling in MPAA rotational flap Lisfranc amputation. The tarsal bones were substantially remodeled after Lisfranc disarticulation. Midfoot Charcot arthropathy causes significant distortion of the bone structure which predisposes to ongoing breakdown. Debridement also provided margin biopsy of the plantar aspect of the cuboid. Residual osteomyelitis was treated with a 6-week course of IV antibiotics

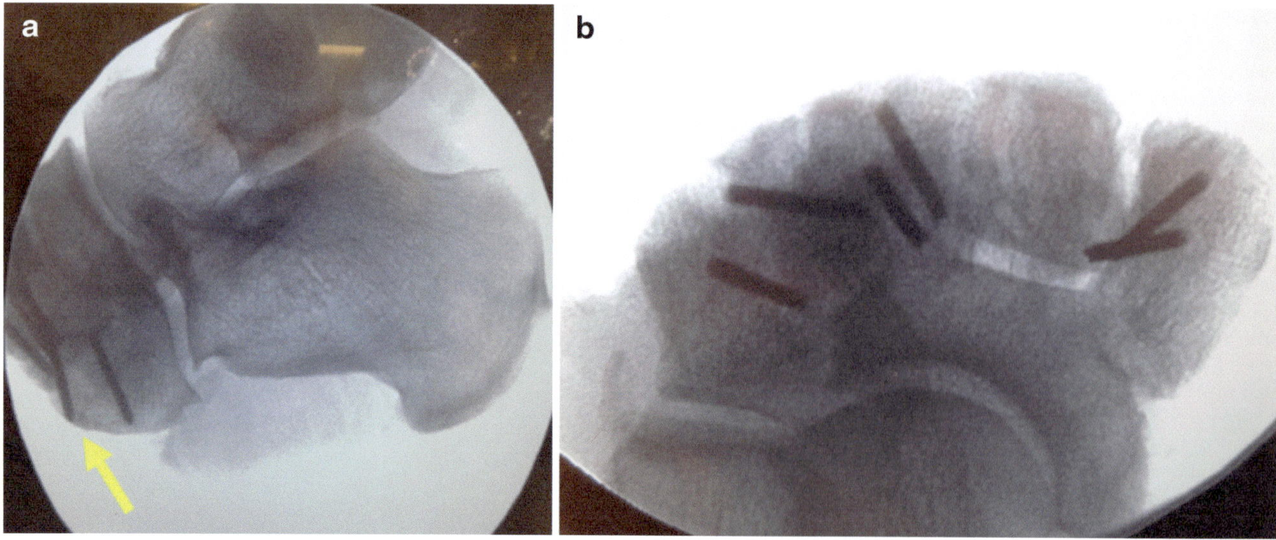

Fig. 19.35 Intraoperative imaging in MPAA rotational flap Lisfranc amputation. (**a**, **b**) Intraoperative imaging is used to assess the contour of the amputation stump. Retained hardware was not retrievable due to broken screws buried in the bone structure. Note the round nature of the plantar leading edge of the cuboid (*arrow*) which was intended to minimize recurrent pressure in this region

Fig. 19.36 Closure of MPAA rotational flap Lisfranc amputation. The flap provided immediate closure of the amputation site and plantar lateral wound defect

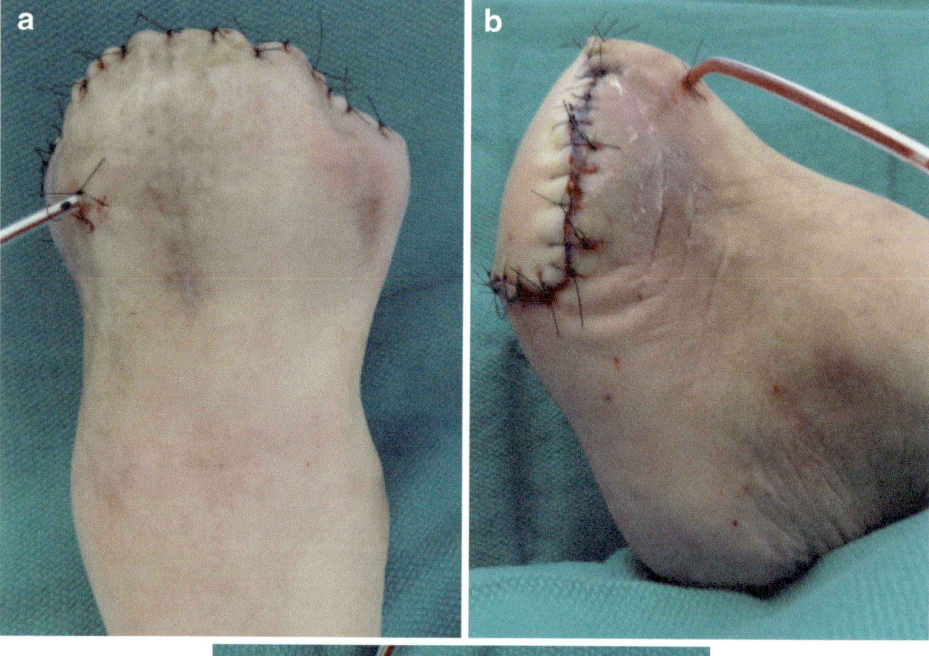

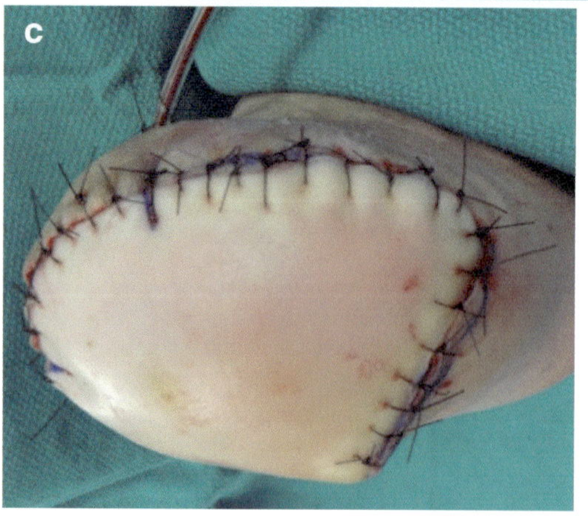

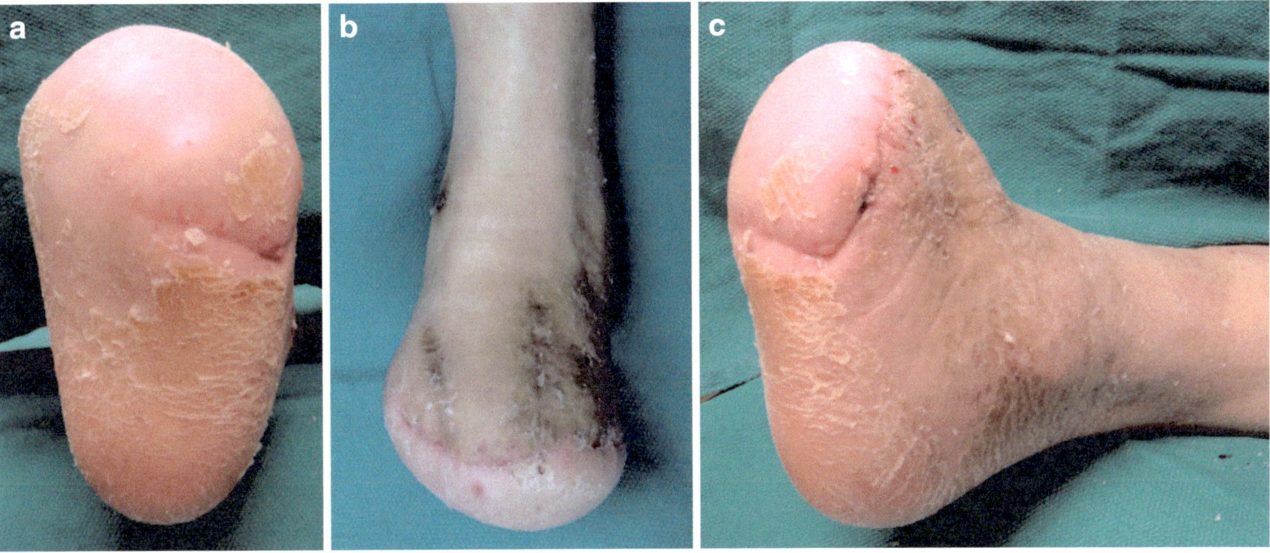

Fig. 19.37 Clinical images of MPAA rotational flap Lisfranc amputation at 10 weeks postoperative with complete healing of the wound

Fig. 19.38 Postoperative radiographs following MPAA rotational flap Lisfranc amputation. (**a**, **b**) Postoperative weight bearing AP and lateral radiographs with the desired rocker bottom contour of the Lisfranc amputation site without plantar, medial, or lateral bone prominence. Note plantar flexion at the ankle (**b**) which was treated with delayed Achilles lengthening

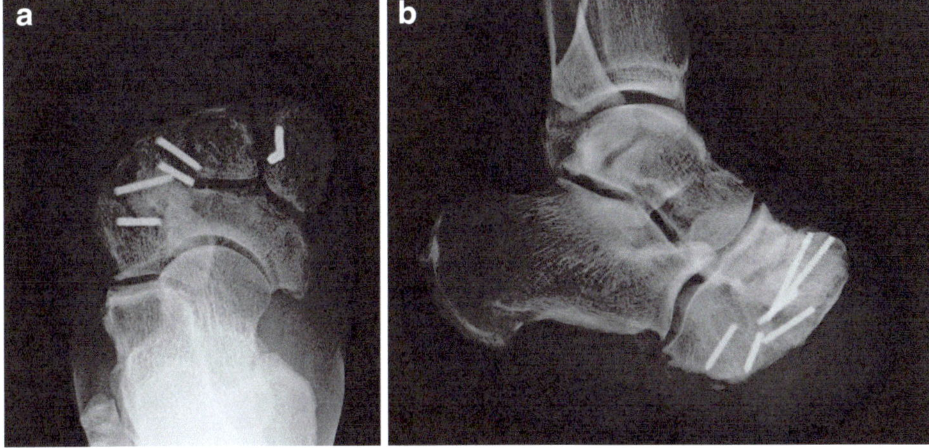

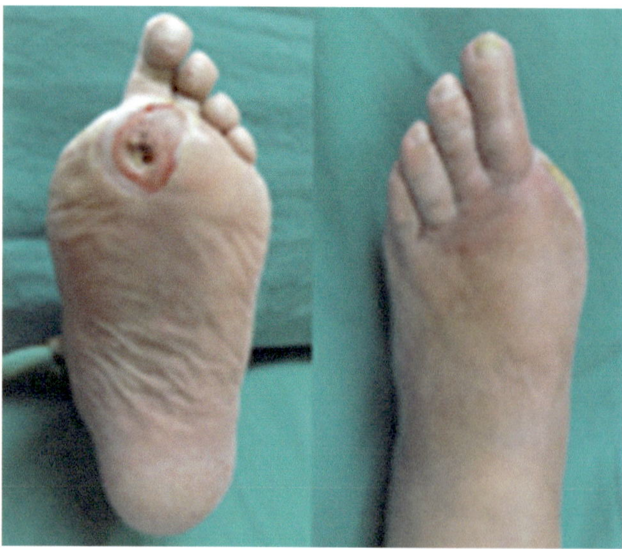

Fig. 19.39 Plantar forefoot wound amenable to V to T plantar flap TMA. This infected plantar second metatarsophalangeal joint ulcer was associated with prior partial first ray amputation

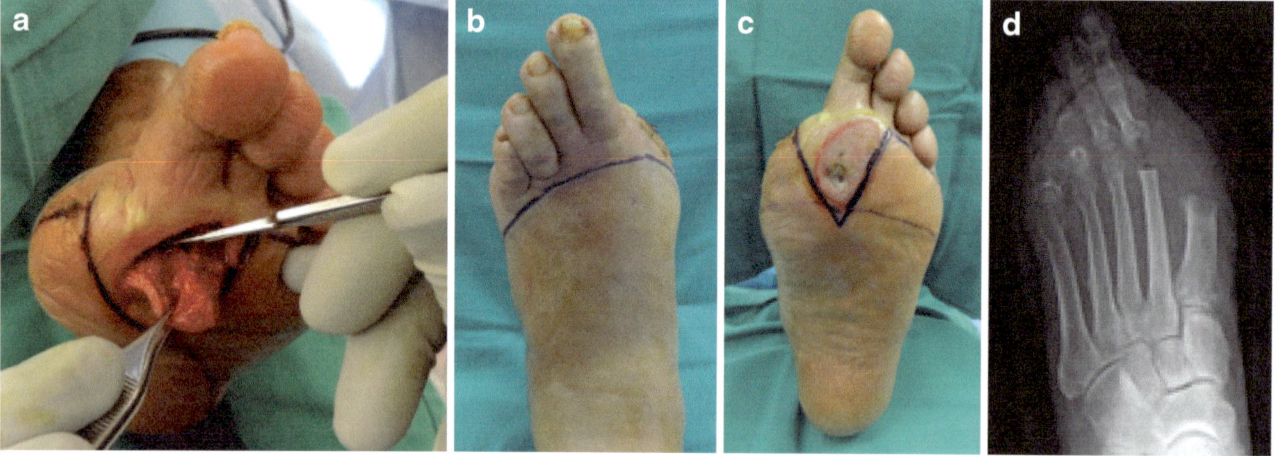

Fig. 19.40 (**a**) Stage 1 surgery for V to T flap TMA involved incision and drainage of infection and wound excision with bone biopsy of the second metatarsal head. (**b, c**) The anticipated incision for conversion to V to T rotational plantar flap TMA is shown. (**d**) Immediate postoperative radiograph with resection of the second metatarsal head and prior partial first ray resection

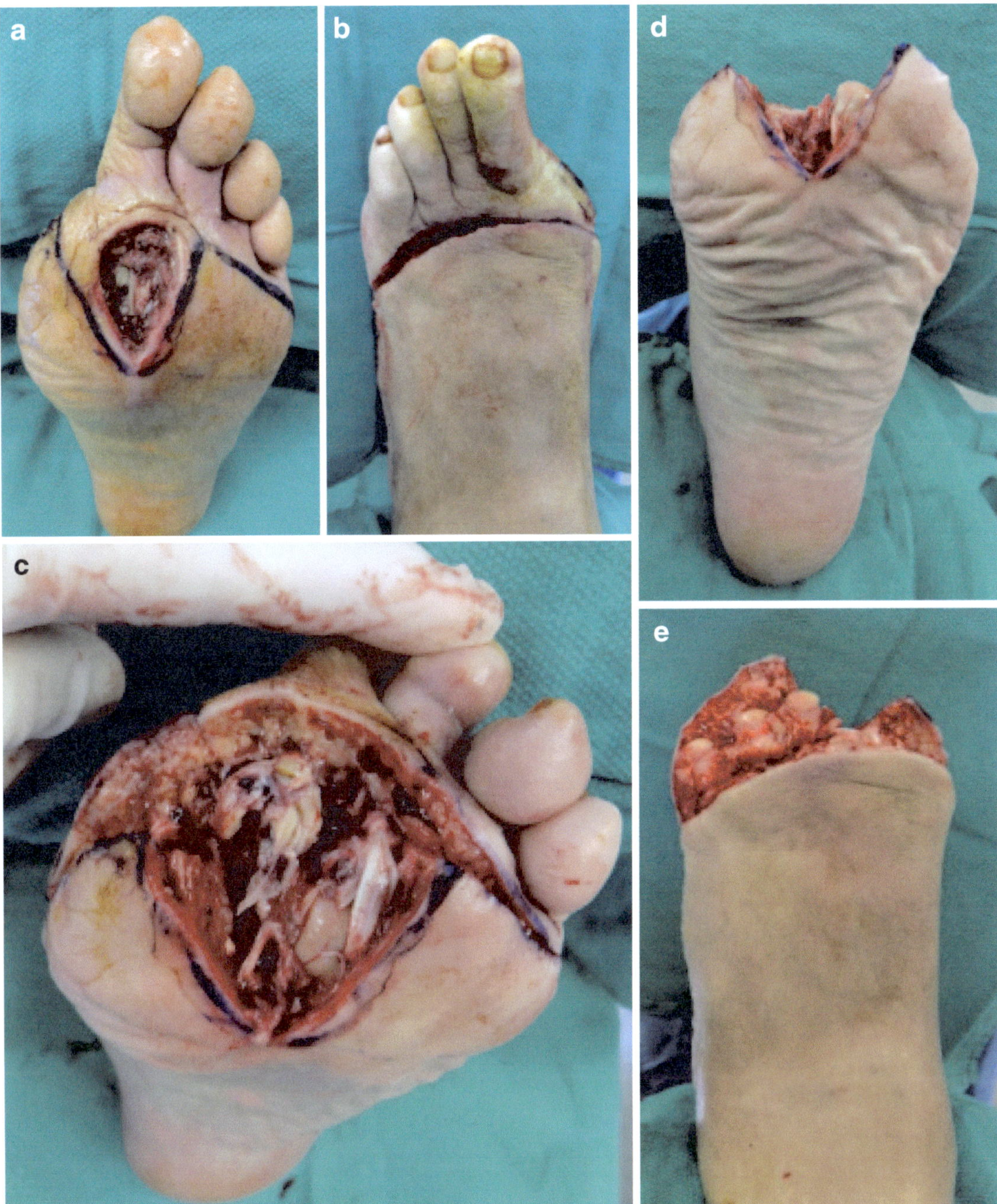

Fig. 19.41 Stage 2 surgery for V to T flap TMA. (**a, b**) Full-thickness incisions were carried down to bone. Containing the amputation at the transmetatarsal level is difficult with larger central plantar soft tissue defects. (**c, d, e**) V-shaped wedge resection of the plantar defect allowed preservation of MPAA and LPAA plantar flaps which converged to produce a V to T flap

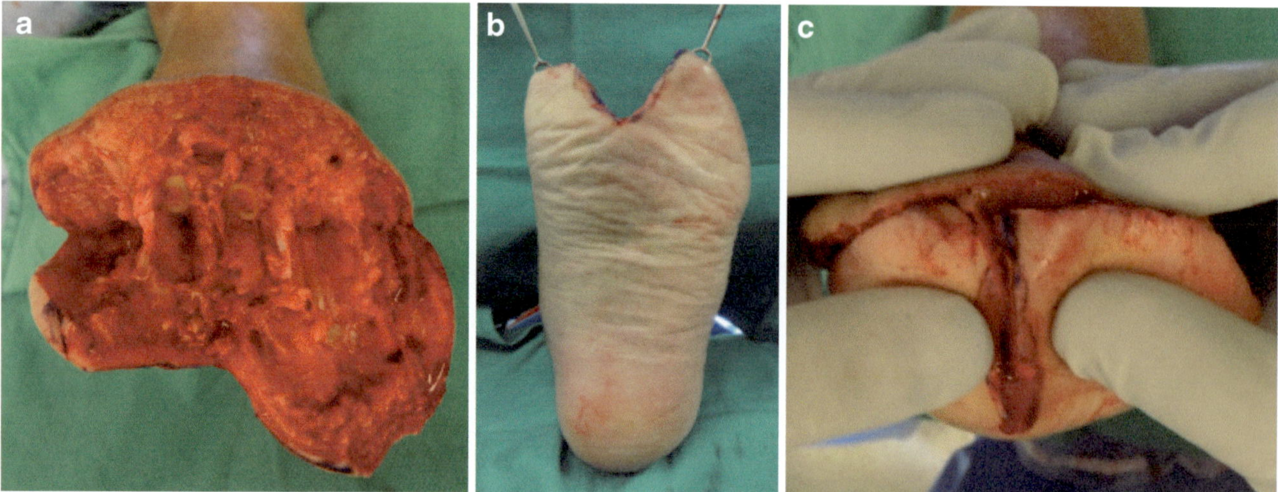

Fig. 19.42 V to T flap closure of TMA wound. (**a**) Intraoperative photos after transmetatarsal resection of the forefoot. The metatarsal bones are cut in line with the dorsal incision. (**b**) Note the preservation of a long plantar flap. (**c**) The plantar flap will be sewn directly to the dorsal flap

Fig. 19.43 (**a**) Postoperative clinical and radiographic imaging in V to T flap TMA. Immediate postoperative photo with V to T closure of the plantar wound defect. Note how the two plantar flaps and transverse dorsal incision close to form a "T." (**b**) Intraoperative imaging demonstrated preservation of a desirable metatarsal parabola and length

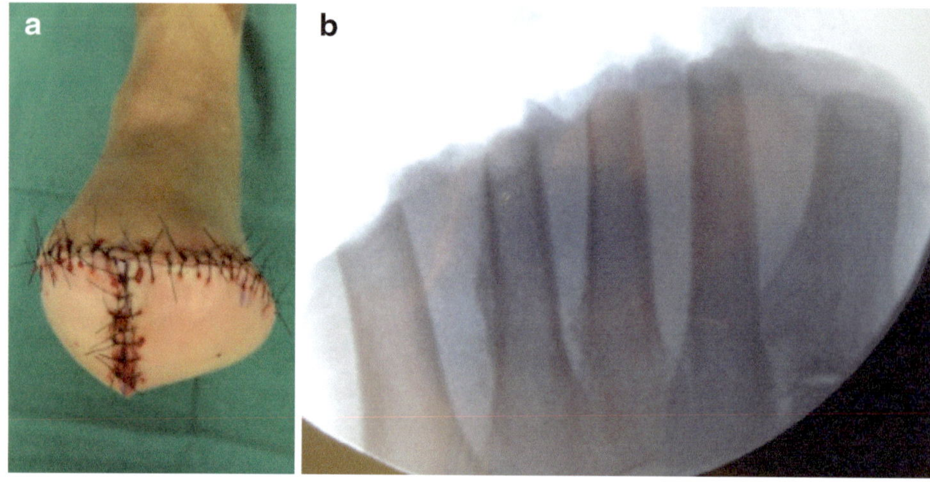

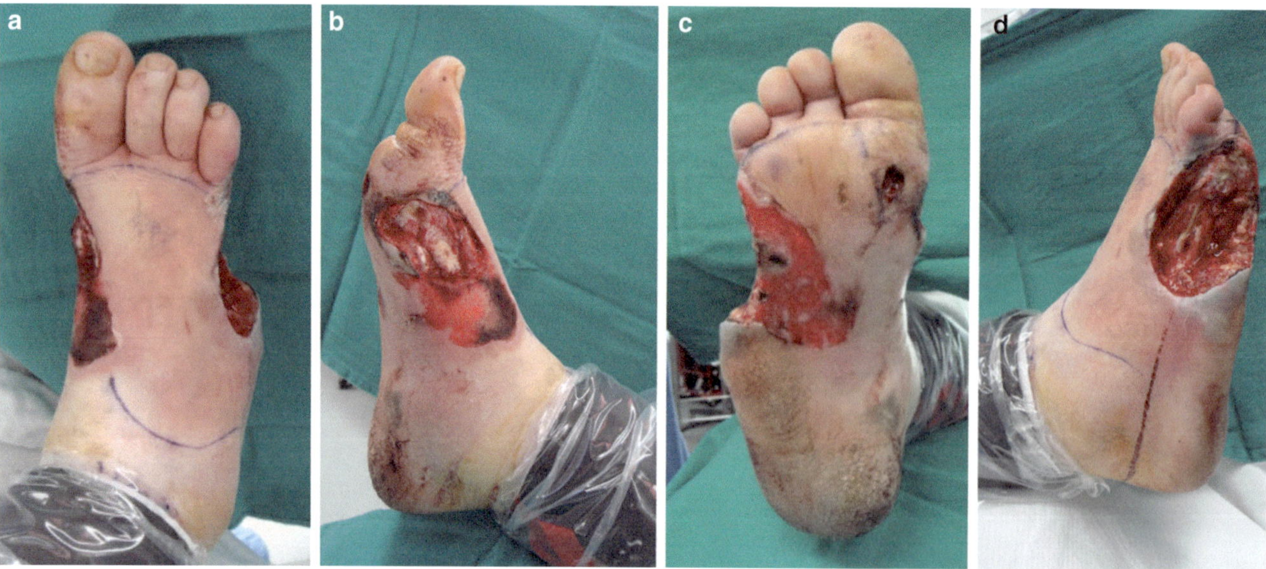

Fig. 19.44 Case presentation of baseball flap midfoot amputation in a diabetic patient with extensive necrosis on the medial and lateral forefoot secondary to frostbite. Stage 1 surgery involved complete open fifth ray amputation for widespread bone exposure, acute soft tissue infection, and osteomyelitis. Frostbite was then allowed to demarcate with extensive soft tissue loss on the medial and lateral forefoot. Dorsal medial and plantar lateral eschars were present in the midfoot with only partial thickness loss. Full-thickness tissue necrosis in these regions would make even Chopart's level amputation challenging. The "baseball flap" midfoot amputation technique was used allowing intact dorsal and plantar tissues to cover the medial and lateral wound defects after bone resection and forefoot amputation

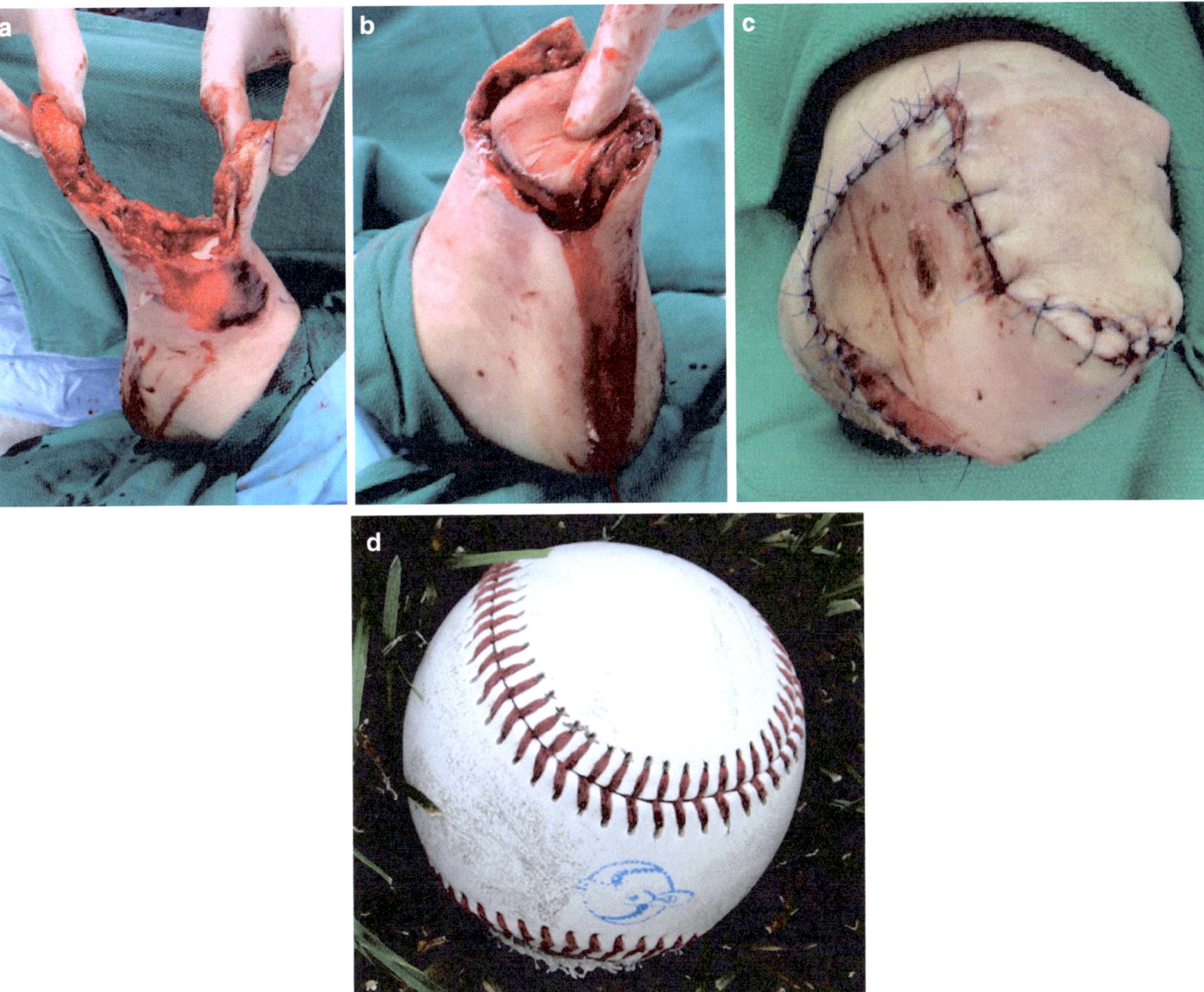

Fig. 19.45 Baseball flap midfoot amputation technique. (**a**) The dorsalis pedis artery angiosome and medial plantar artery angiosome flaps have been preserved in the process of amputating the forefoot. Bone resection was performed near the Lisfranc level. Note the length of the flaps, which can remain viable due to inherent perfusion of the angiosome and direct inflow from the source vessel. (**b**) The flaps were rotated to provide immediate coverage of challenging wounds. (**c**, **d**) The sutured stump resembles a baseball

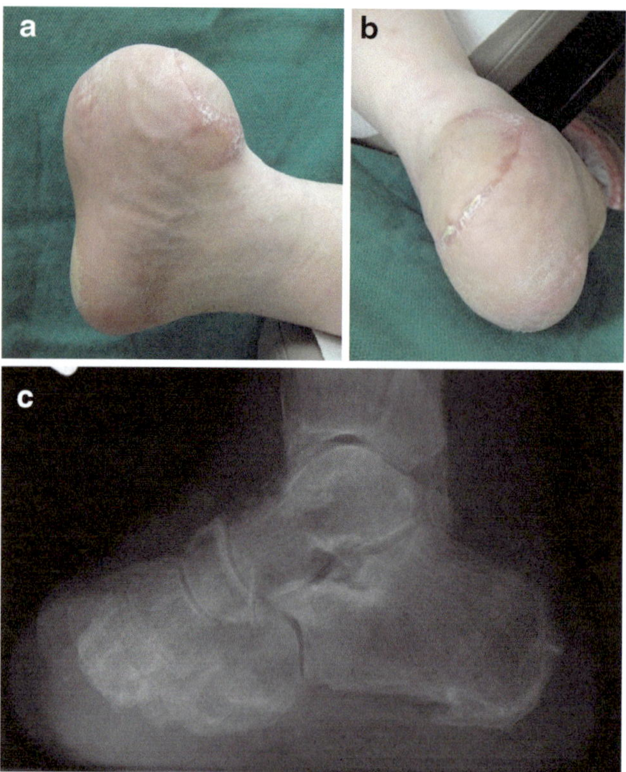

Fig. 19.46 Clinical and radiographic follow-up of baseball flap midfoot amputation. Ten-month clinical photos demonstrate complete healing without wound recurrence. Healing was slow as expected due to the demarcating soft tissue defects dorsal medial and plantar lateral. A weight bearing lateral radiograph demonstrates the level of bone resection including complete fifth ray amputation. Short metatarsal stumps are present but otherwise the foot will function similar to Lisfranc amputation. This weight bearing view highlights the expected inverted nature of the foot without a peroneus brevis tendon. Tendon balancing such as posterior tibial tenotomy and Achilles lengthening are warranted and may be performed in a delayed fashion

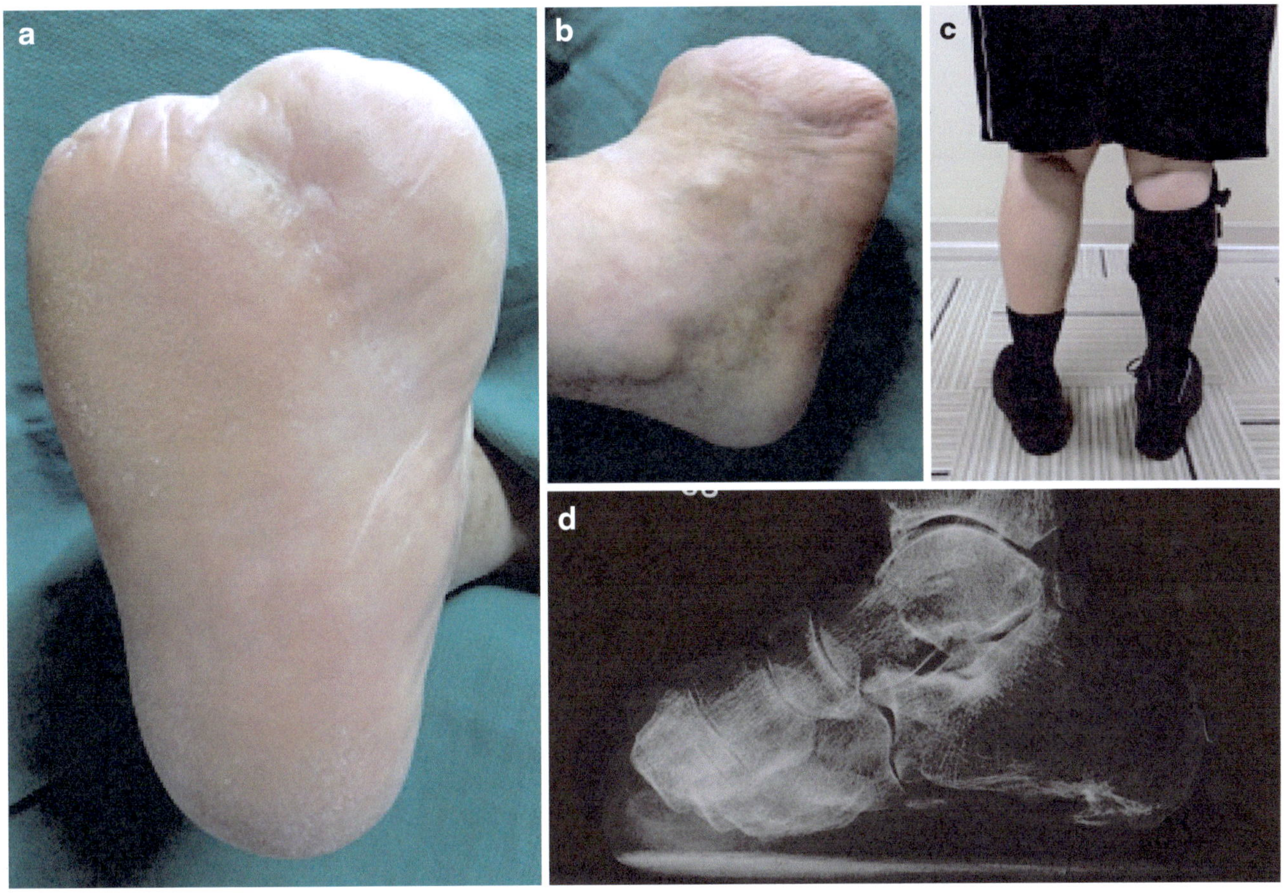

Fig. 19.47 5 year clinical (**a**, **b**, **c**) and (**d**) radiographic results of base-ball flap midfoot amputation. Despite odds in favor of recurrent wound breakdown, this patient has done extremely well and has remained ambulatory using an ankle foot orthotic brace that provides extension of the forefoot lever arm and resistance to inversion forces

Conclusion

Providing a biomechanically functional foot that is free of wounds or infection is the principal goal in the surgical treatment of forefoot osteomyelitis. Ideal procedure selection is dependent on a variety of factors including the size and location of the wound, extent of osteomyelitis, viability of remaining soft tissue, and underlying foot structure. Midfoot amputation at the transmetatarsal level represents a viable limb salvage option when addressing forefoot osteomyelitis associated with diabetes-related wounds, trauma, or vascular insufficiency. Advanced plastic surgical techniques are commonly employed to achieve successful wound closure in cases that would otherwise require more proximal amputation. Lisfranc level amputation is a less functional but sometimes necessary alternative.

References

1. McKittrick LS, McKittrick JB, Risley TS. Transmetatarsal amputation for infection of gangrene in patients with diabetes mellitus. Ann Surg. 1949;130(4):826–40.
2. Brown ML, Tang W, Patel A, Baumhauer JF. Partial foot amputation in patients with diabetic foot ulcers. Foot Ankle Int. 2012;33(9):707–16.
3. DeCotiis MA. Lisfranc and chopart amputations. Clin Podiatr Med Surg. 2005;22:385–93.
4. Early JS. Transmetatarsal and midfoot amputations. Clin Orthop Relat Res. 1999;361:85–90.
5. Attinger C, Venturi M, Kim K, Ribiero C. Maximizing length and optimizing biomechanics in foot amputations by avoiding cookbook recipes for amputation. Semin Vasc Surg. 2003;16(1):44–66.
6. Boffeli TJ, Thompson JC. Partial foot amputations for salvage of the diabetic lower extremity. Clin Podiatr Med Surg. 2013;31:103–26.
7. Hosch J, Quiroga C, Bosma J, Peters EJG, Armstrong DG, Lavery LA. Outcomes of transmetatarsal amputations in patients with diabetes mellitus. J Foot Ankle Surg. 1997;36(6):430–4.

8. Boffeli TJ, Pfannenstein RR, Thompson JC. Radiation therapy for recurrent heterotopic ossification prophylaxis following partial metatarsal amputation. J Foot Ankle Surg. 2015. doi:10.1053/j.jfas.2014.07.010

9. Moore JC, Jolly GP. Soft tissue considerations in partial foot amputations. Clin Podiatr Med Surg. 2000;17(4):631–48.

10. Boffeli TJ, Waverly BJ. Medial and lateral plantar artery angiosome rotational flaps for transmetatarsal and Lisfranc amputation in patients with compromised plantar tissue. J Foot Ankle Surg. 2015. doi:10.1053/j.jfas.2014.12.007

11. Attinger CE, Evans KK, Bulan E, Blume P, Cooper P. Angiosomes of the foot and ankle and clinical implications for limb salvage: reconstruction, incisions, and revascularization. Plast Reconstr Surg. 2006;117:261S–93S.

12. Clemens MW, Attinger CE. Angiosomes and wound care in the diabetic foot. Foot Ankle Clin. 2010;15:439–64.

13. Atway S, Nerone V, Springer KD, Woodruff DM. Rate of residual osteomyelitis after partial foot amputation in diabetic patients: a standardized method for evaluating bone margins with intraoperative culture. J Foot Ankle Surg. 2012;51:749–52.

14. Izumi Y, Satterfield K, Lee S, Harkless LB. Risk of reamputation in diabetic patients stratified by limb and level of amputation. Diabetes Care. 2006;29:366–70.

Troy J. Boffeli and Kevin J. Mahoney

Introduction

Chopart's amputation through the midtarsal joint has limited indications but is an option for unique circumstances involving compromised soft tissues and osteomyelitis of the midfoot tarsal bones that is not amenable to more traditional forefoot amputation techniques. Typical scenarios include large neuropathic midfoot ulceration complicated by tarsal bone osteomyelitis, infected midfoot Charcot arthropathy, widespread gangrene extending into the midfoot, and mangling midfoot injuries. These complex conditions are traditionally treated with leg amputation for which the patient may not be a willing candidate. The surgeon is then left with the difficult decision regarding an acceptable level of amputation that can provide resolution of infection, soft tissue coverage of the wound or exposed bone, prompt healing, and reasonable postoperative weight bearing function.

Skepticism exists regarding the functional benefit of proximal foot amputation. Historically, surgeons have been taught that Chopart's amputation is prone to compromised outcome due to prosthetic challenges, poor function with weight bearing, predisposition to tissue breakdown, and tendency for ankle contracture despite efforts at tendon balancing [1–5]. The conventional wisdom is that potential Chopart's candidates are better off with a leg amputation. For these reasons, many surgeons may forego this level of amputation, while others have limited experience performing this relatively rare operation. However, as energy demands are increased with more proximal amputations, the most distal level of amputation is ideal [4, 6]. Preservation of limb length provides the patient with the highest level of function and, in many cases, earlier weight bearing and

rehabilitation. The short duration of rehabilitation with Chopart's amputation allows quick return to bipedal transfer and weight bearing activities at approximately 6 weeks postop [7]. Advances in below knee prosthetics are praised for providing a high level of function including the ability to run, yet elderly patients may place greater value on independent living, basic in-home activities, and prompt recovery. Recent advances in partial foot prosthetics also allow improved gait and function after Chopart's amputation although not to the point of actual running [8–10]. Minor modifications to the traditional Chopart's amputation technique are intended to improve stump longevity, decrease propensity for contracture, and improve weight bearing function [11].

The traditional Chopart's amputation approach is presented along with modified surgical techniques including angiosome-based rotational flap options for complex plantar wounds. Cases are presented to demonstrate incision planning, surgical technique, bone resection pearls, staging for acute infection, tendon balancing considerations, postop care, and prosthetic options.

Patient Selection Criteria

When selecting the ideal level of amputation, the surgeon should consider the functional goals and priorities of the patient. For many patients, basic daily activities such as standing while taking a shower, midnight trips to the bathroom without a prosthetic leg, and independent transfers are the primary goals. A Chopart's amputation may provide patients with greater independence in comparison to a more proximal level of amputation from this regard. This, of course, is highly dependent on the patient's preoperative condition, comorbidities, goals, and rehabilitation potential, as minimal rehabilitation is necessary in contrast to BKA [7]. The typical patient who presents with foot conditions appropriate for Chopart's amputation may simply be looking for independence with minimal ambulation for their

T.J. Boffeli, D.P.M., F.A.C.F.A.S. (✉) • K.J. Mahoney, D.P.M.
Regions Hospital/HealthPartners Institute for Education and Research, 640 Jackson Street, St. Paul, MN 55101, USA
e-mail: troy.j.boffeli@healthpartners.com; Kevin.j.mahoney@healthpartners.com

© Springer International Publishing Switzerland 2015
T.J. Boffeli (ed.), *Osteomyelitis of the Foot and Ankle*, DOI 10.1007/978-3-319-18926-0_20

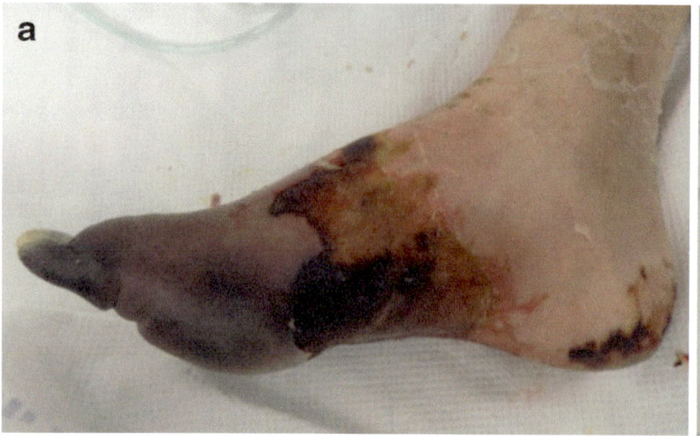 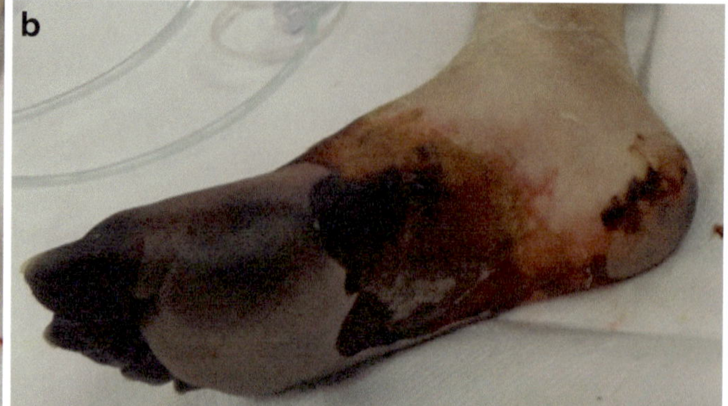

Fig. 20.1 Patient selection criteria for Chopart's amputation. (**a**) Gangrene encompassing the entirety of the forefoot may be considered for Chopart's amputation depending on the viability of the proximal tissue. (**b**) Gangrene and large decubitus ulceration of the weight bearing surface of the heel make leg amputation a better choice as opposed to Chopart's amputation

activities of daily living (ADLs) as opposed to the high level of function that a leg amputation may provide. Other patients have already undergone BKA on the contralateral limb and simply need a weight bearing surface to assist with transfers. The usefulness of the preserved heel with Chopart's amputation should not be underestimated with regard to mobility when laying in bed, especially in patients who have lost the opposite limb. Thorough consideration of an individual patient's situation and practical goals should be considered when deciding on the optimal level of amputation. Adequate circulation is a major factor regarding the decision to perform a Chopart's amputation, which is a concern in patients with diabetes-related wounds and gangrene. For cases involving infection, the residual wound left after surgical debridement oftentimes dictates the level of amputation. Patients with large decubitus heel wounds or extensive gangrene extending into the midfoot and heel are not suitable to Chopart's amputation (Fig. 20.1).

Staged Surgical Approach

Midfoot amputation secondary to acute infection is often performed in a staged manner. The first stage is an incision and drainage procedure or partial foot amputation which is left open for initial management of the infection. Care is taken to completely excise the ulceration while draining any abscess collection, as well as copious irrigation of the wound. A bone biopsy is procured if osteomyelitis is suspected. The second stage is typically performed 3–5 days later allowing the remaining tissues to demarcate and vascular intervention if needed. During the stage 2 operation, Chopart's amputation is performed and closed as outlined below.

Traditional Chopart's Amputation Technique

Dorsal and plantar flaps are created using a fishmouth-type incision with care to ensure tension-free coverage of the amputation stump. The goal of the incision is to preserve as much dorsal and plantar tissue as needed for closure after disarticulation through the talonavicular and calcaneocuboid joints. The medial and lateral apices are near midline just proximal to the level of disarticulation, with the plantar flap being slightly longer to avoid sutures on the weight bearing surface (Fig. 20.2). Incisions are made full thickness down to bone at a 90° angle to the skin surface preserving adequate flap thickness. No attempt is made to preserve the dorsal, plantar, medial, or lateral tendon structures unless planning to transfer the tibialis anterior tendon to the dorsal neck of the talus. Tendons are left in place within the flaps and allowed to scar down where they lay. Patients commonly maintain active dorsiflexion despite loss of insertion of all dorsiflexory tendons (Fig. 20.3). The dorsal flap is raised at the bone level in an effort to preserve a viable and vascularized flap. The Chopart's joint is visualized, and sharp dissection is used to disarticulate at the talonavicular and calcaneocuboid joints (Figs. 20.4 and 20.5). Remodeling of the weight bearing surface of the anterior calcaneus helps to avoid prominent edges that may predispose to future skin breakdown (Fig. 20.6). Interrupted skin sutures are used to close the wound, and deep sutures are not needed or desired (Fig. 20.7). A no-touch suture technique is used to allow minimal handling of the dorsal and plantar flaps. Hash marks are helpful to preplan flap approximation with the expectation that slight puckering will occur due to the plantar flap being longer and broader than the dorsal flap.

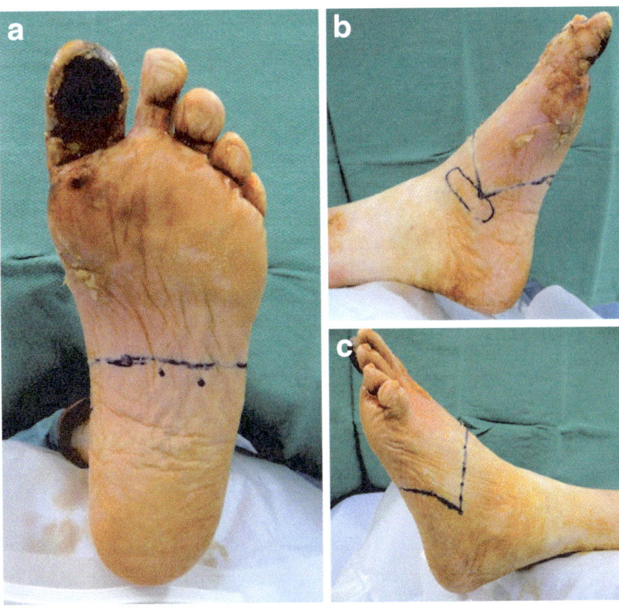

Fig. 20.2 Case 1: Traditional Chopart's amputation technique with standard incision design. Chopart's amputation incisions are drawn at the proximal demarcation of ischemic changes in the midfoot. (**a**) Note extensive gangrene on the plantar hallux with ischemic rubor extending along the medial forefoot despite recent vascular intervention. Localized digital gangrene would normally be treated with first ray amputation or perhaps TMA if not for vascular compromise in the plantar arch. (**b**, **c**)The medial and lateral incision apices are placed midline from dorsal to plantar, with an attempt to have matching dorsal and plantar flaps. The proximal extent of the medial and lateral apices is dictated by the anticipated level of bone resection but typically extend to the midtarsal joint. Note intact and viable tissue on the plantar weight bearing surface of the heel which makes this patient a candidate for Chopart's amputation

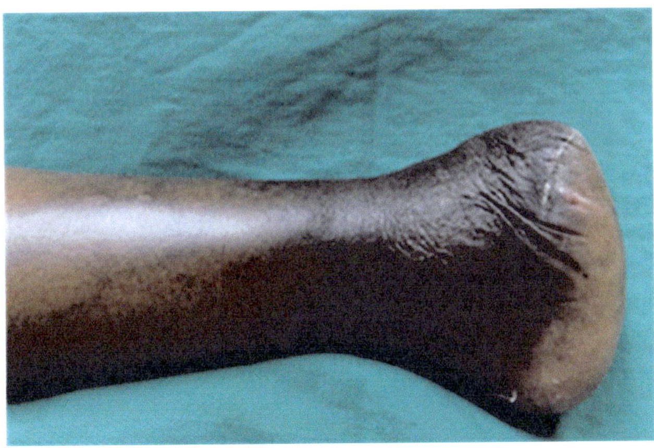

Fig. 20.3 Active ankle dorsiflexion despite loss of the tibialis anterior tendon (TA) with Chopart's amputation. Active dorsiflexion remains despite complete severing of the TA and extensor tendons with Chopart's amputation. No attempt was made to transfer the TA yet active dorsiflexion is commonly seen which is thought to occur secondary to adhesion of the severed anterior tendons to surrounding soft tissues

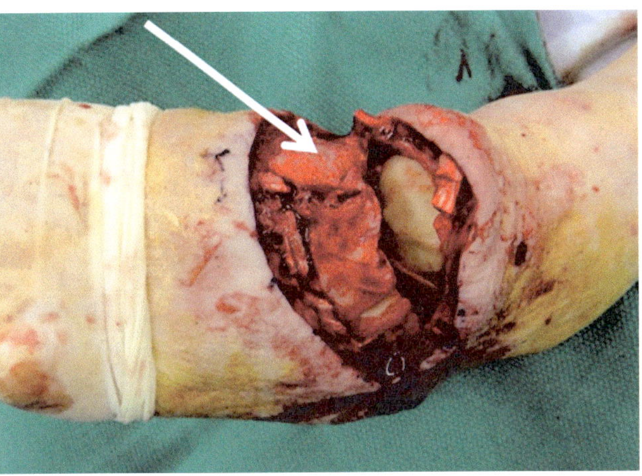

Fig. 20.4 Case 1: Full depth incision to preserve a viable dorsal flap. The dorsal flap was raised off the cuneiforms, cuboid and navicular to accomplish midtarsal joint disarticulation. Note how the exposed tarsal boness (*arrow*) are skeletonized after subperiosteal dissection in an effort to make the flap truly full thickness

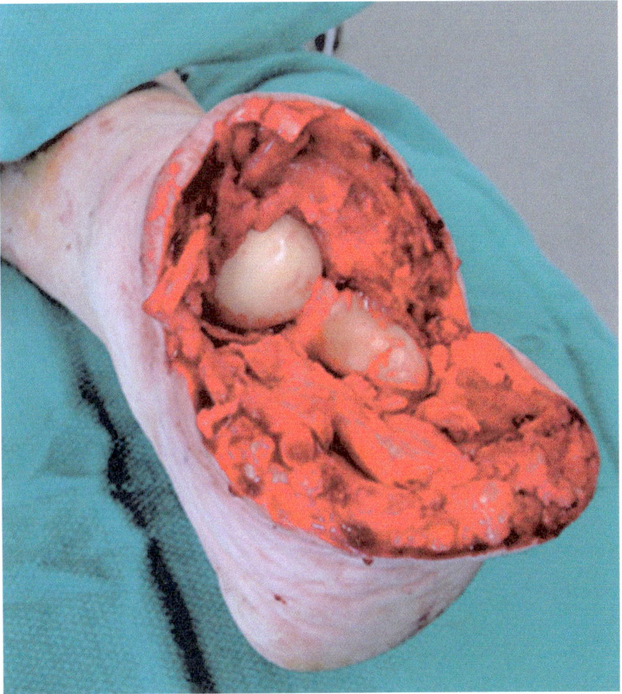

Fig. 20.5 Case 1: Midtarsal joint disarticulation. The plantar flap was incised full depth directly to the tarsal bones. The plantar flap was much thicker than the dorsal flap and included muscle tissue as seen here. Note how the talus was stacked on top of the calcaneus which is the case for all but the most severely pronated foot types. This predisposes to excessive plantar lateral pressure beneath the anterior calcaneus which correlates with the most likely area of breakdown of the Chopart's amputation stump. The cartilage may or may not be removed prior to closure depending on surgeon's preference although we typically leave the cartilage intact

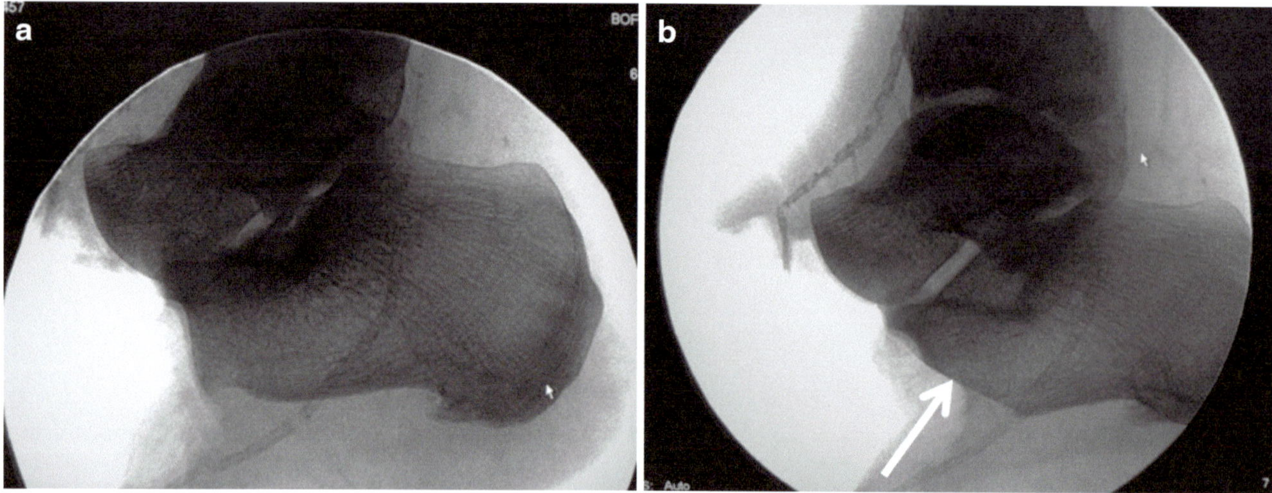

Fig. 20.6 Case 1: Remodeling of the anterior calcaneal weight bearing surface. (**a**) Intraoperative image demonstrated a natural plantar prominence of the anterior calcaneus after removal of the cuboid. The talus bears minimal weight with Chopart's amputation and anterior calcaneal remodeling is helpful to avoid lateral tissue breakdown. The surgeon should assume that the foot will function with maximum plantarflexion of the talus within the ankle joint mortise, and complete loss of calcaneal inclination despite any attempt at tendon balancing. (**b**) The anterior aspect of the calcaneus was remodeled to create a natural plantar rocker bottom contour (*arrow*). The resected portion of the anterior calcaneus was procured for clean margin biopsy

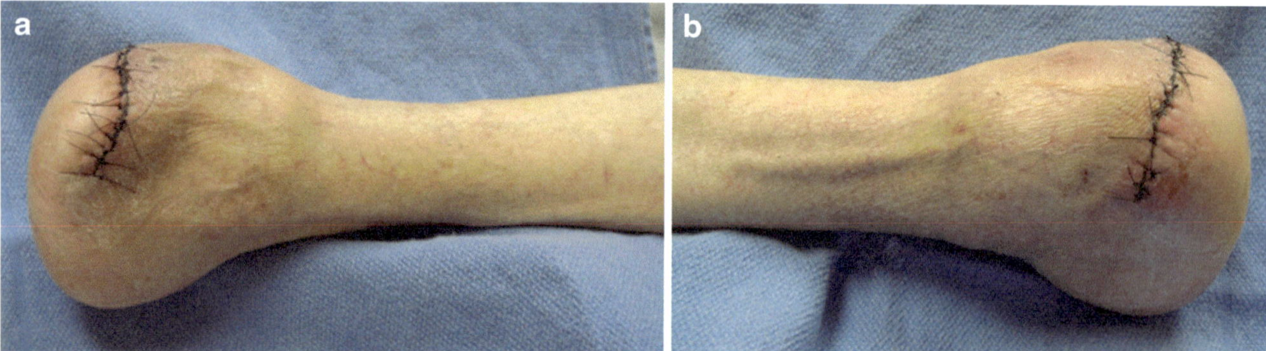

Fig. 20.7 Case 1: Chopart's amputation stump at 2 weeks postoperative. Prompt healing was achieved due to the appropriately selected level of amputation based on local vascularity and tissue quality. The traditional dorsal and plantar flap technique preserved the weight bearing pad of the heel. The short nature of the Chopart's amputation stump allowed bipedal weight bearing for transfer and limited walking with a prosthetic but greatly compromised foot function

Modified Chopart's Amputation Technique (Naviculocuneiform Disarticulation)

Our preferred "Chopart's" amputation technique involves preservation of the navicular provided that the soft tissue flaps can provide adequate coverage of the longer stump. This naviculocuneiform level of amputation is a unique approach that has advantages from a biomechanical standpoint. The traditional Chopart's level of amputation results in complete loss of calcaneal inclination angle, maximum plantarflexion of the talus within the ankle joint mortise, and overload of the lateral column. The head of the talus bears minimal to no weight, and tendon balancing does not actually balance these deformities. Preserving the navicular allows weight transfer through the medial column by extending the reach of the talar head in an attempt to provide improved balance of the amputation stump due to equal length of bone anterior and posterior to the ankle joint. This approach also preserves the insertion of the posterior tibial tendon which could be released if there is concern for inversion deformity. The cartilage on the exposed navicular is left undisturbed although some dorsal remodeling may be necessary to round off the dorsal edge. Figure 20.8 discusses the intended functional benefit of preserving the navicular.

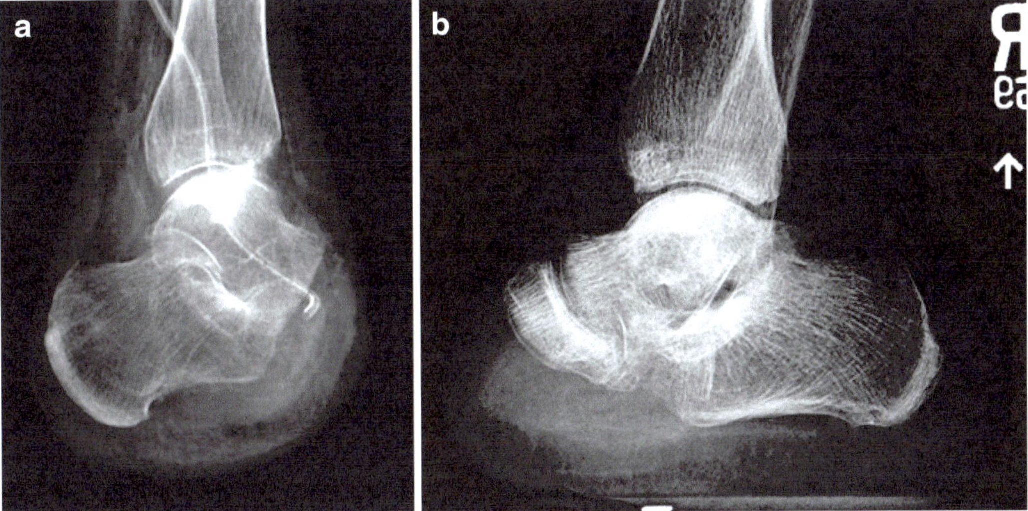

Fig. 20.8 Postoperative radiographs demonstrating traditional and modified Chopart's amputation levels of bone resection. (**a**) The head of the talus does not bear weight after Chopart's amputation, unless the arch was severely pronated prior to surgery. (**b**) Preservation of the navicular creates a rocker bottom forefoot with the intent to decrease lateral stress beneath the anterior calcaneus where tissue breakdown is common following this procedure. Note that the plantar aspect of the distal calcaneus has been remodeled to minimize pressure in this region. Navicular preservation also achieves a fairly similar foot length both in front of and behind the talar dome. This assists with balance of the amputation stump through the ankle and minimizes the expected plantarflexion of the talus which is demonstrated on this weight bearing X-ray

Angiosome-Based Plantar Flap Options

Significant compromise of the plantar soft tissue may suggest that BKA is the better level of amputation, especially when the plantar heel soft tissue is compromised from neuropathic ulceration, gangrene, or decubitus ulceration. Angiosome-based plantar flaps are available which take advantage of direct inflow from the medial or lateral plantar arteries as described in Chap. 19 [12]. Case 2 (Figs. 20.9, 20.10, 20.11, 20.12, 20.13, 20.14, and 20.15) demonstrates our preferred approach to lateral column midfoot ulceration complicated by osteomyelitis of the cuboid which involved a medial plantar artery angiosome (MPAA) rotational flap. The lateral plantar artery angiosome (LPAA) flap allows coverage of wound defects in the medial arch. Combined MPAA and LPAA flaps create a V to T planton flap which are used for central wound defects associated with plantar space infections as shown in Case 3 (Figs. 20.16, 20.17, 20.18, 20.19, and 20.20).

Tendon Balancing and Adjunctive Procedures

Tendon balancing in Chopart's amputation typically involves Achilles lengthening and anterior tibial tendon transfer to the dorsum of the talar neck [11–13]. The primary goal of tendon balancing is to remove the deforming force of the unopposed Achilles tendon. The secondary goal is to preserve active ankle joint dorsiflexion by transferring the tibialis anterior or extensor tendons which has marginal benefit due the ineffective lever arm of the neck of the talus. Less often, an interosseous posterior tibial tendon transfer may be performed with equally limited benefit. Delayed tendon surgery is common when infection is present at the time of amputation.

The author's preference is to perform percutaneous Achilles lengthening (TAL) or complete tenotomy as a staged procedure (Fig. 20.21a). This allows resolution of wounds or infection and the ability to assess whether the patient would benefit from lengthening once they are ambulatory. The procedure can be performed under local anesthesia in an office-based minor procedure room for patients with advanced peripheral neuropathy. Delayed TAL allows immediate weight bearing since there is no risk of over lengthening.

The anterior tibial tendon can be preserved and immediately transferred to the talar neck or dorsal navicular using soft tissue anchors (Fig. 20.21b). Tendon transfer does increase the risk of bone contamination at the clean margin in cases of osteomyelitis. Our preference is to simply cut the anterior tendons and allow natural adherence to surrounding tissues. As discussed earlier, many patients retain some active dorsiflexion following amputation at this level through adherence of the tibialis anterior, extensor, and peroneal tendons to surrounding deep tissues.

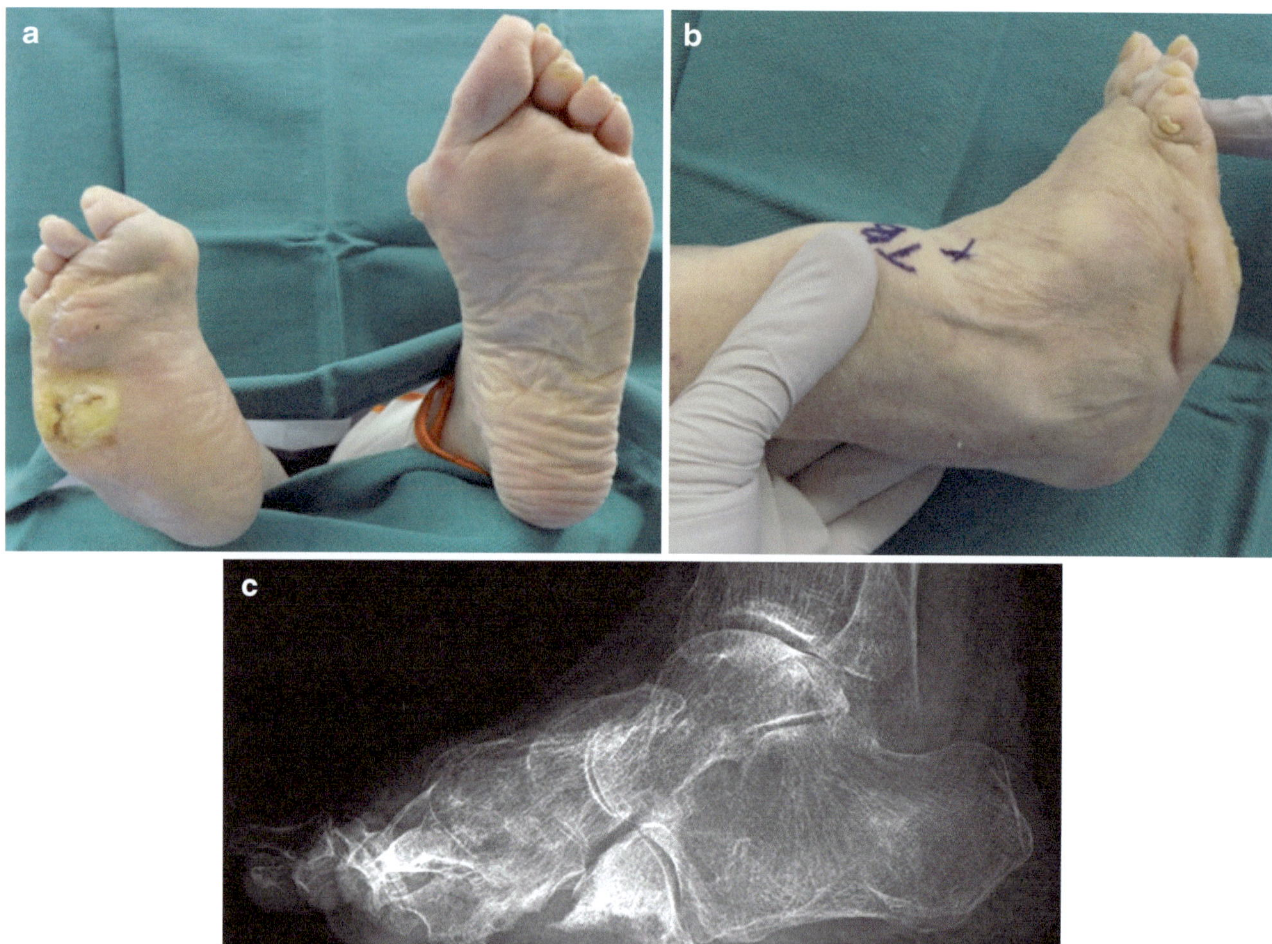

Fig. 20.9 Case 2: Cuboid osteomyelitis secondary to chronic plantar lateral midfoot wound despite numerous prior procedures for residual clubfoot. An elderly female is shown here with short right foot structure associated with residual clubfoot deformity despite surgical treatment in early childhood. Late stage pan metatarsal head resection was performed years later for recurrent forefoot ulcers. (**a, b**) Residual equin-ovarus of the rearfoot and ankle, as well as metatarsus adductus deformity created plantar lateral prominence and chronic ulceration beneath the cuboid bone. (**c**) Chronic osteomyelitis of the cuboid that had been resistant to years of bracing, periodic antibiotic therapy and repeat surgery was treated with Chopart's amputation to preserve a weight bearing limb

The talus will function in maximum plantar flexion within the ankle joint mortise despite any attempt at tendon balancing. Release of soft tissue contracture is therefore of limited benefit but may be useful for recurrent wound breakdown.

Complete release of the posterior tibial tendon may be needed with the modified Chopart's technique as preserving the navicular may predispose to inversion or plantar flexion at the subtalar joint or ankle joint.

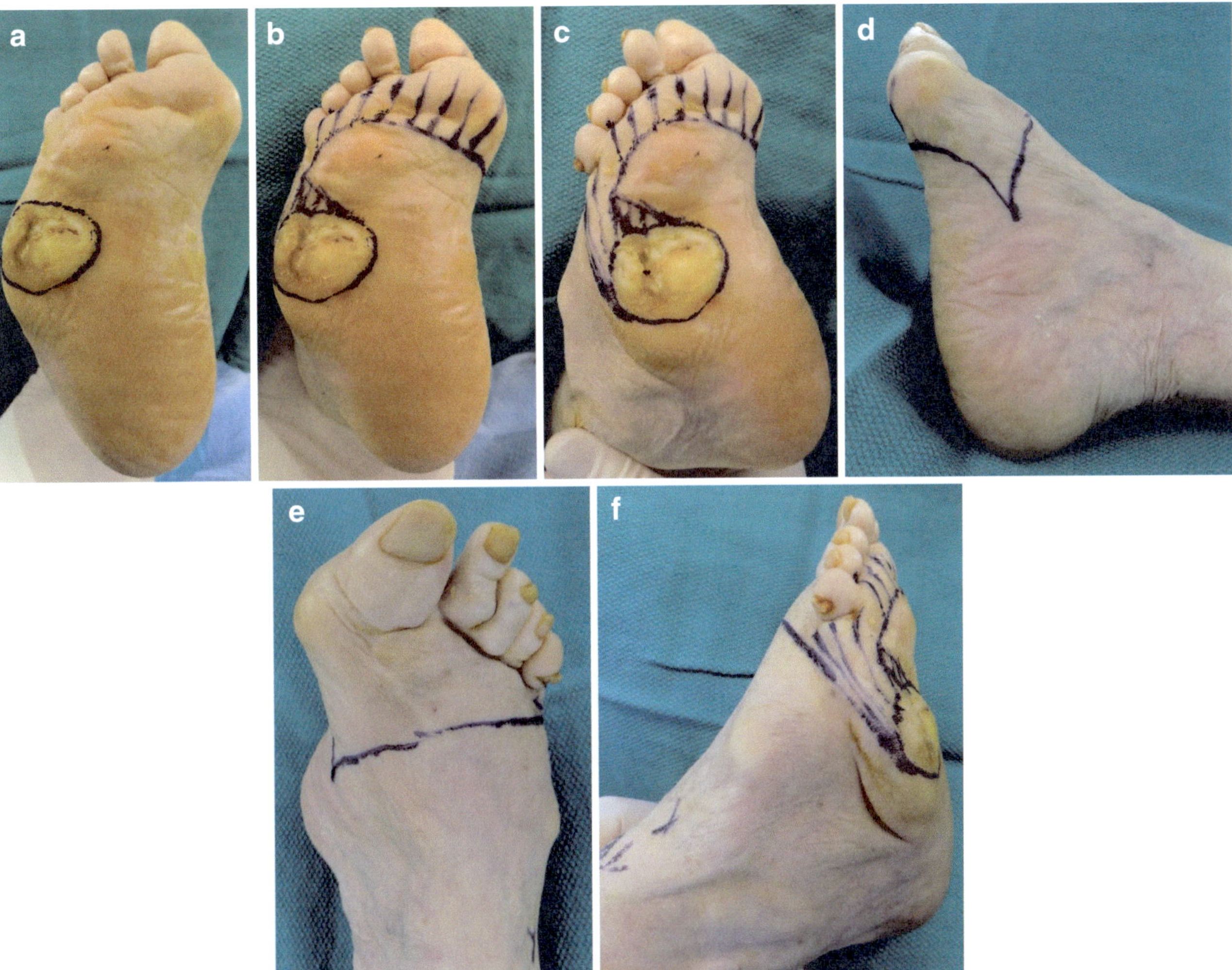

Fig. 20.10 Case 2: Medial plantar artery angiosome (MPAA) rotational flap Chopart's amputation incision design. (**a**) Chronic ulceration beneath the cuboid significantly compromised the traditional Chopart's amputation plantar flap. (**b, c**) The medial plantar artery angiosome flap took advantage of the more distal tissue that remained intact and viable. The hash lines indicate tissue that will be discarded. Note how the plantar flap was drawn quite long in comparison to the traditional Chopart's plantar incision since the flap was expected to shorten with rotation. (**d**) The medial aspect of the plantar flap was drawn in a more traditional manner. (**e & f**) The dorsal incision was made in a standard but slightly more distal fashion due to uncertainty regarding how much plantar coverage would be achieved with the rotational flap

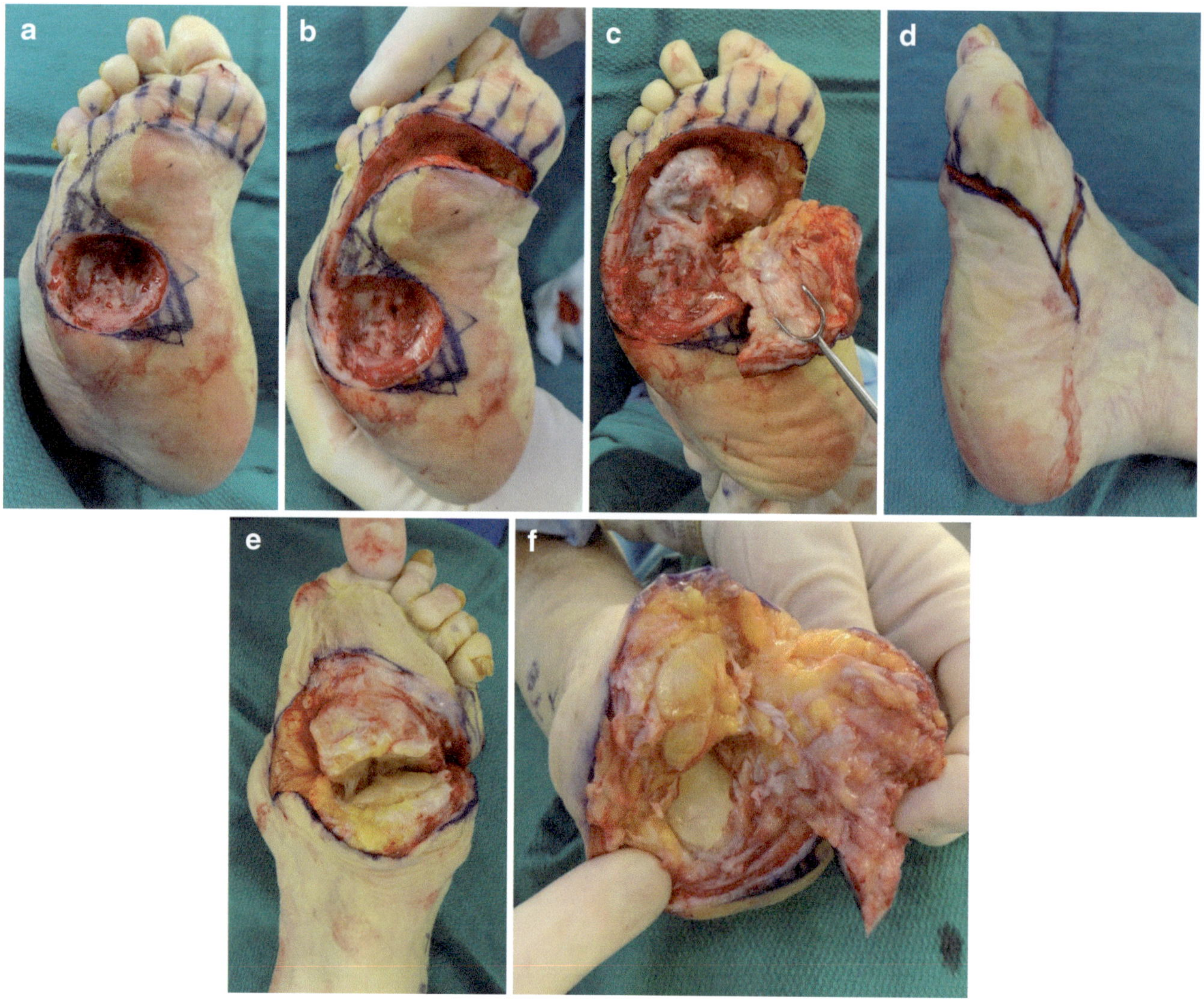

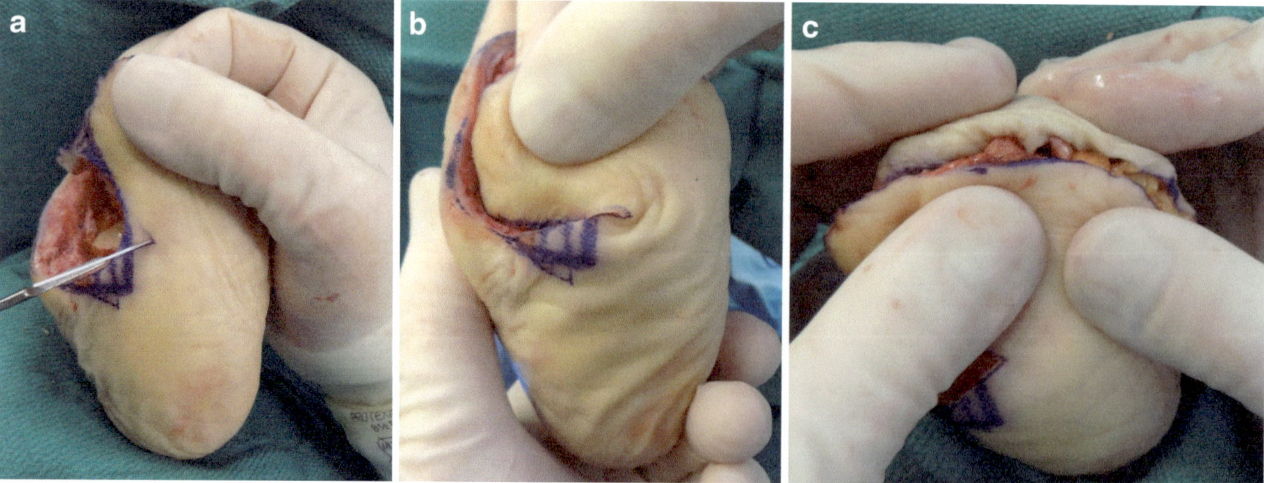

Fig. 20.11 Case 2: Raising the medial plantar artery angiosome rotational flap with disarticulation of the forefoot. (**a**)The plantar ulcer was excised full thickness down to the cuboid. (**b**)The flap incision was then made full thickness down to the metatarsals. The plantar pivot point was left undecided until the forefoot was amputated. Note the different pivot points drawn. (**c**) The flap was raised off of the metatarsal and tarsal bones with care taken to preserve the medial plantar artery. (**d**) The medial aspect of the dorsal and plantar incisions were also made full thickness. (**e & f**) Raising the dorsal flap allowed disarticulation of the forefoot through the calcaneocuboid and naviculocuneiform joints

Fig. 20.12 Case 2: Remodeling of the plantar flap for a custom fit. (**a, b**)The plantar pivot point of the flap was adjusted to provide ideal rotation of the flap. (**c**) The rotated plantar flap matched perfectly with the dorsal flap without tension on the wound

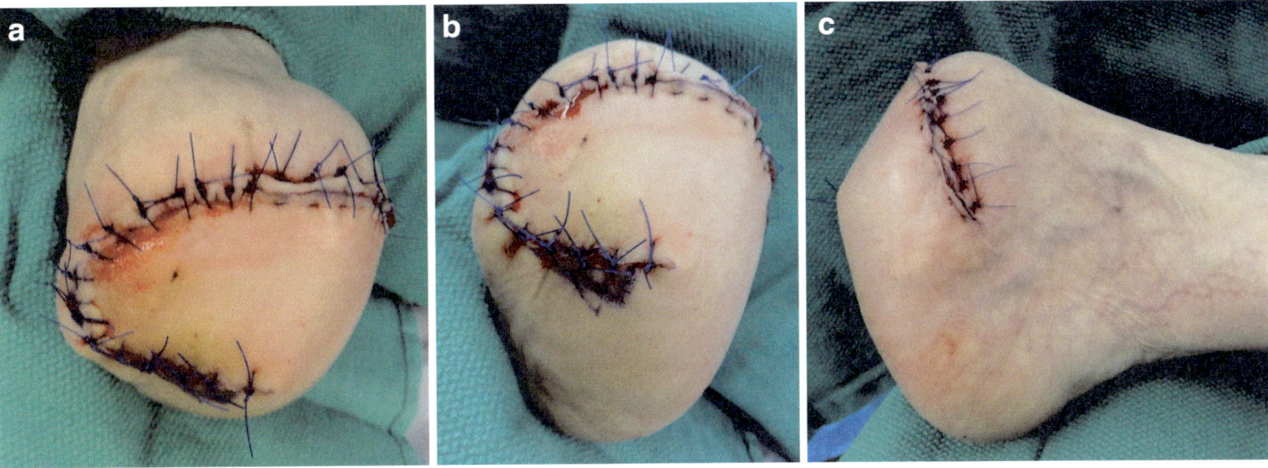

Fig. 20.13 Case 2: Flap closure of modified Chopart's amputation. (**a–c**)Complete coverage with integration of the MPAA rotational flap into the modified dorsal and lateral Chopart's incision technique. Strict non-weight bearing was necessary since the flap incision extended onto the weight bearing surface of the amputation stump

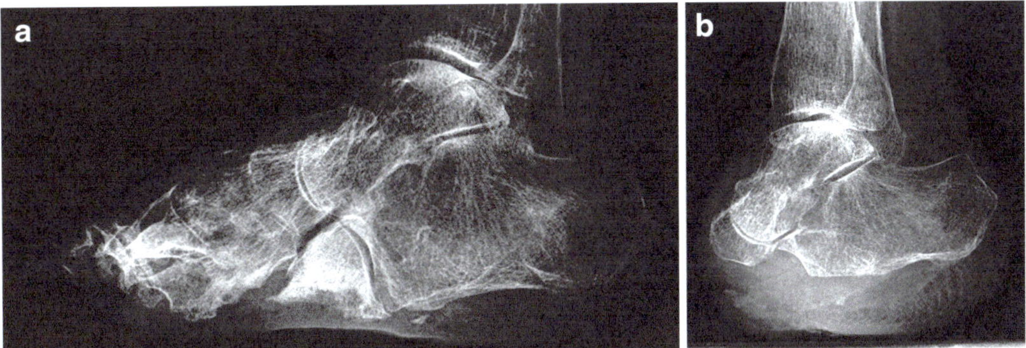

Fig. 20.14 Case 2: Preoperative and postoperative lateral weight bearing (WB) radiographs demonstrating level of amputation and function of the stump after modified Chopart's amputation. Note that the retained navicular allowed functional WB along the medial column and helped to balance forces through the talus with similar length of bone structure on both the anterior and posterior aspects of the ankle joint. The posi- tion of the talus within the ankle mortise is largely unchanged when comparing preoperative (**a**) to postoperative (**b**) lateral WB images. (**b**) The leading edge of the calcaneus has been remodeled along the plantar WB surface. Margin biopsy of the calcaneus was positive for osteomy- elitis which was treated with a six week course of IV antibiotics

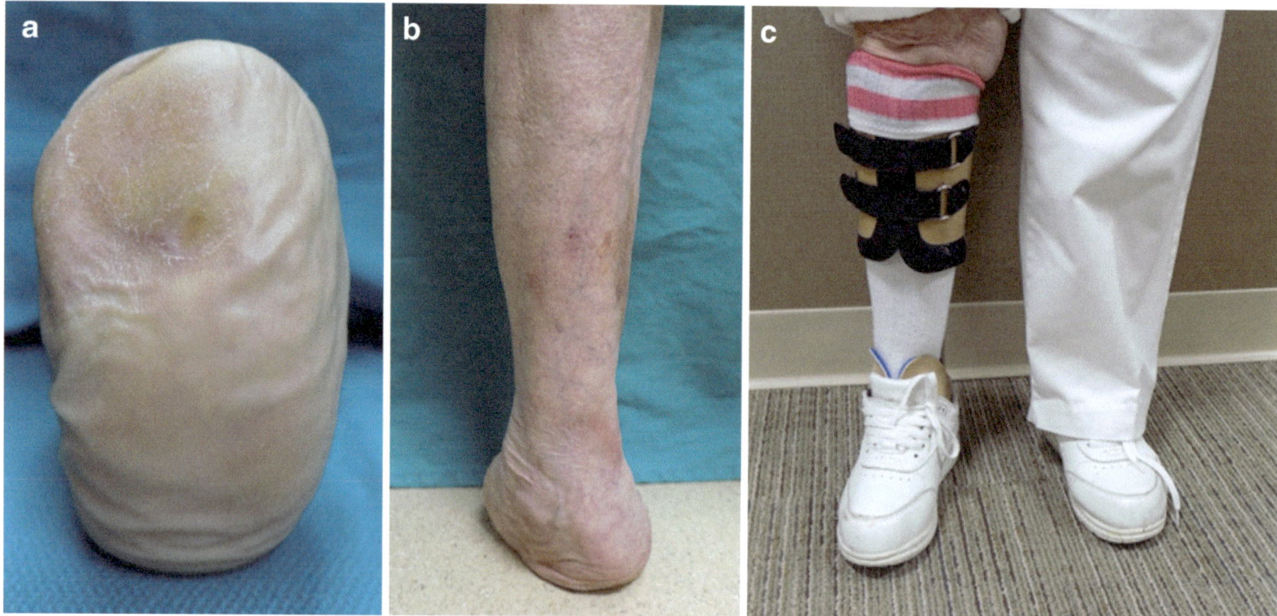

Fig. 20.15 Case 2: 12 months postoperative with complete healing. (**a–c**) Prompt healing allowed full return to activity with near normal gait using a partial foot prosthesis

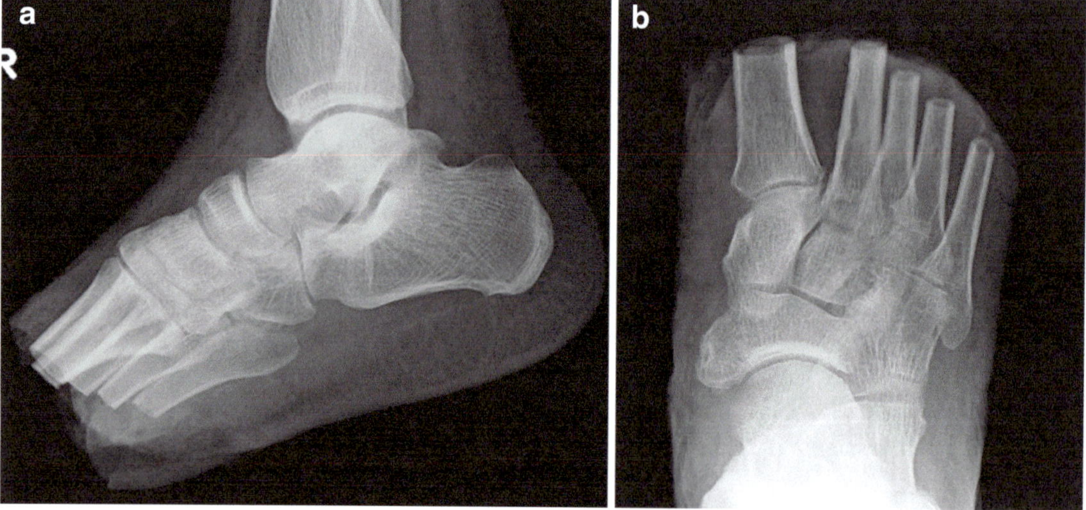

Fig. 20.16 Case 3: Immediate postoperative X-rays following stage 1 open transmetatarsal amputation (TMA). (**a, b**) Open TMA was performed to treat severe planter space infection associated with widespread gangrene and osteomyelitis of the forefoot in a diabetic with end stage renal failure and advanced neuropathy. Note how the soft tissue barely covered the resected metatarsals which typically results in poor healing and recurrent wound breakdown

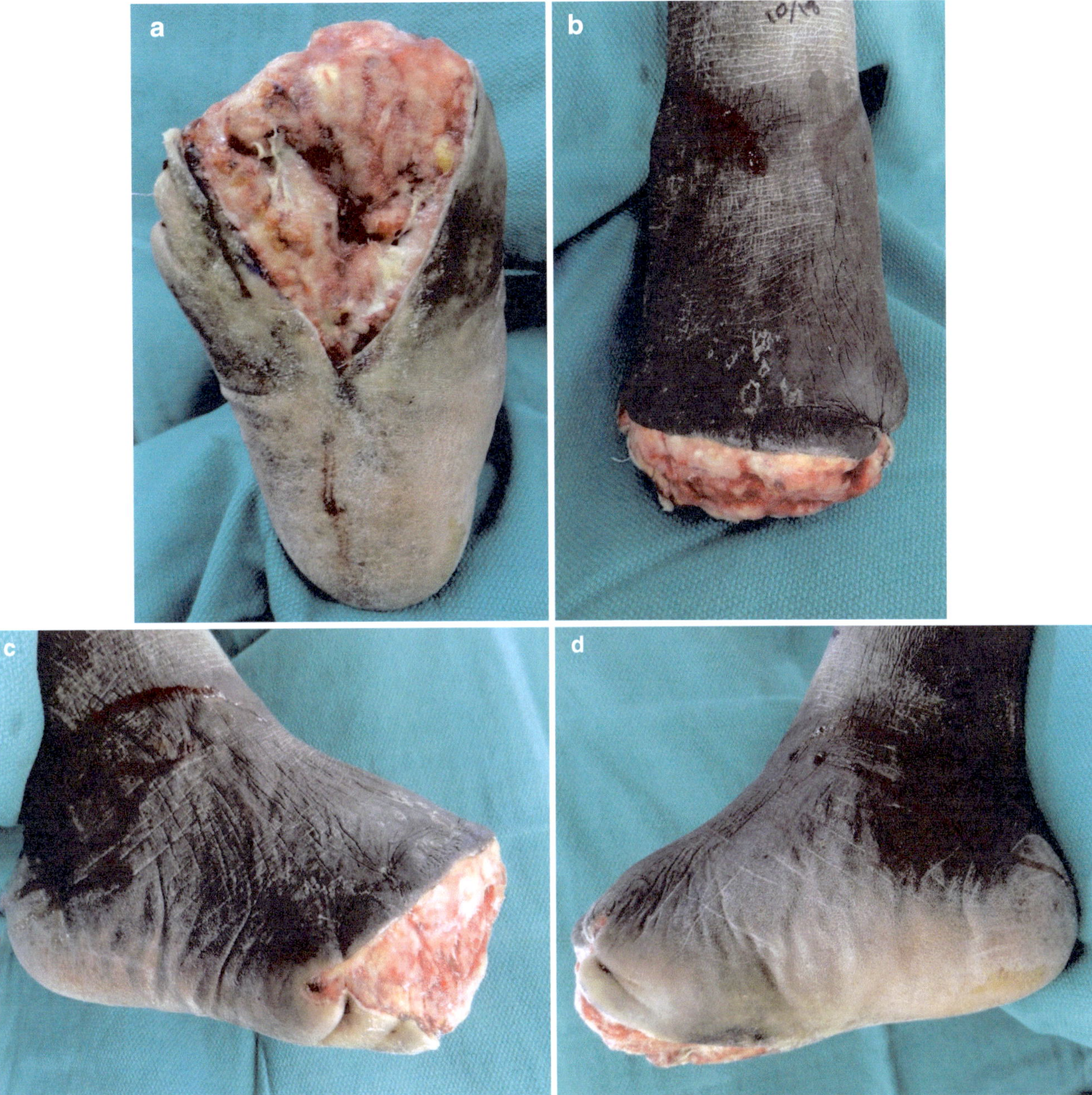

Fig. 20.17 Case 3: Deep space abscess required wide resection of plantar soft tissues. (**a–d**) Stage 1 guillotine type forefoot amputation with wide resection of necrotic and infected tissue through the plantar arch allowed demarcation prior to revision surgery. Reconstructive options were limited including substantial challenges with conversion to Chopart's amputation. Delayed skin grafting was a consideration but poor local tissue quality, chronic edema and history of dialysis predicted high likelihood of poor outcome. Leg amputation is common in this scenario

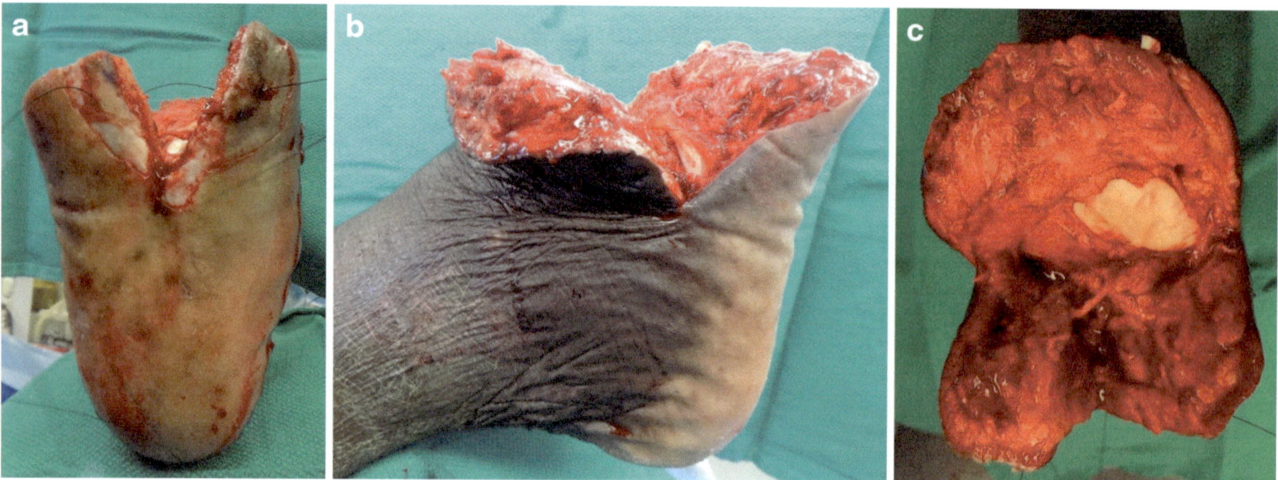

Fig. 20.18 Case 3: Stage 2 surgery involved V to T Plantar flap with conversion to modified Chopart's amputation. (**a**)The plantar soft tissue defect was addressed with a V to T rotational flap. Amputation was performed through the naviculocuneiform joint. Prompt healing of the plantar soft tissue was vital to successful limb preservation. (**b**) Note that the dorsal flap was preserved fairly long since the plantar flap was compromised by tissue loss. (**c**) Note healthy vascularity to the dorsal and plantar soft tissues

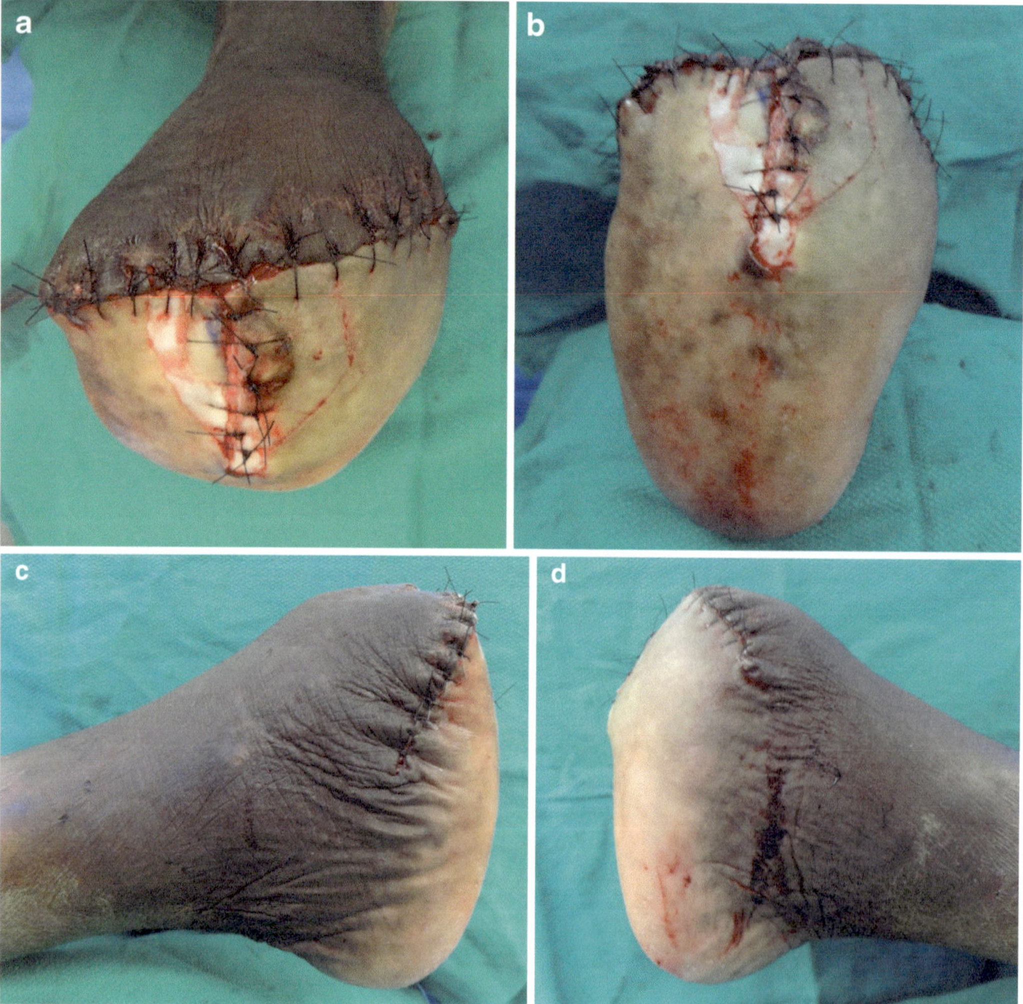

Fig. 20.19 Case 3: V to T flap closure of the plantar wound. (**a–d**) Simple sutures were placed without tension. Note that the transverse wound was near the plantar weight bearing surface due to the short nature of the plantar flap after rotation and closure of the vertical arm of the T. The long dorsal flap wrapped around to the weight bearing surface in this case which is less desirable than wrapping the plantar flap in the dorsal direction

Fig. 20.20 Case 3: Complete healing of the amputation site at ten weeks postop. (**a**–**c**)The plantar aspect of the incision healed uneventfully. Note calloused tissue associated with premature weight bearing and secondary healing. Postop WB lateral X-ray is shown in Fig. 20.8b with preservation of the navicular

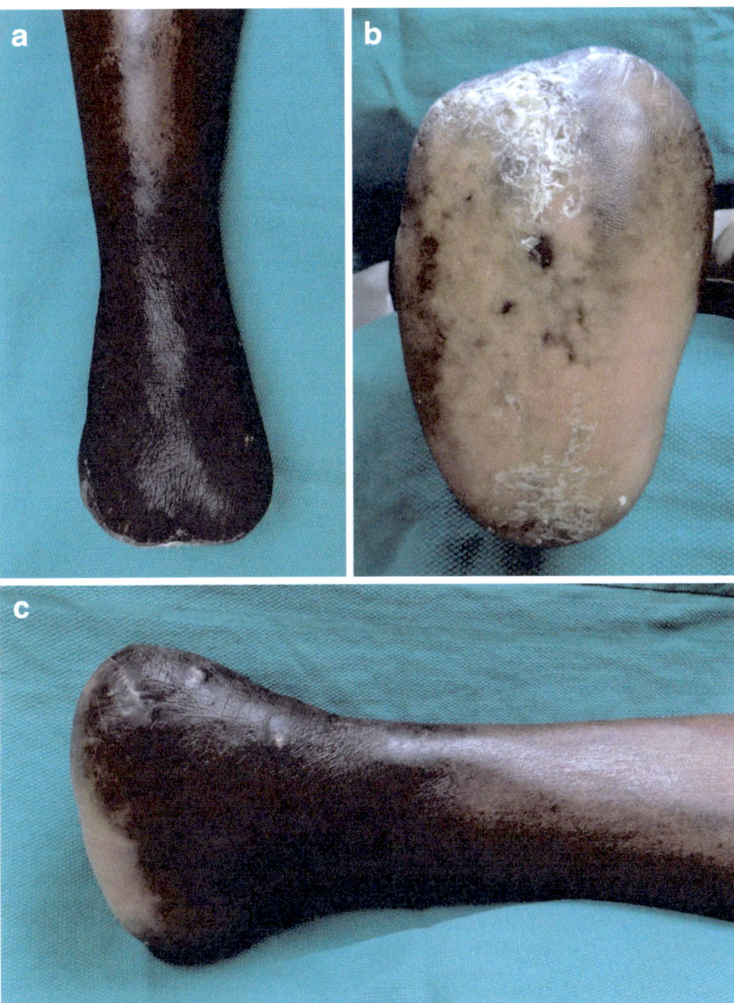

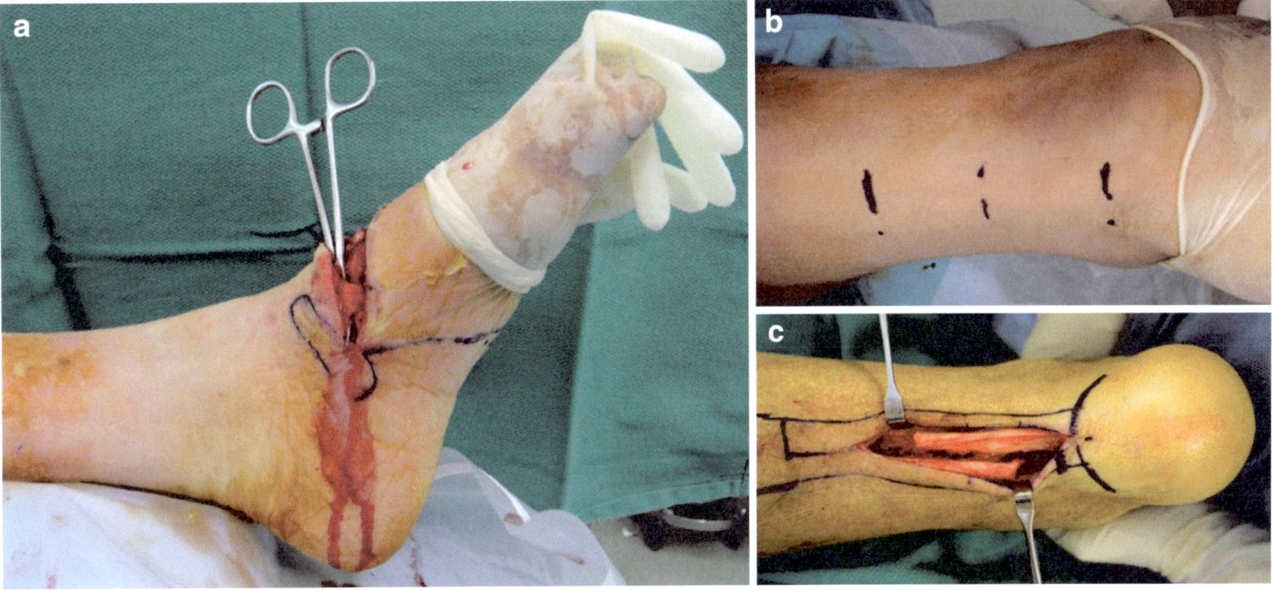

Fig. 20.21 Tendon balancing procedures in Chopart's amputation. (**a**) The dorsal incision in Chopart's amputation is largely made full thickness to bone however an attempt can be made to preserve the tibialis anterior tendon if transfer to the talar neck is desired. The tendon is being isolated here using a hemostat in an effort to preserve the tendon at maximum length. Note that a sterile glove was placed over the necrotic toes in an effort to avoid cross contamination. Achilles tendon lengthening or tenotomy can be performed using a (**b**) percutaneous or (**c**) open approach

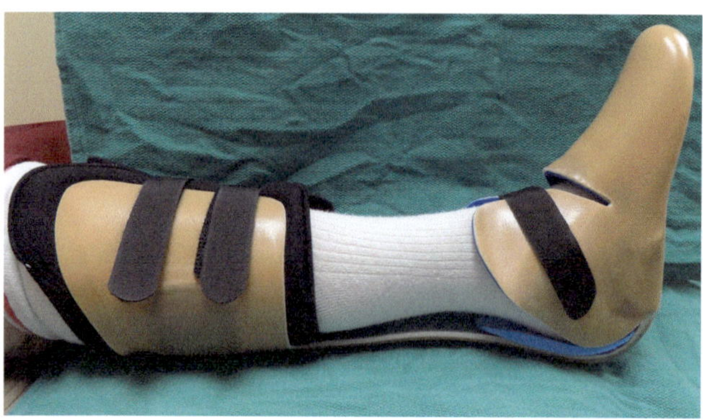

Fig. 20.22 Chopart's amputation partial foot prosthesis. This custom made partial foot prosthesis was designed with a posterior leaf spring made of composite materials which helps to restore reasonable balance and gait despite loss of the forefoot

Postoperative Care

The main goal of postoperative care is resolution of infection and protection of the fragile surgical site. Most patients undergoing partial foot amputation secondary to osteomyelitis have underlying comorbidities that may cause poor soft tissue healing and therefore should be treated with caution. Strict non-weight bearing for 6–8 weeks is the norm. Long-term intravenous antibiotics may or may not be necessary as a surgical cure of forefoot or midfoot osteomyelitis is possible with this level of amputation.

At approximately 6 weeks postoperatively, the patient may begin physical therapy for weight bearing activities provided that the incision is fully healed. The Chopart's amputee may then begin walking in a below knee fracture boot while waiting for partial foot prosthetic fitting. Once the patient is fit with the partial foot prosthesis, they may resume regular activities at approximately 8 weeks postop. This accelerated recovery timeframe assumes prompt healing of the wound but is generally favorable when compared to the rehabilitation process required for BKA.

Partial Foot Prosthetic Options

A custom-made partial foot prosthetic is useful after Chopart's amputation unless the patient's postoperative level of activity is limited to transferring in and out of a wheelchair. Our preferred prosthetic device is a calf offloader, biomechanical composite partial foot prosthesis with full foot lever arm and posterior leaf spring (Fig. 20.22). An alternative brace design is a clamshell type prosthetic device. Advances in prosthetic options for the Chopart's level amputation have helped make proximal foot amputation a more suitable option for a broader patient population due to improved postoperative function.

Conclusion

Osteomyelitis of the midfoot tarsal bones associated with neuropathic ulceration, Charcot arthropathy, and infected gangrene presents the surgeon with a complex decision in terms of ideal level of amputation. Leg amputation remains the primary approach to treating complex midfoot infections associated with nonhealing wounds. For carefully selected patients, Chopart's amputation may provide a greater level of independence in comparison to BKA. Minor modifications to the traditional Chopart's amputation technique are intended to improve the weight bearing function of the stump and decrease the risk of recurrent wound breakdown. Angiosome-based flaps are also useful when the plantar tissue is compromised by chronic wounds or gangrene.

References

1. Krause FG, Pfander G, Henning J, Maziar S, Weber M. Ankle dorsiflexion arthrodesis to salvage Chopart's amputation with anterior skin insufficiency. Foot Ankle Int. 2013;34:1560–8.
2. Liebermann JR, Jacobs RL, Goldstock L, Durham J, Fuchs MD. Chopart's amputations with percutaneous heel cord lengthening. Clin Orthop. 1993;296:86–91.
3. Pinzur MS, Kaminsky M, Sage R, Cronin R, Osterman H. Amputations at the middle level of the foot. J Bone Joint Surg Am. 1986;68:1061–4.
4. Pinzur MS, Sage R, Stuck R, Osterman H. Amputations in the diabetic foot and ankle. Clin Orthop. 1993;296:64–7.
5. Sage R, Pinzur MS, Cronin R, Preuss HF, Osterman H. Complications following midfoot amputation in neuropathic and dysvascular feet. J Am Podiatr Med Assoc. 1989;79:277–80.
6. Waters RL, Perry J, Garland D. Surgical correction of gait abnormalities. Clin Orthop. 1978;131:54–7.
7. Ostojiæ L, Ostojiæ Z, Rupèiæ E, Punda-Bašiæ M. Intermediate rehabilitation outcome in below-knee amputations: descriptive study comparing war-related other causes of amputation. Croat Med J. 2001;42:535–8.
8. Schade VL, Roukis TS, Yan JL. Factors associated with successful chopart amputation in patients with diabetes: a systematic review. Foot Ankle Spec. 2010;3(5):278–84.
9. Baima J, Trovato M, Hopkins M, Delauter B. Achieving functional ambulation in a patient with Chopart amputation. Am J Phys Med Rehabil. 2008;87:510–13.
10. Burger H, Erzar D, Maver T, Olensek A. Biomechanics of walking with silicone prosthesis after midtarsal (Chopart) disarticulation. Clin Biomech (Bristol, Avon). 2000;24:510–6.
11. Letts M, Pyper A. The modified Chopart's amputation. Clin Orthop Relat Res. 1990;256:44–9.
12. Attinger C, Venturi A, Kim K, Ribiero C. Maximizing length and optimizing biomechanics in foot amputations by avoiding cookbook recipes for amputations. Semin Vasc Surg. 2003;16:44–66.
13. Reyzelman A, Hadi S. Limb Salvage with Chopart's amputation and tendon balancing. J Am Podiatr Med Assoc. 1999;89:100.

Troy J. Boffeli and Rachel C. Collier

Osteomyelitis of the calcaneus most commonly results from contiguous spread of infection from an adjacent decubitus heel ulcer. The heel is the second most common site of decubitus ulceration [1, 2] yet relatively few become complicated with infection of the calcaneus. Any neuropathic, ischemic, surgical, or traumatic wound on the heel can result in contiguous spread of infection to the calcaneus; however, decubitus ulceration adds complexity due to a potentially large soft tissue deficit [3, 4]. Hematogenous osteomyelitis is most often encountered in the pediatric population with treatment primarily involving intravenous antibiotics which is covered in Chap. 7. The third potential route of infection is from direct inoculation which is generally caused by puncture wounds to the heel with penetration of a nail or other sharp object directly into the calcaneus. Unlike infected decubitus ulcers, puncture-related wounds are small and largely inconsequential when considering treatment options for the associated osteomyelitis.

The optimal treatment plan for an individual patient with calcaneal osteomyelitis is highly dependent on the extent of bone involvement, size, and location of the soft tissue deficit, local circulation, viability of the surrounding soft tissues, patient age, and anticipated future activity level. Successful treatment typically involves a combined medical and surgical approach although isolated medical treatment is possible depending on the clinical situation. Surgical treatment typically involves excision of the open wound, bone biopsy, debridement of necrotic bone, and advanced closure techniques. Minimally invasive surgery is possible for osteomyelitis associated with small wounds. This chapter will primarily focus on surgical decision making including various approaches to debridement of the calcaneus and wound coverage options.

T.J. Boffeli, DPM, FACFAS (✉)
R.C. Collier, FACFAOM
Regions Hospital/HealthPartners Institute for Education
and Research, 640 Jackson Street, St. Paul, MN 55101, USA
e-mail: troy.j.boffeli@healthpartners.com;
rachel.c.collier@healthpartners.com

When initially developing a treatment plan, the route of infection (hematogenous, direct inoculation, or contiguous spread) can lead to generalized groupings of treatment protocols (Fig. 21.1). Medical management is needed for nearly all cases of calcaneal osteomyelitis regardless of surgical intervention unless the leg is amputated. Conservative surgical approaches such as cortical windowing with internal medullary debridement or wound excision with cortical debridement are preferred when clinically appropriate in an effort to preserve the structure and function of the calcaneus. Partial calcanectomy with flap closure can be a successful limb salvage approach but does not preserve normal foot function [5–15]. Leg amputation remains a viable treatment alternative for advanced osteomyelitis in a non-salvageable limb with extensive tissue loss from decubitus pressure, infection, or gangrene. Table 21.1 provides an overview of the various surgical treatment protocols for calcaneal osteomyelitis. Clinical examples are presented to highlight three different surgical treatment protocols including patient selection criteria, surgical technique tips, staging guidelines, and typical postoperative care plans including postoperative bracing options.

Clinical and Radiographic Workup

A standardized workup for osteomyelitis including probe to bone, vascular status, inflammatory marker labs, and imaging is important for the diagnosis and management of calcaneal osteomyelitis (Fig. 21.2). Radiographic changes generally lag behind the initial development of osteomyelitis by a few weeks. Baseline X-rays early in the course of heel ulceration are helpful for later comparison as anatomy can vary. The opposite heel can also be imaged for comparison as the calcaneus is largely symmetrical in most individuals. A positive probe-to-bone exam or unexplained elevation of inflammatory marker labs raises concern for bone infection at which point advanced imaging or biopsy is helpful to confirm the diagnosis. Advanced imaging such as MRI may have clinical utility even with X-ray changes in an effort to determine the extent of bone infection or involvement of adjacent soft tissues. If the

© Springer International Publishing Switzerland 2015
T.J. Boffeli (ed.), *Osteomyelitis of the Foot and Ankle*, DOI 10.1007/978-3-319-18926-0_21

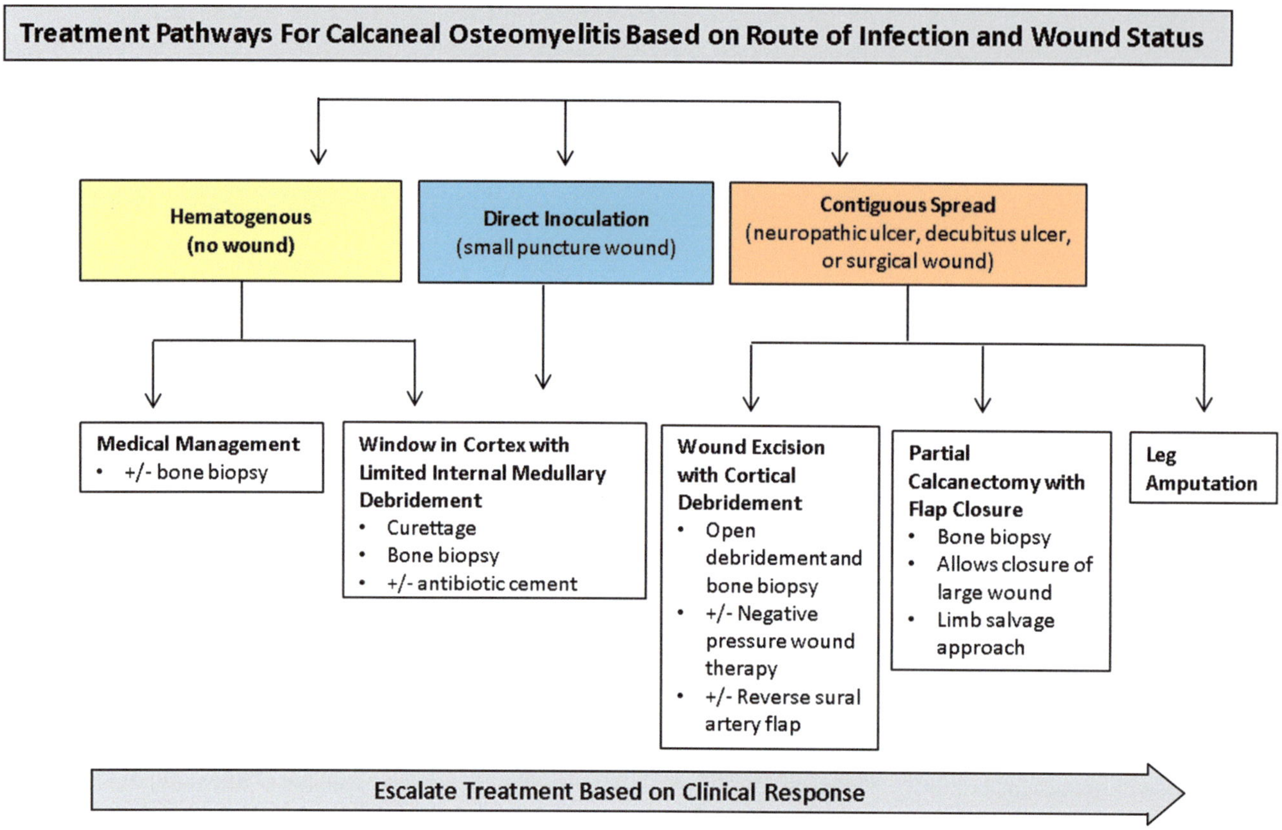

Treatment Pathways For Calcaneal Osteomyelitis Based on Route of Infection and Wound Status

Fig. 21.1 Flow diagram for treatment options based on route of calcaneal osteomyelitis and wound status. Calcaneal osteomyelitis is generally caused by one of three routes of infection including hematogenous, direct inoculation from penetrating trauma, or contiguous spread of infection from adjacent ulceration. Treatment options are dependent on multiple variables including the source of the infection, extent of bone involvement, surrounding soft tissue quality and wound deficit, vascular status, and ambulatory status. The flowchart diagrams our five treatment options which are largely based on route of infection and wound status. Despite surgical intervention, medical management with antibiotics is required in the treatment pathways unless the leg is amputated. This protocol assumes that treatment may be escalated if poor clinical response is encountered

infection extends into the adjacent bones of the rearfoot, limb salvage techniques are likely to fail (Fig. 21.3a). Bone scan and CT are reasonable alternatives for patients unable to undergo MRI. Bone scan is a cost-effective screening method to rule out osteomyelitis, especially in patients with bilateral decubitus heel ulceration (Fig. 21.3b).

Adequate blood flow for healing of the surgical procedure is necessary especially when considering a local flap for closure purposes. The blood supply to the heel is from two source arteries, the lateral calcaneal branch from the peroneal artery and the medial calcaneal branch from the posterior tibial artery [16]. The success of surgical intervention is related to the patency of these two arteries. Patients with non-reconstructible vascular compromise may not be able to successfully heal after foot surgery, and leg amputation may be more prudent for this patient population.

Isolated Medical Management

Medical management of calcaneal osteomyelitis without surgical intervention is feasible under certain circumstances, particularly in hematogenous osteomyelitis which is covered in Chap. 7. Bone biopsy is ideal but not always necessary for patients undergoing medical management which allows culture-specific antibiotic treatment. The trephine or needle bone biopsy technique can be performed as a sterile bedside procedure under local anesthesia, especially in patients with neuropathy. Bone biopsy techniques are covered in Chap. 4. Calcaneal osteomyelitis associated with infected decubitus ulcers, open trauma, and postoperative infections is frequently not amenable to isolated medical management due to wound infection, soft tissue defect, exposed bone, necrotic bone, and soft tissue abscess.

Table 21.1 Treatment protocols for calcaneal osteomyelitis

| | Preservation of functional calcaneus | | | Limb Salvage | Non-salvagable Limb |
	Medical Management	Window in Cortex limited with Medullary Curettage	Wound Excision and Corticotomy	Partial Calcanectomy with Rotational Flap Closure	Leg Amputation
Patient Selection	• Hematogenous osteomyelitis	• Hematogenous osteomyelitis with bone abscess • Medullary infection from penetrating injury	• Contiguous spread from infected local wound • Osteomyelitis from surgical wound (calcaneus fracture ORIF, heel surgery)	• Contiguous spread from necrotic decubitus ulcer • Local soft tissues amenable to flap closure • Current use of limb for transfers or ambulation	• Non-reconstructible vascular compromise • Non-viable peri-wound tissue • Massive edema or lymphedema • Patient who does not use limb to transfer
Soft tissue defect	• None	• Minimal or no wound defect	• Small to moderate decubitus ulcer • Surgical wound dehiscence	• Large posterior or plantar wound defect with bone exposure	• Large wound defect with loss of WB surface • Infected gangrene
Condition and location of of infected bone	• Infected but viable medullary bone	• Medullary bone infection with intact cortical shell	• Broad area of non-viable cortex at base of wound with viable medullary bone	• Widespread infection of calcaneus with healthy peri-wound tissue	• Widespread necrosis of calcaneus • Infection and necrosis spreading into adjacent tissue and bone
Treatment Pearls	• IV followed by PO antibiotics • Monitor infection labs • Consider bone biopsy • Consider blood cultures • Escalate therapy if worsening or recurrent infection	• Allows bone debridement and biopsy without compromising structure of calcaneus • Preserves Achilles tendon insertion • Curettage to healthy, bleeding bone • Consider local antibiotic delivery with beads or cement	• Preserves plantar tuberosity and/or Achilles attachment • Wound excision with debridement of cortex to viable bone • Consider negative pressure therapy or muscle flap with skin graft or reverse sural artery flap for large wound defect	• Wide resection of infected bone creates opportunity for local rotational flap closure • Immediate or staged flap coverage decreases risk of recontamination and re-ulceration • Limb preservation maintains a functional limb to allow transfers and ambulation with an AFO brace	Timely BKA may avoid AKA Staged amputation is common Failure of prior treatment Ambulation with a BK prosthesis is more functional than partial calcanectomy for community ambulators
Antibiotic goal	Isolated medical treatment	Treat residual infection in remaining viable bone, surgery allows shorter antibiotic course and biopsy driven therapy			Long term antibiotics are not needed

BKA below-knee amputation, *AKA* above-knee amputation

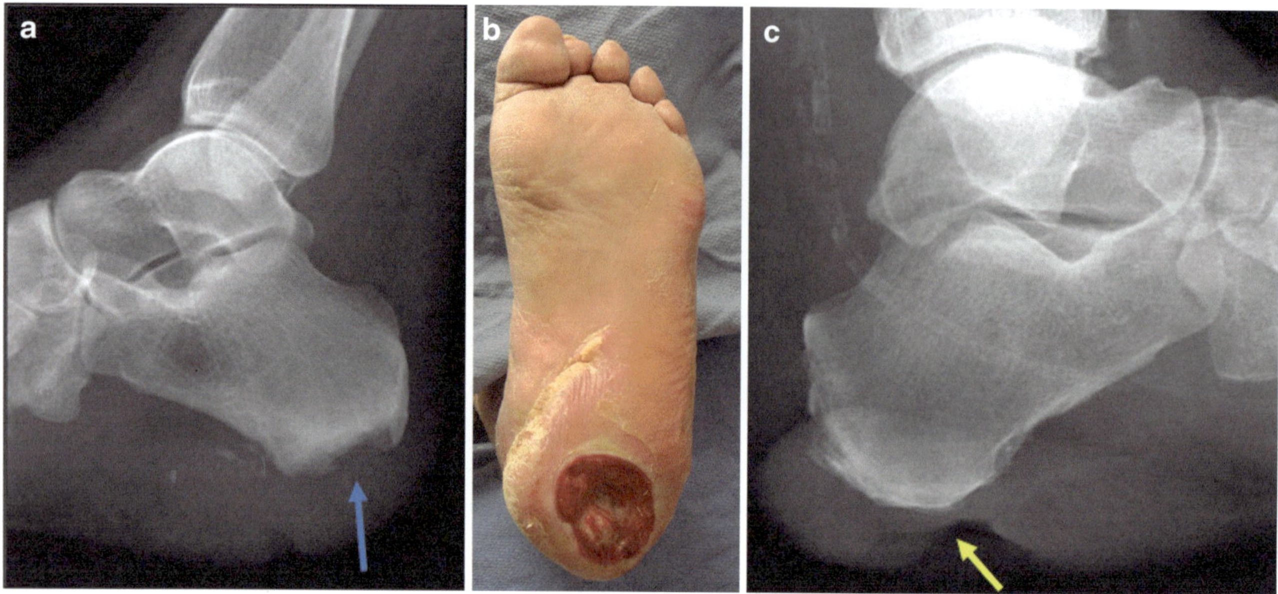

Fig. 21.2 Radiographic evaluation in the workup of calcaneal osteomyelitis. Standard X-rays are the first-line imaging study and should not be skipped for advanced imaging. Our heel X-ray protocol includes four views of the heel which includes the lateral, both obliques, and an axial view. Baseline X-rays for slow-healing wounds are useful for comparison months later if infection develops. Alternatively, bilateral comparison views serve a similar purpose. (**a**) Cortical erosion is typically the first sign of infection as seen here deep to a decubitus ulcer at the apex of the heel (*blue arrow*). (**b**) X-ray findings should be correlated with the clinical picture including location and depth of the wound and clinical signs of infection. (**c**) Note how this large soft tissue defect extends to bone (*yellow arrow*) yet the calcaneus appears relatively normal

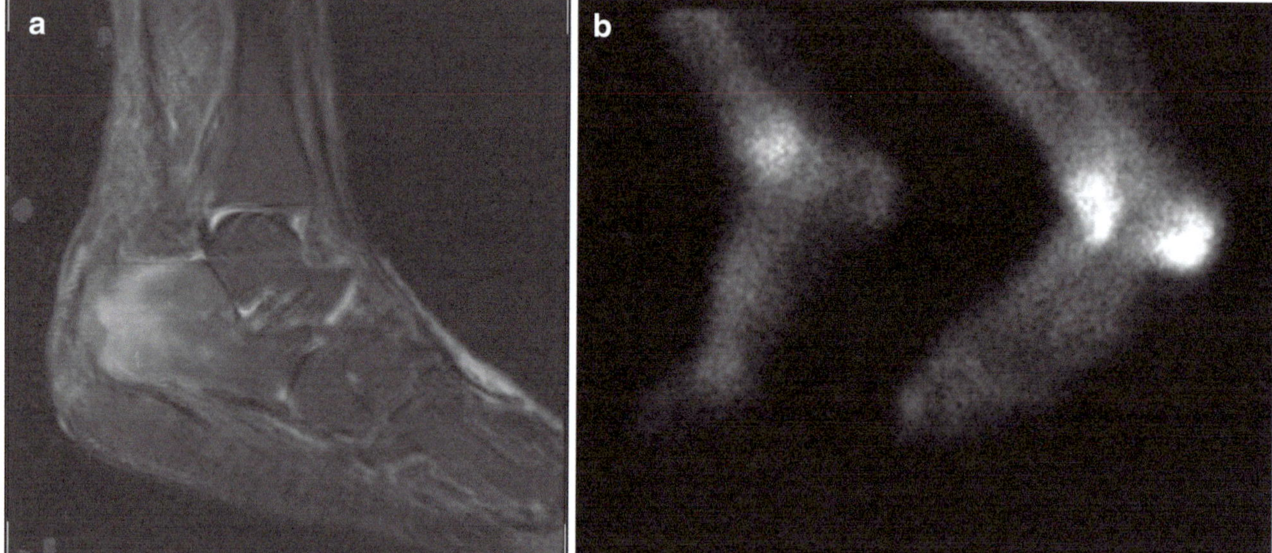

Fig. 21.3 Advanced imaging for diagnosis of calcaneal osteomyelitis and surgical planning. MRI is our go-to advanced imaging modality for calcaneal osteomyelitis. CT and bone scan have clinical utility depending on individual patient circumstances. Advanced imaging can be very sensitive to detect early onset of osteomyelitis but is not entirely diagnostic as false-positive studies are common. Advanced imaging is useful to determine the extent of osteomyelitis; however, bone inflammation as seen on MRI and bone scan can be misleading regarding viability of the involved bone. MRI is useful to evaluate for involvement of the surrounding soft tissues including the plantar arch or proximal leg as well as the subtalar joint, ankle joint, and talus. Infection spreading into these adjacent structures is more likely to be treated with leg amputation as local measures are less effective. (**a**) Once infected, a large portion of the calcaneus will appear inflamed on MRI. Intraoperative assessment of bone viability is important under these circumstances to determine if bone is dead and abscessed or inflamed yet viable. Bone scan has practical implications for screening, especially in patients with bilateral decubitus wound infection. (**b**) Bone scan images suggest unilateral osteomyelitis and decrease the need for bilateral MRI. Bone scan is not as useful for anatomic delineation of infection but is very sensitive for early-onset screening

Cortical Window with Internal Medullary Bone Debridement

Cortical window and medullary bone debridement allows internal medullary debridement of infection with preservation of the structure and function of the calcaneus by preserving the cortical shell which is largely uninvolved in osteomyelitis caused by direct inoculation or hematogenous source. MRI is useful to determine the extent of bone abscess or necrosis; however, it is important to note that inflammation of the medullary bone on MRI does not necessarily indicate dead bone. Infected bone can be preserved as long as it remains viable which is best determined on direct operative inspection. This conservative surgical approach allows decompression of sequestered infection and procurement of tissue for bone biopsy through a small incision.

Patient Selection

Calcaneal osteomyelitis associated with penetrating injuries or hematogenous spread frequently involves medullary bone infection without significant infection of the surrounding soft tissues or cortical bone. Puncture wounds to the heel may violate the cortical bone with implantation of bacteria directly into the medulla of the calcaneus due to the high-impact nature of stepping on a nail [17]. The puncture wound may heal uneventfully while the infection festers deep within the calcaneus with late presentation similar to hematogenous osteomyelitis. Although rare, there is also a potential to develop calcaneal osteomyelitis after injection for plantar fasciitis, and case studies have been described in the literature [18, 19].

Surgical Technique

Typically there is minimal or no wound defect present which allows for ellipse of the small wound or linear incision for exposure to the infected bone as demonstrated in case 1 (Figs. 21.4, 21.5, and 21.6). A medium-sized trephine is used to core out the involved bone or open the cortex (Fig. 21.7). A curette can then be inserted into the canal with the goal to curette to healthy, bleeding bone and procure specimen for biopsy. This technique can be performed in a staged-type manor with the initial surgery involving incision and drainage, bone debridement, placement of antibiotic beads, and wound closure. The stage 2 procedure allows bead removal, repeat debridement, clean margin bone biopsy, and final wound closure (Fig. 21.8a).

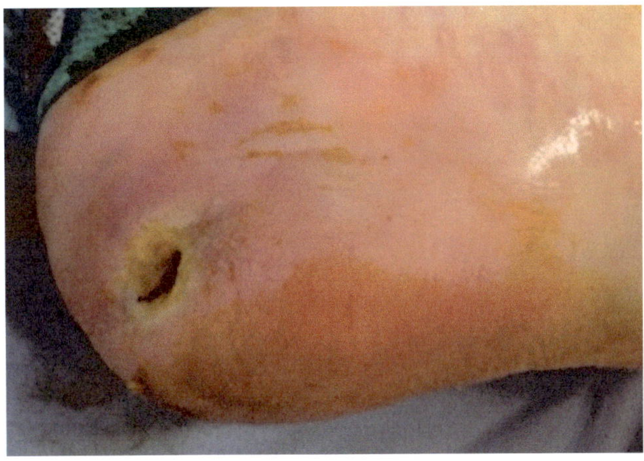

Fig. 21.4 Patient selection for cortical window with internal medullary debridement technique is shown in case 1. This minimally invasive approach is considered in patients with small wounds and localized bone infection associated with penetrating injuries or hematogenous spread of infection. Note the small but penetrating heel wound which probed to bone raising concern for osteomyelitis

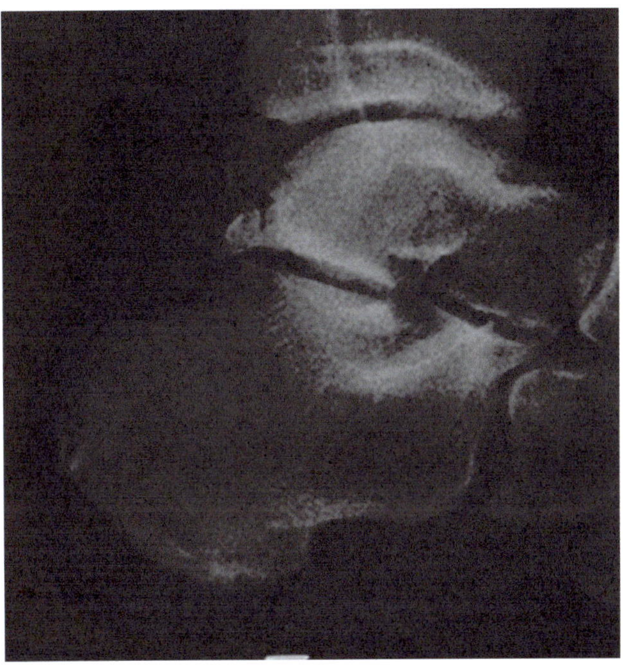

Fig. 21.5 X-ray changes correlate with the location of the small heel wound in case 1. Preoperative radiographs demonstrated lucency and mottling of the posterior aspect of the calcaneal tuberosity which is highly suspicious for osteomyelitis. Elevated ESR and CRP were also consistent with osteomyelitis. MRI followed by bone biopsy and medullary debridement through a cortical window was the next logical step

Bone Grafting of the Defect

Small bone defects can heel secondarily, while large defects may require bone grafting in an effort to minimize the risk of pathologic fracture. Serial negative bone cultures performed during repeat antibiotic bead exchange procedures allow successful bone grafting once culture is negative. Absorbable antibiotic-impregnated calcium sulfate pellets are another option although these are commonly associated with persistent drainage from the surgical wound as the resorbing material is extruded [20–23] (Fig. 21.8).

Postoperative Care

A major benefit of this calcaneus sparing approach is that the Achilles tendon attachment and plantar weight bearing aspect of the heel are not affected. Wound closure is immediate or delayed depending on the clinical situation. The same incision can be used for multiple debridement procedures if a staged approach is needed. Postoperative weight bearing status is

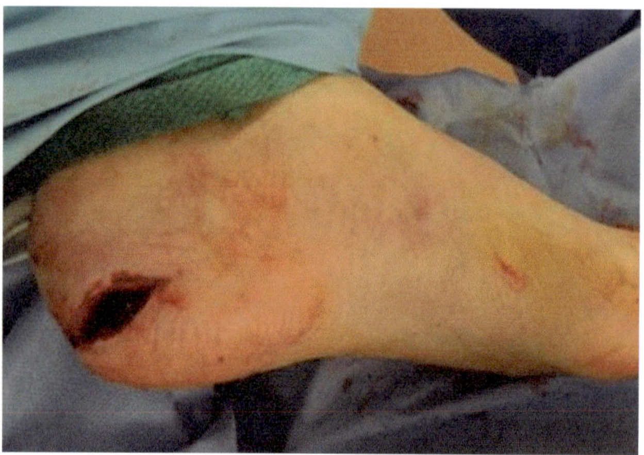

Fig. 21.6 Incision approach in case 1 for biopsy technique through the wound. A 3:1 ellipse of the small wound allowed access for bone debridement and excision of the sinus tract. A linear or oblique incision may be used if there is no soft tissue defect. The incision is kept off of the weight bearing surface and away from the Achilles tendon, sural nerve, and vascular structures where possible. Layered dissection is not necessary or desired since the incision is small and there are no vital structures on the medial, lateral, or plantar aspects of the posterior tuberosity of the heel

determined by the location of the incision and extent of bone debridement. There is risk of pathologic calcaneus fracture from infection or surgical manipulation. It is common to leave stitches in place for up to 6 weeks in the diabetic population if wound healing is delayed (Fig. 21.9). Inflammatory marker labs are monitored to direct the course of antibiotics. Antibiotics are used to treat residual infection as this surgical approach is not intended to be curative in isolation.

Wound Excision with Cortical Debridement

Excision of a decubitus, traumatic, or surgical wound followed by conservative debridement of the underlying cortical bone allows removal of necrotic tissue, debridement of nonviable cortical bone, procurement of bone tissue for biopsy, and exposure of vascular cancellous bone which promotes granulation tissue to allow progressive wound healing. The overall structure of the calcaneus is preserved to maintain heel function. The insertion of the Achilles tendon is preserved when possible although posterior wounds are frequently compromised by exposure and necrosis of the distal Achilles.

This conservative surgical approach takes into account that the remaining calcaneus is infected but still healthy enough to recover with combined medical and conservative surgical management. Local antibiotic delivery is not very practical with this approach due to lack of dead space to accommodate insertion of antibiotic-impregnated beads.

Patient Selection

Calcaneal osteomyelitis associated with contiguous spread of infection from an adjacent decubitus, surgical, neuropathic, or traumatic wound commonly involves a full-thickness soft tissue defect and necrosis of the exposed periosteum and cortical bone. The internal medullary bone

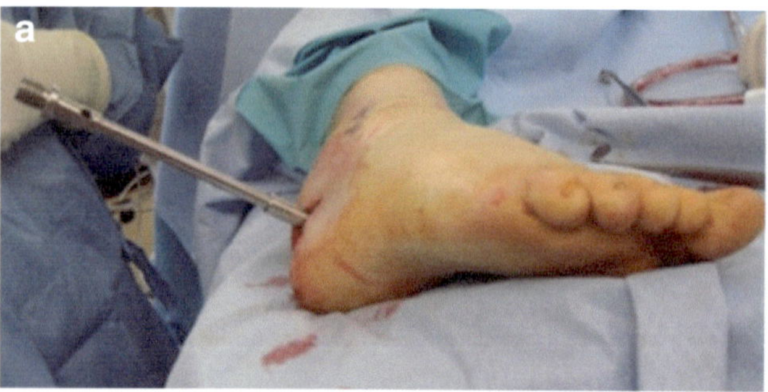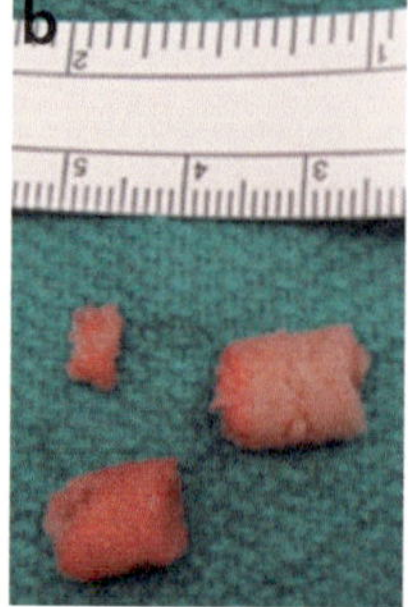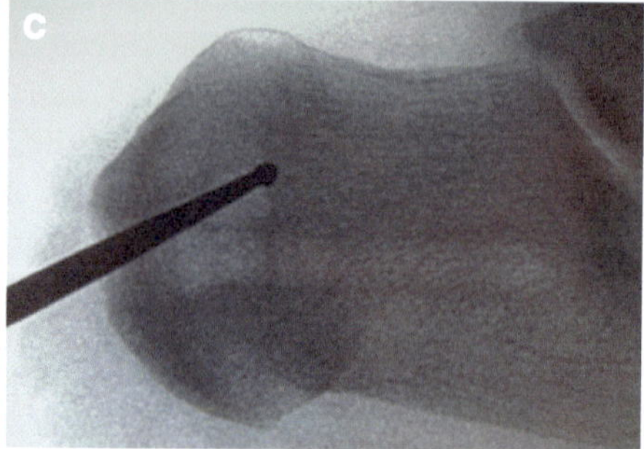

Fig. 21.7 Case 1: Bone debridement and biopsy preferred technique. (**a**) Bone biopsy was obtained with the use of a medium-sized trephine to open the cortex and core out the involved bone and sinus tract. (**b**) This provides bone specimen for biopsy. (**c**) A narrow curette is then passed into the medullary canal allowing debridement to viable, healthy bone as shown in a different patient who developed hardware-related osteomyelitis. Intra-op imaging is used to confirm the location and monitor extent of bone debridement

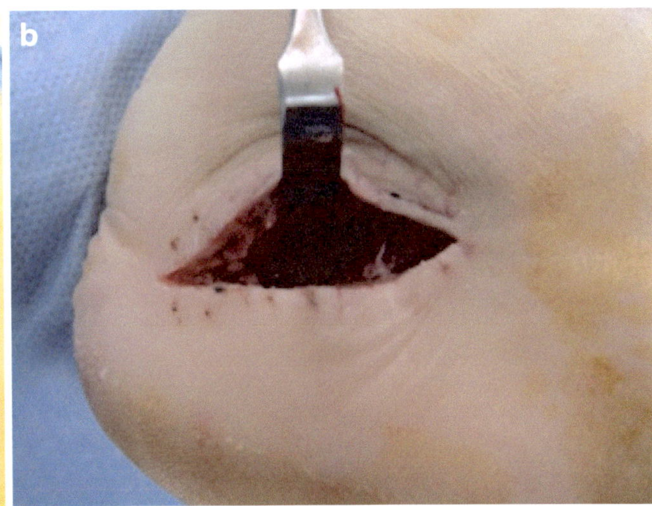

Fig. 21.8 What to do with the bone deficit? (**a**) Staged surgery in case 1 allows insertion of an antibiotic-impregnated cement bead chain and temporary closure of the wound which provides high local levels of antibiotics and serves as a void filler if future bone grafting is planned. Bead removal is performed approximately 2 weeks later which allows repeat biopsy. The same incision can be used for multiple debridement procedures. A dilemma remains regarding the best option for filling of the void at the time of the definitive procedure. (**b**) Stage 2 surgery involves removal of antibiotic beads, and clean margin bone biopsy. The defect could be left as is or the defect could be packed antibiotic-impregnated calcium sulfate pellets which are absorbed slowly but can be associated with persistent wound drainage

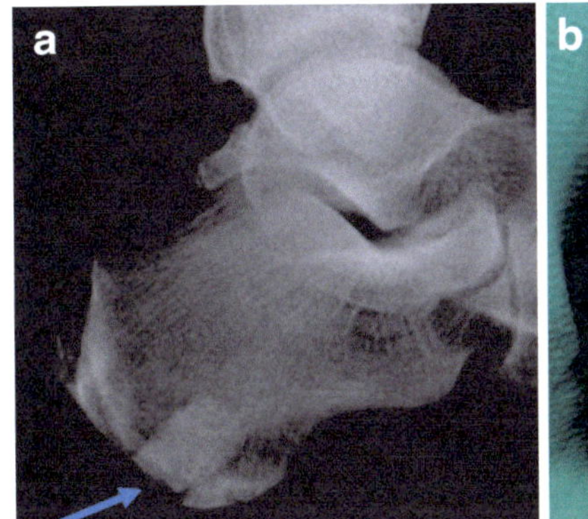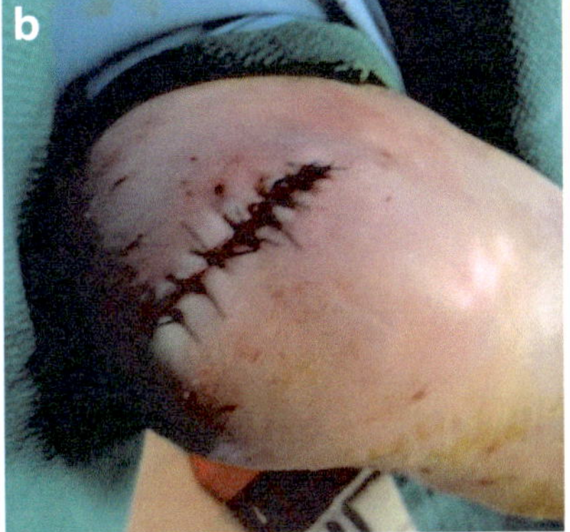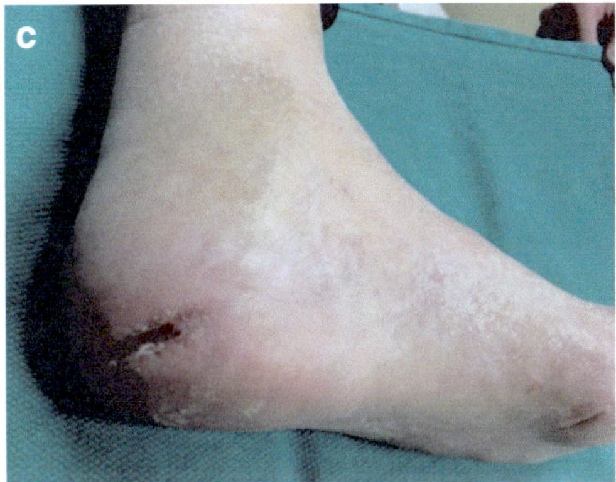

Fig. 21.9 Case 1: Postoperative protocol. Postoperative weight bearing status is determined by the location of the incision and extent of bone debridement. Six weeks of non-weight bearing is the norm given the location of the incision and desire to protect the calcaneus against pathologic fracture. (**a**) Initial postoperative lateral radiograph demonstrating the bone void filler (*blue arrow*). (**b**) Initial intraoperative-closed incision. (**c**) Six weeks postoperative with delayed suture removal and debridement of any dried eschar along the incision

may also be infected but still viable due to the robust internal vascularity of the calcaneus. MRI is useful to determine the extent of infection although the surgeon should be mindful that inflamed bone is not necessarily dead bone. Extensive wounds on the plantar weight bearing surface or necrosis of a broad section of the calcaneus may be more amenable to partial calcanectomy which is discussed later in this chapter.

Surgical Technique

Incision placement will vary based on the wound location and extent of soft tissue involvement. Wound closure may or may not be possible, but 3:1 ellipse of the wound is common, and linear extension may be necessary for adequate exposure. The bed of the wound is often nonviable in patients with osteomyelitis, and wound excision down to bone is the norm.

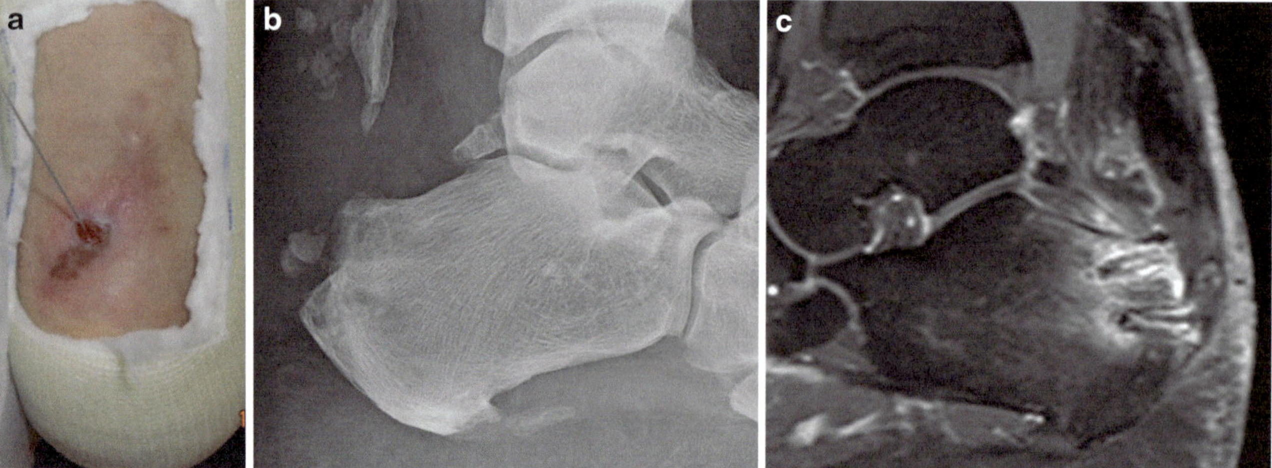

Fig. 21.10 Case 2: nonhealing surgical wound with concern for osteomyelitis. Second-opinion consultation for a nonhealing wound following retrocalcaneal surgery 7 months prior. History of early wound dehiscence with repeat wash out and closure. (**a**) The wound probed to bone raising suspicion for bone infection. (**b**) Radiographs were difficult to interpret given recent surgery and extensive calcifications. (**c**) MRI suggested disease within the Achilles and spread of infection within the calcaneus although false positive is possible with recent tendon and bone surgery. Note anchors present at the site of infection concern. Treatment involved open cortical debridement for removal of infected and prominent bone, removal of residual hardware, bone biopsy, inspection and debridement of the Achilles, and exposure of viable cancellous bone which promotes soft tissue healing

Hardware from previous surgery is removed, assuming the fracture or previous surgical intervention is stable and conversion to external fixation may be necessary. A wide section of cortical bone is encountered with this approach, allowing direct inspection for signs of bone necrosis, abscess, erosion, etc. A rongeur or other bone cutting instrument is used to remove the outer shell of cortical bone, exposing the underlying cancellous bone and procuring bone for biopsy. The intent of bone debridement is to remove the nidus of infection yet preserve a functional calcaneus if possible. The bone is reshaped to minimize the risk of recurrent tissue breakdown. A necrotic Achilles insertion is common with posterior wounds, and salvage of the tendon may not be possible. Normal-appearing, bleeding, viable bone is preserved regardless of what looks abnormal on MRI. Serial debridement every few days or weeks may be necessary to achieve a healthy margin without excessive resection.

Wound Closure Options

Primary wound closure is typically not possible for large ulcers yet prolonged exposure of cancellous bone beyond the course of antibiotic therapy is not likely to be successful. Negative-pressure wound therapy is a common approach to promote formation of granulation tissue over the freshly debrided bone surface which can be covered with a skin graft once the wound granulates to the surface. Local rotational flaps provide better tissue durability on the heel but have limited utility without wide bone resection as in partial calcanectomy. Advanced plastic surgical techniques are possible including a reverse sural artery flap or transpositional muscle flap followed by skin grafting [24–29]. These are fairly invasive options but may be considered depending on the size and location of the wound defect as the sural artery flap or skin graft to the plantar heel may not withstand the stress of walking.

Postoperative Care

Prolonged wound care with an extended period of non-weight bearing may be needed with this approach as complete resolution of the wound may take months. A rigid ankle-foot orthosis (AFO) will be needed in cases where the Achilles tendon cannot be preserved. Delayed flexor hallucis longus tendon (FHL) transfer is an option for selected patients including postoperative calcaneal osteomyelitis secondary to insertional Achilles tendon surgery. Resolution of infection is warranted prior to performing FHL tendon transfer. The surgeon may consider performing repeat bone biopsy prior to undergoing reconstructive tendon surgery.

Case Examples of Wound Excision with Cortical Debridement

Three case examples are shown to demonstrate patient selection criteria, surgical technique, and aftercare. Case 2 involved calcaneal osteomyelitis after repair of an insertional Achilles tendon rupture that developed wound dehiscence postoperatively. The patient underwent wound excision, removal of soft tissue anchors, near-total resection of the Achilles tendon insertion, bone resection and biopsy, and primary wound closure (Figs. 21.10, 21.11, and 21.12). Case 3 involved calcaneal osteomyelitis associated with open reduction and internal fixation of a calcaneal fracture. Treatment consisted of raising the lateral flap, removal of hardware, debridement of cortical bone, bone biopsy, and primary wound closure (Figs. 21.13, 21.14, 21.15, and 21.16). Case 4 involved a decubitus Achilles tendon wound that developed calcaneal osteomyelitis. Treatment involved wide resection of the necrotic Achilles followed by cortical debridement and partial wound closure (Figs. 21.17, 21.18, 21.19, 21.20, 21.21, and 21.22). Bone biopsy-directed post-operative antibiotics were used in each case.

Partial Calcanectomy with Flap Closure of the Wound

Large decubitus heel wounds with associated necrosis and infection of the calcaneus create substantial challenges with regard to limb salvage including resolution of infection and wound coverage with durable soft tissue on the plantar or posterior heel. The extent of bone necrosis and the quality of the surrounding soft tissues need to be considered when selecting the appropriate treatment plan as leg amputation is commonly the most prudent approach. Preservation of the weight bearing calcaneal tuberosity and Achilles insertion is ideal from a functional stand point but is frequently not practical under these circumstances. Eventual limb loss is the norm, and local treatment should take a radical, limb salvage approach. Wide resection of the calcaneal tuberosity creates a fresh margin of viable bone and, more importantly, relaxation of the surrounding tissue which allows local rotational flap closure. Partial calcanectomy should be viewed as a last resort limb salvage approach [5–15] that allows bipedal weight bearing transfer or limited ambulation with a modified ankle-foot orthosis (AFO).

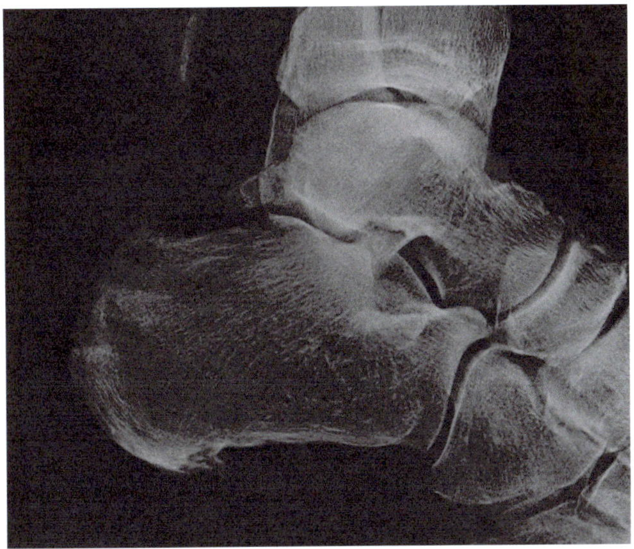

Fig. 21.11 Case 2: initial postoperative lateral radiograph. Intraoperative findings included infection coursing along the bone anchors, and the central portion of Achilles tendon was necrotic. The anchors were removed followed by curettage to debride the anchor holes and procure bone biopsy. The posterior heel was remodeled as shown with the intent to preserve the tuberosity knowing that medical treatment would follow. Only the medial and lateralmost slips of the Achilles tendon remained attached. Bone biopsy revealed chronic osteomyelitis

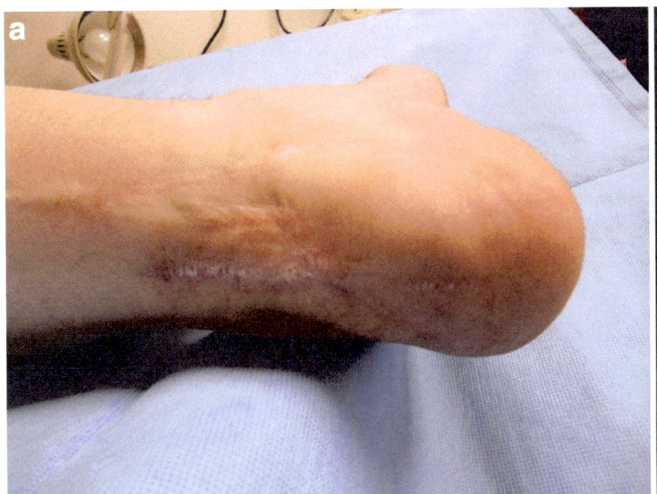
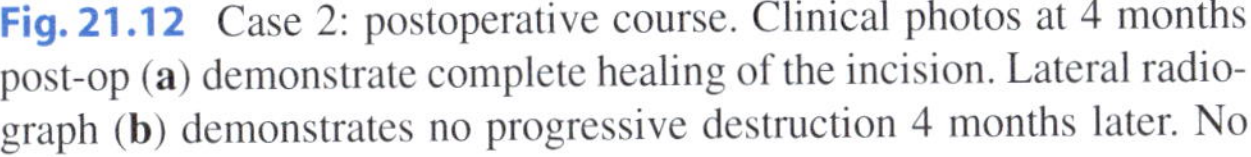
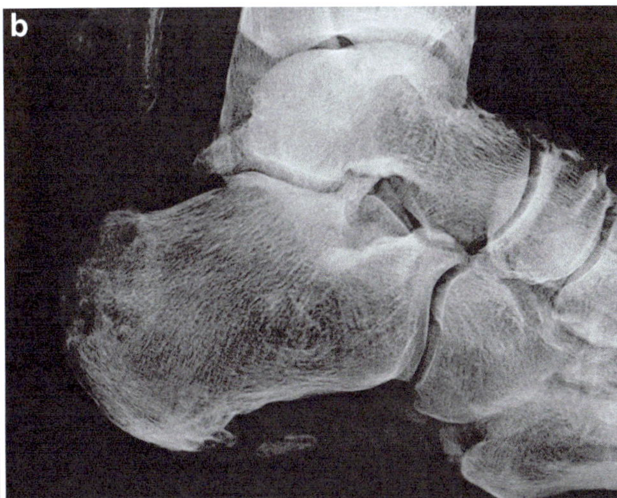

Fig. 21.12 Case 2: postoperative course. Clinical photos at 4 months post-op (**a**) demonstrate complete healing of the incision. Lateral radiograph (**b**) demonstrates no progressive destruction 4 months later. No residual weakness, gait changes, or concern for infection was noted at 11-month follow-up

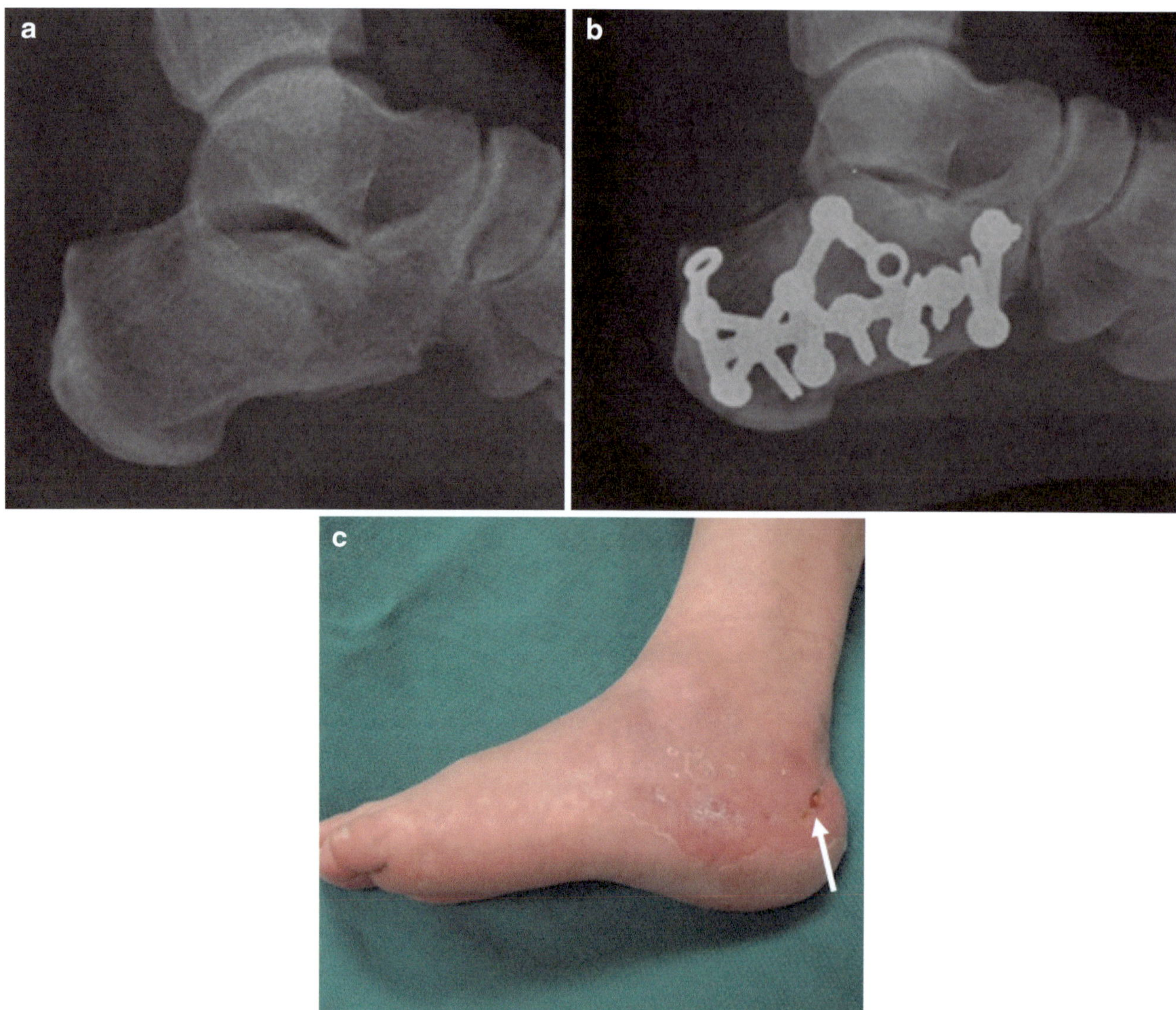

Fig. 21.13 Case 3: infected sinus tract, exposed hardware, and concern for osteomyelitis following calcaneal fracture open repair. (**a**) Preoperative lateral radiograph demonstrates a joint depression intra-articular calcaneal fracture. (**b**) ORIF involved extensile lateral exposure with plate fixation which was delayed for 3 weeks secondary to swelling. (**c**) The tip of the flap failed to heal leading to postoperative infection several months after surgery (*arrow*). Exposed hardware and concern for osteomyelitis was treated with removal of hardware, bone biopsy, cortical bone debridement, and primary closure of the wound

Patient Selection

Appropriate patient selection is critical to successful limb salvage including resolution or suppression of osteomyelitis, successful flap healing, and functional gait or transfer without recurrent tissue breakdown. The typical calcanectomy candidate has a large necrotic posterior or plantar decubitus heel wound, extensive bone infection that is limited to the calcaneus, and viable surrounding soft tissue. Limited ambulation and transfer-only level of activity represents the typical candidate for this technique. These patients are often not ideal candidates for successful prosthetic fitting after limb loss, and therefore partial limb salvage offers a chance to maintain their current level of activity or independent-living status. An active community ambulator who develops a complicated decubitus pressure sore may be better served with leg amputation which allows a more functional gait with the assistance of a lower leg prosthesis. The minimum level of activity to consider for this limb salvage approach is current use of the limb for transfers. Patients who do not utilize the extremity for transfer are better treated with leg amputation which allows prompt healing without the added risks of prolonged antibiotics or staged surgery.

Another important patient selection factor relates to the soft tissue quality surrounding the ulceration. Poor peri-wound tissue, extensive chronic edema, and large wounds that encompass the majority of the plantar heel are indicators of poor results with this approach (Fig. 21.23). A large wound defect after bone resection or extensive soft tissue infection severely compromises potential flap coverage.

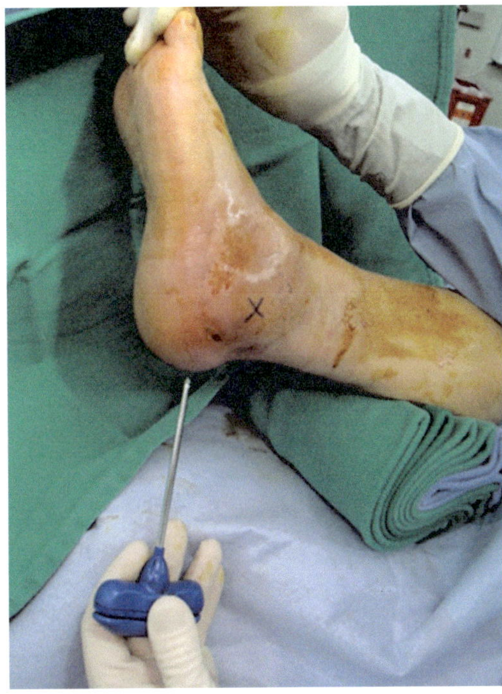

Fig. 21.14 Case 3: bone biopsy considerations. Bone biopsy was initially obtained through a separate incision away from the open wound to minimize the risk of cross contamination. See Chap. 4 for further details on bone biopsy techniques

Infection that courses distally into the plantar arch or proximally along the Achilles with abscess or necrosis into the plantar fascia or proximal leg may be more appropriately treated with leg amputation. Since a larger portion of the calcaneus is likely to be involved with decubitus ulceration, it is imperative to closely evaluate radiographs and MRI to ensure that infection is not crossing into adjacent joints and bony structures. This is another example of when a leg amputation is the better option for the patient. As discussed previously, adequate perfusion is imperative for wound and flap healing purposes.

It is important to note that local rotational flap closure of decubitus ulcer is intended for patients with concomitant calcaneal osteomyelitis. The rotational flap works because of soft tissue laxity that is created at the time of partial calcanectomy. Without wide bone resection, the flap will not advance or rotate appropriately. Patients with decubitus ulceration without osteomyelitis are typically treated with prolonged local wound care, negative-pressure wound therapy, or reverse sural artery flap. Local rotational flaps without calcanectomy are possible, but the donor site defect will likely require skin grafting.

Flap Design and Wound Closure Options

Wound closure options are highly dependent on the size and location of the decubitus ulcer. The decision to attempt flap closure, the ideal flap design, and suitable donor tissue needs to be determined as part of preoperative planning. Stage 1 surgery is ideally limited to excision of the necrotic wound to access the calcaneus for debridement and biopsy. Flap design is determined by the location of the heel decubitus ulceration

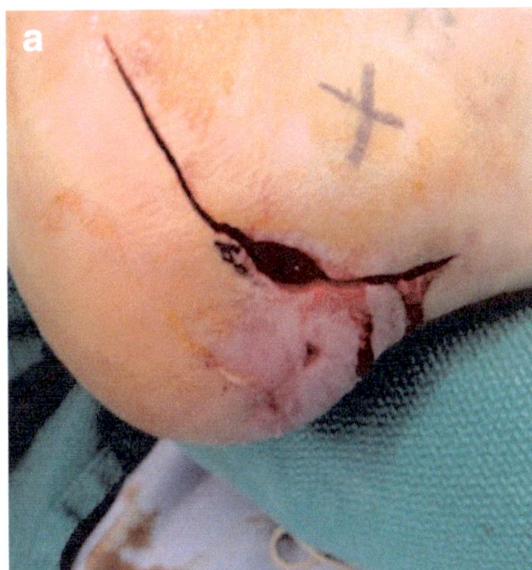
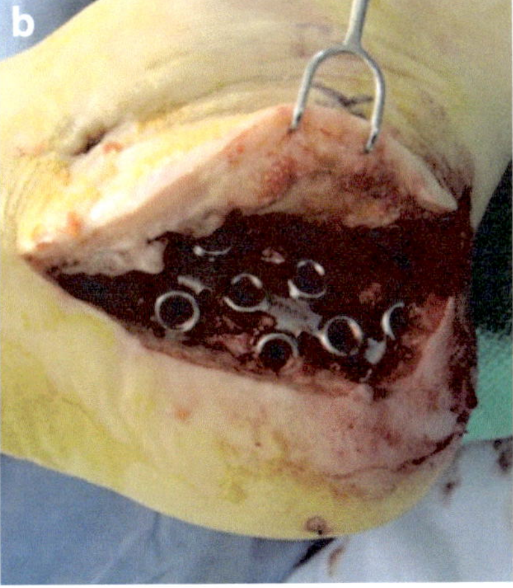
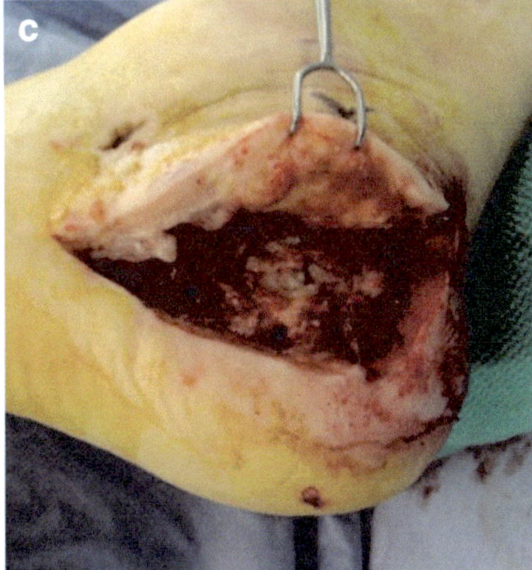

Fig. 21.15 Case 3: hardware removal and cortical debridement. The original flap was raised to allow access for hardware removal and closure of the chronic wound. (**a**) The incision was made full thickness to bone with care to stay perpendicular to the skin edges. (**b**) The flap was raised full thickness with a limited-touch technique. (**c**) Hardware from previous surgery was removed, as the fracture was healed. The lateral cortex was widely exposed for debridement and biopsy

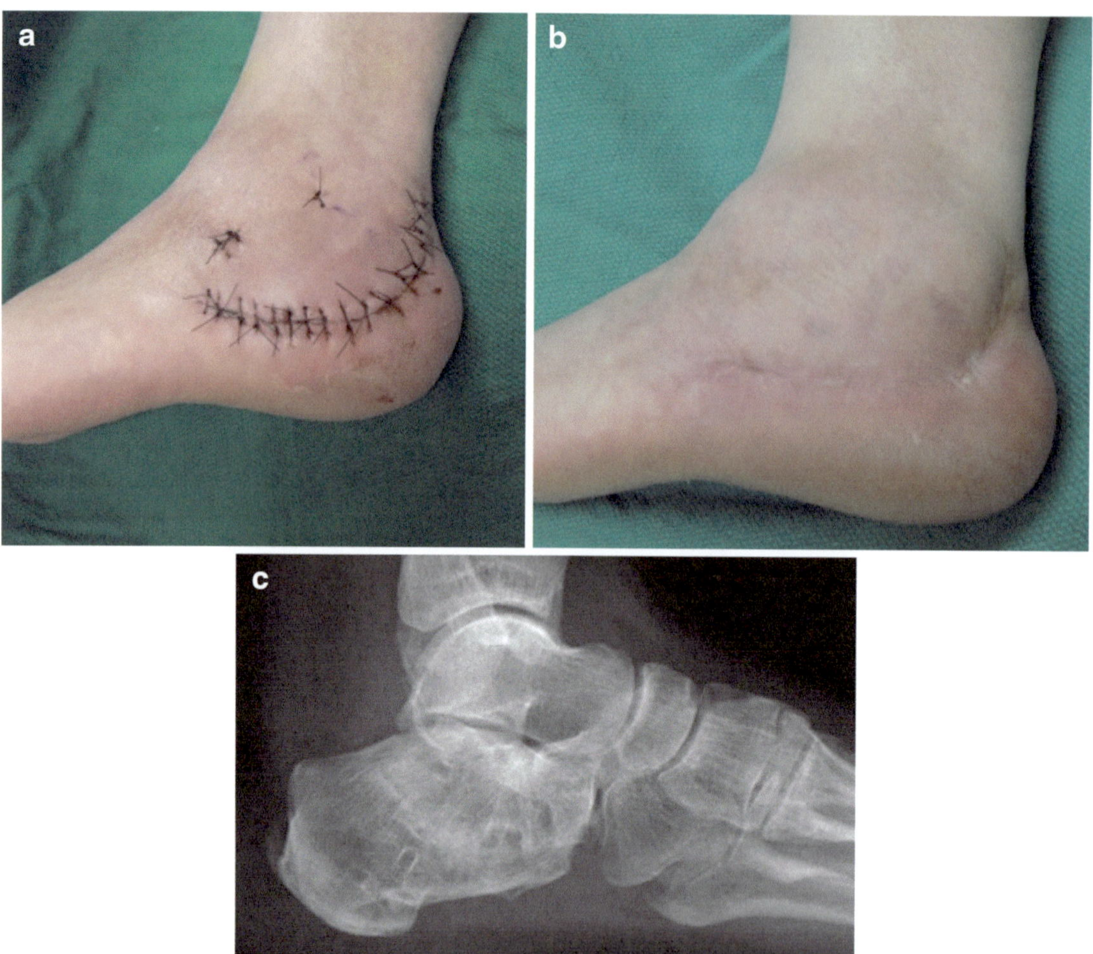

Fig. 21.16 Case 3: postoperative course. Biopsy results revealed acute osteomyelitis on pathologic exam and the bone culture was positive. The patient completed a 6-week course of IV antibiotics at which point labs returned to normal and the wound was resolved. (**a**) Initial postoperative clinical photo demonstrates closure without tension. The patient remained non-weight bearing for a total of 6 weeks. (**b**) Clinical photo at 4 months demonstrates well-healed incisions. (**c**) Lateral radiograph at 4 months demonstrates a consolidated fracture, preservation of calcaneal structure despite debridement, and no concerns of osteomyelitis

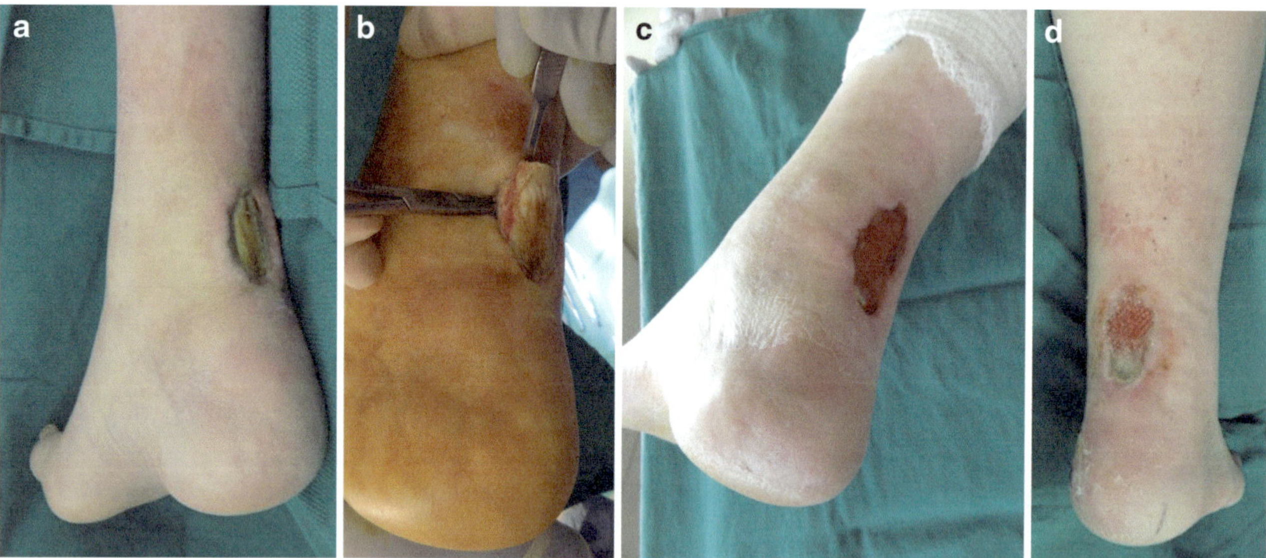

Fig. 21.17 Case 4: diabetic male with decubitus ulcer over the Achilles tendon. (**a**) An exposed and necrotic Achilles tendon associated with posterior decubitus ulceration was excised in an effort to allow progressive granulation of the defect. (**b**) Early attempts to preserve the Achilles failed, and the necrotic tendon was removed for fear of infection spreading into the calf which raises the potential for limb loss. (**c**) Granulation tissue filled the wound promptly after a course of negative-pressure therapy. (**d**) Persistent tendon necrosis at the distal extent of the wound resulted in the eventual development of calcaneal osteomyelitis which was not present on preoperative MRI

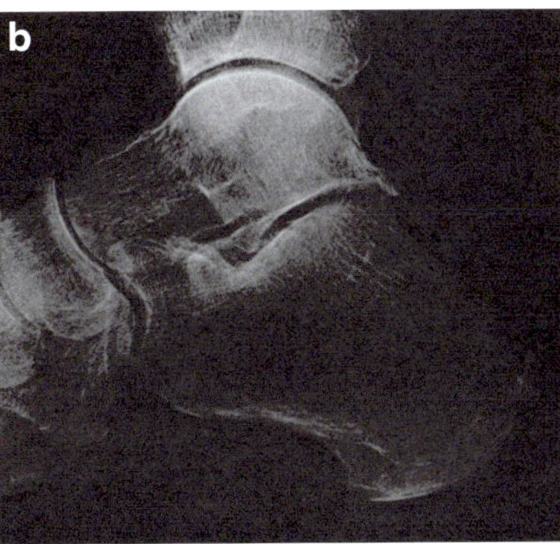
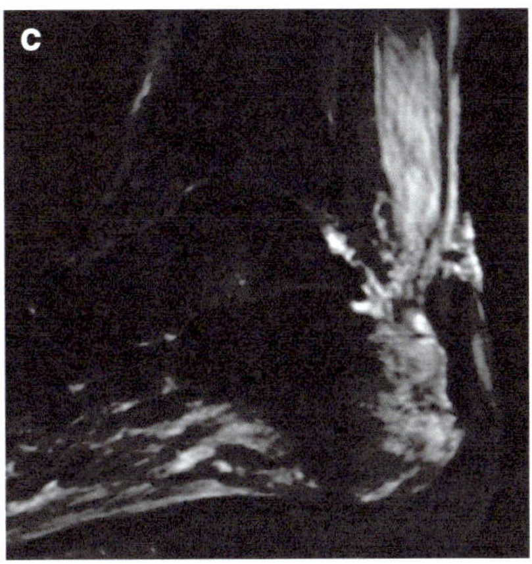

Fig. 21.18 Case 4: X-ray and MRI confirm osteomyelitis of the calcaneus. Comparison of early (**a**) and late (**b**) X-rays suggests osteomyelitis at the Achilles insertion. (**c**) MRI confirms osteomyelitis of the calcaneus which is largely isolated to the posterior tuberosity. Isolated medical management is not likely to be effective under these circumstances due to the persistent sinus tract along the necrotic distal fibers of the Achilles

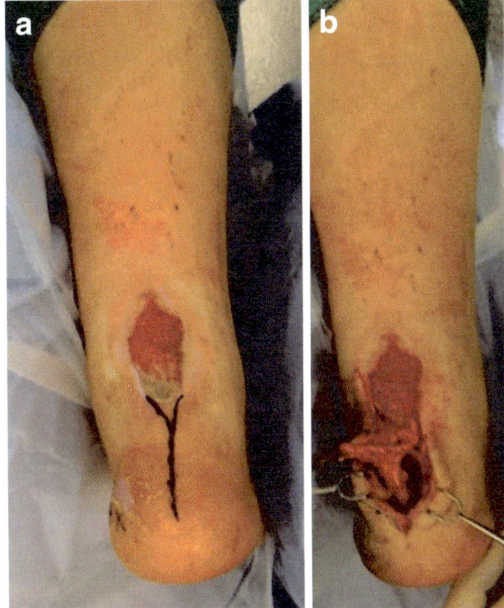

Fig. 21.19 Case 4: single-staged debridement of the calcaneus with partial wound closure. (**a**) A posterior midline calcaneal incision allowed direct access to the Achilles and posterior calcaneus. (**b**) The necrotic Achilles was removed allowing access to the involved bone

and the quality of the surrounding soft tissue. Three zones of decubitus ulcerations have been described [8] which have implications regarding flap planning (Fig. 21.24). Zone 1 is the posterior heel decubitus ulceration which is most often associated with bed sores and is prone to exposure and infection of the Achilles insertion. Zone 2 ulcers are at the apex of the heel at the junction of the posterior and plantar aspects. This appears to be the most common location and is caused by a pressure sore in patients who lay in bed with the foot relaxed in a plantarflexed position. Zone 3 ulcers are located plantarly and are prone to infection extending into the plantar arch. This ulcer location is commonly seen in neuropathic patients with decreased Achilles tendon function (calcaneus gait) or decubitus pressure sores from prolonged sitting in a wheelchair with the foot resting on the ground or on the wheelchair foot rest (Fig. 21.25).

The zone location of the wound and quality of surrounding soft tissues helps to guide the ideal flap closure option. Zone 1 posterior ulcers are amenable to a unilobed rotation flap following the lateral calcaneal artery (Fig. 21.26a, b). Zone 2 junctional ulceration allows elliptical excision of the ulceration with closure of medial and lateral flaps (Fig. 21.26a, c). If MRI demonstrates infection extending into the plantar arch or more proximal into the Achilles, this pattern of incision is amenable to lengthening proximally or distally as needed. The zone 3 plantar ulcer location is least common and is amenable to a posterior unilobed flap (Fig. 21.26a, d).

Surgical Technique

The patient is positioned prone and tourniquet is optional. As with other wound surgeries involving biopsy, preoperative antibiotics are held until cultures are obtained, unless needed for acute soft tissue infection. The ulcer is excised full thickness to bone with care to stay perpendicular to the skin edges. Surgery may be performed staged with the first procedure involving removal of infected tissue, drainage of abscess, and removal of necrotic bone (Fig. 21.27). The second stage is delayed a few days to allow resolution of acute infection at which time partial calcanectomy and flap closure is completed. The flap is then raised off the bone full thickness with a no-touch technique to preserve the viability

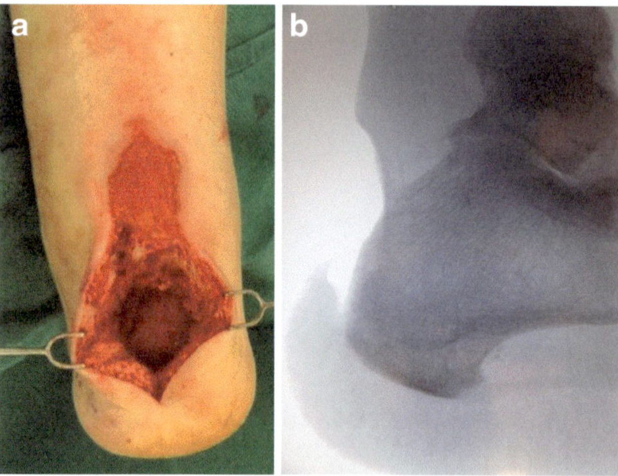

Fig. 21.20 Case 4: cortical debridement of the posterior calcaneus. (**a**) The goal of this approach is to debride a broad area of infected cortex to expose viable cancellous bone. Bone specimens were procured for pathology and culture. (**b**) Adequate debridement without excessive loss of bone structure on the weight bearing aspect of the tuberosity is desired but not always possible

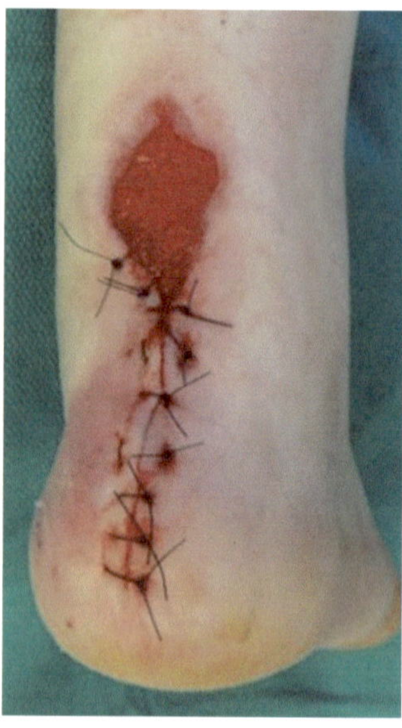

Fig. 21.21 Case 4: partial closure of the distal wound. Primary closure is dependent on the initial wound and quality of the surrounding tissues. A combination of primary closure of the lower portion of the incision and vacuum-assisted wound therapy of the upper wound was utilized. Delayed skin grafting or reverse sural artery flap is indicated for larger wounds

Fig. 21.22 Case 4: postoperative radiograph and clinical photo. (**a**) Note that a large portion of the posterior calcaneus has been removed yet the plantar weight bearing aspect of the tuberosity has been preserved. (**b**) Clinical photo shows complete distal healing with progressive proximal healing 2 months later at which point weight bearing was resumed. Normal plantarflexion strength was found due to flexor substitution

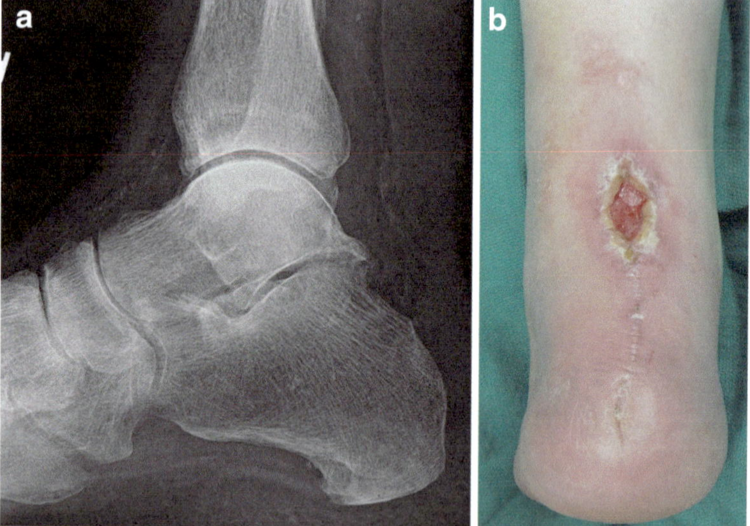

of the flap. It is important to follow the contours of the calcaneus with sharp dissection to avoid the medial neurovascular structures. Zones 1 and 3 involve a unilobed flap technique. Zone 1 is a lateral unilobed flap and zone 3 is a posterior unilobed flap (Fig. 21.26b, d). The traditional unilobe flap is about 75 % the size of the wound defect and maintains a 1:1 flap to length/base width ratio [30, 31]. In our experience, a slightly smaller than traditional flap can be utilized given the significant portion of the heel bone that

is resected as this creates laxity in the soft tissues allowing secondary movement of the surrounding tissue. Zone 2 utilizes an ellipse incision which creates large- and equally sized medial and lateral flaps (Fig. 21.26c). Preparation for bone resection involves osteotomy guidewire placement and intraoperative lateral fluoroscopic imaging to ensure appropriate angle and amount of posterior heel resection to prevent future pressure sores when walking, sitting, wearing a brace, or lying in bed. The extent of bone resection is

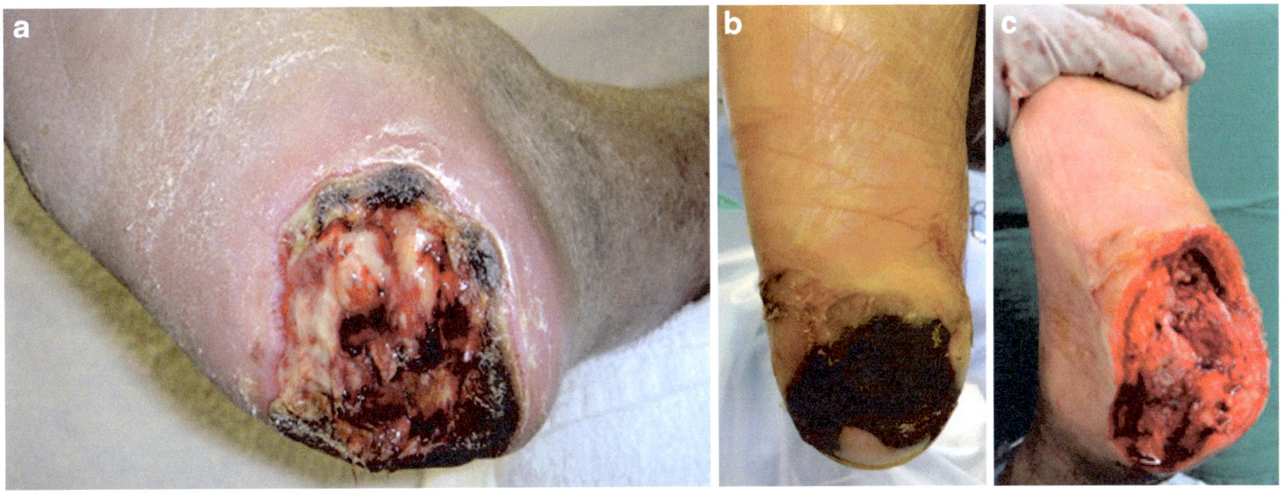

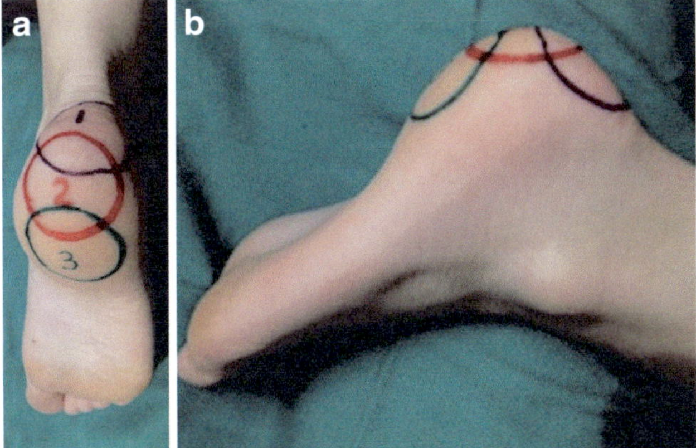

Fig. 21.23 Who is a candidate for limb salvage with partial calcanectomy? (**a**) The tissue quality at the perimeter of the wound is a critical factor regarding the potential for limb salvage with calcaneal osteomyelitis secondary to a large decubitus ulcer. (**b**) Patients with poor local tissue perfusion, uncontrolled edema, and full-depth necrosis of the entire weight bearing surface of the heel are not likely to heal after calcanectomy. (**c**) Gangrenous eschar with undermining and infection spreading into the plantar arch required extensive resection with large soft tissue defect that could not be closed with a local flap. Leg amputation may be the best primary treatment under these conditions

Fig. 21.24 Three zones of decubitus ulceration. Zone 1 is the posterior heel decubitus ulcer location. Zone 2 is an ulceration at the junction or apex of the heel. Zone 3 ulceration is located on the plantar weight bearing surface

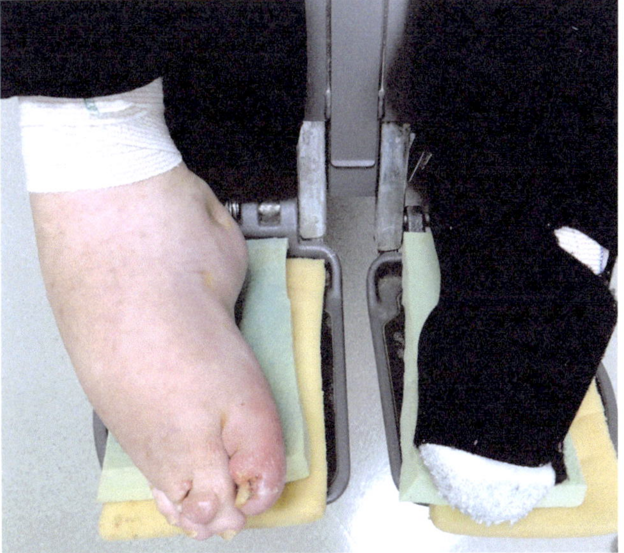

Fig. 21.25 Wheelchair-bound patients are prone to zone 3 plantar heel decubitus ulceration. Sitting in a wheelchair or powerchair predisposes to decubitus pressure on the plantar surface of the heel. Foam pads are applied here for protection, but foot rest modifications are the best preventive approach. Varus contracture also predisposes to lateral foot and ankle decubitus pressure. Uncontrolled edema associated with loss of neurologic tone adds weight to the legs which magnifies this problem

important to allow flap closure of the chronic wound (Fig. 21.28). The technique involves placement of a guide pin that follows an imaginary contour from the posterior aspect of the fibula to the base of the fifth metatarsal with care to stay posterior to the posterior facet of the subtalar joint (Fig. 21.29a). The guide pin is useful to direct the sagittal saw at the desired angle. The surgeon may consider an osteotome for the last portion of the cut as this is often deep within the soft tissues (Fig. 21.29b). After performing the osteotomy, care is taken to smooth rough edges and bony prominences (Fig. 21.29c). This extensive amount of bone resection is what creates laxity in the soft tissues and allows flap closure (Fig. 21.29d). The use of a Hemovac drain is considered to minimize hematoma formation if a large dead space is remaining after the flap is closed. For zone 2 ulcers with medial and lateral flaps, the edges are approximated with simple interrupted sutures. Zones 1 and 3 are with uni-lobed flap; Fig. 21.30 demonstrates our preferred suture technique.

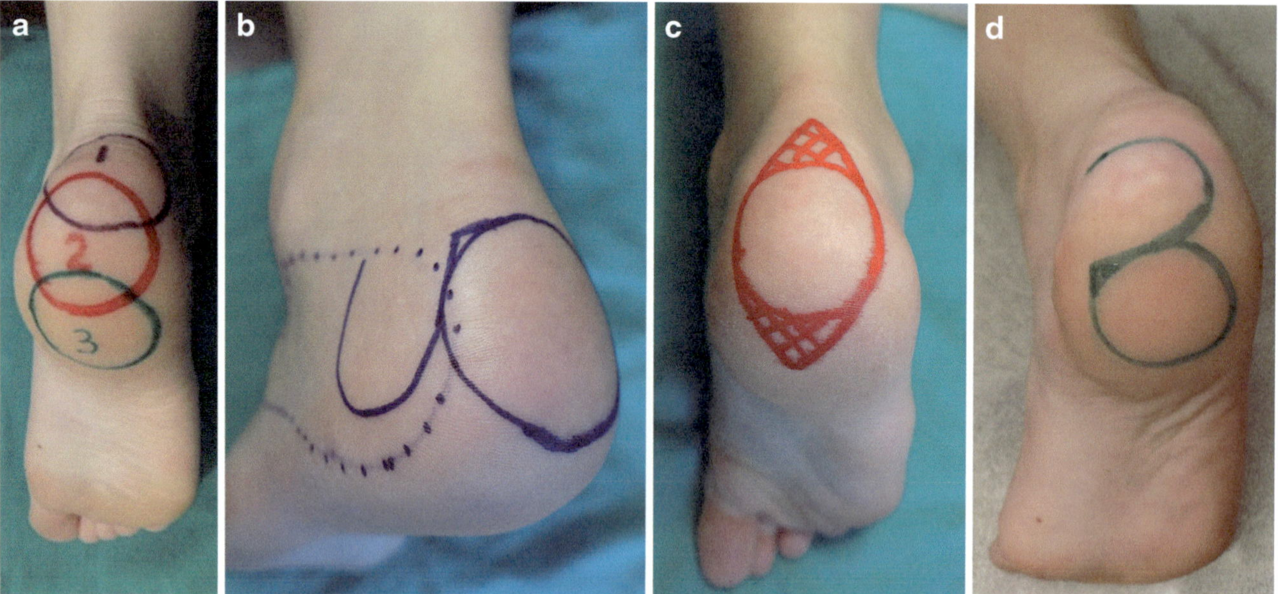

Fig. 21.26 (**a**) Flap planning for calcanectomy based on ulcer zone location. (**b**) The plantar skin remains intact and viable in zone 1 posterior heel decubitus ulceration. The unilobed rotational flap donor site is the lateral heel (*dotted line* is outline of calcaneus) which avoids incision on the intact plantar skin which would be necessary with 3 to 1 elliptical excision and closure. The lateral flap is vascularized by the lateral calcaneal artery, and lateral exposure allows wide exposure for calcaneus resection. (**c**) The zone 2 junction or apical ulcer is most amenable to elliptical excision of the ulcer and closure with available medial and lateral flaps. Note that this incision can be extended proximally or distally as needed for exposure of infection in the plantar arch or leg. (**d**) Zone 3 ulcers are located on the plantar weight bearing surface of the heel where elliptical excision is dangerously close to the lateral plantar artery and nerve. The posterior donor site location for the unilobed flap avoids further violation of the compromised plantar soft tissues

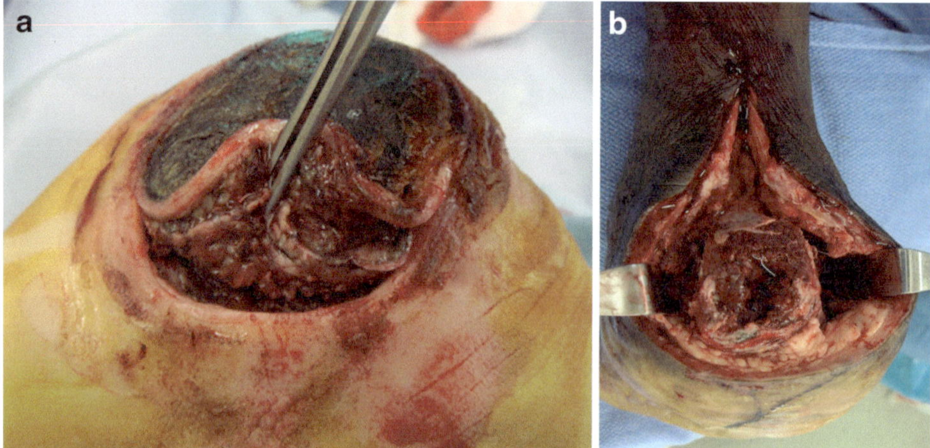

Fig. 21.27 (**a**) Eschar excision involved full-thickness excision to bone with complete resection of the necrotic eschar. A staged procedure is common for soft tissue infection, and open debridement allows stabilization of infection while preparing for the definitive procedure. The decision regarding the opportunity to preserve the Achilles tendon depends on the quality of the tendon and posterior bone. The Achilles tendon is often necrotic and ruptured at the insertion with infected zone 1 ulcers. (**b**) Note how the posterior cortex is no longer intact which was predicted based on X-ray and MRI

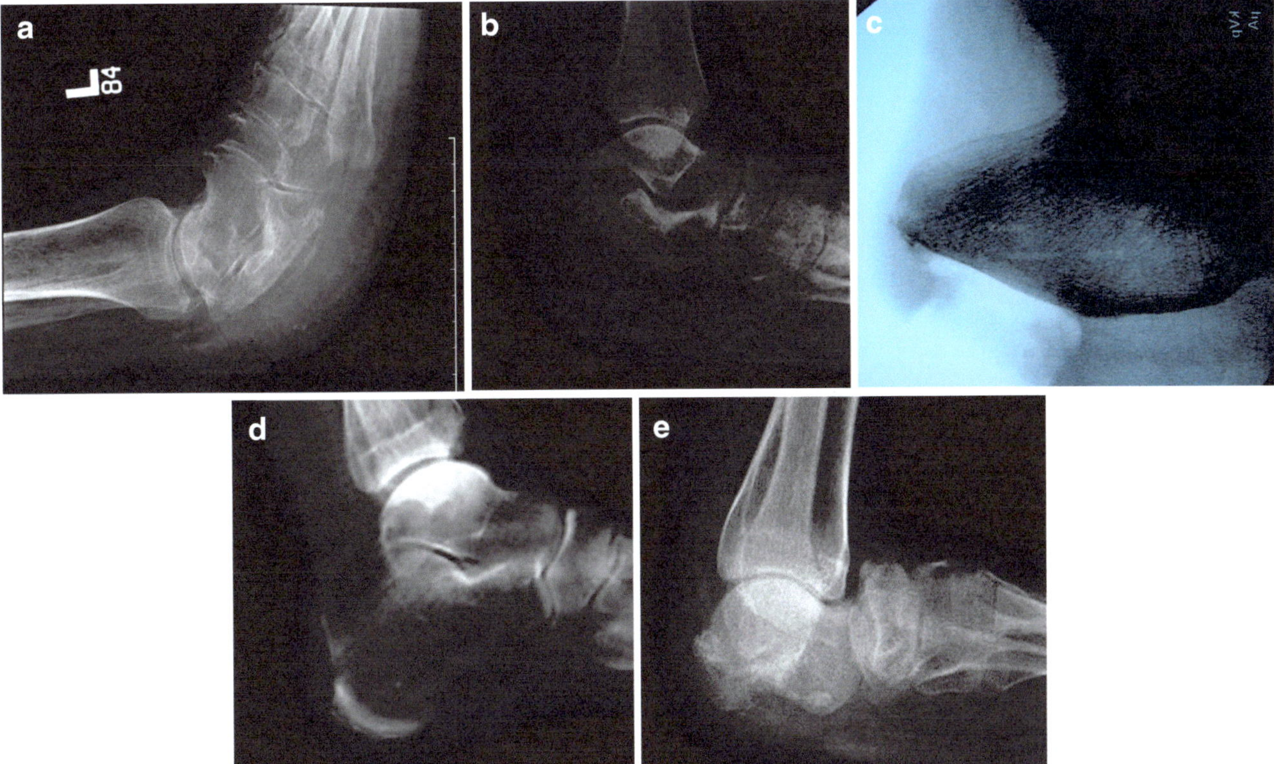

Fig. 21.28 What is the ideal extent of bone resection with "partial" calcanectomy. The extent of bone resection with complicated decubitus ulcers may have more to do with the soft tissue defect, expected wound closure challenges, and the desire to avoid recurrent pressure sores than with the actual condition of the bone. (**a**) Wide resection of the calcaneus allows relaxation of the surrounding soft tissues and also decreases decubitus pressure while lying in bed. (**b**) Our preferred approach involves resecting the posterior portion of the calcaneus to create a natural contour from the posterior tibia, fibula, and talus to the base of the fifth metatarsal. This technique involves sacrificing the attachment of the Achilles tendon which is typically necrotic by the time calcanectomy is being considered. (**c**) Partial calcanectomy with preservation of the Achilles tendon insertion may lead to abnormal prominence on the posterior heel which predisposes to abnormal decubitus pressure and recurrent breakdown. (**d**) Posterior infection of the tuberosity would suggest an abnormal and non-salvageable Achilles. (**e**) Complete calcanectomy is not practical from an exposure standpoint; it also puts neurovascular structures at risk and results in irregularity to the now weight bearing talus

Postoperative Care

A pillow dressing can be applied to the operative extremity to provide continuous off-loading (Fig. 21.31). This encourages the patient and the staff taking care of the patient to maintain continuous off-loading in the immediate postoperative period. Upon preparation for discharge from the hospital, a posterior splint with spacer can be made to ensure appropriate off-loading of the flap and heel (Fig. 21.32). The patient should anticipate complete non-weight bearing for a period of 6 weeks, which is typically the amount of time the sutures are left in place to allow for appropriate healing. Antibiotic therapy is directed by intraoperative cultures which allow ongoing treatment of residual bone infection. This typically involves a 6-week course of IV antibiotics with monitoring of infection labs and clinical progress. Once sutures are removed, the patient will need an ankle-foot orthoses (AFO) for ambulation given the loss of heel height and Achilles tendon function (Fig. 21.33). The rigid AFO is typically a custom-molded calf suspension-type brace with adjustable corset design to accommodate for leg edema with intrinsic accommodation for the loss of heel height.

Case Examples of Partial Calcanectomy Technique

Three case examples are provided that demonstrate decision making and intraoperative technique for partial calcanectomy with a zone 1 posterior heel ulceration demonstrated in case 5

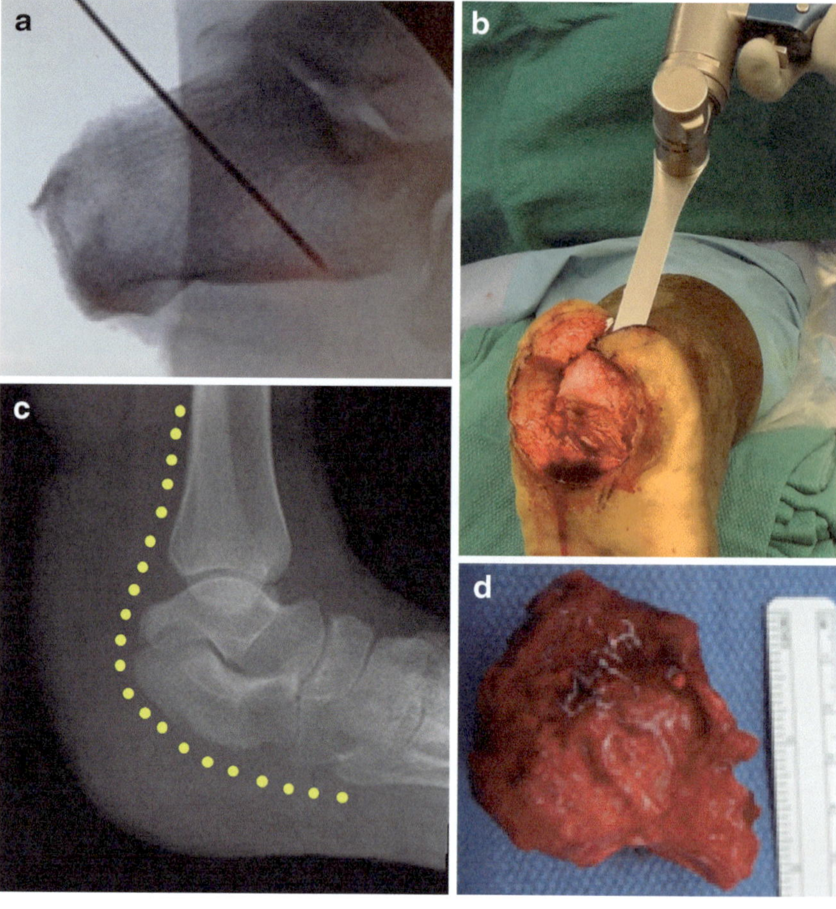

Fig. 21.29 Guide pin technique for ideal level of bone resection. (**a**) A Kirschner wire is placed as an osteotomy guide to ensure that resection achieves the desired result. (**b**) A long saw blade is needed for the osteotomy in order to reach to the plantar cortex although an osteotome can be utilized to finish the plantar aspect of the cut if desired. Care is taken to avoid injury to the medial neurovascular structures which are directly medial along the cut. (**c**) A rongeur and rasp is used to round off the sharp edge around the entire circumference of the osteotomy to prevent future pressure points when lying in bed, walking, or wearing an AFO. (**d**) Note the large portion of calcaneal bone that is resected which allows laxity in the surrounding soft tissues and east of flap closure

(Figs. 21.34, 21.35, and 21.36), zone 2 junctional heel ulceration in case 6 (Figs. 21.37, 21.38, and 21.39), and zone 3 plantar heel ulceration as shown in case 7 (Figs. 21.40, 21.41, 21.42, and 21.43). The goal of a partial calcanectomy is to resect a large portion of bone to allow for soft tissue closure. Healing of the wound during the initial phase of antibiotic therapy decreases the risk of recontamination and reulceration. This is a limb preservation technique which allows a functional limb to allow for transfers and ambulation in an AFO brace as demonstrated by the above case examples.

Leg Amputation for Calcaneal Osteomyelitis

Calcaneal osteomyelitis and associated wound deficits are a challenging and often incurable problem. While attempts should be made to determine if successful limb salvage is possible, this is not always an option and often leg amputation may be the preferred treatment of choice for certain patients. Vascular status has a large impact in the decision process, as patients with non-reconstructible vascular compromise often require leg amputation. Furthermore, leg amputation is often best if the patient has significant nonviable periwound tissue that is unable to be closed with a flap, infected gangrene, or a large wound with necrosis tracking into the plantar arch. Other soft tissue considerations include massive edema or lymphedema that would preclude a limb salvage technique from healing. Activity level also has a role in the decision process. Patients that are nonambulatory and do not utilize the limb for transfer may be better served with leg amputation. Conversely, a younger active patient with a large heel wound may be better with leg amputation as a prosthetic leg may allow a higher level of function when compared to partial calca-

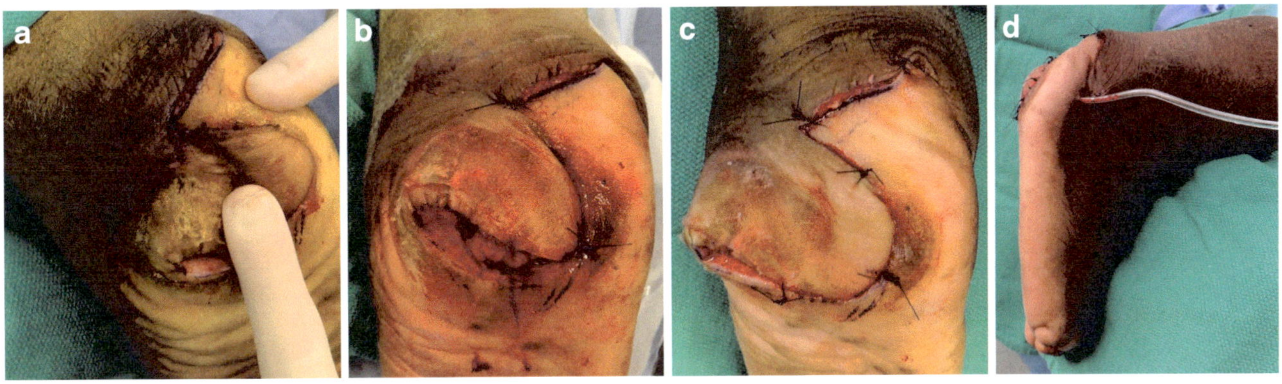

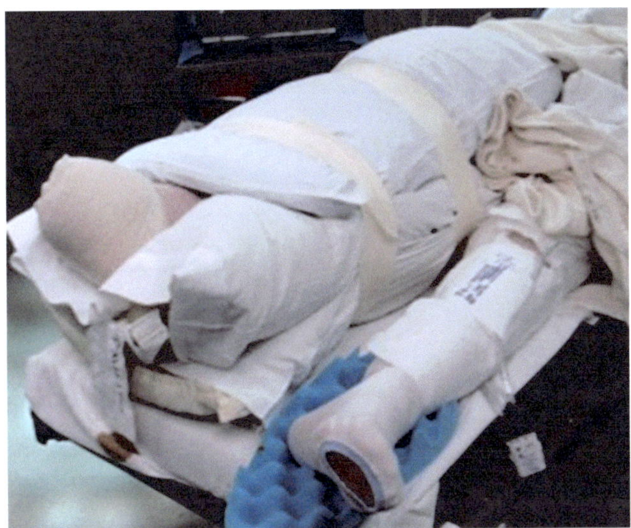

Fig. 21.30 Flap closure of the plantar wound in zone 3 decubitus ulcers. (**a**) The primary unilobed flap is rotated into the defect, and the secondary flap provides coverage of the donor site. (**b**, **c**) Simple interrupted sutures are placed in strategic locations with the wound nearly covered with a few sutures. (**d**) A closed suction drain is common

Fig. 21.31 Post-op flap pillow dressing. A pillow dressing is applied in the operating room which is beneficial to ensure off-loading of the flap while lying in bed. This consists of 3–5 pillows strapped to the leg with tape. The advantage of the pillow dressing over commercially available off-loading devices is that the patient and or other medical staff are not likely to remove the pillow dressing

nectomy. There are significant biomechanical implications with partial calcanectomy with loss of the Achilles, loss of heel height, and need for permanent bracing making minimally active patients the best candidates. Radiographic and advanced imaging has a role in the decision process since widespread necrosis of the entire calcaneus or infection spreading into adjacent soft tissue or bone makes limb salvage techniques less ideal. Lastly, failure of prior attempts at limb salvage may suggest the need for leg amputation.

The decision for timely leg amputation can be important as it may assist the patient in avoiding above-knee amputation versus below the knee in patients with serious infection. In the case of acute infection, staging of the amputation with initial guillotine amputation at the level of the malleolus is common to contain the infection with closed-leg amputation days later. In contrast to limb salvage procedures, long-term antibiotics are not generally needed given the proximal level of amputation performed.

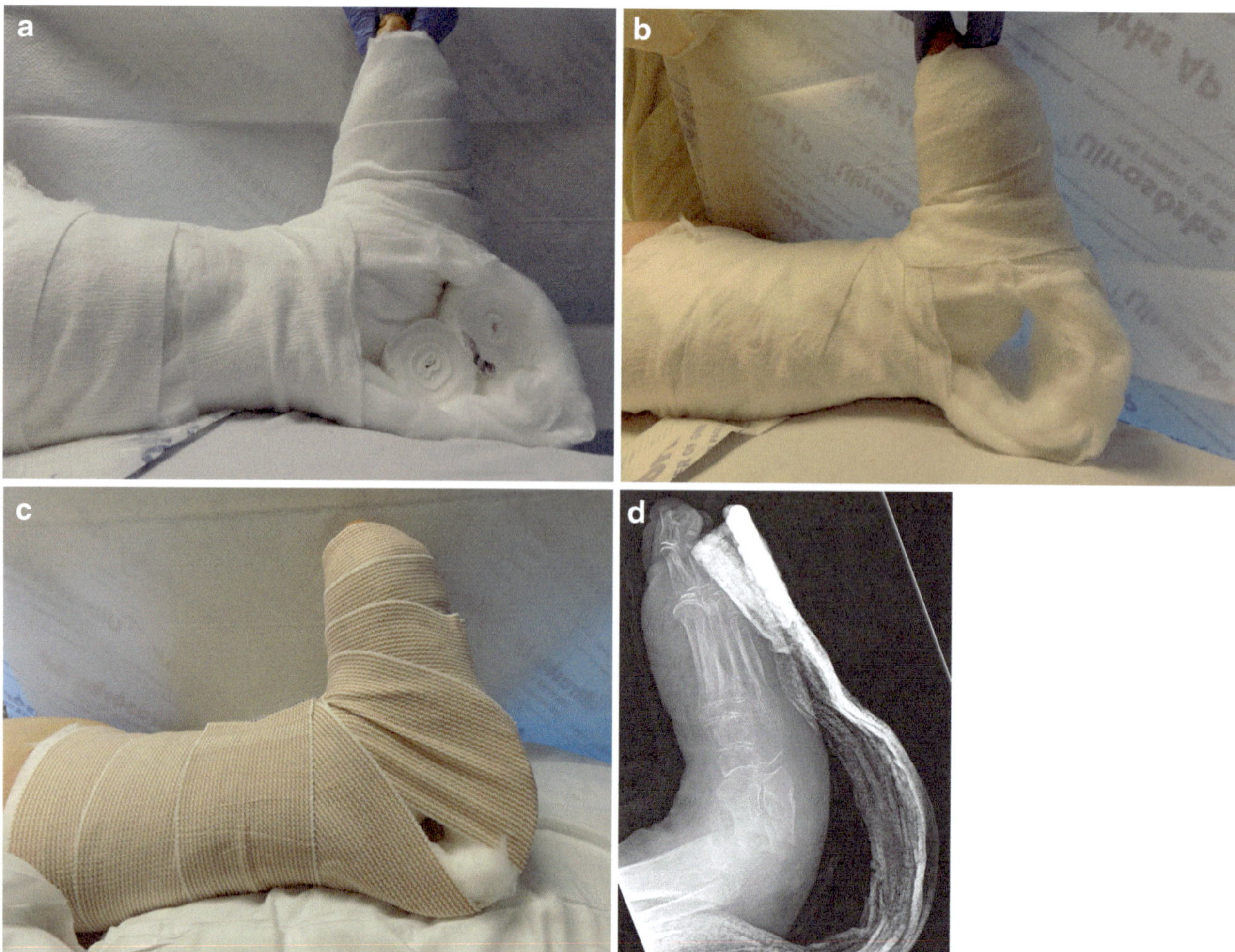

Fig. 21.32 Heel off-loading posterior splint. A posterior splint molded with a spacer at the posterior heel is beneficial for avoiding pressure upon discharge from the hospital. (**a**) Molding the splint with rolls of cast padding placed in the heel area is an easy way to create the spacer, the rolls are then removed (**b**), and wrap is applied (**c**). (**d**) Note how the lateral radiograph demonstrates complete off-loading of the posterior heel and flap while lying in bed

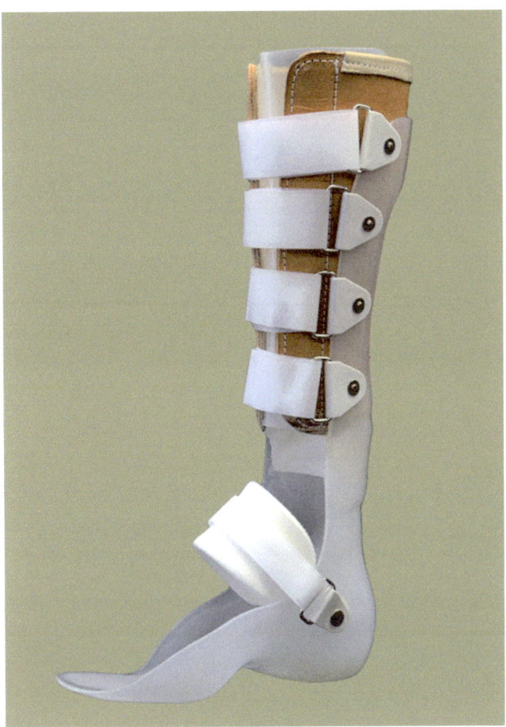

Fig. 21.33 Rigid ankle-foot orthoses bracing is needed for ambulation given the loss of heel height and Achilles tendon function (picture courtesy of Tillges Certified Orthotic Prosthetic Inc., Maplewood, MN)

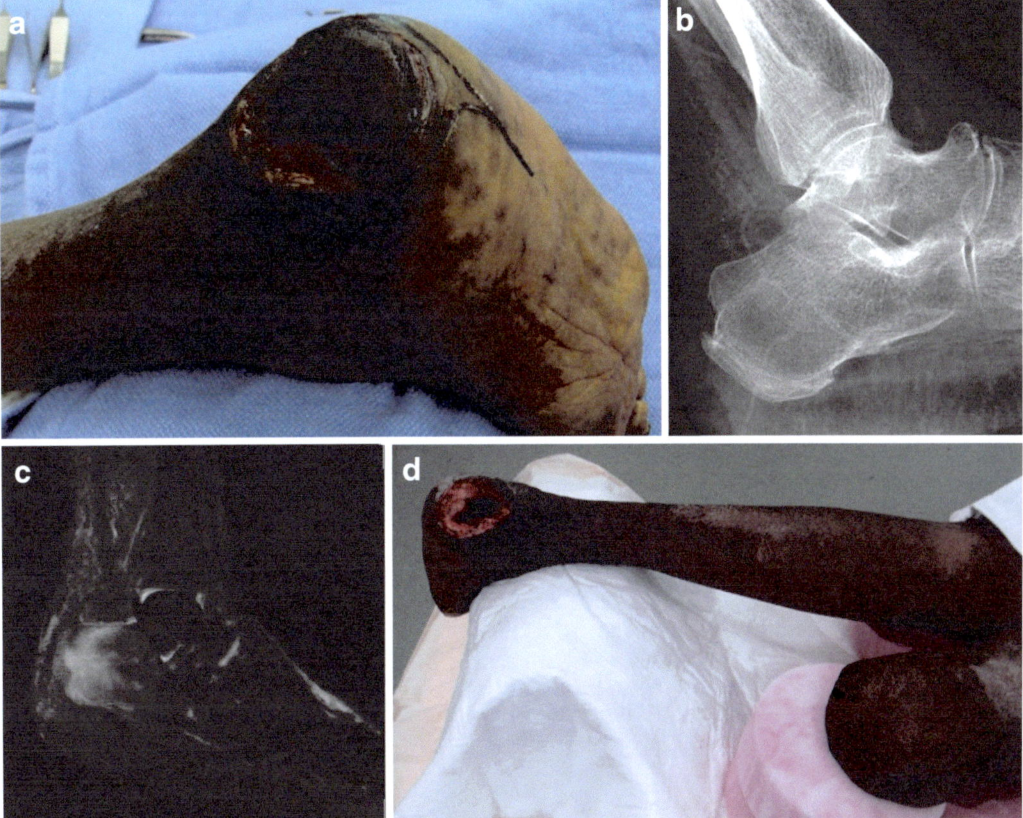

Fig. 21.34 Zone 1 posterior heel decubitus ulceration case 5 example. (**a**) This 89-year-old diabetic female with contralateral leg amputation demonstrates a zone 1 or posterior heel decubitus ulceration which is the most common location for a heel ulcer. (**b, c**) Pre-op labs, X-rays, and MRI confirmed osteomyelitis and abscess surrounding the attachment of the Achilles tendon. (**d**) Given patients contralateral leg amputation and desire to remain living at home with her husband, partial calcanectomy with flap closure was decided as the treatment course

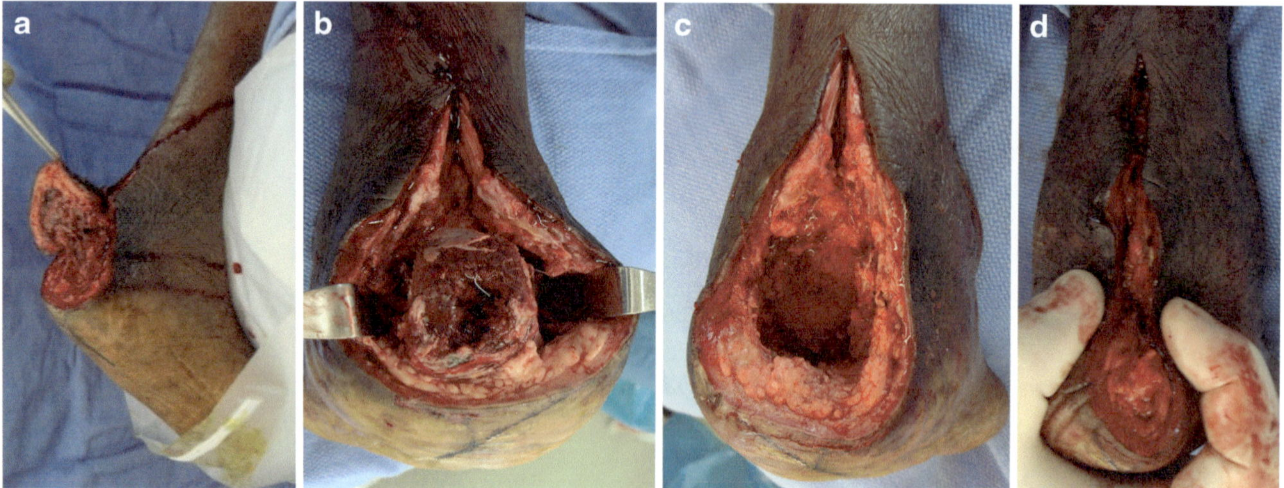

Fig. 21.35 (**a**, **b**) Stage 1 surgery in case 5 involved incision and drainage of the necrotic wound excision of the necrotic, Achilles tendon, and wide bone resection. (**c**) The wound bed looks healthy after debridement despite the original necrotic appearance. (**d**) Note that side-to-side closure was not possible despite extensive calcanectomy. Raising the flap was delayed until the stage 2 procedure which allowed demarcation of the wound

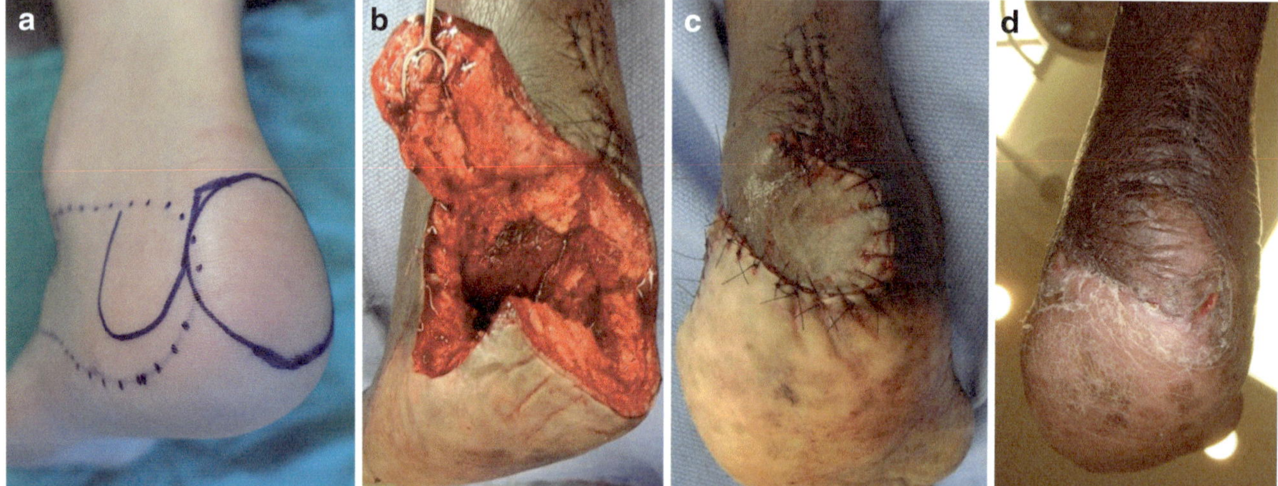

Fig. 21.36 Flap creation and closure for zone 1 decubitus ulceration demonstrated in case 5. (**a**) This zone 1 ulcer location allows use of a lateral-based unilobed flap which is supplied by the lateral calcaneal artery. Note that this flap avoids the intact plantar soft tissues. (**b**) The stage 2 procedure involved creation of the flap and complete wound closure. (**c**) Incision remained well approximated at the initial postoperative visit. (**d**) Six-week postoperative photo demonstrates a well-healed flap. Limb salvage allowed continued independent living despite contralateral leg amputation at 89 years of age

Fig. 21.37 Zone 2 junctional decubitus ulceration case 6 example. (**a**) A 75-year-old diabetic male with a chronic nonhealing junction decubitus ulceration. (**b**) High suspicion for osteomyelitis was based on positive probe to bone, elevated inflammatory marker labs, and positive bone scan despite the X-ray being read as negative. (**c**) Bone scan is our second choice for advanced imaging for patients who cannot undergo MRI

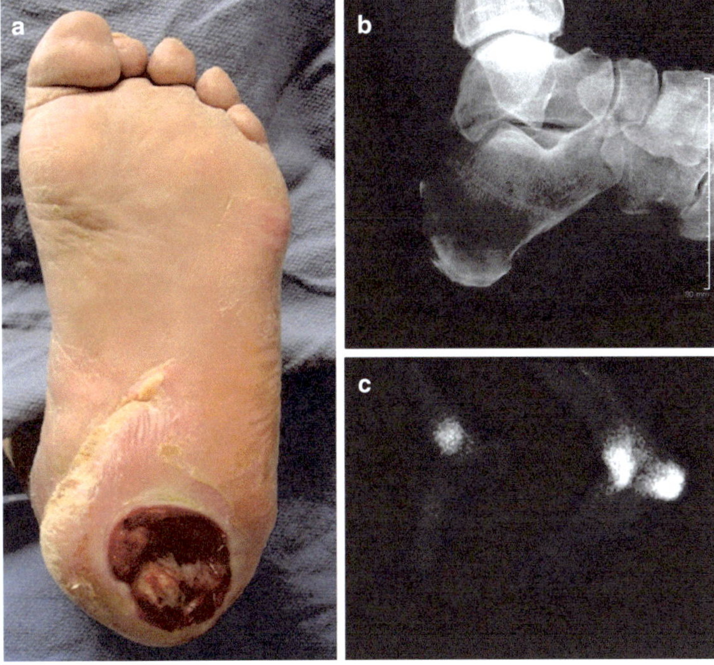

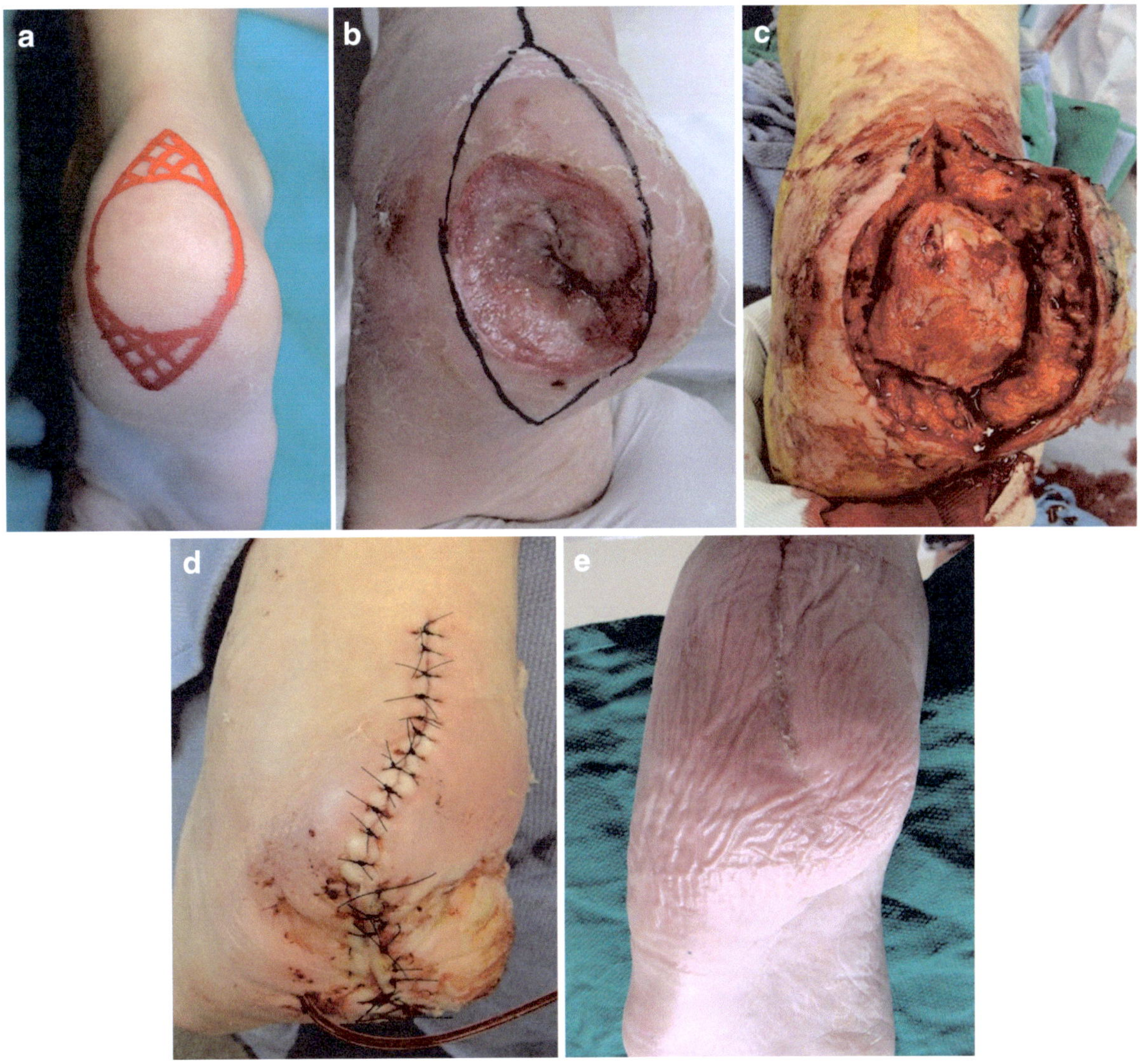

Fig. 21.38 (**a**) Elliptical excision and partial calcanectomy for zone 2 junctional decubitus ulceration in case 6. (**b**) This zone 2 ulcer location is most amenable to an ellipse-type incision. (**c**) Note that incision technique allows adequate exposure of the posterior calcaneus, although portions of good skin are wasted in this incisional technique. (**d**) Primary closure with drain is demonstrated. (**e**) Long-term postoperative clinical photo of well-healed incision

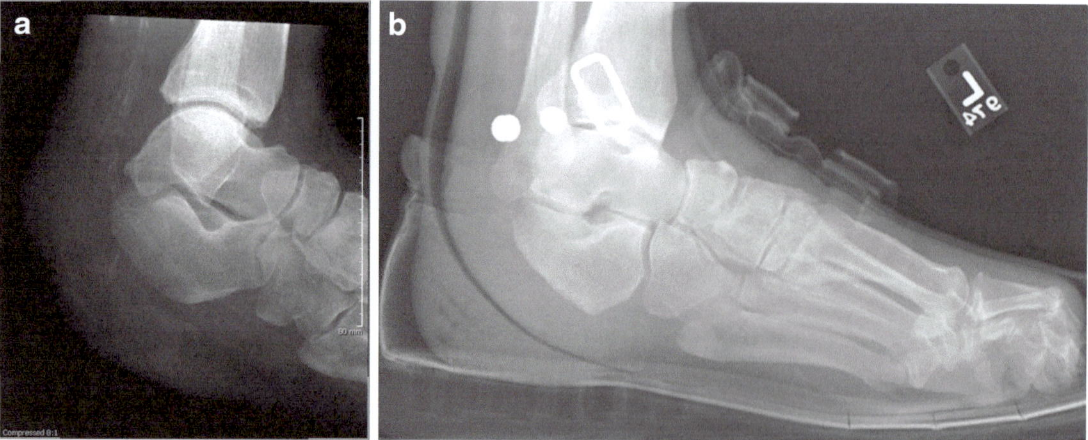

Fig. 21.39 Postoperative course for zone 2 ulceration in case 6. (**a**) Long-term lateral radiograph demonstrates resection that minimized bony prominences. (**b**) Partial calcanectomy results in loss of heel height and Achilles function which is accommodated with the use of a rigid AFO that corrects for loss of heel height; this weight bearing X-ray was taken while wearing the brace and shoe now 8 years after calcanectomy

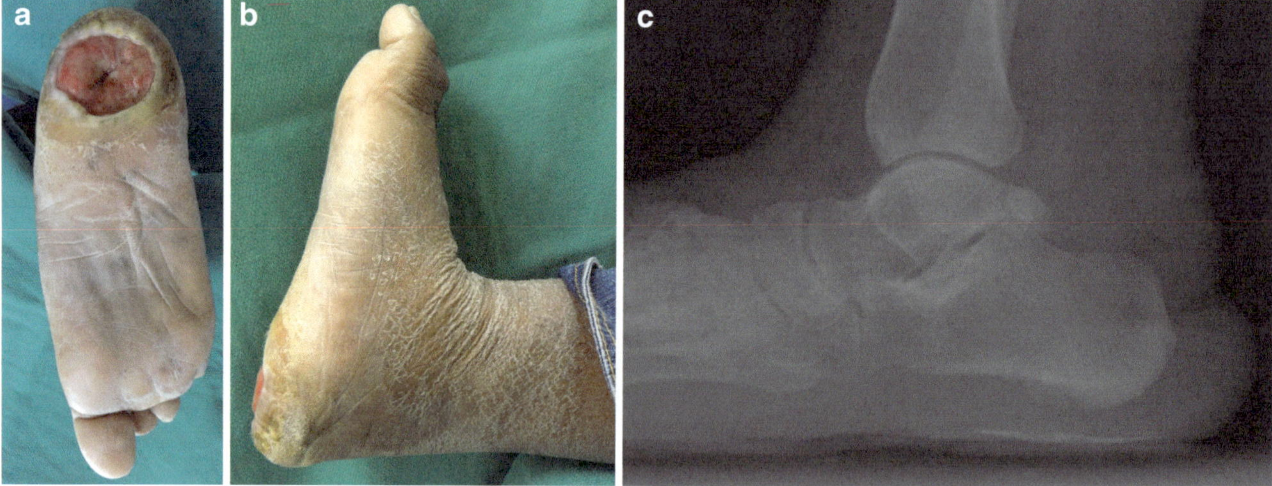

Fig. 21.40 Case 7: Zone 3 plantar heel decubitus ulceration. (**a**) Zone 3 plantar heel ulceration with secondary osteomyelitis was associated with calcaneus gait after walking prematurely following Achilles tendon lengthening. (**b**) Notice the excessive amount of ankle dorsiflexion present. She failed multiple debridements, prolonged negative-pressure wound therapy, and several skin graft trials. (**c**) She presented on referral for calcanectomy after recent MRI demonstrated bone infection yet preoperative lateral imaging demonstrated only subtle cortical changes

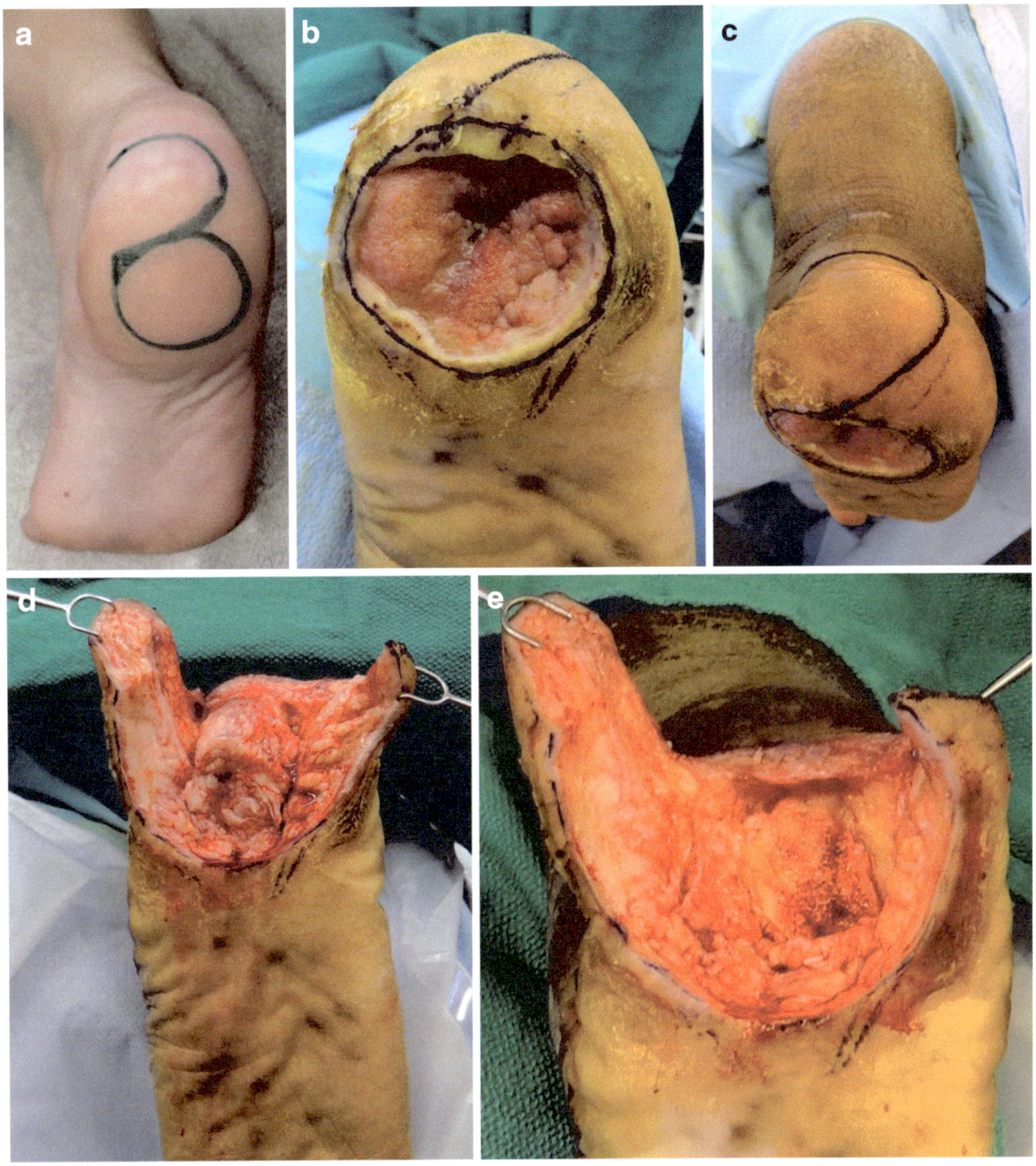

Fig. 21.41 Posterior unilobed flap with partial calcanectomy for zone 3 heel decubitus ulceration demonstrated in case 7. (**a**, **b**) The plantar location of the ulceration allows for a posterior donor site (**c**) for the unilobed flap. (**d**) Note how this flap does not violate the intact plantar skin in the arch and avoids incision where the lateral plantar artery and nerve cross in the plantar arch. Note the extensive calcaneal exposure that is achieved once the flap is raised. (**e**) The posterior flap also provides access for calcanectomy. Resection of the tuberosity creates laxity for flap coverage of the wound

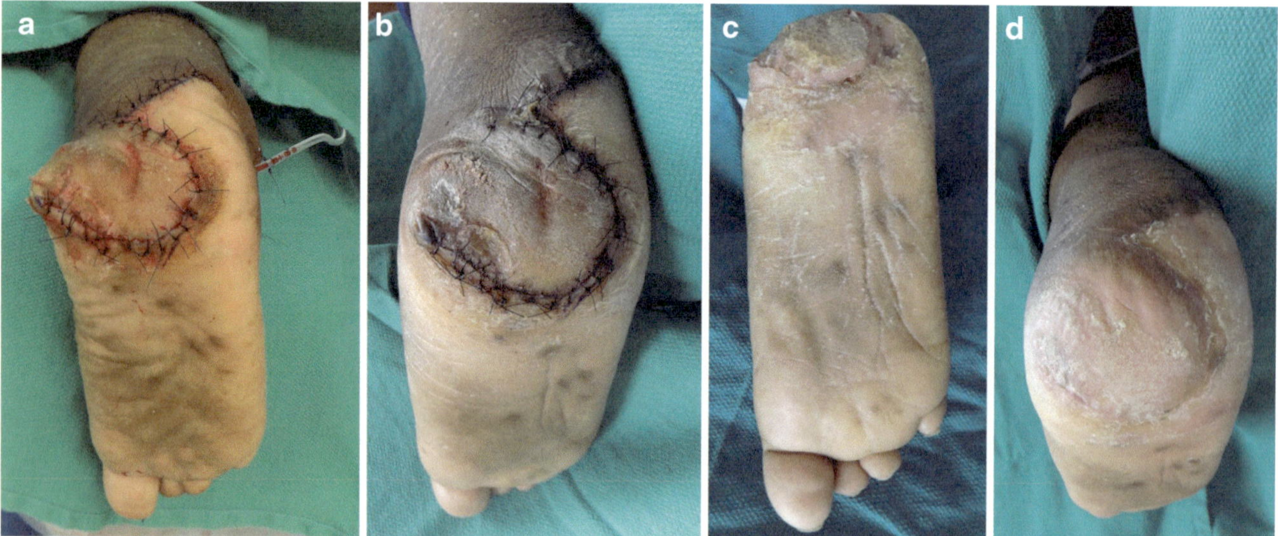

Fig. 21.42 Sequential healing of the zone 3 unilobed flap in case 7. (**a**) Intraoperative photo of closed flap; (**b**) note that it is not uncommon to have a dog ear secondary to hard marginal eschar, flap rotation, and redundant tissue. This will soften, remodel, and flatten with time. (**b**) Two-week postoperative photo (**b**) with sutures intact (**c**). Removal of the sutures and eschar was performed at 6 weeks post-op. At 10 weeks post-op (**d**) skin was soft, edema was well controlled, and patient was able to ambulate with use of an ankle-foot orthoses and custom diabetic shoe. Note that the medial dog ear has resolved

Fig. 21.43 Case 7: Post-op X-rays of zone 3 unilobed flap. (**a**) Postoperative radiographs demonstrate desired level of resection of the posterior calcaneus to remove a large section of infected bone, minimize pressure points to avoid future pressure-related sores, and relax the soft tissues to allow flap closure. (**b**) The calcaneal axial view is helpful to evaluate for medial or lateral prominence

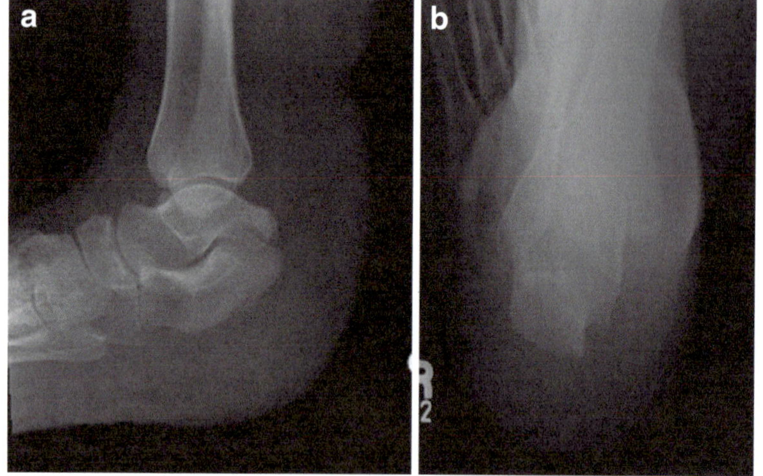

Conclusion

There is no one-size-fits-all approach to surgical treatment of calcaneal osteomyelitis. The optimal treatment protocol is largely determined by the etiology of infection and extent of the soft tissue defect which substantially influences the clinical presentation as detailed in Fig. 21.1 and Table 21.1. The principle treatment goals for calcaneal osteomyelitis are to resolve the bone and soft tissue infection, heal the local wound deficit, maximize postoperative function, and minimize the chance of future breakdown. A poorly planned treatment protocol may likely result in months of expensive treatments, prolonged hospitalization, and multiple operations without achieving the desired goals. Some patients are best treated with leg amputation, and this decision is best made before unnecessary and sometimes harmful interventions are exhausted.

References

1. Cichowitz A, Pan WR, Ashton M. The heel anatomy, blood supply and the pathophysiology of pressure ulcers. Ann Plast Surg. 2009;62:423–9.
2. Randall D, Phillips J, Ianiro G. Partial calcanectomy for the treatment of recalcitrant heel ulcerations. J Am Podiatr Med Assoc. 2005;95:335–41.
3. Coughlin JM, Schon LC. Diabetes. In: Coughlin JM, Saltzman CL, Anderson RB, editors. Mann's surgery of the foot and ankle. 9th ed. Philadelphia: Elsevier; 2014. p. 1385–480.
4. Merlet A, Cazanave C, Dauchy FA, Dutronc H, Casoli V, Chauveaux D, De Barbeyrac B, Dupon M. Prognostic factors of calcaneal osteomyelitis. Scand J Infect Dis. 2014;46:555–60.
5. Fukuda T, Reddy V, Ptaszek AJ. The infected calcaneus. Foot Ankle Clin. 2010;15:477–86.
6. Chen K, Balloch R. Management of calcaneal osteomyelitis. Clin Podiatr Med Surg. 2010;27:417–29.
7. Baravarian B, Menendez MM, Weinheimer DJ, Lowery C, Kosanovich M, Vidt L. Subtotal calcanectomy for the treatment of large heel ulceration and calcaneal osteomyelitis in the diabetic patient. J Foot Ankle Surg. 1999;38:194–202.
8. Boffeli TJ, Collier RC. Near total calcanectomy with rotational flap closure of large decubitus ulcerations complicated by calcaneal osteomyelitis. J Foot Ankle Surg. 2013;52:107–12.
9. Cook J, Cook E, Landsman A, Basile P, Dinh T, Lyons T, Rosenblum B, Giurini J. A retrospective assessment of partial calcanectomies and factors influencing postoperative course. J Foot Ankle Surg. 2007;46:248–55.
10. Han PY, Ezquerro R. Surgical treatment of pressure ulcers of the heel in skilled nursing facilities a 12 year retrospective study of 57 patients. J Am Podiatr Med Assoc. 2011;101:167–75.
11. Lehmann S, Murphy RD, Lawrence H. Partial calcanectomy in the treatment of chronic heel ulceration. J Am Podiatr Med Assoc. 2001;91:369–72.
12. Schade VL. Partial or total calcanectomy as an alternative to below the knee amputation for limb salvage a systematic review. J Am Podiatr Med Assoc. 2012;102:396–405.
13. Smith DG, Stuck RM, Ketner L, Sage RM, Pinzur MS. Partial calcanectomy for the treatment of large ulcerations of the heel and calcaneal osteomyelitis. J Bone Joint Surg. 1992;74:571–6.
14. Walsh TP, Yates BJ. Calcanectomy: avoiding major amputation in the presence of calcaneal osteomyelitis–a case series. Foot (Edinb). 2013;23:130–5.
15. Woll TS, Beals RK. Partial calcanectomy for the treatment of osteomyelitis of the calcaneus. Foot Ankle Int. 1991;12:31–4.
16. Attinger CE, Evans KK, Bulan E, Blume P, Cooper P. Angiosomes of the foot and ankle clinical implications for limb salvage: reconstruction, incisions and revascularization. Plast Reconstr Surg. 2006;117:2615–935.
17. Laughlin RT, Reeve F, Wright DG, Mader JT, Calhoun JH. Calcaneal osteomyelitis caused by nail puncture wounds. Foot Ankle Int. 1997;18:575–7.
18. Giduma R, Evanski P. Calcaneal osteomyelitis following steroid injection: a case report. Foot Ankle. 1985;6:44–6.
19. Wronka KS, Sinha AM. Calcaneal osteomyelitis following steroid injection for plantar fasciitis: a case report. Foot Ankle Spec. 2012;5:253–5.
20. McKee MD, Wild LM, Schemitsch EH, Waddell JP. The use of an antibiotic impregnated osteoconductive, bioabsorbable bone substitute in the treatment of infected long bone defects: early results of a prospective trial. J Orthop Trauma. 2002;16:622–7.
21. Sangray B, Malhotra S, Steinbury JS. Current therapies for diabetic foot infections and osteomyelitis. Clin Podiatr Med Surg. 2014;31:57–70.
22. Coughlin M, Grimes JS, Kennedy MP. Coralline hydroxyapatite bone graft substitute in hindfoot surgery. Foot Ankle Int. 2006;27:19–22.
23. Lee MC, Tashjian RZ, Eberson CP. Calcaneus osteomyelitis from community-acquired MRSA. Foot Ankle Int. 2007;28:276–80.
24. Al-Qattan MM. The reverse sural artery adipofasciomuscular flap for the reconstruction of a heel sinus with underlying calcaneal osteomyelitis. Ann Plast Surg. 2007;58:688–90.
25. Attinger C, Cooper P. Soft tissue reconstruction for calcaneal fractures or osteomyelitis. Orthop Clin North Am. 2001;32:135–70.
26. Chen SL, Chen TM, Chou TD, Chang SC, Wang HJ. Distally based sural fasciomusculocutaneous flap for chronic calcaneal osteomyelitis in diabetic patients. Ann Plast Surg. 2005;54:44–8.
27. Ghods M, Grabs R, Kersten C, Chatzopoulos PP, Geomelas M. A modified free muscle transfer technique to effectively treat chronic and persistent calcaneal osteomyelitis. Ann Plast Surg. 2012;68:599–605.
28. Xu XY, Zhu Y, Liu JH. Treatment of calcaneal osteomyelitis with free serratus anterior muscle flap transfer. Foot Ankle Int. 2009;30:1088–93.
29. Yildirim S, Gideroğlu K, Aköz T. The simple and effective choice for treatment of chronic calcaneal osteomyelitis: neurocutaneous flaps. Plast Reconstr Surg. 2003;111:753–60.
30. Dockery GL. Advancement and rotational flaps. In: Dockery GL, Crawford ME, editors. Lower extremity soft tissue and cutaneous plastic surgery. Philadelphia: WB Saunders; 2006. p. 129–46.
31. Schrudde J, Petrovici V. The use of slide-swing plasty in closing skin defects: a clinical study based on 1308 cases. Plast Reconstr Surg. 1981;6:182–6.

Osteomyelitis of the Distal Fibula Associated with Lateral Ankle Decubitus Ulceration

Ryan R. Pfannenstein, Kevin J. Mahoney, and Troy J. Boffeli

Introduction

Osteomyelitis of the distal fibula is typically associated with contiguous spread of infection from an adjacent decubitus ulceration overlying the lateral ankle. The soft tissues overlying the distal fibula are relatively thin which increases the likelihood of bone exposure once the decubitus wound eschar sloughs [1]. Wide exposure of cortical bone at the base of the wound is not conducive to progressive formation of granulation tissue, and local infection including osteomyelitis is a common late-stage sequelae [2]. The residual wound defect significantly compromises the ability to successfully resolve osteomyelitis as the fibula frequently remains chronically exposed. Infection may spread proximally along the peroneal tendons or penetrate deep into the ankle joint, which is difficult to control and frequently results in leg amputation.

Osteomyelitis of the distal fibula less commonly occurs due to direct inoculation associated with open ankle fracture, complications associated with surgical repair of ankle fracture, or secondary infection associated with venous stasis ulceration [3]. Neuropathic ulcers are not common at this location although neuropathy plays a role in decubitus pressure sores. Hematogenous osteomyelitis is less common in the distal fibula, but festering ankle joint sepsis can spread to the adjacent fibula, tibia, or talus.

The lateral malleolus is a common location for decubitus pressure sores associated with prolonged bed rest, surgery, or hospitalization with reports of up to 12 % of all decubitus ulcerations occurring at this location [4–6]. Patients with severe hip and knee contracture are particularly at risk of lateral ankle pressure sores if they can only be positioned in the lateral decubitus position [1]. Decubitus pressure can also occur when sitting in a wheelchair with the lateral ankle resting against the leg rest (Fig. 22.1). Early recognition that pathologic pressure is occurring while in the wheelchair is critical since not all lateral ankle pressure sores occur while in bed. Patients with equinovarus contracture of the foot and ankle associated with neuromuscular diseases such as stroke or cerebral palsy are particularly at risk for ankle-foot orthotic (AFO)-related lateral ankle pressure sores as fibular prominence is accentuated by inversion contracture (Fig. 22.2). Early intervention involves brace modifications and attempts to reduce spasticity through medical interventions. Surgical treatment involving Achilles, posterior tibial, and flexor tendon lengthening may be helpful to allow AFO bracing in the neutral position, reduction of fibular prominence, and improved patient mobility [7].

Treatment protocols for osteomyelitis of the distal fibula are not well described in the literature. Osteomyelitis is largely a late-stage presentation which commonly results in failure to heal a decubitus ulcer despite months of expensive wound care. The late-stage development of bone exposure and resultant osteomyelitis of the fibula is difficult to predict in the early stages of wound management. Full-depth compromise of the overlying soft tissue is likely the main determining factor since the bone becomes immediately exposed when a truly full-thickness eschar finally sloughs after months of monitoring. Factors that lead to poor wound healing, including poor nutrition, circulatory compromise, and edema, further predispose to soft tissue infection and resultant osteomyelitis. Early intervention for lateral malleolar decubitus ulceration primarily involves off-loading, local wound care, edema control, and vascular intervention if needed. Surgery is primarily considered once the underlying bone becomes exposed or when early signs of infection develop. Consideration of surgical treatment for equinovarus contracture deformity can also be considered early in the course of treating pressure sores.

R.R. Pfannenstein, D.P.M., F.A.C.F.A.S. (✉)
K.J. Mahoney, D.P.M. • T.J. Boffeli, D.P.M., F.A.C.F.A.S.
Regions Hospital/HealthPartners Institute for Education and Research, 640 Jackson Street, St. Paul, MN 55101, USA
e-mail: ryan.r.pfannenstein@healthpartners.com;
kevin.j.mahoney@healthpartners.com;
troy.j.boffeli@healthpartners.com

© Springer International Publishing Switzerland 2015
T.J. Boffeli (ed.), *Osteomyelitis of the Foot and Ankle*, DOI 10.1007/978-3-319-18926-0_22

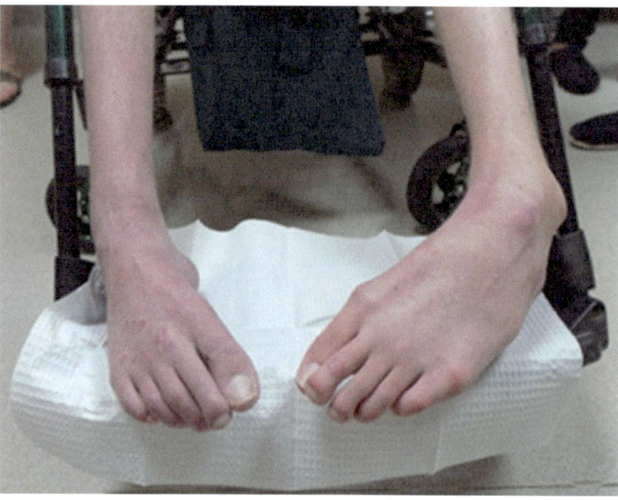

Fig. 22.1 Wheelchair-related lateral ankle decubitus pressure sores. Nonambulatory patients likely spend more hours of the day in a wheelchair or motorized powerchair than in bed which increases the risk of wheelchair-related foot and ankle pressure sores. Contracture of the lower extremity associated with neuromuscular conditions creates lateral prominence which further predisposes to lateral pressure from the foot rest

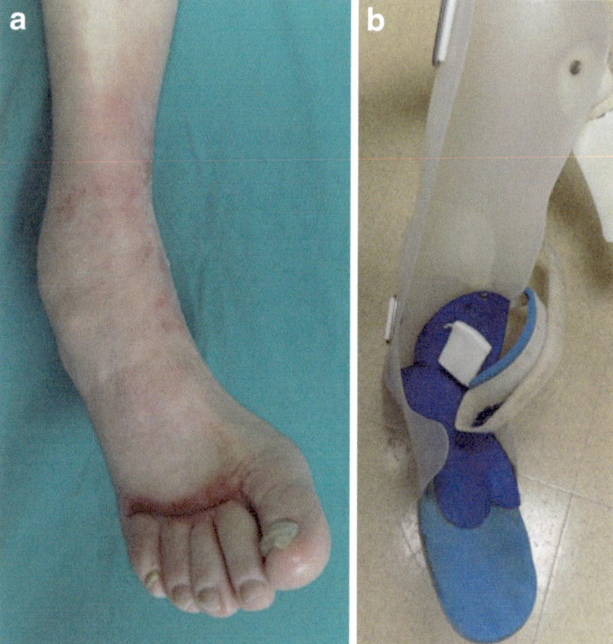

Fig. 22.2 Lateral ankle pressure sores associated with ankle-foot orthotic (AFO) bracing. AFO bracing is commonly employed for foot and ankle weakness or contracture deformity. (**a**) Neuromuscular disorders like stroke, cerebral palsy, and traumatic brain injury commonly result in plantar flexion and inversion deformity at the ankle which creates lateral malleolar prominence and is a source of pressure associated with AFO bracing. (**b**) The brace is intended to maintain positioning at the foot and ankle which naturally applies pressure in the region of the lateral malleolus. Early intervention with brace modifications is helpful, but medical or surgical treatment to reduce spastic contracture may be necessary

Conservative surgical intervention is not likely to cure osteomyelitis of the distal fibula since infection can be extensive throughout the lateral malleolus and wound defects are difficult to close primarily. Wide resection of the distal fibula may be the most prudent approach for patients confined to a wheelchair as extensive resection of bone allows mobility of the surrounding tissue which aids in primary closure. Complete distal fibulectomy is less practical for ambulatory patients as this is likely to destabilize the ankle and results in exposure of the ankle joint, talus, and tibia which may lead to contiguous spread of infection [8]. Successful wound healing is a critical aspect of successful surgical management for osteomyelitis of the distal fibula since prolonged bone exposure following bone resection often leads to persistent infection. Our preferred surgical approach involving wound excision, lateral cortical debridement of the distal fibula, bone biopsy, and advanced wound closure techniques including negative-pressure wound therapy (NWPT) or local flap closure of the wound is the focus of this chapter. Extensive soft tissue loss can also be treated with various musculocutaneous pedicle flaps or free muscle flaps followed by skin grafting [9–17]. Wide resection of the infected wound and distal fibula with delayed fusion of the ankle is discussed in Chap. 10.

Natural Progression of Lateral Ankle Decubitus Ulceration with Late-Stage Development of Osteomyelitis

Lateral ankle pressure sores typically follow a natural healing progression from initial decubitus insult to eventual healing that may be protracted for perhaps 1 year in duration depending on the size and stage of ulceration and effectiveness of off-loading. The superficial skin may initially form a blister while the compromised deeper soft tissues eventually become a black, leathery eschar that remains firmly attached to the underlying tissue and bone. Minimal topical care or debridement is necessary during the early phase of eschar formation or maturation since the eschar serves as a natural barrier to infection. It is important to minimize edema in the extremity and protect the peripheral tissues against ongoing decubitus pressure. Antibiotics are not necessary or helpful during this stage, and expensive wound care treatments are of little value while the eschar remains intact. Assessment of extremity circulation may identify the need for vascular intervention which is more useful at this early stage rather than later when the wound becomes compromised with infection. The patient may remain ambulatory for lateral malleolar decubitus ulcers since mobility minimizes the risk of ongoing decubitus pressure. Non-bed-related sources of decubitus pressure should be rectified including pressure while sitting in a wheelchair and ill-fitting AFO braces.

Debridement of the eschar eventually becomes necessary during the course of eschar maturation. Blistering of the superficial skin may occur early, and loosely adhered tissue can be removed once the blister becomes dessicated. Deep debridement is otherwise delayed until the edges of the eschar become softened, macerated, and delaminated months into the healing process. Granulation tissue around the margin of the eschar is frequently noted at this time. The central aspect of the eschar typically remains firmly attached to the deep periosteum and should be left in place as a natural barrier to infection. The ideal healing process would involve progressive formation of granulation tissue as the eschar delaminates from the peripheral margin toward the center of the wound [18]. Epithelialization at the intact skin margin and simultaneous circumferential contraction toward the center of the wound allows progressive healing. Normal healing takes months and frequently more than 1 year for large wounds. The central aspect of the eschar eventually softens or "ripens" to the point where it is no longer advantageous and should be removed. A soft, necrotic, and foul-smelling eschar eventually becomes a harbinger for bacteria and may predispose to the onset of infection. This slow approach to eschar removal can oftentimes be performed in the office and without anesthesia provided that only necrotic and loose tissue is removed. Final eschar excision may require an operating room procedure for patients with intact sensation. Our routine is to begin hydrating or enzymatic debriding agents once granulation tissue is exposed around the peripheral margin of the eschar or when the eschar is completely removed.

Complete eschar removal finally allows assessment of the depth of necrosis and potential exposure of the fibula. The distal fibula is oftentimes covered with nonviable slough which represents unhealthy periosteum and devitalized fibrotic tissue. The fibula may become exposed but is frequently not yet infected at the time of complete eschar removal. Lateral malleolar decubitus wounds differ from heel decubitus wounds in that the heel has a thick pad of compartmentalized fat separating the superficial skin from the deep bone allowing greater healing potential once the eschar is removed.

Early workup for osteomyelitis is typically not necessary since osteomyelitis is more likely to develop over time once the eschar sloughs. Assessment of probe-to-bone status, baseline inflammatory marker labs, and X-rays are oftentimes obtained at this point. The patient may still be months away from the onset of fibular osteomyelitis, but consideration could be given to early decortication and rotational flap coverage of the wound. This decision is oftentimes based on the size of the wound, the extent of bone exposure, the quality of the surrounding tissue, and the relative health of the patient. The typical patient with a lateral malleolar decubitus ulcer is not a great surgical candidate, yet waiting for infection to develop may compromise the healing potential of this potentially life-altering situation. One year of wound treatment can be very disheartening and frustrating for an ambulatory patient who is unwilling to accept the risk of potential limb loss. Wheelchair-bound patients may be more amenable to a wait-and-see approach. Ultimately, the decision for early surgical intervention is difficult since flap surgery puts adjacent tissue at risk and surgery may expose uninfected bone to potential contamination.

Diagnosis of Distal Fibular Osteomyelitis

Standard X-rays are not very effective at identifying early onset of osteomyelitis in the distal fibula. Erosion of the lateral cortex is typically the first finding yet the cortex on the distal fibula is relatively thick, and it may take months to see radiographic signs of cortical erosion (Fig. 22.3). Abnormality of the overlying soft tissue due to the leathery eschar or sloughing tissue also changes the appearance of bone density on X-ray. Serial MRIs during a 12-month course of wound monitoring is not practical or cost-effective. MRI is typically reserved for patients with high suspicion for osteomyelitis with desire to evaluate the extent of infection and to rule out soft tissue abscess, ankle joint sepsis, and involvement of the tibia or talus. The diagnosis of osteomyelitis is best made by evaluating the entire clinical picture including local wound appearance, probe-to-bone status, infection marker labs, and X-rays. An abrupt jump in erythrocyte sedimentation rate (ESR) from a baseline normal value to a high double-digit

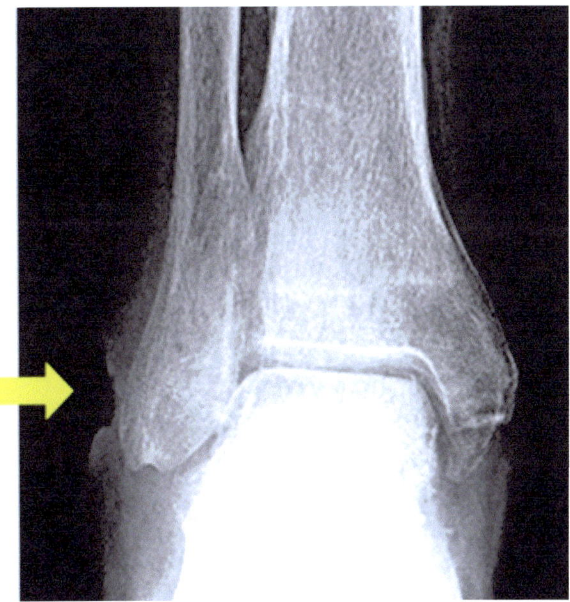

Fig. 22.3 Radiographic evaluation for osteomyelitis. X-rays are not very sensitive at detecting early onset of osteomyelitis in the distal fibula, but periosteal reaction or cortical erosion may eventually become apparent. Early X-rays are primarily useful for late-stage comparison once osteomyelitis develops. The lateral cortex is the most likely location for osteomyelitis associated with decubitus ulceration. Note the obvious soft tissue deficit over the distal fibula which interferes with assessment of bone density

value raises suspicion for new onset of osteomyelitis; however, this approach can be misleading since an elevated ESR is not specific to the ankle condition, which makes baseline lab values clinically useful.

Osteomyelitis typically occurs from contiguous spread of infection from the overlying decubitus wound. Lack of clinical signs of wound infection therefore would suggest the absence of osteomyelitis. Chronic wounds that are covered in slough are always contaminated with bacteria, and wound culture is not an accurate way to identify infection or causative organisms. Bone biopsy is ultimately the ideal diagnostic test to identify osteomyelitis which is discussed in Chap. 4. The primary risk of bone biopsy when wounds are present is that violation of the cortex exposes the cancellous bone to potentially contaminating organisms. Festering and untreated osteomyelitis, on the other hand, will likely preclude progressive wound healing despite costly and burdensome wound care, thus making bone biopsy a valued test despite inherent risks.

Bone scan should be considered for patients unable to undergo MRI and is more cost-effective than bilateral MRI for patients with bilateral involvement. A negative bone scan largely rules out osteomyelitis with the exception that severe arterial insufficiency could lead to a false negative bone scan. MRI is useful from a surgical planning standpoint regarding extent of incision and drainage procedures, ideal location of bone biopsy, involvement of adjacent bone structures, and involvement of the peroneal tendons. The lateral ankle tendons are commonly exposed within a chronic lateral malleolar ulcer and oftentimes become diseased or infected. The peroneal tendon sheath can also become a pathway for spread of infection into the leg or foot. The peroneal tendons can be

inspected at the time of surgery but avoiding interruption of the tendon sheath is desirable if the tendons appear uninvolved on MRI. Findings on MRI consistent with inflammation within the distal fibula should not be automatically interpreted as necrotic or dead bone. Direct visualization of bone viability at the time of surgery allows for surgeon judgment regarding the potential to preserve the distal fibula with conservative lateral cortical debridement and postoperative antibiotic therapy. It is desirable to preserve a functional lateral malleolus unless the bone is truly dead and necrotic [8]. CT is a third option for advanced imaging although MRI and bone scan may have greater clinical utility.

Tendon Lengthening Options for Neuromuscular Contracture of the Foot and Ankle

Surgical treatment of equinovarus contracture deformity may be necessary for AFO-related lateral malleolar ulcers in patients with contracture associated with neuromuscular disorders. Tendon lengthening procedures allow proper positioning in the brace which ultimately reduces lateral ankle decubitus pressure [7]. The posterior tibial tendon is lengthened to reduce varus contracture of the foot and ankle. For ambulatory patients, a sliding Z-lengthening procedure allows side-to-side repair after lengthening. Nonambulatory patients with chronic edema and expected permanent use of AFO bracing can be treated with a smaller, almost percutaneous incision and complete posterior tibial tenotomy (Fig. 22.4). Equinus ankle contracture is addressed with

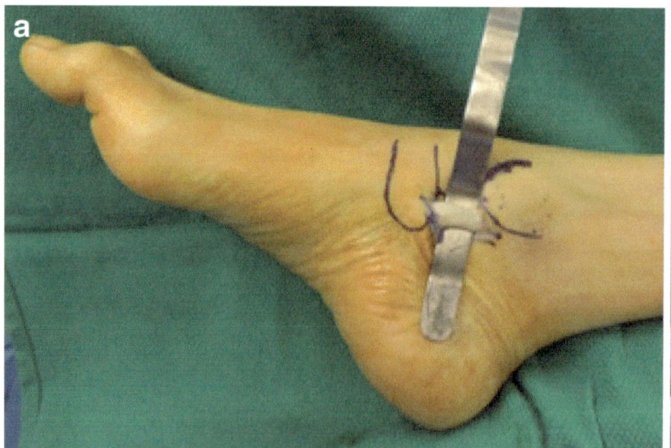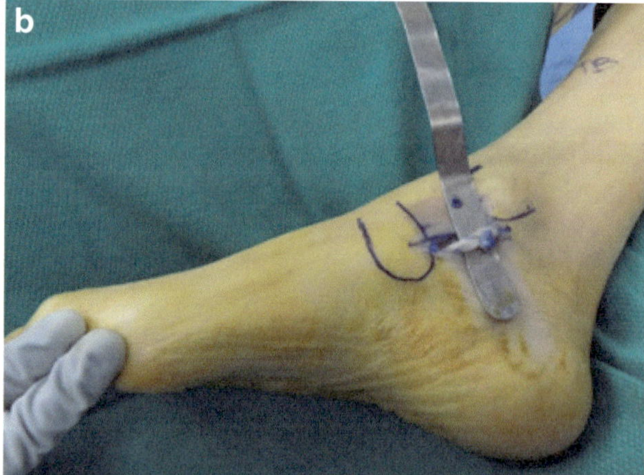

Fig. 22.4 Open Z-lengthening of the posterior tibial tendon to treat inversion contracture deformity. (**a**) Posterior tibial tendon Z-lengthening or tenotomy was performed through a small open incision extending from the tip of the medial malleolus to the navicular tuberosity. The posterior tibial tendon is fairly subcutaneous at this location, and the incision is safely away from the posterior tibial nerve and artery. Tendon contracture makes for easy palpation of the tendon for incision placement. (**b**) A sliding Z-lengthening tendon release was performed followed by side-to-side repair

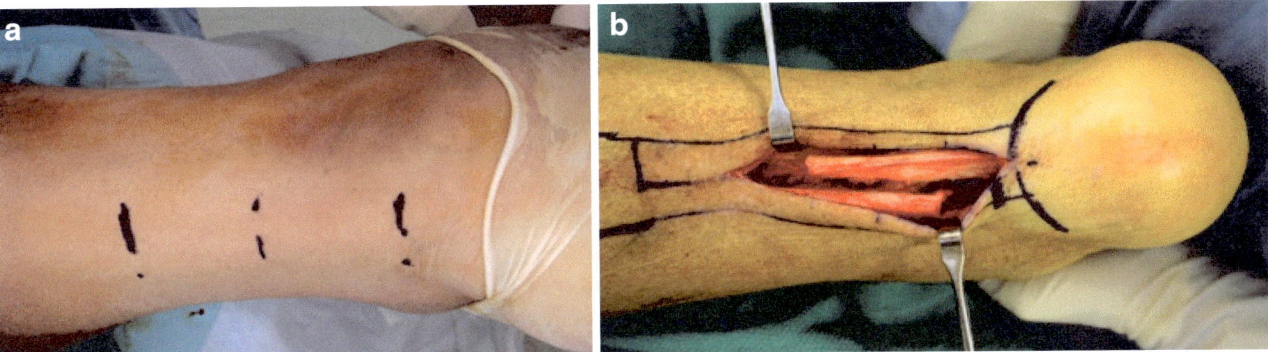

Fig. 22.5 Achilles tendon lengthening to treat ankle equinus. (**a**) Incisions are shown for minimally invasive triple hemisection Achilles lengthening. (**b**) Open Achilles Z-lengthening allows more controlled lengthening with direct suturing at the desired tendon length

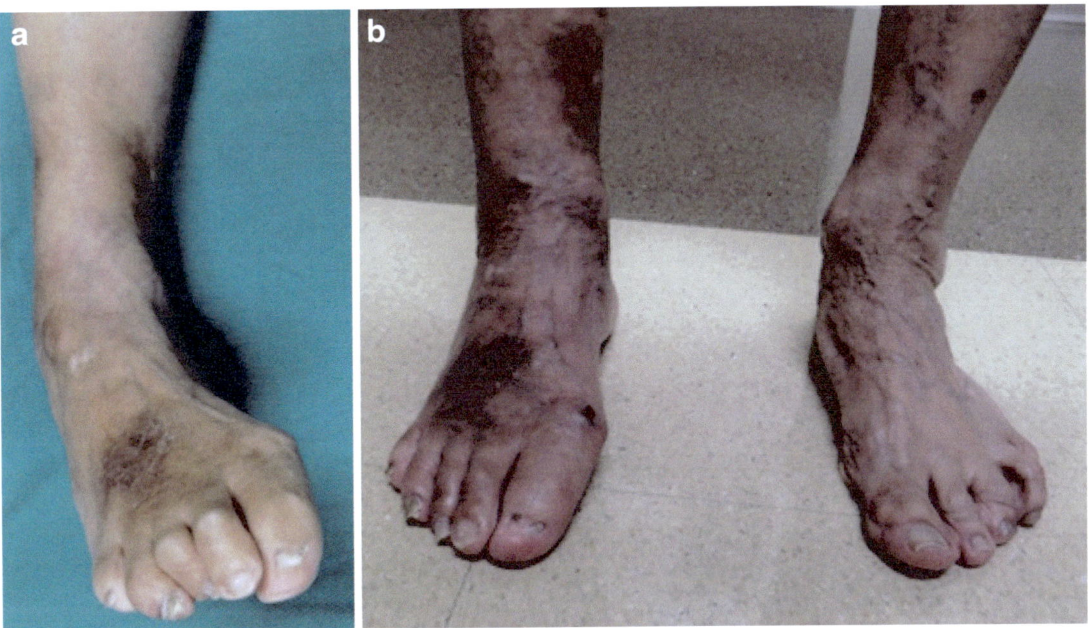

Fig. 22.6 Soft tissue release of ankle and digital contracture associated with stroke. (**a**) This foot was partially supple when relaxed but severely plantarflexed and inverted when weight bearing forces stimulated spasticity. This created a dilemma when attempting to brace the limb in the neutral position. (**b**) Six-week post-op clinical result is shown with the right foot now resting flat on the ground. She regained active ankle dorsiflexion at the ankle and no longer suffered with toe contracture. Intentional weakening of the spastic posterior tibial, Achilles, and flexor tendons allowed fairly normal function of the anterior tibial and extensor tendons which were previously overpowered by posterior contracture. Surgical intervention oftentimes allows ambulation without an AFO which further alleviates pressure on the lateral malleolus

Achilles tendon lengthening (TAL) which can be performed using multiple small incisions or as an open procedure (Fig. 22.5). The minimally invasive triple hemisection TAL does not allow suturing of the tendon; however, this may be desired in conditions involving spasticity to ensure that the tendon is adequately lengthened. Over lengthening is less of a concern since postoperative use of a rigid AFO is likely under these circumstances. Open Achilles Z-lengthening allows direct suturing at the desired tendon length but is less desirable when the local soft tissue is compromised by uncontrolled edema or when adjacent ulceration predispose to cross contamination. Figure 22.6 highlights the effectiveness of soft tissue release in patients with neuromuscular contracture.

Wound Excision and Lateral Cortical Debridement

Surgical treatment of osteomyelitis of the distal fibula may be performed in a staged manner, yet single-stage wound excision, bone resection, and flap closure are common. Staged surgery is useful for acute soft tissue infection with the first stage involving wound excision, lateral decortication of the distal fibula, bone biopsy, inspection and debridement of the peroneal tendons, drainage of local abscess, and open packing of the wound. Lateral malleolar ulcerations commonly demonstrate significant undermining of the wound margins. Following excision of the undermined tissue, the subsequent wound may be too large for primary or local flap closure (Fig. 22.7). Negative-pressure wound therapy (NPWT) is an option provided that infection is under control and necrotic tissue has been removed [18–20]. A short course of NPWT assists in determining the patient's ability to form granulation tissue. Staged surgery also allows vascular intervention if necessary prior to the definitive procedure. The stage 2 procedure can be performed days, weeks, or even months later [21]. Large wounds are challenging to cover with local flaps since adjacent tissue has limited coverage capabilities. NPWT is commonly employed after surgical debridement. In our experience, exposure of the cancellous bone within the distal fibula oftentimes stimulates robust granulation tissue in a previously nonhealing wound. Healing by secondary intention is possible under these circumstances as demonstrated in Case 1 (Figs. 22.8, 22.9, 22.10, 22.11, and 22.12).

Local Flap Closure Options for Lateral Malleolar Wounds

Local rotational and advancement flap closure of lateral malleolar wounds is possible depending on the size of the wound and condition of the surrounding tissue. One advantage of flap surgery is that raising the flap provides broad access for incision and drainage procedures, bone debridement, and peroneal tendon exploration. Compromised perfusion, uncontrolled edema, continued decubitus pressure, and inflexibility of the local tissue due to induration or ankle joint contracture may preclude success with local flap surgery. Case 2 (Figs. 22.13, 22.14, 22.15, and 22.16) highlights the surgical technique for unilobed flap closure of a medium-sized wound defect following wound excision and lateral cortical debridement of the distal fibula. Case 3 (Figs. 22.17, 22.18, and 22.19) shows an advancement flap technique that provided broad access for bone debridement and single-stage closure of a smaller wound defect.

Musculocutaneous Flaps

For cases involving larger wounds which are not amenable to local flaps, musculocutaneous flaps provide an alternative treatment option. Multiple options for soft tissue coverage with intrinsic muscle flaps have been described including using the abductor hallucis brevis, abductor digiti minimi, flexor digiti minimi, flexor digitorum brevis, and the extensor digitorum brevis [14–17]. Intrinsic muscle flaps mini-

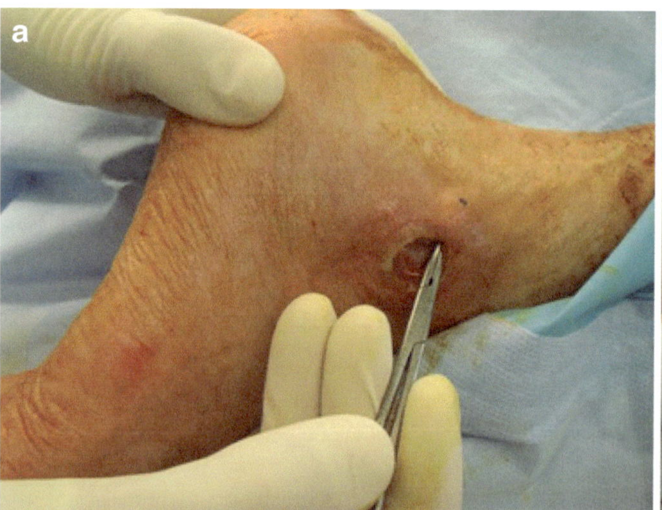
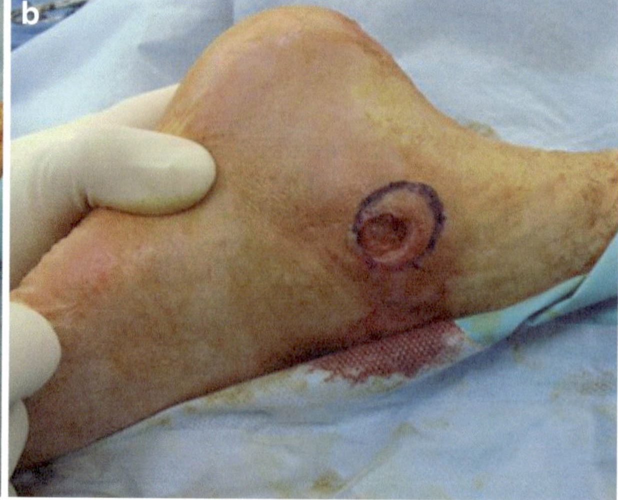

Fig. 22.7 Soft tissue undermining associated with lateral malleolar decubitus ulceration. The soft tissues covering the lateral malleolus are relatively mobile which predisposes to undermining at the wound margin. (**a**) A seemingly small ulcer can result in widespread exposure of the distal fibula and peroneal tendons. The undermined pocket is also a harbinger for bacterial colonization. (**b**) Surgical treatment often involves excision of the undermined wound margin which is not likely to reattach or contribute to healing. Excision enlarges the soft tissue defect which can create coverage challenges

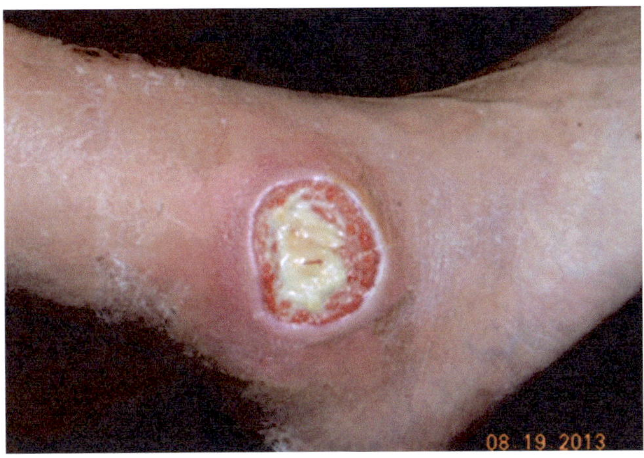

Fig. 22.8 Case 1: Lateral ankle decubitus ulceration with secondary osteomyelitis of the distal fibula. Extensive lateral ankle decubitus ulceration treated conservatively for the past 8 months. The nonviable, black eschar recently sloughed free exposing a nonviable wound bed with exposure of the lateral malleolus. Note that the peripheral margin contains granulation tissue that had formed in the preceding 2–3 months beneath a slowly delaminating eschar. The ability to form granulation tissue is a critical factor that differentiates healers from nonhealers. This large, full-thickness wound was highly prone to infection, and osteomyelitis was likely either present or inevitable

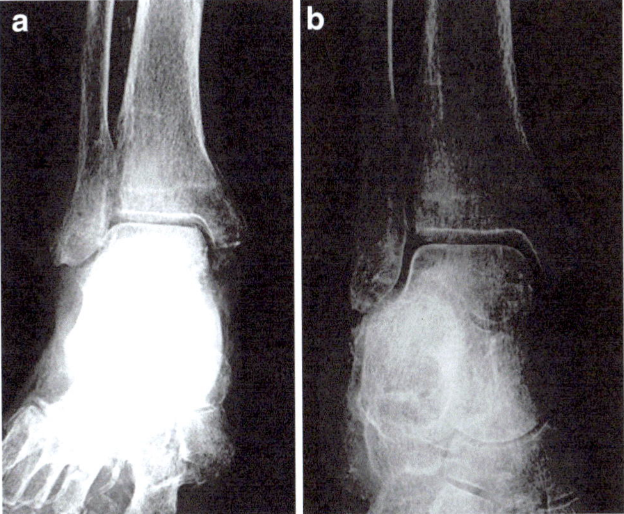

Fig. 22.9 Preoperative and postoperative radiographs in Case 1. (**a**) Preoperative X-rays were fairly unremarkable. The soft tissue defect was predictably over the most prominent aspect of the distal fibula. Surgical treatment involved excision of the fibrotic base of the wound, lateral decortication of the distal fibula, bone biopsy, and negative-pressure wound therapy. (**b**) Note how conservative removal of the lateral cortex made the lateral malleolus less prominent yet the ankle joint complex remained intact, without destabilizing or exposing the ankle joint

mize donor site morbidity compared to extrinsic muscle flaps or free flaps, although coverage is limited by the relatively small size of the intrinsic muscles. Pedicled flaps, such as the reverse sural flap as well as multiple free flap options, have historically provided effective coverage of larger lower-extremity wounds [9–14] as described further in Chap. 10.

Distal Fibulectomy

Complete excision of the distal fibula is perhaps the most expeditious treatment approach for nonambulatory patients with complicated lateral malleolar wounds. Destabilization of the ankle joint is less concerning for patients who are confined to a wheelchair but is the primary reason that we attempt to preserve a functional lateral malleolus in patients who ambulate or are capable of bipedal transfer. Case 4 is a paraplegic patient with prior ankle fracture and complicated lateral ankle pressure wound. Treatment involved excision of the lateral ankle ulceration, removal of infected hardware, and complete resection of the lateral malleolus (Figs. 22.20, 22.21, 22.22, 22.23, and 22.24).

Postoperative Care

Surgical treatment of osteomyelitis of the distal fibula is typically performed as an inpatient procedure, and the patient may remain hospitalized while waiting for the stage 2 procedure. A short hospital stay is also common after flap surgery in order to provide aggressive edema control, minimize hematoma formation, allow strict bed rest, and start preliminary IV antibiotic therapy. Confirmed osteomyelitis is commonly treated with 6 weeks of IV antibiotic therapy since surgery is typically not curative when attempting to preserve a functional lateral malleolus. The decision regarding duration of antibiotics is oftentimes based on clinical assessment of wound healing while monitoring of infection marker labs can also be clinically useful. Avoidance of ongoing decubitus pressure remains a challenge, especially while on bed rest after surgery. A well-padded posterior splint can be designed to off-load the posterior calcaneus and lateral malleolus. A flap pillow dressing is also useful as described in Fig. 22.25. Flap sutures are commonly left in place for approximately 4–6 weeks since delayed healing is the norm. Following flap surgery, a period of non-weight bearing is required as undo tension across the flap will likely result in flap failure. Continued measures to control edema should be instituted upon discharge from the hospital. Repeat bone biopsy is commonly performed with staged surgery. Postoperative stabilization of the foot and ankle against inversion contracture is helpful to avoid tension on the flap. Concomitant tendon surgery may be delayed until infection clears.

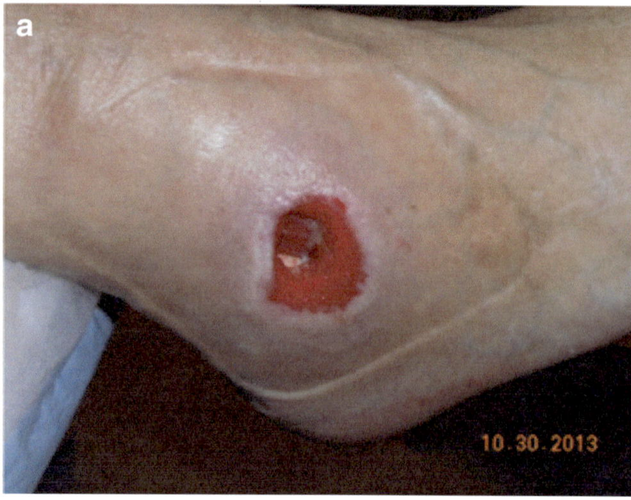
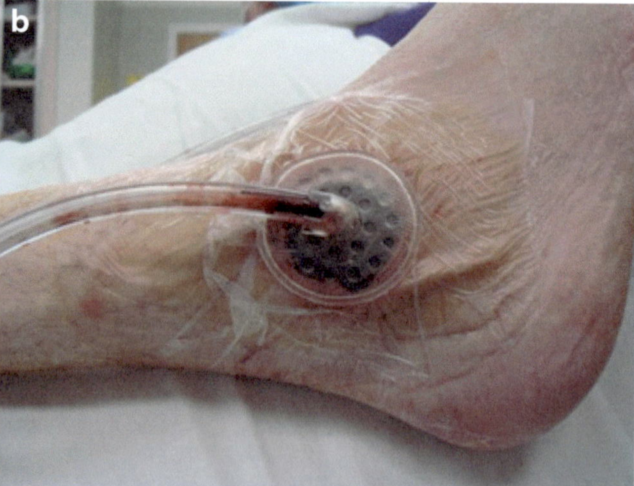

Fig. 22.10 Interval healing after 10 weeks of postoperative negative-pressure wound therapy in Case 1. (**a**, **b**) Healthy granulation tissue had formed which now covered the exposed cancellous bone. Bone debridement to expose viable medullary bone stimulated the formation of granulation tissue which was an advantage over attempting to preserve the nonvascular cortical bone. The overall surface area of the wound had also decreased which was the combined result of wound contracture and progressive epithelialization at the wound margin

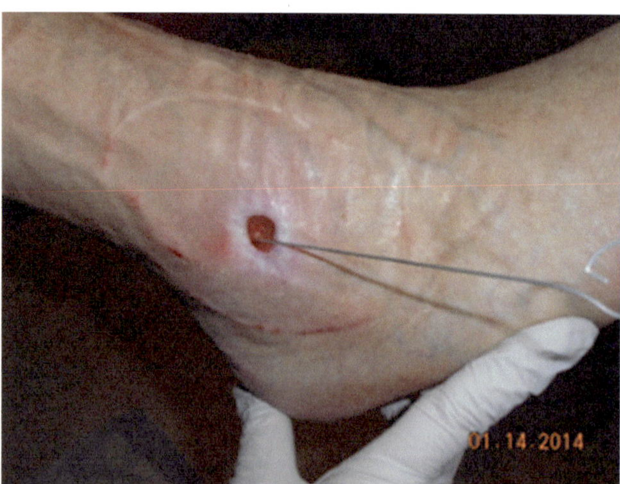
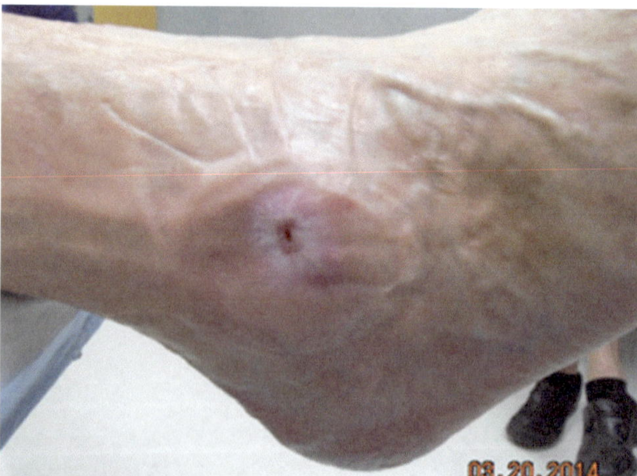

Fig. 22.11 Clinical photograph 5 months after surgery in Case 1. Progressive healing was noted with a healthy, granular wound bed. The probe-to-bone test demonstrated significantly less undermining and no bone exposure

Fig. 22.12 Near-complete wound healing at 8 months post-op in Case 1 without recurrent infection or progression of osteomyelitis. The wound was almost completely healed, and no signs of residual infection were noted

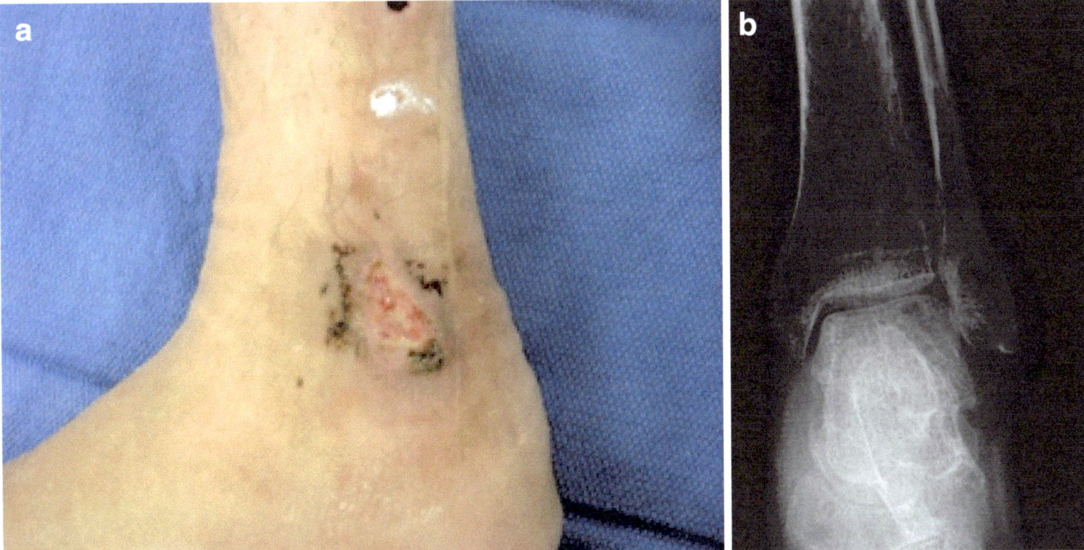

Fig. 22.13 Case 2: Lateral ankle decubitus ulceration with secondary osteomyelitis of the distal fibula. (**a**) Worsening lateral malleolar ulcer with recurrent soft tissue infection. Undermining of the wound margins was noted with a deep-probing sinus tract. (**b**) X-rays were inconclusive for osteomyelitis

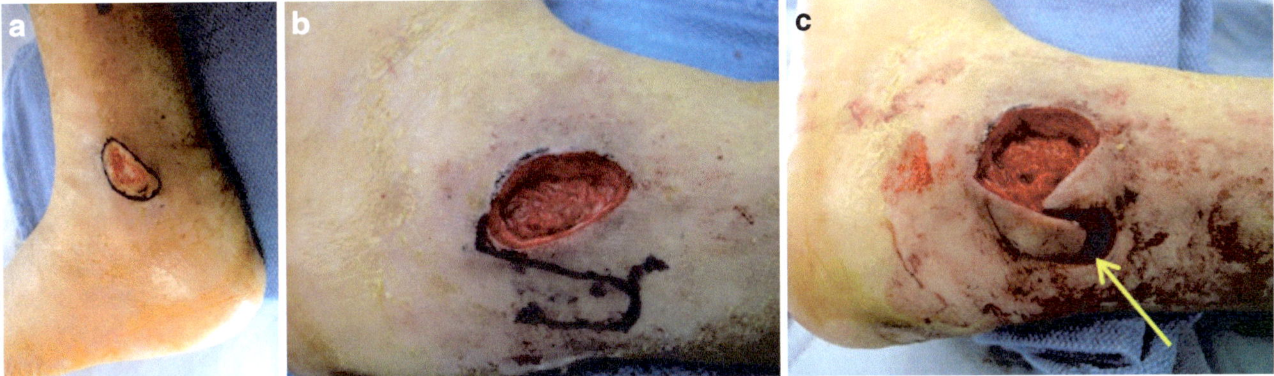

Fig. 22.14 Surgical treatment in Case 2 involved a unilobed flap and conservative bone debridement. (**a**) Full-thickness excision of the wound including the undermined tissue margins, sinus tract, and nonviable tissue. (**b**) A distally based oblong unilobed flap is shown just posterior to the fibula. (**c**) Raising the flap full depth resulted in retraction of the flap (*arrow*). Inversion contracture of the ankle accentuates tension on the lateral skin creating further difficulty with flap coverage. The flap length was intentionally designed to be 100 % or greater than the length of the wound defect to accommodate for anticipated retraction

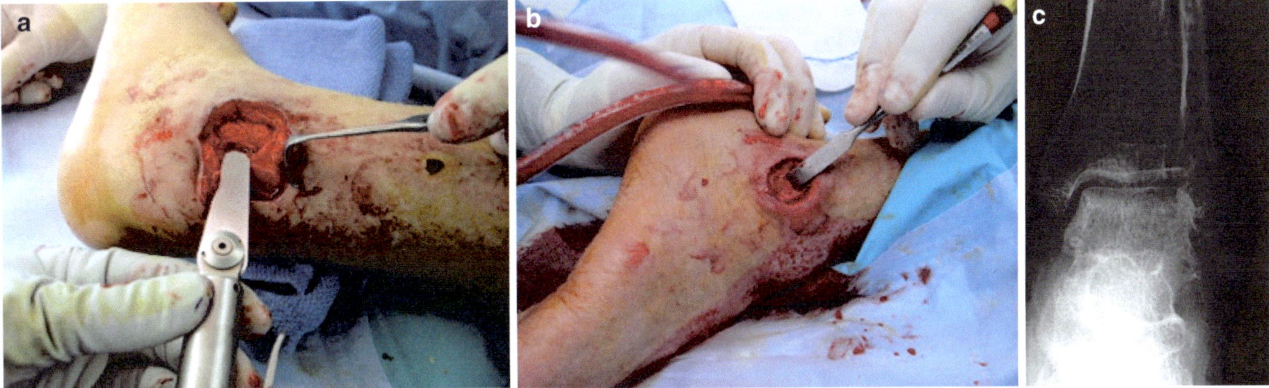

Fig. 22.15 Lateral cortical debridement of the distal fibula in Case 2. (**a**) Corticotomy was performed with a bone saw, with the intent to remove the infected lateral cortical bone, expose the viable underlying cancellous bone, procure bone biopsy specimen, and minimize bone prominence. Note how the posterior flap allowed broad access for bone resection. (**b**) Bone debridement may also be performed with an osteotome. (**c**) Postoperative radiograph demonstrating partial resection of the distal fibula

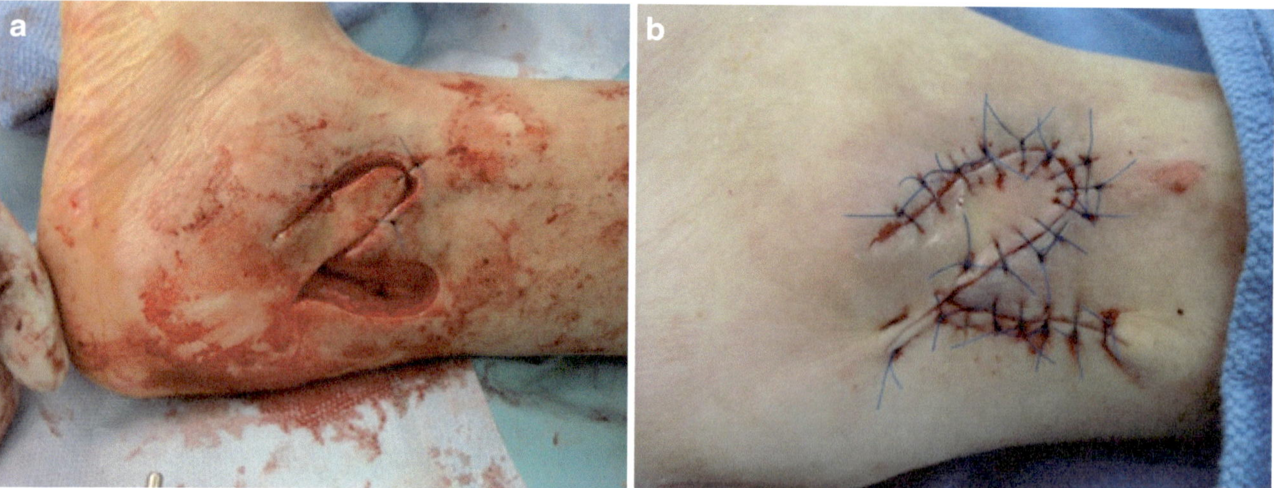

Fig. 22.16 Rotation of the unilobed flap and primary closure of the donor site in Case 2. (**a**) A single stitch was used to stretch the flap back to anatomic length. (**b**) Simple sutures were placed to evenly distribute tension across the flap and close the donor site

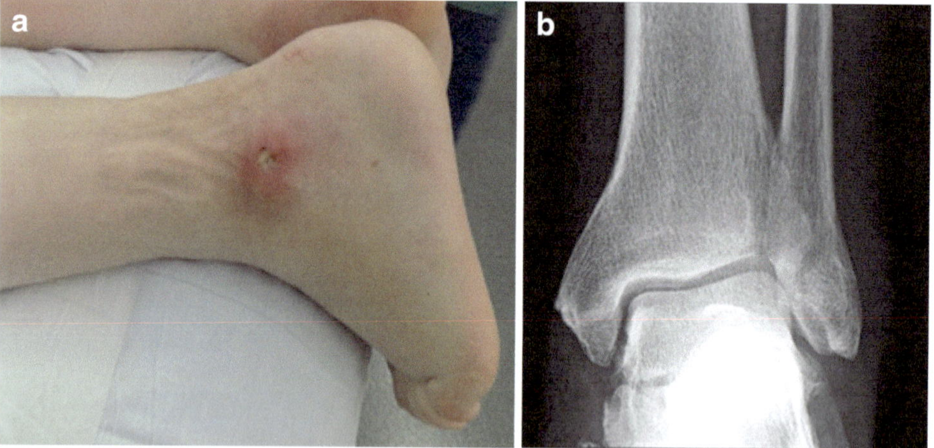

Fig. 22.17 Case 3 with small but undermined lateral malleolar pressure sore leading to bone exposure. (**a**) This small lateral malleolar pressure sore seems innocuous and would be treated conservatively if not for underlying bone infection. (**b**) Preoperative X-rays were relatively unremarkable, and diagnosis was made by bone biopsy

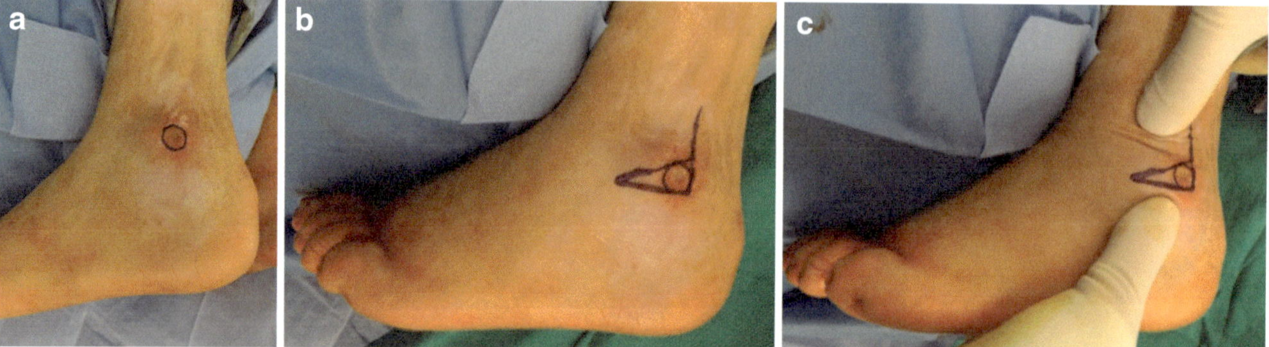

Fig. 22.18 Advancement flap in Case 3. (**a, b**) An advancement flap allowed excision of the wound, exposure of the distal fibula for debridement of the lateral cortex, and immediate coverage of the exposed cancellous bone. Note how simple excision of the small wound would not provide access for bone resection although an elliptical excision could be extended proximally along the fibula. (**c**) Mobility of the flap and surrounding tissue was tested prior to raising the flap

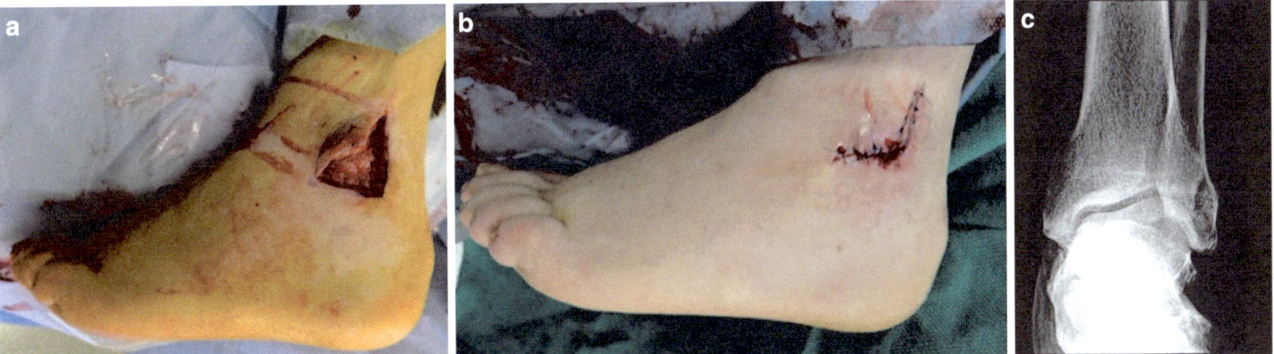

Fig. 22.19 Advancement flap wound closure in Case 3. Decortication was performed with a rongeur preserving the bulk of the lateral malleolus. (**a**) The proximal arm of the flap can be extended proximally for wide exposure if intraoperative inspection identifies proximal abscess or wide necrosis of the fibula. Undermining of the flap and wound margins improves tissue mobility and allows secondary movement of the surrounding tissue which takes tension off of the flap. (**b**) Advancement and closure of the flap provided immediate coverage of exposed bone with viable tissue. (**c**) Postoperative X-ray with preservation of a functional lateral malleolus

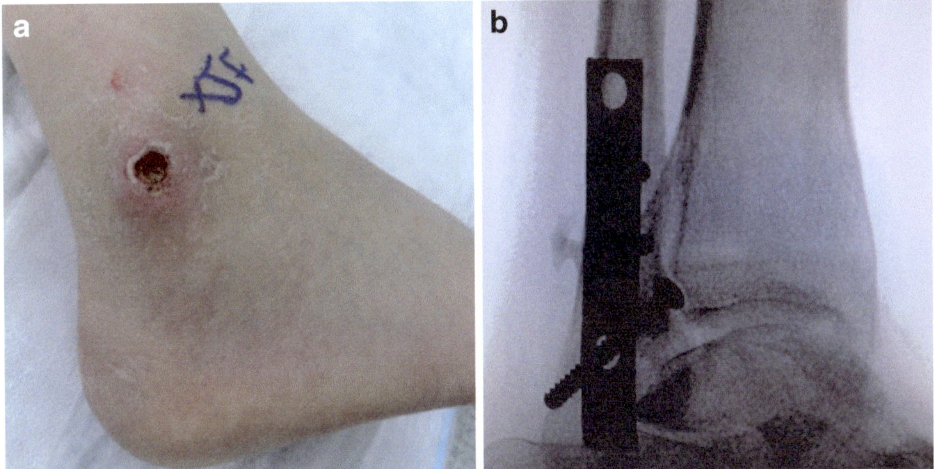

Fig. 22.20 Case 4: Paraplegic male with exposed hardware and osteomyelitis associated with chronic lateral ankle ulceration. (**a, b**) Full-thickness lateral ankle decubitus wound with exposed orthopedic hardware and suspected osteomyelitis of the distal fibula

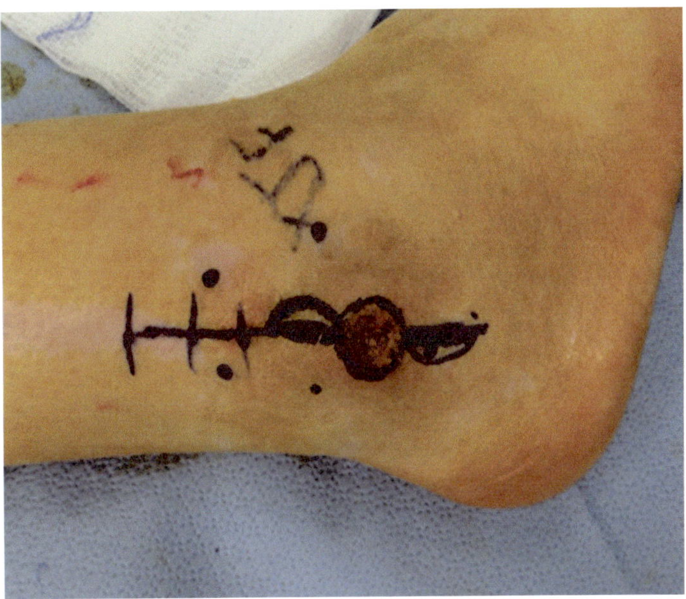

Fig. 22.21 Incision plan for wound excision and hardware removal in Case 4. Skin plasty incision plan for excision of the wound allowed exposure for hardware removal and wide resection of the infected distal fibula

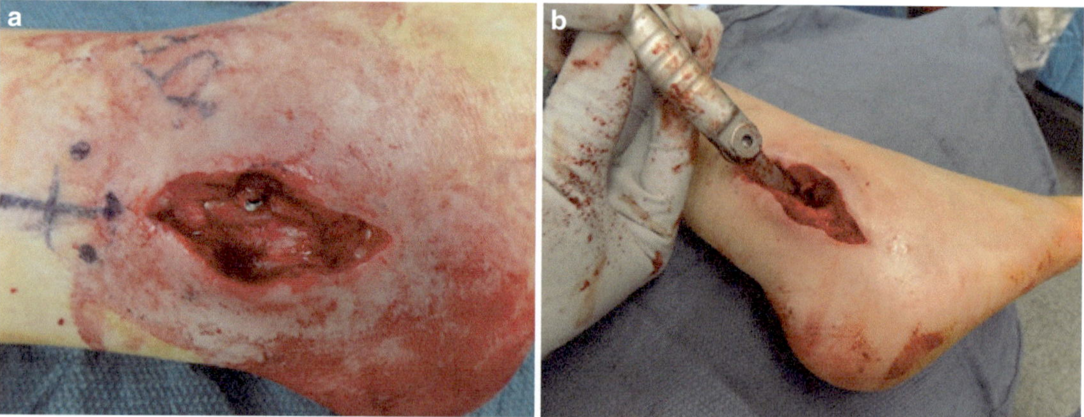

Fig. 22.22 Exposure of infected distal fibula and hardware in Case 4. (**a**) Wound excision allowed wide exposure to the fibula and underlying hardware. (**b**) A sagittal saw was used to resect the distal fibula

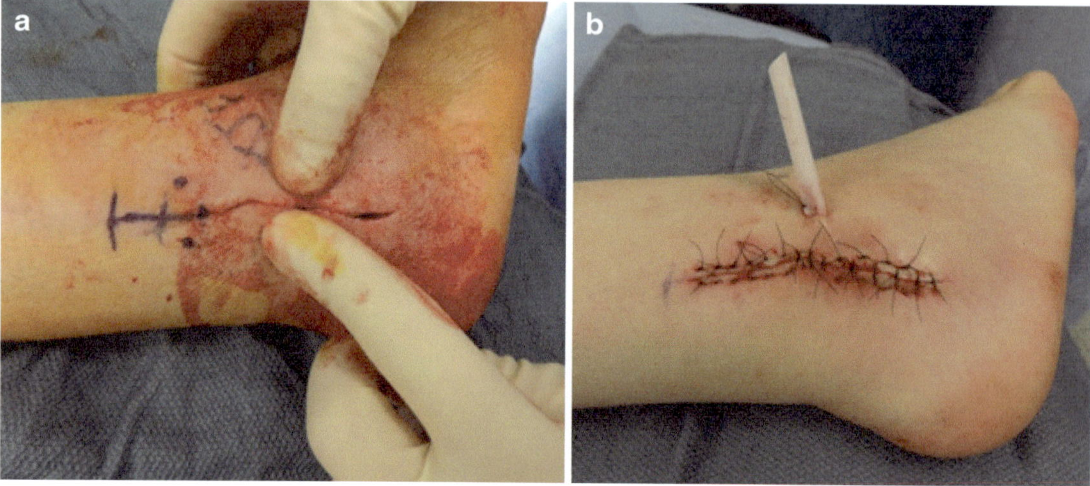

Fig. 22.23 Closure of wound under minimal tension in Case 4. (**a**) Note how the incision was approximated with little tension. (**b**) Simple interrupted sutures and drain placed for primary closure with single-stage surgery

Fig. 22.24 Postoperative radiograph in case 4 demonstrating level of fibulectomy with beveled cut to minimize lateral pressure. Note exposure to the ankle joint which could lead to complications if the wound failed to heal primarily or if there was residual infection. Preservation of the lateral malleolus is less important if the limb is not being used for ambulation or transfer. Wide resection also makes the limb easier to brace but may predispose to further contracture in patients with spastic neurologic conditions

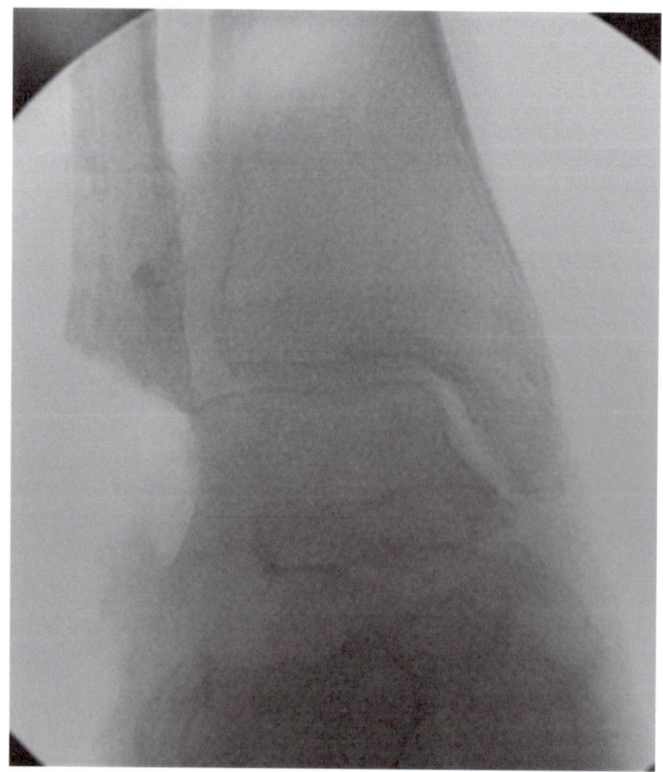

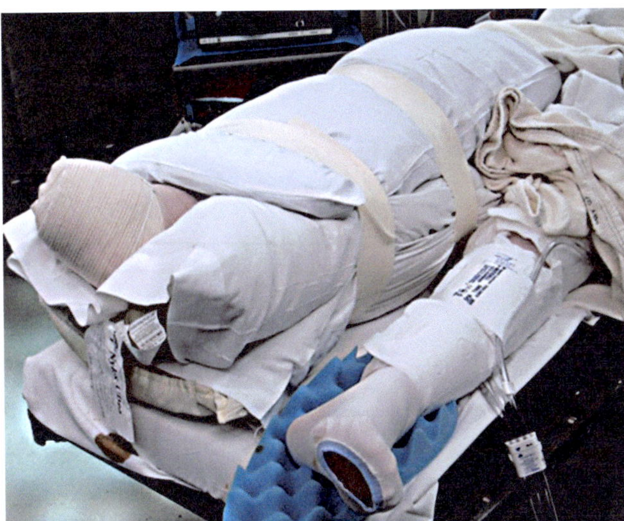

Fig. 22.25 Flap pillow dressing. Postoperative off-loading of lateral malleolar flaps is a challenge both while hospitalized and upon discharge to home or a nursing facility. Commercially available removable foam devices work well when used as indicated. Unfortunately, these devices are oftentimes removed by facility staff or patients resulting in direct pressure on the flap while lying in bed. Posterior splints are commonly fabricated; however, these are made of hard casting materials and may cause pressure elsewhere. Flap surgery does not typically require cast immobilization or ankle dorsiflexion although inversion contracture of the ankle does place unwanted stress on the flap. The flap pillow dressing is a cost-effective alternative. This is constructed with four hospital pillows. While not very comfortable for sleeping, hospital pillows provide effective off-loading of the heel and ankle. Two stacked pillows are placed posterior to the calf, and one pillow is placed on each of the medial and lateral sides. Tape or self-adherent elastic wrap is then placed from the knee to the ankle holding the pillows in place. This intentionally bulky "dressing" protects against pressure no matter how the patient is positioned in bed. The bulk of the dressing also suggests the need for strict bed rest, intentionally indicating that weight bearing is not desired. Patients and facility staff are less likely to remove the pillow dressing as compared to a removable foam pad. An order is written for the dressing to be changed only by the surgical team

Conclusion

Osteomyelitis of the distal fibula associated with lateral malleolar decubitus ulceration presents the surgeon with a complex decision-making process. If left untreated, bone involvement may lead to extensive infection and ultimately predispose the patient to limb loss. Early surgical intervention with excision of the wound eschar, lateral cortical debridement of the distal fibula, and bone biopsy allows prompt diagnosis and aggressive medical management. Advanced wound closure options are commonly employed including advancement and rotational flaps as well as NPWT. Wide resection of the distal fibula is ideally reserved for advanced infection or when preservation of ankle stability or function is not a primary concern.

References

1. Fisher AR, Wells G, Harrison MB. Factors associated with pressure ulcers in adults in acute care hospitals. Adv Skin Wound Care. 2004;17:80–90.
2. DeFranzo AJ, Argenta LC, Marks MW, Molnar JA, David LR, Webb LX, Ward WG, Teasdall RG. The use of vacuum-assisted closure therapy for the treatment of lower-extremity wounds with exposed bone. Plast Reconstr Surg. 2001;108:1184–91.
3. Mendonca DA, Cosker T, Makwana NK. Vacuum-assisted closure to aid wound healing in foot and ankle surgery. Foot Ankle Int. 2005;26:761–6.
4. Yoshiko T, Zenzo I, Fumihiro M, Katsunori F, Tetsuya N, Hiroyuki K, Masahiko Y. Location-dependent depth and undermining formation of pressure ulcers. J Tissue Viability. 2013;22:63–7.
5. VanDenKerkhof E, Friedberg E, Harrison M. Prevalence and risk of pressure ulcers in acute care following implementation of practice guidelines: annual pressure ulcer prevalence census 1994–2008. J Healthc Qual. 2011;33(5):58–67.
6. Barrois B, Labalette C, Rousseau P, Corbin A, Colin D, Allaert F, et al. A national prevalence study of pressure ulcers in french hospital inpatients. J Wound Care. 2008;17(9):373–6. 378–9.
7. Boffeli T, Collier R. Minimally invasive soft tissue release of foot and ankle contracture secondary to stroke. J Foot Ankle Surg. 2014;53:369–75.
8. Bozkurt M, Yavuzer G, Ergin E, Kentel B. Dynamic function of the fibula. Gait analysis evaluation of three different parts of the shank after fibulectomy: proximal, middle and distal. Arch Orthop Trauma Surg. 2005;125:713–20.
9. Rautio J, Asko-Seljavaara S, et al. Suitability of the scapular flap for reconstructions of the foot. Plast Reconstr Surg. 1990;85:922–8.
10. Lamberty B, Cormack G. The antecubital fascio-cutaneous flap. Br J Plast Surg. 1993;36:428–33.
11. Koshima I, Saisho H, et al. Flow-through thin latissimus dorsi perforator flap for repair of soft-tissue defects in the legs. Plast Reconstr Surg. 1999;103:483–1490.
12. Ohta M, Ikeda M, et al. Limb salvage of infected diabetic foot ulcers with free deep inferior epigastric perforator flaps. Microsurgery. 2006;26:87–92.
13. Ozkan O, Coskunfirat O, et al. Reliability of free-flap coverage in diabetic foot ulcers. Microsurgery. 2005;25:107–12.
14. Fitzgerald O'Connor E, Vessely M, et al. A systematic review of free tissue transfer in the management of non-traumatic lower extremity wounds in patients with diabetes. Eur J Vasc Endovasc Surg. 2011;4:391–9.
15. Suk Oh T, Seung Lee H, et al. Diabetic foot reconstruction using free flaps increases 5 year survival rate. J Plast Reconstr Aesthet Surg. 2013;66:243–50.
16. Attinger C, Ducic I, Cooper P, et al. The role of intrinsic muscle flaps of the foot for bone coverage in foot and ankle defects in diabetic and non diabetic patients. Plast Reconstr Surg. 2002;110:1047–54.
17. Attinger C, Ducic I, Zelen C. The use of local muscle flaps in foot and ankle reconstruction. Clin Podiatr Med Surg. 2000;17:681–711.
18. Morykwas M, Argenta L, et al. Vacuum assisted closure: a new method for wound control and treatment: animal studies and basic foundation. Ann Plast Surg. 1997;38:553–62.
19. Lee HJ, Kim JW, Oh CW, et al. Negative pressure wound therapy for soft tissue injuries around the foot and ankle. J Orthop Surg Res. 2009;4:14.
20. Bollero D, Carnino R, Risso D, et al. Acute complex traumas of the lower limbs: a modern reconstructive approach with negative pressure therapy. Wound Repair Regen. 2007;15:589–94.
21. Janis JE, Kwon RK, Attinger CE. The new reconstructive ladder: modification to the traditional model. Plast Reconstr Surg. 2011; 127(Suppl):S205–12.

Index

© Springer International Publishing Switzerland 2015
T.J. Boffeli (ed.), *Osteomyelitis of the Foot and Ankle*, DOI 10.1007/978-3-319-18926-0